Hypospadiology

Amilal Bhat
Editor

Hypospadiology

Principles and Practices

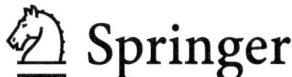

Editor
Amilal Bhat
Bhat's Hypospadias and Reconstructive Urology
Hospital and Research Centre
Jaipur, Rajasthan, India

ISBN 978-981-16-8394-7   ISBN 978-981-16-8395-4 (eBook)
https://doi.org/10.1007/978-981-16-8395-4

© The Editor(s) (if applicable) and The Author(s), under exclusive license to Springer Nature Singapore Pte Ltd. 2022
This work is subject to copyright. All rights are solely and exclusively licensed by the Publisher, whether the whole or part of the material is concerned, specifically the rights of translation, reprinting, reuse of illustrations, recitation, broadcasting, reproduction on microfilms or in any other physical way, and transmission or information storage and retrieval, electronic adaptation, computer software, or by similar or dissimilar methodology now known or hereafter developed.
The use of general descriptive names, registered names, trademarks, service marks, etc. in this publication does not imply, even in the absence of a specific statement, that such names are exempt from the relevant protective laws and regulations and therefore free for general use.
The publisher, the authors and the editors are safe to assume that the advice and information in this book are believed to be true and accurate at the date of publication. Neither the publisher nor the authors or the editors give a warranty, expressed or implied, with respect to the material contained herein or for any errors or omissions that may have been made. The publisher remains neutral with regard to jurisdictional claims in published maps and institutional affiliations.

This Springer imprint is published by the registered company Springer Nature Singapore Pte Ltd.
The registered company address is: 152 Beach Road, #21-01/04 Gateway East, Singapore 189721, Singapore

The book is dedicated to the patients of Hypospadias.

Foreword

It is my pleasure and honor to introduce "Hypospadiology: Principles and Practices" to all those called upon to treat hypospadias. The book has been edited by Dr. Amilal Bhat, an eminent Hypospadiologist, Pediatric Urologist and Educator, and one of the foremost authorities on Hypospadias.

The challenge of hypospadias correction has always tested the ingenuity of surgeons. Although many of the older methods have been discredited and discarded, the diversity of current practice procedures suggests that the perfect operation has yet to be devised. The average hypospadias surgeon concentrates on mastering a basic arsenal with a certain number of flexible options.

Evidently, there have been important advances during the past 50 years, and the results now obtained would be the envy of older surgeons. The problems do not stop with the completion of an apparently successful surgery. I know of no surgery that can quite humble a surgeon as much as hypospadias and with its list of complications, most infuriating when they occur years later.

There was undoubtedly a need for a comprehensive text dealing with all aspects of abnormal development and its consequences as well as giving guidance on methods of surgical correction. Dr. Amilal Bhat is to be congratulated on assembling a distinguished and expert team to fulfill this requirement.

H. S. Asopa
Association of Surgeons of India
Chennai, Tamil Nadu, India

International Society of Hypospadias and Intersex Disorders
Delhi, India

Royal College of Surgeons of England
London, UK

S N Medical College & Hospital
Agra, India

M L B Medical College
Jhansi, India

Asopa Hospital & Research Centre
Agra, India

Foreword

It is a great pleasure to write the foreword of Professor Amilal Bhat's textbook on hypospadias surgery. Professor Bhat has developed great skills in urogenital surgery in children in India and more precisely in Jaipur, Rajasthan. His hypospadias surgery experience is well known around the world, and his recruitment of pediatric urological patients is amazing.

With elegance and intelligence, Professor Amilal Bhat managed to gather world experts in hypospadiology in this textbook. As a result, most aspects of this common and complex genital anomaly are covered and will allow the reader to update his/her knowledge.

Never forget that Hypospadias is a development arrest of the tissues forming the ventral aspect of the genital tubercle. Having this definition in mind, one can better understand the frequent obstacles and complications met in this surgery even in the best hands. Hypospadiology should no longer be confined to surgery only. It should be a joint approach with pediatric endocrinologists, geneticists, molecular biologists, psychologists, urogenital surgeons and, of course, children and parents. Although most hypospadias have not identifiable underlying disorders, every effort should be made to understand the causes of this malformation. The "masculinization window" (6–16 weeks of gestation) is a critical period of genital construction, and many factors can affect it.

The recent years have also put under light the indications of hypospadias surgery, particularly in the most distal ones. The hypospadiologists should humbly review their results and always question the indications and the management of their patients. Should all hypospadias be treated is a common debate raised in international meetings as well as the psychological consequences of this surgery.

Tubularization of the urethral plate (Thiersch-Duplay-TIP), as shown in this book, is very popular among surgeons dealing with hypospadias. Hypospadiologists should, however, question the quality of ventral tissues located distal to the ectopic meatus used for the reconstruction of the missing urethra. Hypoplastic tissues (do not forget the above definition of Hypospadias) do not grow at the same pace as the rest of the genital tubercle. This explains the significant rate of late complications (mostly urethral stenosis) met with these techniques. An easy-to-learn operation does not mean a good operation in terms of long-term results. Alternatives exist, and the reader should always remember this.

So enjoy this great textbook and many congratulations again to Professor Amilal Bhat for this achievement.

Pierre D. E. Mouriquand
University Department of Paediatric Uro-Genital Surgery
Lyon, France

Preface

Hypospadiology Principles and Practices

With the inception of hypospadias science and the term "Hypospadiology" by John Duckett in 1982, there have been many advancements in hypospadias surgery. Over the years, Hypospadiology has developed, expanded, matured, and established a diverse body of knowledge and proficiency. Some of the procedures performed demand a high level of skill and expertise. These should be performed in well-developed centers having sub-speciality knowledge and surgical expertise. It is encompassing a better understanding of the anatomy of the hypospadiac penis and chordee correction. Hypospadias surgery needs perfection in implementation of surgical principles. Even a single missed step of precaution leads toward the path of complications. The management of these patients' necessitates the need for state-of-the-art surgery to have optimal results. Hypospadiology is coming up as a separate speciality in present-day surgery. This inspired me to pursue writing a book on the speciality with the title "Hypospadiology: Principles and Practices." Book chapters have been organized around pertinent clinical questions, especially chordee correction, utilizing the principles of urethral plate preservation, spongioplasty, and management of variants of hypospadias like female hypospadias, Mega-meatus intact prepuce, penile torsion, and iatrogenic hypospadias with a discussion on imaging in hypospadias with special mention of sono-elastography. The discussed text is based on various randomized controlled trials and prospective observational studies. It contains tables that summarize important studies and figures that illustrate algorithms with the best management options and expected results. Evidence for optimal patient management is an indispensable and unique resource for Hypospadiologists, Pediatric Urologists, Pediatric Surgeons, General Urologists, and plastic surgeons with an inclination toward Pediatric Urology, as well as fellows and residents in training. Though utmost care has been taken to avoid repetition of the text and achieve clarity in all topics, there may be some overlap and differing views on the choice of techniques by different authors. The editor would like to express a deep sense of gratitude for the outstanding work by all the contributors in the production of this innovative textbook. I wish to convey my thanks to Mr. Naren Agarwal, Mr. Gaurav Singh, Mr. Kumar Athiappan from Springer

Nature, who has been the pillar of support in bringing this book to life with incredible efficiency, from its production to its delivery. Finally, I would like to thank all my family members for their wonderful and uninterrupted support.

Jaipur, India   Amilal Bhat

Contents

1. **Hypospadias History: The Long Way to Perfection** 1
   Sameh Shehata

2. **Hypospadias Embryology, Etiology, and Classification** 9
   M. S. Ansari, Prabhu Chakravarthy, and Priyank Yadav

3. **Anatomy of the Penis in Hypospadias**...................... 17
   Anil Takvani

4. **Penile Anthropometry**.................................... 31
   Mahakshit Bhat and Amilal Bhat

5. **General Considerations in Hypospadias Surgery** 41
   Amilal Bhat and Nikhil Khandelwal

6. **Chordee Correction in Hypospadias Repair** 55
   Amilal Bhat and Mahakshit Bhat

7. **Management of Distal and Mid-Penile Hypospadias**.......... 79
   Ujwal Kumar, Vikash Singh, and Amilal Bhat

8. **Modified Tubularized Incised Urethral Plate Urethroplasty** ... 101
   Amilal Bhat

9. **Single Stage Repair in Proximal Hypospadias**............... 113
   Pramod P. Reddy and Mahakshit Bhat

10. **Tubularized Incised Urethral Plate Urethroplasty in Severe Hypospadias**... 135
    Amilal Bhat

11. **Spongioplasty in Hypospadias Repair** 143
    Amilal Bhat

12. **Flaps and Grafts in Hypospadias Repair** 165
    Octavio Herrera and Mohan S. Gundeti

13. **The Surgical Approach to Two-Stage Hypospadias Repair** 187
    Christopher J. Long, Aseem R. Shukla, and Mark R. Zaontz

14. **Modifications in Inner Prepucial Flap Repair of Hypospadias** 201
    Amilal Bhat

15	**Management of Chordee Without Hypospadias** . . . . 215 Amilal Bhat	
16	**Management of Female Hypospadias** . . . . 231 Amilal Bhat, Akshita Bhat, and Madhu Bhat	
17	**Management of Megmeatus Intact Prepuce/Concealed Hypospadias**. . . . . 243 Amilal Bhat	
18	**Management of Penile Torsion in Hypospadias and Isolated Penile Torsion** . . . . 255 Amilal Bhat	
19	**Management of Iatrogenic Hypospadias** . . . . 275 Amilal Bhat, Nikhil Khandelwal, and Akshita Bhat	
20	**Acute Postoperative Complications of Hypospadias Repair**. . . . 283 Amilal Bhat	
21	**Late Postoperative Complications of Hypospadias Repair**. . . . . 295 Amilal Bhat	
22	**Management of Hypospadias Cripple**. . . . . 315 Amilal Bhat	
23	**Management of Hypospadias in Patients with Disorders of Sexual Development (DSD)** . . . . 333 P. Ashwin Shekar and Amilal Bhat	
24	**Management of Penoscrotal Transposition with or without Hypospadias**. . . . . 349 Amilal Bhat and Akshita Bhat	
25	**The Prepuce and Prepucioplasty in Hypospadias** . . . . 363 Amilal Bhat, Mahakshit Bhat, and Nikhil Khandelwal	
26	**Dressing in Hypospadias Repair** . . . . 381 Arun Chawla and Anupam Choudhary	
27	**Psychosocial, Sexual Function, and Fertility in Hypospadias**. . . 389 Sudhindra Jayasimha and J. Chandrasingh	
28	**Current Status Evaluation of Hypospadias Repair Results** . . . . 401 M. A. Baky Fahmy	
29	**Radiological Evaluation of Hypospadias Patients** . . . . 409 Aparna Prakash, Mahakshit Bhat, and Amilal Bhat	
30	**Evolutions in Hypospadiology and Current Status of Tissue Engineering** . . . . 423 Priyank Yadav and Martin A. Koyle	
31	**Variables in Hypospadias Repair** . . . . 431 Amilal Bhat	

About the Editor

Amilal Bhat is an eminent hypospadiologist, pediatric urologist, and educator of international fame. Dr. Bhat has dedicated his life to hypospadiology and pediatric urology. He has developed six new operative techniques in pediatric urology, three of which have been featured in the Campbell's Textbook of Urology. He has been an operating faculty in various international and national workshops on hypospadias. Dr. Bhat has also been a panelist and guest speaker at many international and national conferences and workshops. He has been a prominent educator and has spent 30 years as a consultant urologist, pediatric urologist, hypospadiologist, and a teacher with tenure of more than 10 years as a professor and subsequently as principal and dean of Dr. S.N. Medical College Jodhpur. He is the recipient of many appreciation awards for development of urology and services to society.

List of Contributors

M. S. Ansari Division of Pediatric Urology, Sanjay Gandhi Postgraduate Institute of Medical Sciences, Lucknow, India

P. Ashwin Shekar Consultant Urologist, Department of Urology, Sri Sathya Sai Institute of Higher Medical Sciences, Puttaparthi, India

M. A. Baky Fahmy Pediatric Surgery, Al-Azhar University, Cairo, Egypt

Akshita Bhat Department of Surgery, Sawai Man Singh Medical College, Jaipur, Rajasthan, India

Amilal Bhat Bhat's Hypospadias and Reconstructive Urology Hospital and Research Centre, Jaipur, Rajasthan, India

Department of Urology, Jaipur National University Institute for Medical Sciences and Research Centre, Jaipur, Rajasthan, India

Department of Urology, Dr. S.N. Medical College, Jodhpur, Rajasthan, India

Department of Urology, S.P. Medical College, Bikaner, Rajasthan, India

P.G. Committee Medical Council of India, New Delhi, India

Academic and Research Council of RUHS, Jaipur, Rajasthan, India

Madhu Bhat Department of obstetrics and Gynecology, S.M.S. Medical College, Jaipur, India

Mahakshit Bhat Department of Urology, National Institute of Medical Sciences Medical College, Jaipur, Rajasthan, India

Prabhu Chakravarthy Division of Pediatric Urology, Sanjay Gandhi Postgraduate Institute of Medical Sciences, Lucknow, India

J. Chandrasingh Division of Adolescent and Pediatric Urology, Department of Urology, Christian Medical College, Vellore, Tamilnadu, India

Arun Chawla Department of Urology and Renal Transplant, Kasturba Medical College, Manipal Academy of Higher Education, Manipal, Karnataka, India

Anupam Choudhary Department of Urology and Renal Transplant, Kasturba Medical College, Manipal Academy of Higher Education, Manipal, Karnataka, India

Mohan S. Gundeti Pediatric Urology (Surgery), MFM (Ob/Gyn) and Pediatrics, The University of Chicago Medicine & Biological Sciences, Chicago, IL, USA

Pediatric Urology, Comer Children's Hospital, Chicago, IL, USA

Octavio Herrera Class of 2021, Pritzker School of Medicine, University of Chicago, Chicago, IL, USA

Sudhindra Jayasimha Division of Adolescent and Pediatric Urology, Department of Urology, Christian Medical College, Vellore, Tamilnadu, India

Nikhil Khandelwal Department of Urology, Vijayanagar Institute of Medical Sciences, Bellary, Karnataka, India

Martin A. Koyle University of Toronto & Hospital for Sick Children, Toronto, ON, Canada

Ujwal Kumar Department of Urology, IMS, BHU, Varanasi, Uttar Pradesh, India

Christopher J. Long Division of Urology, Department of Surgery, The Children's Hospital of Philadelphia, Perelman School of Medicine, University of Pennsylvania, Philadelphia, PA, USA

Aparna Prakash OK Diagnostic and Research Centre, Jaipur, Rajasthan, India

Department of Radiology, SMS Medical College, Jaipur, Rajasthan, India

Pramod P. Reddy Division of Pediatric Urology, Cincinnati Children's, Univ. of Cincinnati College of Medicine, Cincinnati Children's Hospital Medical Center, Cincinnati, OH, USA

Sameh Shehata Department of Pediatric Surgery, University of Alexandria, Alexandria, Egypt

Aseem R. Shukla Division of Urology, Department of Surgery, The Children's Hospital of Philadelphia, Perelman School of Medicine, University of Pennsylvania, Philadelphia, PA, USA

Vikash Singh Maa Rajwati Hospital Pvt Ltd, Varanasi, Uttar Pradesh, India

Anil Takvani Takvani Kidney Hospital, Junagadh, Gujarat, India

Priyank Yadav Division of Pediatric Urology, Sanjay Gandhi Postgraduate Institute of Medical Sciences, Lucknow, India

Division of Pediatric Urology, The Hospital for Sick Children, University of Toronto, Toronto, ON, Canada

Mark R. Zaontz Division of Urology, Department of Surgery, The Children's Hospital of Philadelphia, Perelman School of Medicine, University of Pennsylvania, Philadelphia, PA, USA

Hypospadias History: The Long Way to Perfection

Sameh Shehata

1.1 Introduction

The first documentation of hypospadias as a congenital anomaly was done by Heliodorus, Antyllus, and Galen during the first and second centuries AD. Descriptions to original attempts at hypospadias repairs during this time period have been found in Roman, Greek, and Egyptian manuscripts. The term (hypospadias) was first used by Gallen, Fig. 1.1, [1, 2].

1.2 The Past; Initial Attempts

Galen (130–199 AD), the most influential physician of his era and the personal treating physician to many of the Roman emperors and also to the gladiators of Rome, described repair as a partial amputation of the penis to the level of the urethral opening, and in order to simulate a glanular shape, he added a conical incision. In order to achieve hemostasis, compression, vinegar, or cautery were used as necessary [2, 3]. Similar technique was proposed by two alexandrine surgeons, Heliodorus and Antyllus (first century AD).

During the middle ages, The Islamic physician, Albucasis of Cordoba (936–1013), contributed to many important medical texts (Fig. 1.2), he re-described the technique of partial amputation of the penis beyond the hypospadiac meatus, which may be the only technique of hypospadias repair with zero incidences of fistula [1, 2, 4].

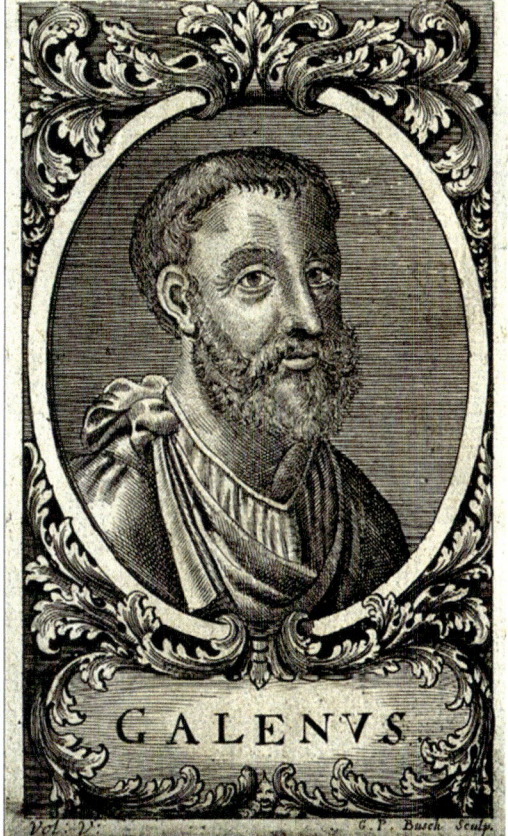

Fig. 1.1 "The Roman physician Claudius Galen in the second century AD" Wikipedia.org

S. Shehata (✉)
Department of Pediatric Surgery, University of Alexandria, Alexandria, Egypt

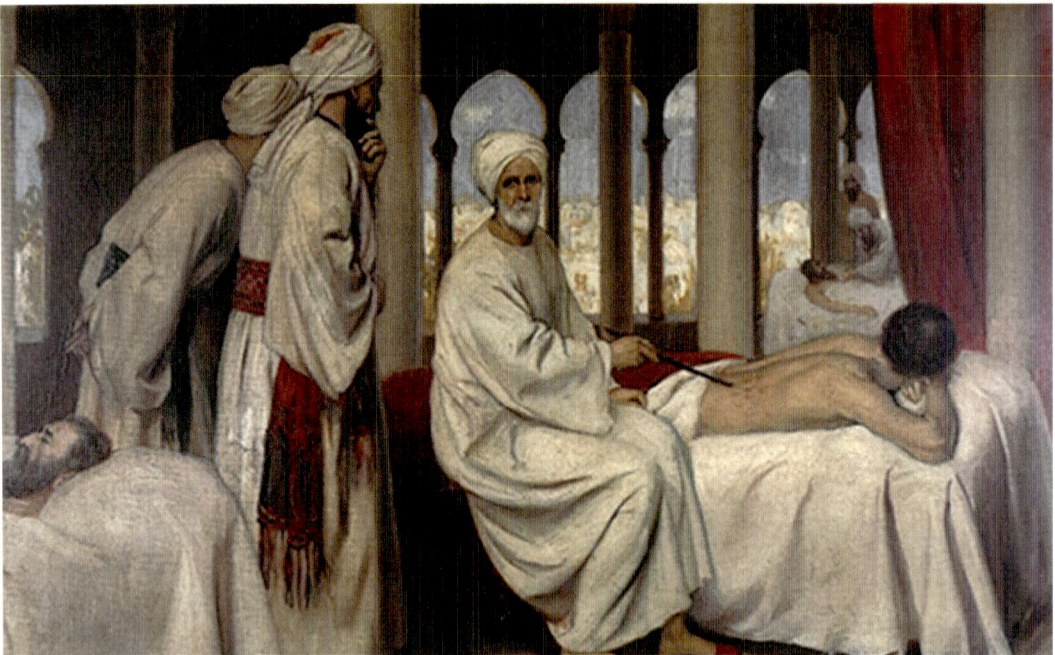

Fig. 1.2 Albucasis blistering a patient at the hospital in Cordoba, courtesy commons. wikipedia.org

Serefeddin Sabuncuoglu, (1385–1468), Fig. 1.3, one of the most eminent surgeons of the Ottoman Empire, was convinced by Albucasis recommendations and practiced surgery in what is known now as Northern Turkey. He described a technique quite similar to that of Albucasis, but he added the importance of adding a catheter in the urethra to sustain patency. He also highlighted the expectation of profuse bleeding from this procedure and the importance of controlling bleeding with cautery. Sabuncuoglu's texts included many drawings of surgical techniques and instruments [1, 2, 4].

The nineteenth century has witnessed the appearance of many new techniques and concepts; some were sound and contributed to the progress forward, while others were inhumane and absolute failures. Dupuytren described a change of the canalization concept. The canal formed was treated with a hot wire, and after healing of resulting inflammation, he recommended keeping the new canal open with elastic tubes.

In 1838, Dieffenbach pierced the glans to the level of the urethral meatus and inserted a tube in between until the neourethra was covered by the normal epithelium [6].

1.3 Canalization

The Renaissance period showed a radical change of concept and thought from the partial penectomy to a more sound technique of canalization by Amatus Lusitanus from Portugal (1511–1568). He described a procedure for canalization to repair proximal hypospadias in a 2-year-old boy; he created a channel reaching distally to the glans using a silver cannula [1, 3, 5].

1.4 Tubes, Catheters, and Diversion

Albucasis from Cordoba (963–1013) used a solid metal rod to avoid stricture formation after the treatment of imperforated urinary meatus. He removed and reintroduced the rod to allow the child to pass urine intermittently [1–3].

Serefeddin Sabuncuoglu (fifteenth century) used a sound with a patent lumen. This was very

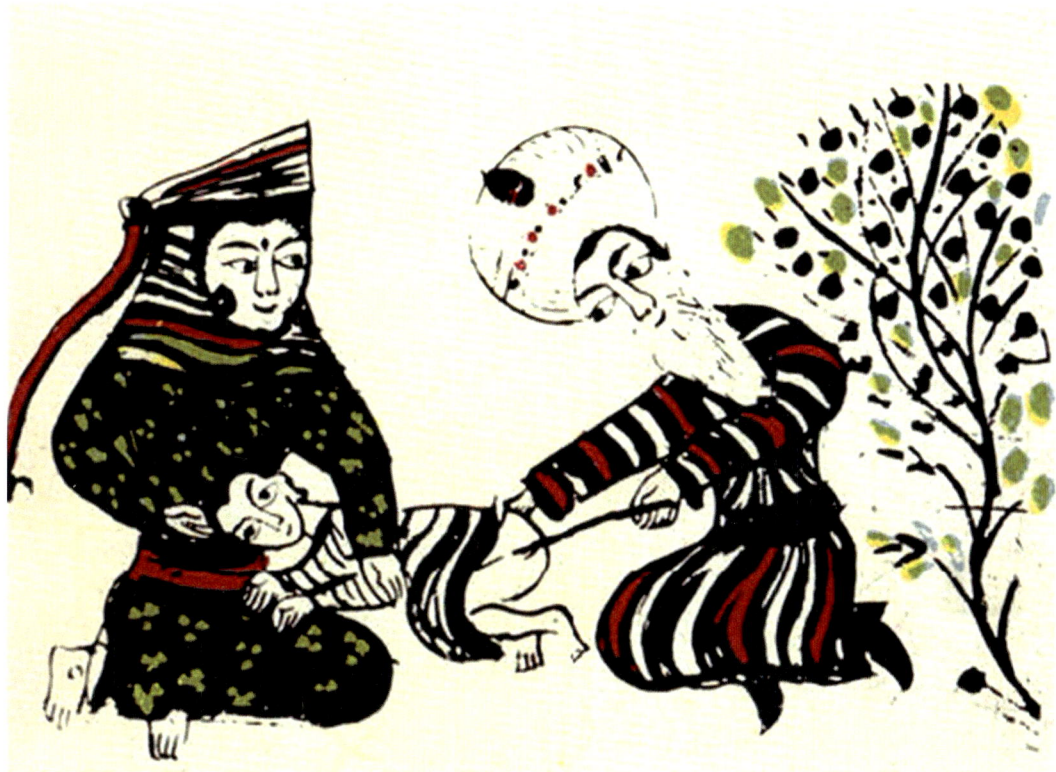

Fig. 1.3 Serefeddin Sabuncuoglu. Wikimedia commons

useful for children, enabling them to pass urine through it instead of removing it many times during the day [1]. In the 1950s and the 1960s, urine was diverted using perineal urethrostomy.

More recently, a simple method, "Silastic tubing placed into the bladder through the repair allowing a constant flow from the catheter into the diaper," which was suggested by Duckett and Snyder [7].

1.5 Penile Curvature

"Galen and Oribasus" specifically described the chordee by stating that "the curvature of the penis prevents its normal urine stream from being directed forwards and precludes normal sexual intercourse [1–3]." Some other terms have also been used to describe the abnormal bending of hypospadias. (1842) and Mayo used the terms ventral curvature or ventral deformity. Nesbit, in his important article on hypospadias in 1941, used the term ventral curvature [8, 9].

"Clinton Smith was the first surgeon to use the term chordee in the description of hypospadias." He used the term congenital chordee to distinguish it from the chordee associated with gonorrhea common at that time [1]. Ambroise Pare (1510–1590), the famous French surgeon of the French Royalty, emphasized the importance of penile curvature and its effect on hindering the generation of children, and he highlighted the importance of the deliberate division of the chordee. Jean Fernel treated the chordee of Henry II, King of France, in 1547, who had been married for ten years with no children. After the successful surgery, he fathered ten children [10].

In 1707, P. Dionis (1643–1718), a well-known French anatomist and surgeon described the importance of the repair of the associated chordee. Dionis correctly described two inconveniences to the patient with hypospadias, which is the inability to void in a forward direction and the inability to ejaculate semen properly into the vaginal canal. In 1842, Mettauer suggested creating subcutaneous incisions to treat skin tethering. Although this was a very correct and logic concept for the mid-nineteenth century, it was overlooked for a long time before being accepted [8].

Penile curvature can be treated in the majority of cases by using skin degloving; in cases that cannot be corrected by skin degloving alone, two approaches emerged, dorsal shortening (plication) and ventral lengthening. In 1965, Nesbit explained the technique of excising elliptical segments of the dorsal tunica albuginea to correct ventral curvature. In 1994, Duckett and Baskin suggested the technique of plication of the dorsal shaft by creating two incisions and closing the edges together, achieving shortening the dorsal shaft without the need to remove tunical tissue. Baskin and colleagues documented a scantiness of neurovascular tissue in the dorsal midline of the penis. As a result, most dorsal plications are preferably performed now at the dorsal midline position of the penis [11].

For more severe cases, dorsal plication is not enough alone; for these cases, to achieve ventral lengthening, transverse incisions are made, in the ventral tunica albuginea, these can be closed vertically. Another option was to cover the incisions in tunica albuginea free dermal skin grafts or tunica vaginalis, and this has evolved more recently to corporotomies without grafting. Perovic from Yugoslavia in 1998 presented the "penile disassembly" procedure for the treatment of severe chordee and also for glans tilt and curvatures that are located distally [12].

1.6 Artificial Erection

In 1974, Gittes and McLaughlin popularized the "artificial erection test" by injecting saline solution following applying a tourniquet at the base of the penis. This was a real milestone in the management of penile curvature [13].

1.7 The Importance of the Prepuce (Preputial Flaps)

Weller Van Hook, a distinguished Chicago surgeon, described for the first time the principle of urethroplasty using a tubularized pedicle flap of preputial skin. An important principle was used by many surgeons afterward. In 1970, Hodgson continued tubularizing the preputial skin pedicled on its blood supply. He describes transillumination to demonstrate the course of dorsal vessels and allow transfer of the preputial flap from dorsum to ventral aspect; he used a buttonhole technique. Asopa described the "transverse preputial flap urethroplasty" based on the dorsal blood supply of the penis, and he also retained the continuity of the urethral plate [5, 14].

Moving towards (reconstruction of a new urethra) Liston, a London surgeon, in 1838, reported successful hypospadias repair using a preputial flap. Mettauer, an American surgeon, described a similar repair in 1842. He wrote extensively on urethral anomalies, including hypospadias and epispadias. Mettauer also made the important observation that most of the chordee are caused by skin tethering; consequently, he advised correction of chordee by successive subcutaneous incisions till the penis is straightened (degloving) [3, 8].

In 1980, Duckett described the pedicled tubularized preputial flap as a one-stage correction for proximal hypospadias. Asopa popularized his double-face prepuce flap to create the neourethra and to cover the ventral skin deficiency [15].

1.8 Penile Shaft Tubularization

Modern hypospadiology began in 1869 when German surgeon, Karl Thiersch from Leipzig, described the technique of "tubularization of the penile shaft skin" for the treatment of epispadias. Theophile Anger, his student, from Paris described his concept to repair penoscrotal hypospadias successfully and presented it in a surgical meeting. Anger was the real designer of the modern repair techniques in hypospadias surgery [1].

Duplay in 1880 reported his technique where he wrapped the urethral plate around a catheter; he did not suture the skin edges together but covered it with skin. This concept of creating an incomplete new urethra was later popularized in the 1940s by Denis Browne (the buried strip). He secured the skin edges with glass or glass beads [1, 3].

Encouraged by improvement in the results, other surgeons in 1874 refined these techniques, including Nove-Josserand, Duplay, and Ombredanne. Duplay described three steps for hypospadias repair; correction of ventral curvature, urethroplasty with penile skin flaps, and joining of the neourethra with the hypospadiac meatus [1].

An alternative approach for the one-stage correction of proximal hypospadias was described by Koyanagi, where he tubularized a lateral penile shaft skin for urethroplasty. Koyanagi described the use of lateral penile shaft skin and prepuce from both sides for the creation of neourethra. This was later modified by Snow, Emir, Hayashi and Hadidi [16, 17].

1.9 Meatus Based Flaps (Flip-flaps)

In 1917, Bevan described a meatal-based rectangular flap and transferred it through the glanular tunnel to treat distal hypospadias. This was the prototype of flip-flap techniques. The use of metal-based flap has been very popular for more than 80 years. Bouisson used a rotated local pedicled scrotal flap to create the anterior part of the neourethra with a technique. Mathieu used the same technique for distal hypospadias in 1932, although the principle was explained earlier by Wood in 1875, Ombredanne in 1911, and Bevan in 1917.

Horton and Devine (1959) created a flip-flap from the ventral skin of the shaft based on the urethral meatus to be joined to a triangular glanular flap to form the distal segment of the urethra [18–20].

In 1965, Mustarde merged the two techniques, Bevan rectangular flap technique and the glanular flap technique. Instead of incising the glans, he passed the tube through a glanular channel [3, 18].

1.10 Free Grafts

Different tissues have been proposed as grafts with varying success. A totally different approach was the use of different types of free grafts, Nove-Josserand in 1897, used a free graft from the thigh; the graft was placed through a trocar, and canalization was done to create a neourethra [21]. Initially, full-thickness skin grafts were used from non-hair-bearing areas, but this resulted in a lot of scarring and contracture. Subsequently, bladder mucosa was introduced by Memmelaar in 1947and by Marshall and Spellman in 1955. This method was popularized by Hendren and Reda (1986) and Ransley et al. [22–24].

The use of buccal mucosa was described by Humby in 1941 and Mirabet in 1964, but popularized by Duckett, Dessanti et al, and Ransley from the UK but did not gain widespread use until the 1980s and the 1990s where it has proved to be the most successful free graft on the long-term [25, 26].

Devine harvested grafts from preputial skin, which yielded much better results as it was pliable, thin, and hairless, the proximal anastomosis was made oblique in order to avoid stenosis, and the glans was tunneled to create the distal anastomosis. Skin cover was done using penile or scrotal skin, and the diversion was made using perineal urethrostomy [27].

1.11 Ventral Skin Coverage

Many of the operations used for hypospadias repair resulted in ventral skin deficiency, especially those cases with significant chordee. Several tissues have been used for the coverage of the resultant ventral defect. In 1870 Moutet, the ventral penile skin deficiency over the neourethra was covered by bi-pedicled suprapubic abdominal skin flaps.

Wood, in 1875, introduced the concept of the buttonhole within the preputial flap in order to cover the ventral defect of the penile shaft and the raw surface of the neourethra. The buttonhole principle had originally been described by Thiersch in epispadias surgery to cover the dorsal shaft defect.

Rosenberg, Landerer, and Bidder described the technique of "burying" the ventral part of the penis into the scrotum and sutured the resulting skin edges. During the second stage, they divided the penoscrotal fusion where it was possible to cover the ventral defect by lateral flaps from the penile shaft [28]. Blair and Byars in 1938 and Byars in 1955 used the model of dorsal preputial flaps "Byars flaps" to treat ventral skin deficiency [29].

1.12 The Importance of the Covering Layer

The importance of the intervening second layer for the prevention of urethra-cutaneous fistula was recognized, and many tissues he has been used in this respect, including ventral Dartos, dorsal Dartos, de-epithelialized flaps. In 1994, Snow suggested using tunica vaginalis as an additional protective layer to cover the urethra to minimize fistula formation [30, 31]. Another important tissue for the coverage of the neourethra is the tissue that normally surrounds the urethra; namely, corpus spongiosum; Yerkes and colleagues described the technique of spongioplasty using the distal spongiosum as a protective vascularized layer, Bhat described double breasting Spongioplasty as a protective second layer [32, 33].

1.13 Repair Without Urethroplasty

Beck and Hacker described an interesting technique for the distal hypospadias with no chordee. They mobilized the urethra and advanced it into the glans either by tunneling or by incision and reconstruction of the glans [34].

Duckett described the meatal advancement and glanuloplasty "MAGPI" for coronal and subcoronal hypospadias. The basis of this technique is a modification of the Heineke–Mikulicz principle [35, 36]. A longitudinal incision is created from the meatus through the distal glans groove. This incision is closed in a horizontal manner, followed by the ventral glanuloplasty [13, 14].

1.14 The Urethral Plate

Glenister was the first to describe the "urethral plate" which he defined as "an outgrowth from the anterior walls of the urogenital sinus." Paul and Kanagauntheram described the urethral plate as "the moist pink gutter of a mucus membrane with well-defined mucocutaneous line and extended from the urethral orifice to the base of the glans." John Duckett used the term urethral plate to describe the characteristic skin and tissue derived from the corpus spongiosum which is located distal to the urethral meatus in patients with hypospadias and reaches to the ventral side of the glans [14, 37].

Care has been directed to the cosmetic appearance of the meatus, and improvements were sought in order to imitate the vertical slit-like normal meatus, as many of the previous techniques resulted in unsightly oval or fish mouth meatus. Zaontz described the incision of the glans groove followed by Tubularization in the Glans approximation procedure (GAP) [38].

Snodgrass described the use of tubularized incised plate urethroplasty (TIP) for distal hypospadias without chordee. This was based on the assumption that the midline incision of the urethral plate heals by epithelialization and not by scarring, and this allowed widening of the urethral plate to allow for adequate urethroplasty without the need for other tissues. The technique gained wide popularity and this led to trials of extending the indications for more proximal and redo cases [39, 40].

1.15 The Present; Established Concepts

At the present time, and in the author's opinion, there are well-established rules and guidelines for the successful correction of hypospadias.

- Most cases of hypospadias have some degree of chordee even distal and minor ones; chordee can be present without hypospadias.
- An artificial erection test is very important before and after correction to check for the complete correction of chordee.
- Chordee less than 30 degrees can be corrected with dorsal plication at the midline.
- Chordee more than 30 degrees will need ventral lengthening plus dorsal plication.
- The best graft material is the inner prepuce, followed by buccal mucosa.
- The second vascular layer covering urethroplasty is very important to minimize fistula formation.
- Excellent functional and cosmetic outcome is expected in distal hypospadias in one stage.
- For proximal hypospadias, either one-stage or two-stage procedures are optional; results are inferior to distal hypospadias.
- Complete lack of tension is very important in urethroplasty and other suture lines.

1.16 The Future; Technology and Innovation

An interesting innovation recently was the use of computer technology and artificial intelligence in classifying hypospadias and predicting prognosis by comparing anatomical variables such as meatal location, quality of the urethral plate, glans size, and ventral curvature as predictors for postoperative outcomes [41].

The long history of hypospadias repair gives us a lot of important lessons. It shows the contribution of pioneers to the progress and evolution of the current understanding of this common and complex malformation. The importance of accurate recording and comparison of data is the only way to reach evidence-based conclusions when comparing different treatment options. It is very interesting to see how science progresses based on previous experiences and a better understanding of the underlying anatomy and embryology.

References

1. Smith ED. The history of hypospadias. Pediatr Surg Int. 1997;12(2/3):81–5.
2. Lambert SM, Snyder HM, Canning DA. The history of hypospadias and hypospadias repairs. Urology. 2011;77(6):1277–83.
3. Hadidi AT. History of hypospadias: lost in translation. J Pediatr Surg. 2017;52(2):211–7.
4. Kendirci M, KadioĐlu A, Boylu U, MiroĐlu C. Urogenital surgery of the 15th century in Anatolia. J Urol. 2005;173(6):1879–82.
5. Hadidi AT, Lambert SM, Snyder HM, Canning DA, Fernandez N, Lorenzo AJ, et al. The island tube and island Onlay hypospadias repairs offer excellent long-term outcomes: a 14-year follow-up. J Urol [Internet]. 1994;172(1):464–5. https://doi.org/10.1016/S0022-5347(17)55288-X.
6. Dieffenbach JF. Guerison des fentes congenitales de la verge, de l'hypospadias. Gaz Hebd Med Chir. 1837;5:156–8.
7. Duckett JW. Transverse preputial island flap technique for repair of severe hypospadias. J Urol. 1980;167(2):1179–82.
8. Mettauer JP. Practical observations on those malformations of the male urethra and penis, termed hypospadias and epispadias, with an anomalous case. Am J Med Sci. 1842;4(7):43–57.
9. Nesbit RM. Congenital curvature of the phallus: report of three cases with description of corrective operation. J Urol. 1965;93(2):230–2.
10. Pare A. The workes of that famous Chirurgion Ambrose Parey. London: Th: Cotes and R. Young 1634.
11. Baskin LS, Duckett JW. Dorsal tunica albuginea plication for hypospadias curvature. J Urol [Internet]. 1994;151(6):1668–71. https://doi.org/10.1016/S0022-5347(17)35341-7.
12. Perovic SV, Radojicic ZI. Vascularization of the hypospadiac prepuce and its impact on hypospadias repair. J Urol. 2003;169(3):1098–101.
13. Gittes RF, McLaughlin AP. Injection technique to induce penile erection. Urology. 1974;4(4):473–4.
14. Baskin LS, Ebbers MB. Hypospadias: anatomy, etiology, and technique. J Pediatr Surg. 2006;41(3):463–72.
15. Duckett JW. Transverse preputial island flap technique for repair of severe hypospadias. 1980. J Urol. 2002;167(2 Pt 2):1179–82.
16. Ben YS, Ksia A, Ben FM, Messaoud M, Laamiri R, Belhassen S, et al. Intérêt de la technique de Koyanagi dans le traitement de l'hypospadias posterieur chez l'enfant. African J Urol. 2018;24(4):331–5.

17. Emir H, Jayanthi VR, Nitahara K, Danismend N, Koff SA. Modification of the Koyanagi technique for the single stage repair of proximal hypospadias. J Urol. 2000;164(3 3 II):973–6.
18. Hamdy MH. Modification of the "Mustardé-Mathieu" and "Horton-Devine" urethroplasty in the management of hypospadias. Br J Plast Surg. 1987;40(5):494–6.
19. Chigot PL, Lisfranc RQA. Traitement chirurgical de l'hypospadias (procédé de Mathieu modifié) [surgical treatment of hypospadias (Mathieu's modified procedure)]. Ann Chir. 1965;19(11):738–50.
20. Klimberg IWR. A comparison of the Mustardé and Horton-Devine flip-flap techniques of hypospadias repair. J Urol. 1985;134(1):103–4.
21. Vejvalka JFL. Bemerkungen über die Technik der Uberbrückungsplastik bei der Methode nach Nové-Josserand; vorläufige Mitteilung [Technic of bridge plastic surgery in Nové-Josserand's method; preliminary report]. Z Urol. 1957;50(6):338–43.
22. Memmelaar J. Use of bladder mucosa in a one-stage repair of hypospadias. J Urol. 1947;58(1):68–73.
23. Hendren WH, Reda ER. Bladder mucosa graft for construction of male urethra. J Urol [Internet]. 1986;136(1 Part 1):192. https://doi.org/10.1016/S0022-5347(17)44793-8.
24. Ransley PG, Duffy PG, Oesch ILHD. Autologous bladder mucosa graft for urethral substitution. Br J Urol [Internet]. 1987;59(4):331–3. Available from: https://pubmed.ncbi.nlm.nih.gov/3580773/
25. Snodgrass WT, Elmore J, Snyder H, Mokhless IAS, Kryger J. Initial experience with staged buccal graft (Bracka) hypospadias reoperations. J Urol. 2004;172(4 II):1720–4.
26. Baskin LS, Duckett JW. Buccal mucosa grafts in hypospadias surgery. Br J Urol. 1995;76(6):23–30.
27. JR. S. Hypospadias repair with preputial free inlay graft urethroplasty. J Urol. 1966;96(1):73–9.
28. Kuznetsov IL. Treatment of hypospadias in children. Vestn Khir Im I I Grek. 1987;138(5):87–90.
29. Nosti JC, Davis JW. Treatment of hypospadias by the Byars technique. Plast Reconstr Surg. 1973;52(2):128–31.
30. Snow BW. Use of tunica vaginalis to prevent fistulas in hypospadias surgery. J Urol. 1986;136(4):861–3.
31. Tabassi KT, Mohammadi S. Tunica vaginalis flap as a second layer for tubularized incised plate urethroplasty. Urol J. 2010;7(4):254–7.
32. Yerkes EB, Adams MC, Miller DA, Pope JC IV, Rink RC, Brock JW. Y-to-I wrap: use of the distal spongiosum for hypospadias repair. J Urol. 2000;164(5):1669.
33. Bhat A, Bhat M, Kumar R, Bhat A. Double breasting spongioplasty in tubularized/tubularized incise plate urethroplasty: a new technique. Indian J Urol. 2017;33(1):58–63.
34. Atala A, Kolon T, Kurzrock E. Urethral mobilization and advancement for midshaft to distal hypospadias. J Urol. 2002;168(2):1738–41.
35. Duckett JW. MAGPI (meatoplasty and glanuloplasty). A procedure for subcoronal hypospadias. Urol Clin North Am. 1981;167(5):2153–6.
36. Duckett JW, Snyder HM. The MAGPI hypospadias repair in 1111 patients. Ann Surg. 1991;213(6):620–5.
37. Hayashi Y, Kojima Y. Current concepts in hypospadias surgery. Int J Urol. 2008;15(8):651–64.
38. Zaontz MR, The GAP. (Glans approximation procedure) for glanular/coronal hypospadias. J Urol [Internet]. 1989;141(2):359–61. https://doi.org/10.1016/S0022-5347(17)40766-X.
39. Snodgrass W. Tubularized, incised plate urethroplasty for distal hypospadias. J Urol [Internet]. 1994;151(2):464–5. https://doi.org/10.1016/S0022-5347(17)34991-1.
40. Bhat A, Sabharwal K, Bhat M, Saran R, Singla M, Kumar V. Outcome of tubularized incised plate urethroplasty with spongioplasty alone as additional tissue cover: a prospective study. Indian J Urol. 2014;30(4):392–7.
41. Fernandez N, Lorenzo AJ, Rickard M, Chua M, Pippi-Salle JL, Perez J, et al. Digital pattern recognition for the identification and classification of hypospadias using artificial intelligence vs experienced Pediatric urologist. Urology [Internet]. 2020;147:1–6. https://doi.org/10.1016/j.urology.2020.09.019.

Hypospadias Embryology, Etiology, and Classification

M. S. Ansari, Prabhu Chakravarthy, and Priyank Yadav

Abbreviations

GMS score	Glans, urethral meatus and shaft score
hCG	Human Chorionic Gonadotropin
IHC	Immunohistochemistry
SHBG	Sex Hormone Binding Globulin

2.1 Introduction

Hypospadias is a common congenital malformation affecting one in 250 boys. It has the dubious distinction of being one of the most common surgical conditions in pediatric urology and yet having the least consensus on approach to treatment. Concepts in hypospadias are still evolving. For a greater part of the last century, surgeons focused on devising newer surgical techniques for hypospadias based on permutation and combination of different flaps, grafts, and other tissues. In the recent years, an increasing emphasis was laid on understanding the pathogenesis of hypospadias from the genetic level to embryogenesis in order to understand why there is an arrest in development and how to correct it in the most anatomically appropriate way. The prevailing ideas on the development of urethra itself were challenged and then changed as more evidence emerged from the use of newer techniques such as immunohistochemistry. To understand the nature of defect in hypospadias and the cause of deformities associated with it, an understanding of normal and abnormal penile development is essential. A knowledge of genetic and non-genetic factors that influence the development of the male urethra is also equally important in hypospadiology. Hypospadias is a spectrum of arrested development that requires careful assessment and individualized treatment based on how severe the defect appears and thus it is necessary to classify it appropriately so that clinical decisions can be tailored to meet the requirements of individual cases.

2.2 Normal Penile Development and Embryology of Hypospadias

The differentiation of external genitalia into male and female types starts after the appearance of Leydig cells at 9 weeks of gestation and subsequent surge in testosterone. Till that period, the external genitalia are represented by an indifferent genital tubercle lying above the urogenital membrane that itself is flanked by urogenital folds and further by labioscrotal folds. The genital development up to this point is androgen independent and is same in male as well as female

M. S. Ansari (✉) · P. Chakravarthy · P. Yadav
Division of Pediatric Urology, Sanjay Gandhi Postgraduate Institute of Medical Sciences, Lucknow, India

fetuses. Under the influence of testosterone, the genital tubercle and urogenital folds form the penis while the labioscrotal folds form the scrotum (Fig. 2.1). That this process is androgen driven is indicated by the presence of androgen receptors on penile skin, prepuce, urethra, as well as corporal tissues [1]. The skin of the penis is an ectodermal derivative while the mesoderm gives rise to the corporal bodies and endoderm forms the urethra. By 16 weeks, fusion of the urethral folds is usually complete and by 18 weeks, the penile development is also over.

The development of male urethra is complex and proceeds differently in the glans and the penile shaft. The most recent hypothesis which explains urethral development is the "double zipper" hypothesis by Li et al. (2015) [3]. According to this hypothesis, an initial "opening zipper" is responsible for distal canalization of the otherwise solid urethral plate and forms the urethral groove. Using immunohistochemistry (IHC) markers such as Ki67 and Caspase 3, the authors found that the canalization process is associated with increased cellular proliferation and there is complete lack of apoptosis. Subsequently, a "closing zipper" causes fusion of the margins of the urethral groove and proceeds from proximal part of the penis towards glans penis. The development of glanular urethra is slightly different. Previously, it was thought that the ectodermal cells from skin invaginate into the glans to form the distal urethra. This theory was proposed by Glenister and remained popular for decades [4]. IHC markers such as cytokeratin 7, FoxA1 (endodermal urothelial markers), and cytokeratin 10 (ectodermal marker), when applied to human fetal penile specimens, indicate towards an endodermal origin of the entire urethra right up to the meatus [2]. The glanular urethra develops due to direct canalization of the urethral plate and epithelial remodeling within the glans.

The preputial development begins around 12 weeks of gestation from the *preputial placode*, an epithelial thickening that appears on the dorsal surface of the developing penis near the proximal edge of the corona [2]. Lateral to that, *preputial laminar processes* extend ventrally on both sides, to fuse in the midline. The preputial placode soon delaminates from the epidermis, separated from it by mesenchymal cells. The prepuce grows distally to cover the glans as well as ventrally, fusing in the midline at the preputial frenulum around the time of fusion of urethral folds. Near birth, the preputial lamina that separates the glans from prepuce canalizes to create a preputial space and allow retraction of the prepuce. Till it canalizes, it remains as an adherent structure that causes physiological adhesion of prepuce over glans. In case of hypospadias, ventral fusion of prepuce does not take place and it grows excessively dorsally leading to "hooded" appearance.

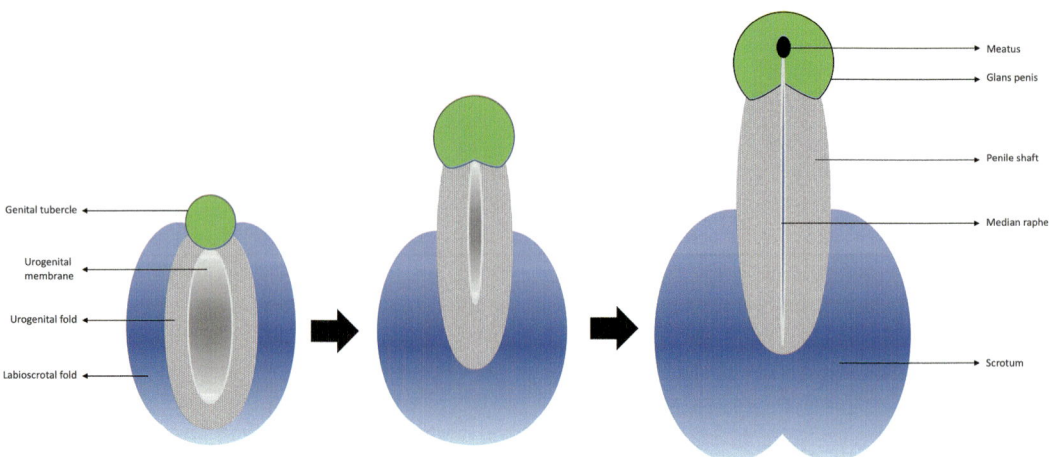

Fig. 2.1 Development of male external genitalia from the indifferent stage

In children with hypospadias, the type of lesion depends on the stage of development that is arrested. An early arrest, typically associated with severe deficiency of testosterone or testosterone resistance, is associated with female like external genitalia with small phallus, proximal meatus, and bifid scrotum. Late arrest may manifest as a mild variety—coronal or glanular hypospadias. Besides genetic susceptibility, hormonal influence plays a crucial role in pathogenesis of hypospadias. The development of male external genitalia is largely dependent on hormonal sufficiency and insufficient androgens or androgen resistance causes lack of midline fusion of urethral and scrotal folds leading to incomplete masculinization and hence, hypospadias. The most common location of hypospadiac meatus is at the coronal sulcus which is also the junction of two different canalization processes of the urethra. All types of hypospadias are typically associated with a ventrally deficient prepuce, barring few exceptions. Downward curvature or "chordee" is the consequence of abortive development of ventral structures rather than any fibrosis. Hence, the urethral plate is preserved for urethral reconstruction wherever possible without compromising the correction of curvature.

2.3 Etiology of Hypospadias

The arrested development in hypospadias is thought to be multifactorial. The proposed etiologies involve feto-maternal factors, genetic factors, and environmental factors. It has been seen that monozygotic twins and boys born out of assisted reproductive technology have a higher risk of hypospadias.

2.3.1 Feto-maternal Factors

Premature birth and low birth weight are commonly associated with both hypospadias and cryptorchidism. Placental insufficiency and intrauterine growth restriction too predispose to hypospadias. The human chorionic gonadotropin (hCG) produced by the placenta in the early part of gestation is vital for sustaining pregnancy. Since hormone production from pituitary is minimal during early pregnancy, placental hormones like hCG are vital for genital development and placental insufficiency causes multiple growth aberrations including hypospadias and stunted growth. Maternal smoking, diabetes mellitus, pregnancy induced hypertension, and preeclampsia are also associated with hypospadias due to their effect on placental function and various other effects on the developing fetus. Diabetes mellitus before gestation carries a higher risk of congenital defects including hypospadias than gestational diabetes. A hypoandrogenic state as well as a hyperoestrogenic state can lead to hypospadias. Examples of the hyperoestrogenic states include maternal obesity and maternal exposure to diethylstilbestrol. The risk of hypospadias also increases in mothers at extremes of their reproductive age, i.e. younger than 20 and older than 40. It is likely that hormonal disruption at those ages plays a causative role since the women in their early and late reproductive ages are more susceptible to such disruption. This is also true for other congenital defects. Another belief is that between age 20 and 40, the natural checks are more robust that normally eliminate the fetuses with birth defects and hence mothers in this group have lower risk of having boys with hypospadias. Increasing age is associated with other factors as well which increases the risk of hypospadias such as increased organochlorine pesticide concentration in adipose tissue, increased births and fertility treatments. Rural residence and consanguinity are other risk factors thought to predispose to hypospadias although the evidence is weak.

With preoperative hormonal stimulation, the results of surgery in proximal hypospadias show significant improvement than otherwise and may indicate role of androgens in severe hypospadias [5]. Non-genetic causes of disorders of sexual differentiation that are associated with reduced level of androgens also lead to arrest in development and lead to hypospadias, particularly proximal hypospadias.

2.3.2 Genetic Factors

Familial clustering of hypospadias occurs in about 10% and monogenic inheritance only accounts for a minority of cases. In a recent study by Nerli et al. (2018), out of 234 boys with hypospadias operated over a 10-year period, 9% reported having an additional family member with hypospadias [6]. The risk of hypospadias in the relatives is directly proportional to the severity of hypospadias in index case. In a recent study by Johnson et al. (2020), 60 boys with proximal hypospadias were assessed and 28% among those were found to have genetic abnormalities [7]. The type of familial clustering indicates a multifactorial etiopathogenesis and it is likely that a combination of genetic susceptibility and hypoandrogenic state tips the balance in favor of arrested development of urethra. More than 100 syndromes have been described in association with hypospadias, the well-known ones being Denys–Drash Syndrome and Androgen Insensitivity Syndrome. Androgen receptor gene mutations as well as 5-alpha reductase gene mutations (that affects conversion of testosterone to dihydrotestosterone) are commonly found in boys with hypospadias, usually in association with unilateral or bilateral undescended testes. The expression of estrogen dependent gene ATF3 on prepuce is upregulated in patients with hypospadias [8].

Several genes related to phallus development are important in the pathogenesis of hypospadias. Homeobox genes A and D regulate the development of the phallus and their knock-out induces hypospadias like defect in mice [9]. Polymorphisms of FGF8, FGF10, and FGFR2 also increase the risk of hypospadias in men [10]. Genes such WT1, SOX9, and GATA4 are important for testicular development which secondarily influences genital development and mutations of these genes are associated with severe grades of hypospadias [11]. Another gene that may play a role in pathogenesis in hypospadias is testosterone biosynthesis genes MAMLD1 which is important for testosterone synthesis at the time of genital development [12].

2.3.3 Environmental Factors

Chemicals and hormones that come in contact with the mother or the developing fetus can become an etiological factor for hypospadias. This is because urethral closure is highly dependent on the hormonal milieu. Pesticides, plastics, and soya diet increase the risk of hypospadias. The risk due to oral contraceptives is, however, less certain. Energy drinks taken during pregnancy may affect the normal estrogen metabolic pathway. Cocoa consumption increases the risk of hypospadias and testicular cancer. Artificial sweeteners increase the levels in insulin which reduces the level of sex hormone binding globulin (SHBG) in women, predisposing their male children to hypospadias. Other chemicals such as phytoestrogens, epichlorohydrin, atrazine, and furans also predispose to hypospadias via various pro-oestrogenic or antiandrogenic effects. Hence, they are also referred to as xenoestrogens. Higher incidence of hypospadias is also seen when pregnant mothers are on a vegetarian diet, probably indicating the role of phytoestrogens. Iron supplementation too is thought to be a predisposing factor. It is hypothesized that the environmental factors such as synthetic estrogens exert their effect through various epigenetic mechanisms such as altering DNA methylation leading to developmental reprogramming [13]. Effects may also take place via nongenomic mechanisms by binding to estrogen or androgen receptors. Gene polymorphisms involving steroid receptor genes may increase susceptibility to environmental factors. Other environmental substances with estrogenic activity that are ingested such as pesticides on fruits and vegetables have also been implicated in hypospadias. Besides, increasing parity and higher maternal age have also been noted in some of the studies [14].

Assisted reproductive technologies such as intracytoplasmic sperm injection and invitro fertilization too are associated with an increased risk of hypospadias, though the risk with invitro fertilization is lower compared to the former. Antiepileptic drugs such as valproic acid are associated with increased risk while evidence is lacking for other drugs such as antibiotics, antidepressants, and antihistaminics for playing etiological role in hypospadias.

2.4 Classification of Hypospadias

Hypospadias has been classified in different ways but most of these are purely anatomical classifications, primarily taking into account the location of the meatus (Fig. 2.2).

2.4.1 Anatomical Classification

In one of the earliest classifications, Brown (1936) categorized hypospadias into glanular, subcoronal, midshaft, penoscrotal, midscrotal, and perineal [15]. Smith (1938) categorized hypospadias into first degree (corona to distal shaft), second degree (distal shaft to penoscrotal junction), and third degree (penoscrotal junction to perineum) [16]. Schaeffer and Erbs (1950) classified hypospadias as glanular, penile, and perineal [17]. Avellán (1975) classified hypospadias in Swedish boys as glanular, penile, and penoperineal/perineal (with or without bulb) [18]. Similarly, Hadidi (2004) also classified hypospadias simply as glanular, penile, and proximal [19]. A major limitation of such systems was that they did not take into account the degree of curvature or the actual location of aberration. Many boys with hypospadias may have a meatus that is near the glans but only a thin membrane covers the urethra ventrally indicating that the actual level of spongiosum divarication is much proximal. This level is indicated by the junction of two lines drawn along the inner and outer prepuce [20]. The severity of hypospadias as such may be best identified during surgery when it is possible to assess the inner penile tissue and assess the hypoplastic urethral tissue [21]. In 1996, Duckett proposed that the classification of hypospadias must be done after degloving and releasing the curvature [22]. He classified hypospadias as anterior, middle, and posterior hypospadias and his method of classification after release of curvature made the diagnosis of hypospadias more precise. In another system of classification, Orkiszewski (2012) divided hypo-

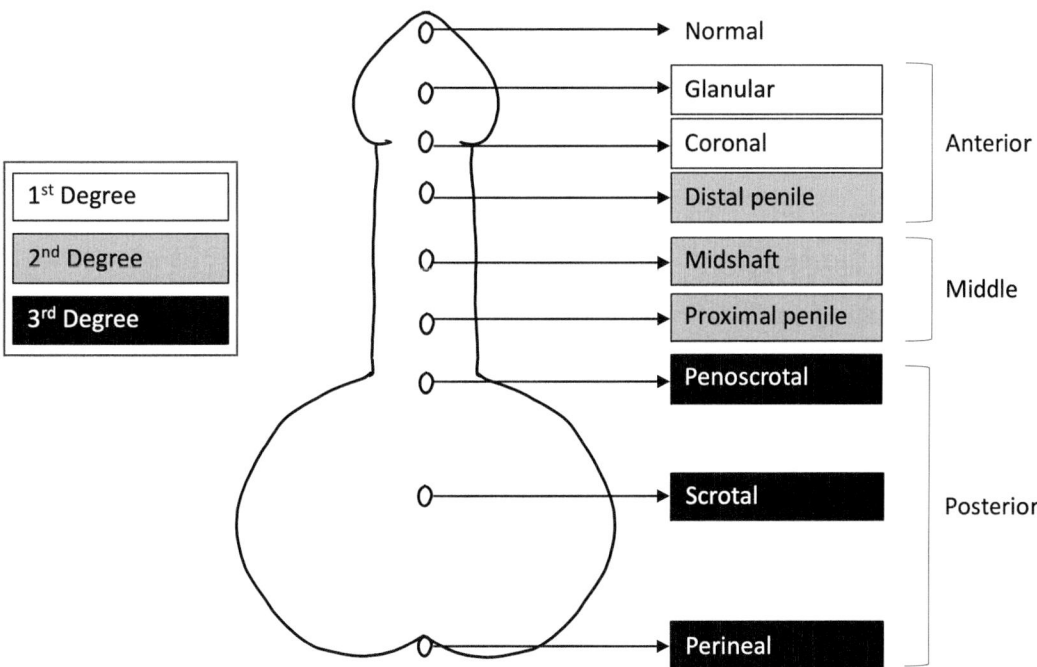

Fig. 2.2 Clinical classification of hypospadias

spadias into two types: penile and proximal [23]. The distinction was made by a horizontal line at the level of upper pubis, with the child in supine position. Penile hypospadias was further subclassified as glanular, distal third, mid shaft, and proximal third, while proximal hypospadias was further subclassified as scrotal and perineal. Importantly, this classification was based on the position of divarication of corpus spongiosum rather than the location of meatus as in Duckett's classification. However, several important aspects that are determinants of success in hypospadias were still not addressed. These include details about glans (grooved or flat), prepuce (partial or complete), urethral plate (width and presence of fibrosis), and degree of curvature. In order to overcome these limitations, Merriman et al. (2013) proposed the GMS score (Table 2.1) [24]. The highest score in this system is 12 and a higher score indicates more severe hypospadias. The authors reported that for a GMS score 6 or less, the complication rate was 5.6% while that for a score greater than 6 was 25%. Thus, it is the first classification system that makes it possible to report the severity objectively which may allow comparisons between different surgeons/centers performing hypospadias repair. In a detailed application of the score subsequently, the authors reported that boys who had a ventral curvature more than 60 degrees and underwent single-stage repair were 27 times more likely to develop a fistula than those without chordee [25]. On multivariate analysis, meatus location was not found significant implying that hypospadias has to be evaluated completely rather than the meatus location alone.

A limitation of the GMS classification system is that the associated scrotal anomalies are not incorporated into the system. Scrotal anomalies may range from a penoscrotal transposition to completely bifid scrotum. The impact of scrotal anomaly on outcome of hypospadias repair is debatable and it does not hinder the tubularization of the urethra. Further, this classification system does not take into account the mega-meatus intact prepuce variant which has an entirely different appearance from classical hypospadias.

2.4.2 Etiological Classification

Albers et al. (1997) proposed an etiological classification for severe hypospadias with an aim to standardize the diagnostic approach to children with hypospadias [26]. Using clinical assessment, ultrasonography, karyotyping, and endocrine evaluation in 33 boys, they found that 21 boys did not have any identifiable etiology whereas in 12 boys, the causes that were found were Anti-Mullerian hormone deficiency (1), Drash syndrome (3), partial androgen insensitivity (2), gonadal dysgenesis (1), chromosomal aberration (1), 5-alpha reductase deficiency (1), true hermaphroditism (2), and XX-male syndrome (1). They proposed a step ladder approach for diagnosis of the specific etiology to avoid unnecessary testing in all patients. It was seen that a descended testis decreased the possibility of finding an etiology and hence further investigation. Further, ultrasonography and genitography were recommended in all boys with severe hypospadias to find additional abnormalities, particularly Mullerian structures, which would need removal at the time of hypospadias repair. Similarly, SHBG was found useful as a tool to assess androgen receptor function. Normally, its levels decrease on administration of androgens

Table 2.1 GMS scoring system

		Score
Glans score (G)	Glans good size; healthy urethral plate, deeply grooved	1
	Glans adequate size; adequate urethral plate, grooved	2
	Glans small in size; urethral plate narrow, some fibrosis or flat	3
	Glans very small; urethral plate indistinct, very narrow or flat	4
Meatus score (M)	Glanular	1
	Coronal sulcus	2
	Mid or distal shaft	3
	Proximal shaft, penoscrotal	4
Shaft score (S)	No chordee	1
	Mild (<30 degrees) chordee	2
	Moderate (30–60 degrees) chordee	3
	Severe (>60 degrees) chordee	4

but this effect is blunted or lost with varying degrees of androgen resistance. Patients with gonadal dysgenesis and those with Drash syndrome need close follow-up for development of gonadal tumors and Wilms' tumor, respectively.

2.5 Conclusion

Hypospadias results from arrested development of the urethra along with associated abnormalities of the penile shaft and scrotum leading to the classical appearance ectopic (proximal) meatus, ventral curvature, and hooded prepuce. The development of glanular urethra occurs in a single step via cavitation while the rest of the urethra develops in two steps via "double zipper." The junction of these two parts of urethra, the corona, is the commonest location of hypospadias. The etiology of hypospadias is thought to be multifactorial, with placental insufficiency, endocrine factors, genetic factors, and exposure to environmental agents such as phytoestrogens and pesticides playing a possible role. Purely anatomical classifications of hypospadias that are usually based on location of the meatus alone are insufficient for clinical decision-making. An objective assessment of the defect in hypospadias not only leads to better clinical decision-making but also allows comparison between different centers and surgeons.

References

1. Kim K, Liu W, Cunha GR, Russell DW, Huang H, Shapiro E, et al. Expression of the androgen receptor and 5α-reductase type 2 in the developing human fetal penis and urethra. Cell Tissue Res. 2002;307(2):145–53.
2. Liu X, Liu G, Shen J, Yue A, Isaacson D, Sinclair A, et al. Human glans and preputial development. Differentiation. 2018;103:86–99.
3. Li Y, Sinclair A, Cao M, Shen J, Choudhry S, Botta S, et al. Canalization of the urethral plate precedes fusion of the urethral folds during male penile urethral development: the double zipper hypothesis. J Urol. 2015;193(4):1353–9.
4. Glenister TW. The origin and fate of the urethral plate in man. J Anat. 1954;88(3):413–25.
5. Chua ME, Gnech M, Ming JM, Silangcruz JM, Sanger S, Lopes RI, et al. Preoperative hormonal stimulation effect on hypospadias repair complications: meta-analysis of observational versus randomized controlled studies. J Pediatr Urol. 2017;13(5):470–80.
6. Rajendra BN, Shridhar CG, Shivayogeeswar EN, Murigendra BH, Neeraj SD. Familial aggregation of hypospadias in south Indian population. Res J Congenit Disease. 2018;1(2):02.
7. Johnson EK, Jacobson DL, Finlayson C, Yerkes EB, Goetsch AL, Leeth EA, et al. Proximal hypospadias-isolated genital condition or marker of more? J Urol. 2020;204(2):345–52.
8. Liu B, Wang Z, Lin G, Agras K, Ebbers M, Willingham E, et al. Activating transcription factor 3 is up-regulated in patients with hypospadias. Pediatr Res. 2005;58(6):1280–3.
9. Morgan EA, Nguyen SB, Scott V, Stadler HS. Loss of Bmp7 and Fgf8 signaling in Hoxa13-mutant mice causes hypospadias. Development. 2003;130(14):3095–109.
10. Beleza-Meireles A, Lundberg F, Lagerstedt K, Zhou X, Omrani D, Frisén L, et al. FGFR2, FGF8, FGF10 and BMP7 as candidate genes for hypospadias. Eur J Hum Genet. 2007;15(4):405–10.
11. Huang B, Wang S, Ning Y, Lamb AN, Bartley J. Autosomal XX sex reversal caused by duplication of SOX9. Am J Med Genet. 1999;87(4):349–53.
12. Chen Y, Thai HTT, Lundin J, Lagerstedt-Robinson K, Zhao S, Markljung E, et al. Mutational study of the MAMLD1-gene in hypospadias. Eur J Med Genet. 2010;53(3):122–6.
13. Kalfa N, Philibert P, Baskin LS, Sultan C. Hypospadias: interactions between environment and genetics. Mol Cell Endocrinol. 2011;335(2):89–95.
14. Raghavan R, Romano ME, Karagas MR, Penna FJ. Pharmacologic and environmental endocrine disruptors in the pathogenesis of hypospadias: a review. Curr Environ Health Rep. 2018;5(4):499–511.
15. Browne D. An operation for hypospadias. Lancet. 1936;1:141.
16. Smith CK. Surgical procedures for correction of hypospadias. J Urol. 1938;40:239.
17. Schaefer AA, Erbes J. Hypospadias. Am J Surg. 1950;80(2):183–91.
18. Avellán L. The incidence of hypospadias in Sweden. Scand J Plast Reconstr Surg. 1975;9(2):129–39.
19. Hadidi A. Classification of hypospadias. In: Hadidi AT, Azmy AF, editors. Hypospadias surgery, an illustrative guide. Berlin: Springer-Verlag; 2004. p. 79–82.
20. Catti M, Demède D, Valmalle A-F, Mure P-Y, Hameury F, Mouriquand P. Management of severe hypospadias. Indian J Urol. 2008;24(2):233–40.
21. Snodgrass W, Macedo A, Hoebeke P, Mouriquand PDE. Hypospadias dilemmas: a round table. J Pediatr Urol. 2011;7(2):145–57.
22. Duckett JW. Hypospadias. In: Gillenwater JT, Grayhack JT, Howard SS, Duckett JW, editors. Adult and pediatric urology. 3rd ed. St Louis: Mosby Year Book; 1966. p. 2550–65.

23. Orkiszewski M. A standardized classification of hypospadias. J Pediatr Urol. 2012;8(4):410–4.
24. Merriman LS, Arlen AM, Broecker BH, Smith EA, Kirsch AJ, Elmore JM. The GMS hypospadias score: assessment of inter-observer reliability and correlation with post-operative complications. J Pediatr Urol. 2013;9(6):707–12.
25. Arlen AM, Kirsch AJ, Leong T, Broecker BH, Smith EA, Elmore JM. Further analysis of the Glans-Urethral Meatus-Shaft (Gms) hypospadias score: correlation with postoperative complications. J Pediatr Urol. 2015;11(2):71.e1–5.
26. Albers N, Ulrichs C, Glüer S, Hiort O, Sinnecker GH, Mildenberger H, et al. Etiologic classification of severe hypospadias: implications for prognosis and management. J Pediatr. 1997;131(3):386–92.

Anatomy of the Penis in Hypospadias

Anil Takvani

3.1 Introduction

Hypospadias is the second most frequently occurring congenital condition in infants, only to be preceded by undescended testis [1], with an incidence of approximately 1% [2]. Hypospadias is defined as an abortive development of the corpus spongiosum, urethra, and ventral prepuce with an arrest of the normal embryological correction of ventral penile curvature [3]. The Greek physician Galen should be credited for coining the term "Hypospadias" in the second century Common Era [4]. Hypospadias means rent or fissure underneath which has originated from the Greek words hypos meaning "under'" and spadon meaning "rent/fissure". It is an abnormality of the anterior urethra and penile development. The urethral opening (meatus) is abnormally located on the ventral surface of the penis proximal to the tip of the glans while the glans is splayed open. The urethral opening can be located as proximal as up to the perineum. The prepuce of the hypospadiac penis is deficient ventrally, casting a hooded appearance on the dorsal aspect [5]. Hypospadiac penis is commonly associated with a ventral curvature called "chordee".

Embryological Basis of Hypospadiac Phallus The constellation of anatomical anomalies in hypospadias includes—an abnormal urethral opening; ventral curvature of the penis; an incomplete prepuce; rotation of the penis; abnormal raphe, disorganized corpus spongiosum and penile fascia. Urethral development occurs between 8 and 20 weeks of gestation. Therefore, hypospadias occurs due to the abortive development of the urethra during this phase of intrauterine life.

The genes in the Y chromosome direct the development of testes from the undifferentiated gonads. The testes secrete testosterone, which along with its active metabolite dihydrotestosterone, acts on the undifferentiated genital structure to give rise to the male phenotype. After that, the undifferentiated genital structure develops into male genitalia by the orderly occurrence of the following events. First, the genital tubercle elongates to form the phallus. Second, the primary urethral groove also elongates along with the developing phallus, and the genital swellings develop into scrotal folds. As further development occurs, the urethral groove coalesces in the midline from proximal to the distal end, forming the urethra. The line of union of the urethral folds is represented as the median scrotal raphe. An ectopic urethral opening leads to hypospadias when the fusion of the urethral folds in the midline does not occur. The distal anterior urethra is thought to be developed by the proximal invagination of ectodermal cells from the summit of the glans, which canalizes to join at the corona glandis with the distal limit of urethra formed from the closure of the urethral groove. The higher

A. Takvani (✉)
Takvani Kidney Hospital, Junagadh, Gujarat, India

incidence of subcoronal hypospadias can be explained by this theory very well.

The above-mentioned theory of the urethral development by fusion of the urethral folds in the midline has been challenged in recent years. As it is not possible to explain the whole spectrum of hypospadias with this zipper theory. Baskin (2000) projected another version of this theory stating that urethral folds merge to form a seam of the epithelium, which is then transformed into mesenchyme, and this subsequently canalizes by apoptosis or programmed cell resorption [6]. Theoretically, the epithelium seam also develops at the glandular level, and therefore, the endoderm differentiates into ectoderm with subsequent canalization by apoptosis.

Regarding prepucial development, prepuce first appears as a skin fold at the dorsal aspect of the penis at the corona level. It then grows circumferentially, finally merging at the ventral aspect over the fused urethral groove. Failure of fusion of the urethral grooves in hypospadias impedes this process leading to a dorsal hooded prepuce. Occasionally, a variant of glandular hypospadias may have an intact prepuce called "Megameatus Intact Prepuce". One can miss this subtle anomaly if the prepuce is not fully retracted during neonatal circumcision.

Ventral penile curvature or chordee is frequently associated with severe hypospadias and pronounced in the proximal forms of hypospadias. Several theories explain the origin of penile curvatures, such as abnormal urethral plate development, dysplastic mesenchymal tissue at the urethral meatus, and dorsoventral corporal disproportion [7, 8]. The ventral penile curvature at the 16th week of foetal development resolves during the 20th and 25th weeks [7]. An arrest of the embryonic development at some point during this process may cause persistence of this curvature. Moreover, the urethral defect is related to thinning and hypo development of the corpus spongiosum and other ventral structures that lead to penile disproportion and curvature. These factors may be interlinked and impact the final severity of curvature in these patients [9].

3.2 Anatomy of Normal and Hypospadiac Penis

Meatus The urethral meatus of a normal newborn penis is positioned slightly on the ventral surface of the glans and is slit-like. The abortive urethra of hypospadias can terminate at any point proximal to its usual location on the tip of the glans penis. The urethral opening (meatus) of hypospadias is usually splayed. Most commonly, the transverse type of meatus is observed in hypospadias (Fig. 3.1a). Another common type is the pinpoint type of meatus, surrounded by a fibrous ring (Fig. 3.1b) that can cause meatal

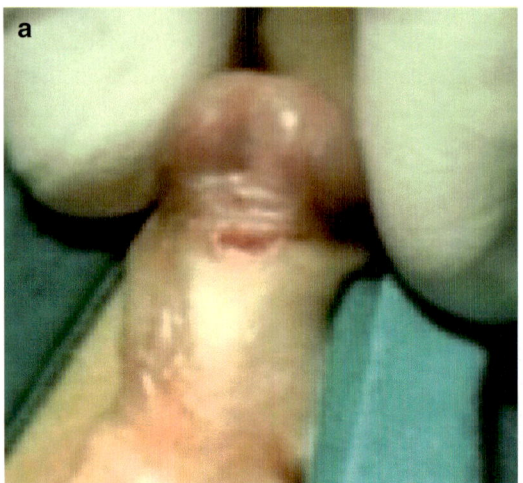 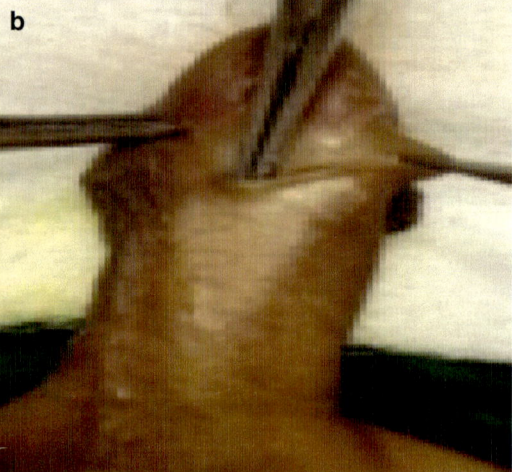

Fig. 3.1 Configuration of the meatus, (**a**)—Transverse form, (**b**)—Pinpoint meatus with fibrous ring

stenosis and consequent difficulty in passing urine. There may be an elevation (bridge) distal to the meatus [9]. The meatal calibre of the hypospadiac penis is inadequate in comparison to that of a normal penis. A study by Avellan demonstrated that meatal calibre was inadequate in 91% of the patients with glanular hypospadias, which is a common type of hypospadias [10].

Glans and Urethral Plate in Distal Hypospadias Usually, the spongiosum extends distally to form the glans and protects the ends of corpora cavernosa, offering a cushioning effect. The urethral meatus is positioned slightly in the ventral surface of the glans like a slit guarded by two tiny labia on either side. The glans edges extend from the penile shaft forming a rim called the corona glandis. In hypospadias, glans appears abnormally globular. Hadidi et al. classified the glans penis in hypospadias anatomically into three categories based on the degree of clefting and other urethral plate characteristics [9].

Cleft glans: A deep groove in the middle of the glans with adequate clefts, the narrow urethral plate, and the projecting glans tip (Fig. 3.2a).

- Incomplete cleft glans: This has a variable degree of glans split, a shallow glanular groove, and a varying degree of urethral plate projection (Fig. 3.2b).
- Flat glans: The urethral plate ends short of the glans penis; absent glanular groove (Fig. 3.2c).

The size of the glans in a patient with hypospadias is generally smaller than the glans of a normal child of a similar age. Snodgrass et al. reported that the width of the glans was less than normal newborn with distal and the majority of those with proximal hypospadias. They showed that the average maximum glans diameters were significantly different in controls (normal), distal and proximal hypospadias (14.3, 14.8, and 12.9 mm, respectively). In their study, the mean age of controls was lower than those with hypospadias; some boys with distal and most boys with proximal hypospadias had smaller glans diameter of <14 mm. The size of the glans did not correlate with increasing age in patients with distal or proximal hypospadias at 3–24 months of age [11]. A recently published article by Abass et al. gave objective anatomical criteria to differentiate flat glans from cleft glans (Fig. 3.3). Three anatomical points (A, B, C) were marked on the glans along the line of the urethral plate extending from the tip of the glans to its junction with the corona. The first point "A" is marked at the distal end of the urethral plate groove; second point "B" is marked at the most prominent knob-like projection of the glans; third point "C" is marked at the lowest end of the urethral plate at the glans/coronal junction. The ratio of AB/BC < 1.2 is considered flat glans, whereas AB/BC >1.2 is regarded as wide and grooved urethral plate [12].

Hypospadias represents hypoplasia of the tissues forming the ventral aspect of the penis

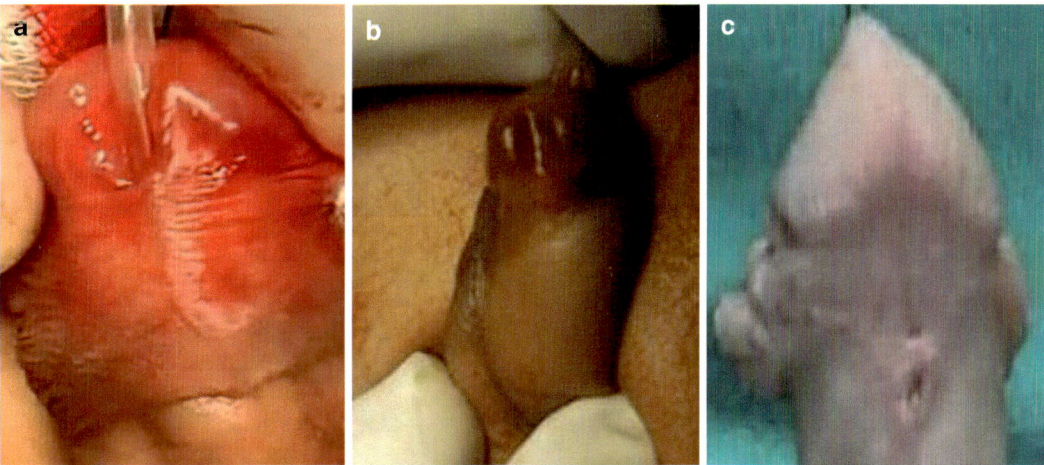

Fig. 3.2 Anatomical classification of glans, (**a**)—Cleft glans, (**b**)—Incomplete cleft glans, (**c**)—Flat glans

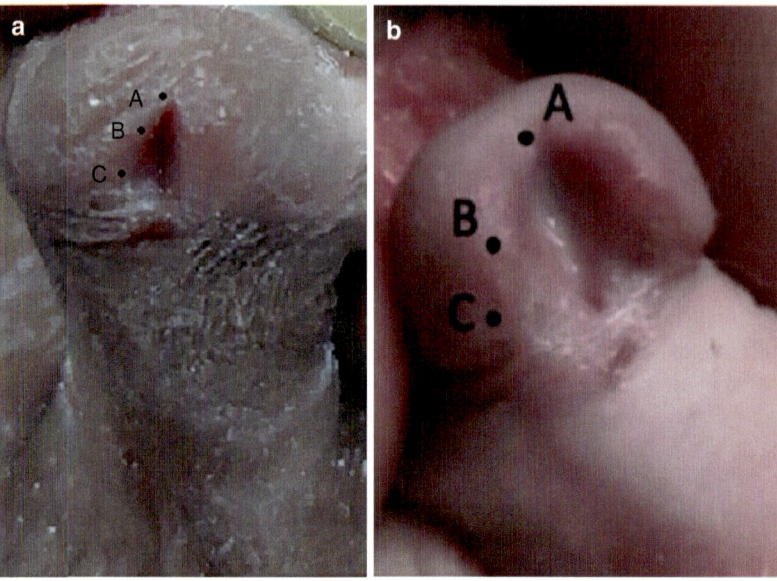

Fig. 3.3 POST score: Plate Objective Scoring Tool, (**a**)—Poor plate, (**b**)—Grooved better plate

POST AB/BC <1.2   POST AB/BC ≥1.2

beyond the division of the corpus spongiosum, which involves the urethra, the corpus spongiosum, and ventral prepuce. Mouriquand et al. described anatomical defects of hypospadias as a ventral triangular defect, the apex of which is at the division of the corpus spongiosum, sides are two pillars of atretic spongiosum and base is formed by the glans. Contents of this triangle starting from the glans tip as an apex proceeding proximally in sequence are wide open glans, the urethral plate extending from the apex of the glans to the ectopic urethral meatus, the ectopic urethral meatus, and a segment of variable length of the atretic urethra (not surrounded by any spongiosum) which starts at the point of division of the corpus spongiosum. Based on this anatomical finding, they divided hypospadias broadly into two types: one where the corpus spongiosum divides distally with little or no chordee in the erect penis and second where the corpus spongiosum divides proximally, with a significant degree of chordee and marked hypoplasia of the tissues forming the ventral radius. The base of this triangle is formed mainly by the urethral plate with a smaller contribution from the open glans (Fig. 3.4). The urethral plate is a strip of mucosa extending from the ectopic meatus towards the glans. The width of the urethral plate varies in each patient. A pinkish appearing urethral plate suggests the well-vascularized plate and is well-supported underneath by abortive spongiosal

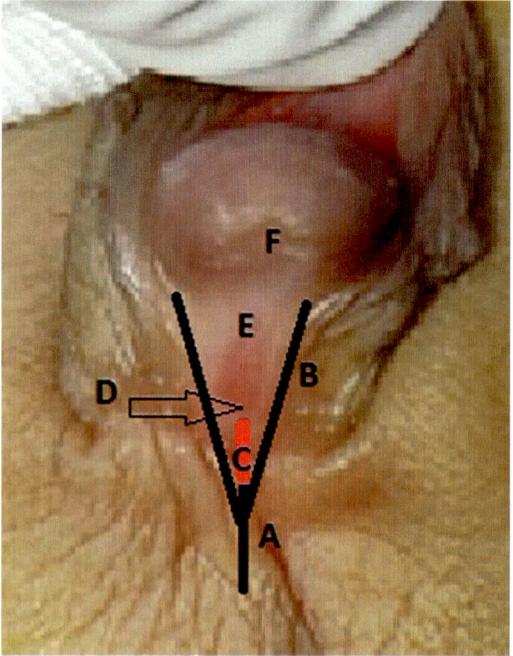

Fig. 3.4 (**a**)—Normal urethra, (**b**)—Divergent corpus spongiosum, (**c**)—Hypoplastic urethra, (**d**)—ectopic meatus, (**e**)—urethral plate

tissue. The poor urethral plate can be recognized by its pale appearance and narrow width with lots of tethering and a skinny strip of underlying spongiosal tissue. According to Bhat et al., divergent corpus spongiosum on either side of the urethral plate extends into the glans. They recommend an oblique incision at 45 degrees to separate the glans wings, creating healthy thick glans wings with an intact spongiosum [13].

Penile Shaft A normally developed penile shaft comprises three erectile bodies, the two corpora cavernosa, and a corpus spongiosum. These erectile columns are enveloped by fascial layers, nerves, lymphatics, and blood vessels. The skin forms the outer cover and is distensible, expandable, and hairless. The two suspensory ligaments composed predominantly of elastic fibres support the penis at its base [14]. In hypospadias, some parts of the urethra and corpus spongiosum are deficient. As we have read in the previous paragraph, urethral plate varies in its thickness and width. The corpus spongiosum thins out as it travels distally underneath the urethral plate. The spongiosum of hypospadiac patients is divergent in disposition, and the bulk of it lies lateral and posterior to the urethral plate.

Layers of the penis: Layers of the penis from inside out are; Tunica albuginea, Buck's fascia (deep fascia of the penis), Dartos (superficial fascia), and skin (Fig. 3.5).

Tunica Albuginea The paired corpora cavernosa contain erectile tissue surrounded by tunica albuginea, the dense fibrous sheath of connective tissue. It is made up of two layers; inner circular and outer longitudinal. The tunica albuginea of the corpora cavernosa turns thicker ventrally where it forms a groove to accommodate the corpus spongiosum. The corpus spongiosum is also surrounded by tunica albuginea, but it is thinner and more elastic to allow for the discharge of ejaculate through the urethra [15]. The corpus spongiosum is single and lies in the ventral

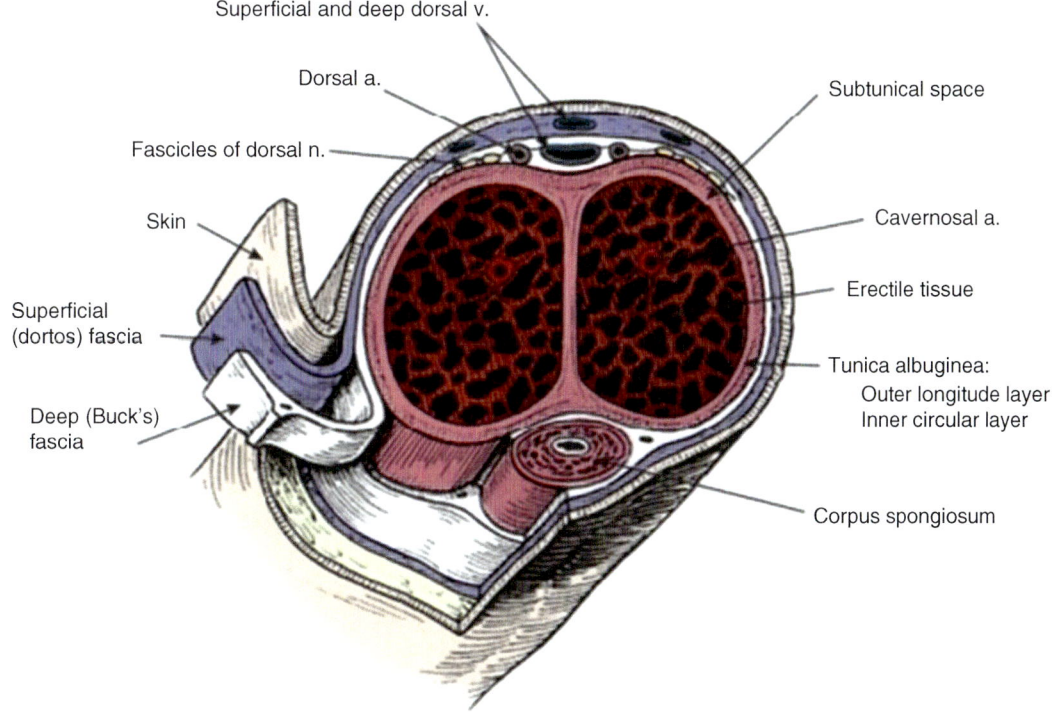

Fig. 3.5 Skin, Dartos fascia, Buck's fascia dissected away from the longitudinal layer of tunica albuginea in a layer-wise fashion

groove between the two corpora cavernosa; the urethra traverses through the corpus spongiosum (Fig. 3.5).

In hypospadias surgery, spongioplasty is a relatively newer concept. Sound knowledge of the surgical anatomy of the layers of the penile shaft is essential to avoid damage to the spongiosum and the urethral plate, as the procedure of spongioplasty entails complete mobilization and medialization of spongiosum as available to cover the neourethra completely. This involves sharply incising Buck's fascia proximal to the hypospadiac urethral opening and a dissection commencing from the lateral border of the divergent spongiosum to the urethral plate medially. The plane of dissection is kept between Buck's fascia and the longitudinal layer of the corpus cavernosa [13].

(Fig. 3.6).

The spongioplasty serves three goals [16]:

- Achieves better correction of penile curvature.
- Lands the glans a more rounded contour.
- Reduces the risk of fistula.

Studies by Hayashi et al. suggest that spongiosum dissection and spongioplasty decrease the curvature of the penis, avoiding dorsal conciliation in a significant number of patients with mild to moderate curvature associated with hypospadias [17]. **In addition, fistula development can be averted through anatomical wrapping of corpus spongiosum** in "Y to I" fashion without causing residual or recurrent curvature. Furthermore, it reconstructs a nearly normal urethra with the spongiosum around in some cases [18].

In 2014, Bhat et al. classified hypospadias spongiosum anatomically; depending on the appearance and vascularity, three types were recognized: (Chap. 11, Figs. 11.2, 11.3, and 11.4):

- Poorly developed—Thin spongiosal tissue with decreased vascularity; the diameter of the neourethra covered by spongiosum after spongioplasty was less than the proximal healthy urethra.
- Moderately developed—Average thickness with normal vascularity of spongiosal tissue; the diameter of the neourethra covered by spongiosum after spongioplasty was almost equal to that of the proximal healthy urethra.
- Well-developed—Thick spongiosum with good vascularity of spongiosal tissue; the diameter of the neourethra covered by spongiosum was greater than that of the proximal healthy urethra [13].

Knowledge of the surgical anatomy of the tunica albuginea is necessary while correcting ventral curvature of the penis associated with hypospadias by ventral corporotomies. Pippi Salle et al. described cuts in the longitudinal layer of the tunica albuginea in an elliptical fashion at the level of maximum curvature, taking care not to cut the circular layer of the tunica albuginea. Inner circular fibres of tunica albuginea form a pinkish layer around the corpora cavernosa, and care is taken not to enter into the spongy tissue. According to them, in full-thickness corporotomy, the defects in the tunica albuginea need to be repaired with either free grafts or pedicle flaps. Few hypospadias surgeons prefer to make multiple superficial cuts into the outer longitudinal layer to correct the chordee termed "fairy cuts".

Buck's Fascia The three erectile bodies are covered by the deep fascia of the penis, which is called Buck's fascia, and it is a strong fascial layer that is immediately superficial to the tunica

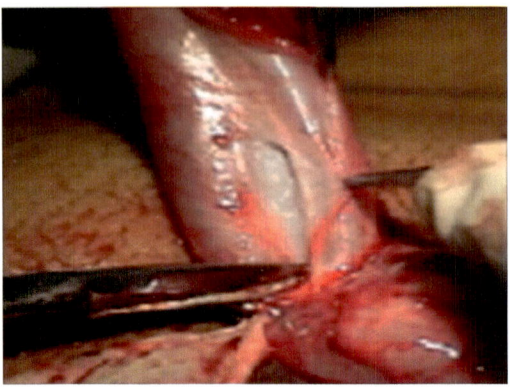

Fig. 3.6 Courtesy Dr. Amilal Bhat creation of plane proximal to meatus between tunica and Buck's fascia to mobilize the corpus spongiosum

albuginea. Proximally Buck's fascia is continuous with the deep fascia of the muscles covering the crura and bulb of the penis. The Buck's fascia surrounds the corpora cavernosa and splits to contain the corpus spongiosum separately. Buck's fascia encompasses the deep dorsal vein, paired dorsal arteries, and branches of the dorsal nerves on the corporal dorsal surface. Anatomical knowledge of Buck's fascia is crucial in hypospadias surgery. While degloving the penis, the dissection plane is deep to the dartos fascia and superficial to Buck's fascia. In Nesbitt's plication, dissection is carried out under Buck's facia and over the tunica albuginea of corpora cavernosa. It takes care to avoid injury to the artery, veins, nerves, and branches running within Buck's fascia [19]. In most cases, hypoplastic Buck's fascia and dartos fascia are responsible for the curvature in patients with hypospadias.

Penile Skin and Dartos Fascia The skin of the penis is continuous with the lower abdominal wall and distally merges with the smooth, hairless skin covering the glans. At the distal-most end, skin gets folded on itself to form the prepuce (foreskin) at the corona, covering the glans. The smooth muscles profusely present in the subcutaneous connective tissue of the penis and scrotum of normal boys are known as the dartos muscles, and connective tissue is known as the dartos fascia. It continues into the perineum combining with the superficial perineal (Colles) fascia, The dartos fascia is loosely attached to the skin and Buck's fascia on the penile shaft. It contains superficial arteries, veins, lymphatics, and nerves of the penis. There is a third layer known as tela subfascialis; dissection in this plane separates dartos from the underlying Buck's fascia without damaging vascular and lymphatic supplies of skin and dartos [14]. In patients with hypospadias, dartos fascia has fewer hypoplastic smooth muscles replaced by fibrous bands containing connective tissues responsible for a certain degree of ventral curvature and penile torsion associated with hypospadias. The ventral penile skin is thinned out and deficient in hypospadias.

The Prepuce An ectopic urethral meatus on the ventral shaft of the penis and arrest in ventral preputial formation with excess foreskin on the dorsal penile surface are predominant among many preputial malformations of hypospadias [20]. This dorsal excess gives glans of hypospadias a hooded appearance that may accentuate the degree of penile chordee (curvature). In mild forms of hypospadias, the urethral meatus is not affected and resides in its normal position on the glans, with the only abnormality being the deficiency of ventral prepuce. In hypospadias, the prepuce has a hump and two lateral edges fixed laterally because of deficiency of skin ventrally. Cunha et al. hypothesized that failure to form the urethra within the glans is linked to a ventral deficit in the prepuce. Megameatus Intact Prepuce is a rare hypospadias variant wherein the prepuce grows in a normal circumferential manner. The urethral defect is diagnosed after neonatal circumcision or in the initial infant years when the physiological preputial adhesions resolve spontaneously [21]. Outwardly, it is a deformation of the glanular urethra that involves complex remodelling of the canalized urethra plate and midline mesenchymal confluence, leading to an enlarged calibre urethral meatus (mega meatus) with the development of normal prepuce [22].

Knowledge of the surgical anatomy of the prepuce is crucial in achieving good outcomes of hypospadias surgeries as this skin is in abundance, hairless, and distensible. Now we know the prepuce is the highly vascularized foreskin that overlies the glans and is continuous with the shaft of the penis [22]. Prepuce can be released through circumferential incision before preparing a flap. The arteries mostly come in the prepuce proximally along the shaft and less often from the coronal sulcus region. Most cases of hypospadias, regardless of severity, are associated with a prepuce that could be sufficient to create an onlay or neourethra to bridge the gap caused by deficient urethra on correcting the ventral curvature and also to cover the repair with skin. A major part of the success depends on three anatomical findings:

- A sufficiently lengthy inner layer of the prepuce.
- The adequate epithelial surface of the prepuce.
- An appropriate and adequately vascularized subcutaneous tissue is present amidst the external and internal layer of the prepuce.

Radojicic and Perovic classified the hypospadias prepuce based on anatomical characteristics and vascularization. Based on the predominant morphological characteristics and abnormalities, they classified the prepuces into six groups—A: "monk's hood" or one-humped; B-cobra eyes or "2 humped", C; normal (intact), D; flat, E; V-shaped and F; collar-scarf. In addition to this, based on the presence of well-developed blood vessels, prepuces were further classified as well vascularized and poorly vascularized for the creation of vascularized flaps. Prepuces with a favourable vascular pattern were types 1 to 3 (1: A & B; 1 predominant blood vessel, 2: C & D; two predominant blood vessels, and 3: E & F; H-like form, respectively) and prepuces with an unfavourable vascular pattern, where type 4 (G & H; net-like structure) [23] (Fig. 3.7).

Arterial Supply of Penile and Preputial Skin The skin of the penis receives asymmetrical blood supply [24] arising from the left and right superficial external pudendal arteries, branches of the femoral artery. The superficial external pudendal arteries divide into dorsolateral and ventrolateral branches, which enter the superficial penile fascia (Colle's fascia) dorso-lateral and ventrolateral, respectively (Fig. 3.8a). These four arteries contain numerous collaterals that together generate a fine subcutaneous/subdermal arterial plexus (Fig. 3.8b). Next, the blood supply to the ventral penile skin is received from the posterior scrotal artery, a superficial branch of the deep internal pudendal artery [24]. Finally, the frenulum gets the blood supply from the dorsal artery of the penis, the branches of which curve around the distal shaft on either side of the penis entering the glans and the frenulum ventrally.

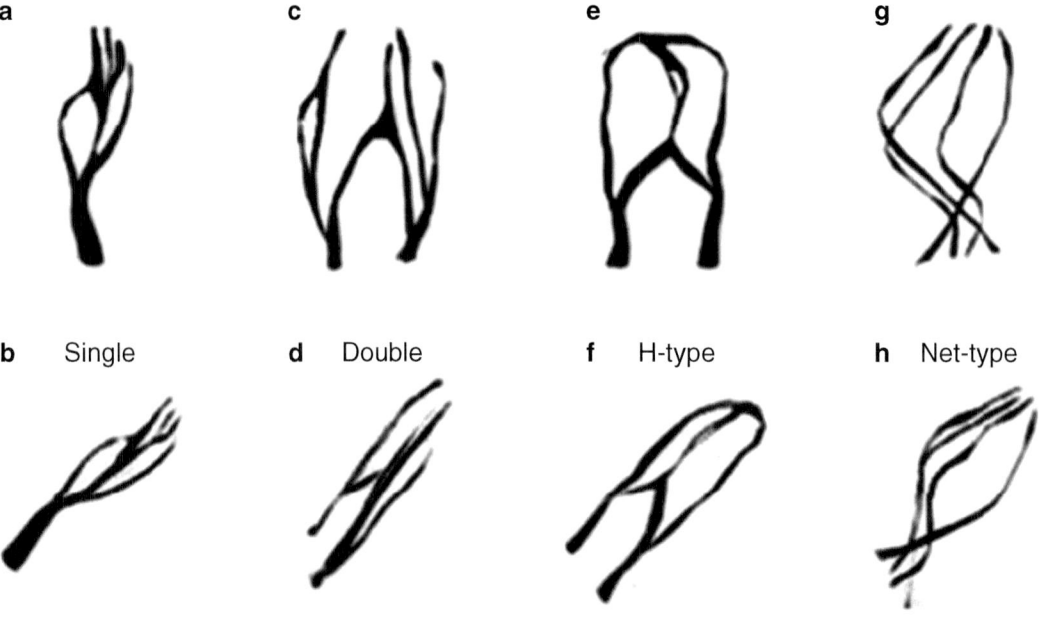

Fig. 3.7 3D reconstruction of 4 different arterial systems in the hypospadiac preputial flap. (**a** and **b**)—Single artery predominant. (**c** and **d**)—2 arteries predominant. (**e** and **f**) H type arch artery. (**g** and **h**)—no predominant artery but the net-like system with fewer distal branching

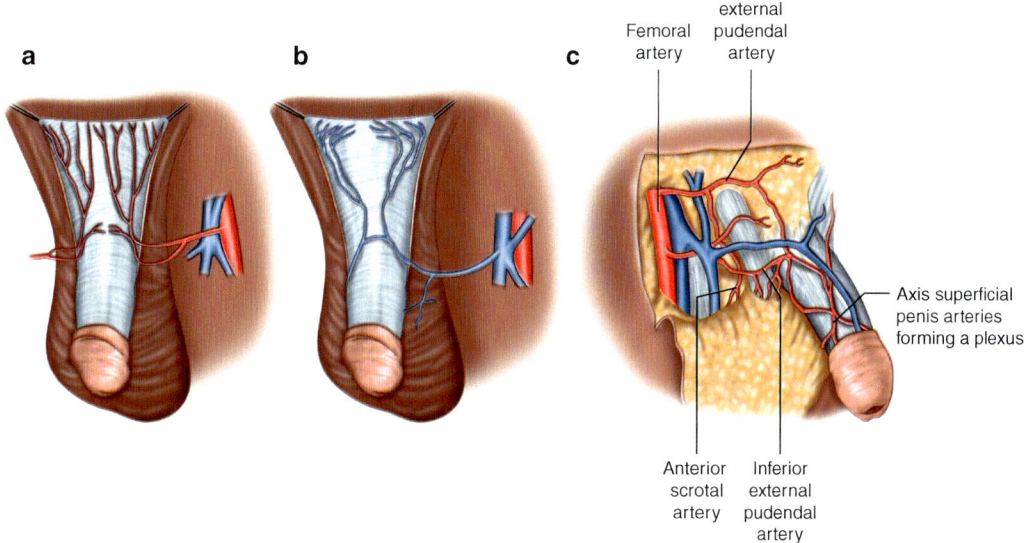

Fig. 3.8 (**a**)—Arterial Supply of the prepuce, (**b**)—Venous drainage of the prepuce, (**c**)—Arterial network around the penis

Based on the predominance of blood vessels, S V Perovic et al. classified preputial vascularization in hypospadias cases into four groups: 1; 43% chiefly had one blood vessel predominance, 2; 12% had two blood vessels, 3; 14% had an H-like formation with communication between two well-developed blood vessels, and 4; 29% showed a net-like structure without the presence of predominant vessels [25] (Fig. 3.7).

This vascular anatomical classification is based on the transillumination technique, which was confirmed to be precise and easy to perform. Yucel et al. reported the pattern of the preputial blood vessels in children with hypospadias and healthy children with the assistance of transillumination, arterial methylene blue injection, and 3-dimensional (3-D) reconstruction of serial histological sections targeting the arterial vessels [26]. They observed that about 50% of children with hypospadias presented a net-like arterial system, which was predominant in severe cases of hypospadias. Other than for milder cases of hypospadias, most hypospadias procedures make use of the prepuce. The blood supply to the prepuce in the area of the proposed flap follows the contour of the skin by doubling back at the preputial ring [27]. The dissection of the pedicle containing the blood supply to the inner prepuce is done with care, preserving the vascularity of the flap.

Zhao et al. further divided the total prepuce blood supply into superficial vessels and deep vessels. According to them, the deep vessels were usually on or leaned towards the middle line. In prepuce proximally, the deep vessels traverse axially and are oriented horizontally as they travel distally (Fig. 3.8a). In a peduncle inner preputial skin flap, dissection to be carried out in a deep layer of the superficial fascia and the skin at the junction of the inner and outer prepuce constitutes a peduncle of the skin flap. For the rest of the skin, blood supply is preserved in the superficial layer of the superficial fascia. Thus, there can be a ramus communicans between the superficial and deep layers of the superficial fascia [28].

The Arterial Supply of Deep Structures of the Penis The blood supply to the deep structures of the penis is derived from the internal pudendal artery. These are three paired arteries supplying blood to the penis through the dorsal, cavernosal, and bulbourethral arteries. The artery of the bulb (bulbourethral artery) penetrates through Buck's fascia to supply the bulb of the penis and the penile urethra. The dorsal artery of the penis lies between the dorsal nerve and the deep dorsal vein and eventually arborizes into circumflex branches in the glans penis. The cavernosal artery is generally a single artery, arising on either side and passes through the crus of the corpus cavernosum, and travels along the length of the penile shaft branching into the helicine arteries that form an integral element of the erectile apparatus. (Fig. 3.8c) [14, 22].

Venous Drainage of the Penis Venous drainage is less well-organized (Fig. 3.8b) and is not analogous to the arterial supply, unlike other places in the body [27]. Various minor veins present in the prepuce link the superficial dorsal veins from the dartos fascia indefinitely. The superficial veins merge at the base into a single superficial dorsal vein which drains into the saphenous vein through the superficial external pudendal veins. Only a single deep dorsal vein travels along with the dorsal arteries and nerves in Buck's fascia above the tunica albuginea. The emissary's veins traverse obliquely through tunica albuginea enabling compression during erections for penile tumescence. The deep dorsal vein receives drainage from the distal two-thirds of the corpora cavernosa via emissary's veins, and circumflex veins drain the corpus spongiosum. Emissary's veins are the veins that traverse obliquely through the tunica albuginea, allowing them to be compressed during erections for penile tumescence. The deep dorsal vein then drains to the periprostatic plexus [29].

Lymphatic Drainage of the Penis The lymphatic drainage system of the penis runs parallel to the venous system, wherein the superficial system cascades into the skin and a more in-depth system into the glans and the corporal bodies. The lymph capillary network originates within the skin, mucosa, submucosa of the urethra, septum of the glans, and tunica albuginea of the corpora cavernosa. The glans skin consists of a bi-layered lymphatic network located within the stratum papillare and the stratum reticulare with free communication between the two networks. These networks travel parallel to the skin and orient radially from the urethral meatus that merges and forms one network at the corona while passing through the inner and outer prepuce. The skin of the penile shaft is sequestered with distinct layers of lymphatics coursing within the papillary and reticular layers of the skin. In addition, a distinct systema lymphaticum exists within the fascia and tunica albuginea. The systema lymphaticum drains into the frenulum and unites at the corona; further, extending proximally below Buck's fascia terminating in the nodes of the femoral triangle [14].

Neuroanatomy of Hypospadias Penis Penile innervations consist of the dorsal, cavernosal, and perineal nerves. Dorsal nerves arising from the pudendal nerves and travel within Buck's fascia with the dorsal arteries and veins constitute the sensory innervations of the penile skin [15]. Despite its nomenclature, it is important to note that the nerves do not lie directly within the dorsal midline but rather extend from the 11 and 1 o'clock positions laterally to the junction of the cavernosa and spongiosum on each side [30]. Few nerves are present at the 12 o'clock position, and they do not send perforators deep through the tunica albuginea to the corpora cavernosa [14]. Baskin et al. have modified their approach to correcting penile ventral curvature associated with hypospadias based on these anatomical studies. Previously tunica albuginea plication was popularized [19, 30]. According to Baskin et al., in the procedure of tunica plication for ventral curvature correction, it is impossible to lift the neurovascular bundle that wraps around the shaft of the penis within Buck's fascia without damaging few nerve fibres. Therefore, they recommended penile straightening by placing rows of plication sutures at the 12 o'clock position in a nerve-free area. Also, this position has the thickest tunica and hence the strongest portion to hold the stitches in place. It was also noticed that nerve distribution in hypospadias glans was less extensive than in the normal penis [31–34].

Histology of Urethral Plate, Abortive Corpus Spongiosum, and Ventral Curvature (Chordee) In hypospadias, urethral development is an arrest resulting in an open urethral plate deficient corpus spongiosum, which is divergent on either side of the urethral plate [35].

The urethral plate is thought to be a continuation of the urogenital sinus that extends from the base to the glans tip [5]. In the study by Baskin and his group, both the urethral plate and the skin expressed cytokeratin [14]. According to them, this pattern is consistent with the urethra forming as an extension of the urogenital sinus. Hayashi et al. reported that the source of the urethral plate and the underlying tissue were the same as that of urethral mucosa and corpus spongiosum, respectively, that cannot form the lumen nor conceal the urethra [36]. They stated the urethral plate is well vascularized, has muscular backing, and is capable of glands formation. It is richly innervated by the dorsal nerves that distribute completely around the corporal bodies.

Baskin proposed that the glands underneath the urethral plate are an abortive attempt at the urethral formation in hypospadias. They stated all the components of a normal urethral spongiosum are present in the hypospadiac penis with some abnormal organization of glands, smooth muscle, vessels, and nerves. These findings indicate that abnormal cellular signalling could be a possible causative factor of hypospadias [3, 35]. For a long, the urethral plate and the underlying spongiosum were predicted to be responsible for ventral curvature of the penis in patients with hypospadias [31]. Because of that, they were excised to correct the curvature (chordee). Currently, there is a shift in the paradigm of our understanding of the histological anatomy of the abortive urethral plate and the corpus spongiosum.

Snodgrass et al. carried out a histological study in subepithelial biopsy samples of the urethral plates in boys undergoing TIP repairs. The findings of this study showed well-vascularized connective tissues underneath the urethral plate, comprising collagen and smooth muscles scattered along with blood vessels and nerves. The histological features did not display any evidence of fibrous bands or dysplastic tissues [37]. Erol et al., in anatomical studies of the urethral plate and the tissue underneath, showed the presence of large blood vessels, glands, and muscles under the plate and suggested that this well-developed tissue corresponds to the corpus spongiosum. Hayashi et al. using transmission electron microscopy, reported that structures under the urethral plate were similar to corpus spongiosum and are composed of myelinated nerves, unmyelinated nerves, smooth muscle cells, and capillary vessels. They also observed the distinctive feature of the vessels of the cavernosal sinus, which implies that the origin of the tissue beneath the urethral plate is the same as the corpus spongiosum [36].

In histological studies of hypospadias, Erol et al. stated that collagen intensity under the urethral plate was similar to that in the normal region [38]. They concluded that the urethral plate and underlying tissue, akin to spongiosum, were not a cause of curvature in patients with hypospadias. Baskin et al. proposed that incision into the urethral plate and the glans results in the opening of the large endothelial sinuses from which the epithelial growth factors (keratinocytic growth factor) are liberated and encourage tissue repair. Keratinocytic growth factor stimulates the immediate restoration of the skin and urothelium after tissue injury [39, 40]. These ultrastructure findings of the hypospadiac urethral plate may help explain the technique of tubularized incised plate urethroplasty as described by Snodgrass et al. [40].

Against these observations, Hayashi et al. observed that immunohistochemical staining showed collagen subtype I in all tissues underneath the urethral plate instead of collagen subtype III, indicating the absence of distensible elastic tissue in urethral plate and underlying tissues and could be one of the causes of penile curvature. They concluded that the tissue beneath the urethral plate originated from the corpus spongiosum, and it might affect ventral penile curvature to some degree. According to them, although the procedure of dorsal plication could resolve penile curvature without division of the urethral plate and removal of the tissue beneath the plate in a considerable number of patients with hypospadias, careful long-term follow-up is essential as there can be delayed failure or recurrence of the ventral curvature [36].

Anatomy of Urogenital Anomalies Associated with Hypospadias The penile raphe is generally situated in the ventral midline. However, in hypospadias, it branches proximal to the hypospadiac meatus into two limbs that end distally into the glans. The area between two limbs can predict the extent of hypoplastic defect in the corpus spongiosum and ventral fascia. Next is penile torsion; the incidence of penile torsion with hypospadias is underreported; hence its prevalence is unpredictable. Few studies have reported penile torsion ranging from 15° to 180° concurrent with hypospadias [41]. Penile torsion was commonly found in patients with anterior hypospadias (distal and mid penile), while it was less common in patients with posterior hypospadias. In the study by Bhat et al., 31.6% overall incidence of penile torsion was reported. It was more common in distal (68.9%) than with proximal (10.34%) hypospadias [42]. They said that in the majority of patients, the direction of congenital penile torsion is counter-clockwise (to the left) (Fig. 3.9), observed right-to-left ratio was 1:3 with the occurrence of right-sided torque of 29.3%. Several theories explain the occurrence of torsion and claim torsion to occur due to the abnormal attachments of the dartos fascia, Buck's fascia, and the skin [43].

The size of the hypospadias penis is normal in a majority of patients. However, hypospadias in patients with disorders of sex development constitutes a different category. Avellán found inadequate penile size in 3% of his patients with severe forms of hypospadias; half of them had associated chromosomal anomalies [10].

In the majority of the patients with hypospadias (90%), the scrotum is normal, but proximal hypospadias not infrequently presents with partially bifid or completely bifid scrotum. In very few cases, it can be associated with penoscrotal transposition, a condition in which the scrotal skin surrounds the root of the penis to a variable extent. A different degree of penoscrotal transposition has been reported in patients with hypospadias in literature [10].

Most hypospadiac patients have normal testes in the scrotum. Retractile or undescended testes may be encountered in 10% of patients with hypospadias, usually in proximal forms with almost 3% incidence in cases of distal hypospadias [10]. Patients with hypospadias associated with bilateral undescended/absent scrotal testis should undergo chromosomal and hormonal analysis, as well as ultrasound to exclude disorders of sex differentiation (DSD). An inguinal hernia with or without hydrocele can be there with hypospadias.

Avellan found some infrequent congenital anomalies of underdevelopment of the prostate and absence of the internal sphincteric mechanism in severe perineal hypospadias patients [10]. Occasionally, difficulty encountered in catheterization of some patients of severe forms of hypospadias (proximal penile, penoscrotal, and perineal) could be because of enlarged utricle or verumontanum. Cystoscopy might be needed in such circumstances to catheterize under vision.

The majority of hypospadiac patients have no other renal anomalies. However, rarely there may be pelvic ureteric junction obstruction, vesicoureteric reflux, a double ureter, renal agenesis, and ectopic kidney.

3.3 Anogenital/Anoscrotal Distances and Severity of Hypospadias

Anogenital distance (AGD) is the distance from the anus centre to the base of the penis, and anoscrotal distance (ASD) is the distance from the centre of the anus to the junction between the smooth perineal skin. The scrotal skin is smaller in patients with hypospadias in comparison to regular counterparts. Both are

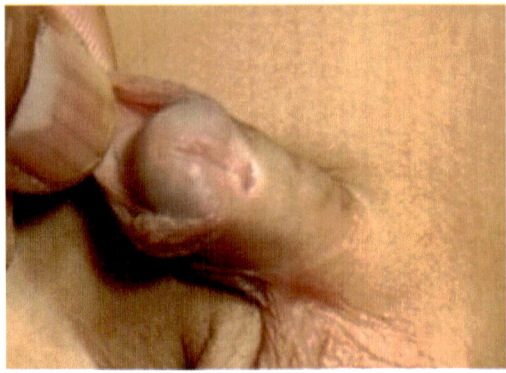

Fig. 3.9 Left side torsion of penile shaft associated with distal hypospadias

recognized markers of in utero androgen action; poor expression of androgen leads to severe male genital malformation. A study by Cox et al. evaluated the relationship between the severity of hypospadias and AGD/ASD. In their study, the median AGD for normal participants was 74.0 mm, and for patients with hypospadias, it was 72.3 mm. The median ASD for normal participants was 42.3 mm, and for hypospadias, it was 39.4 mm. The shorter AGD and ASD are seen in more severe hypospadias and suggest severely affected androgen production. They hypothesized that mild forms of hypospadias occur due to different aetiology affecting at a later stage of development and are not due to reduced androgen exposure in the male programming window between the eighth and 14th weeks' gestation [44].

3.4 Summary

Hypospadias is a congenital anomaly with the clinical appearance of a ventrally lying urethral meatus on the penis or more proximally on the scrotum/perineum, depending on its severity. It involves complex disarray of developmental malformations ranging from non-development of the distal urethra and the underlying spongiosum to the ventral curvature of the penis and hooded prepuce. A thorough understanding of the anatomy of the hypospadias is of prime importance in understanding the severity of hypospadias, availability of tissues like the urethral plate, spongiosum, preputial and penile skin important for selecting a procedure from various techniques of repair which has been classically described. The hypospadias repair is a meticulous procedure that, if not adequately performed, might result in recurrence of chordee, fistula formation, and crippled hypospadias, decreasing the success rate of subsequent repair, which in turn, causing significant physical and mental morbidity to the patient. Anatomical knowledge is pivotal for communicating to parents, deficiencies present in hypospadias, possible procedures, and outcomes.

References

1. Bouty A, Ayers KL, Pask A, Heloury Y, Sinclair AH. The genetic and environmental factors underlying hypospadias. Sex Dev. 2015;9(5):239–59.
2. Hadidi AT. History of hypospadias: lost in translation. J Pediatr Surg. 2017;52(2):211–7.
3. Baskin LS, Ebbers MB. Hypospadias: anatomy, aetiology, and technique. J Pediatr Surg. 2006;41(3):463–72.
4. Laios K, Karamanou M, Androutsos G. A unique representation of hypospadias in ancient Greek art. Can Urol Assoc J. 2012;6(1):E1–2.
5. Van der Horst HJR, de Wall LL. Hypospadias, all there is to know. Eur J Pediatr. 2017;176(4):435–41.
6. Baskin LS. Hypospadias and urethral development. J Urol. 2000;163(3):951–6.
7. Barcat J. Current concepts in of treatment. In: Horton CE, editor. Plastic and reconstructive surgery of the genital area. Boston, MA: Little Brown; 1973. p. 249–62.
8. Jordan GH, McCammon KA. Surgery of the penis and urethra. In: Wein AJ, Kavoussi LR, Novick AC, Partin AW, Peters CP, editors. Campbell's urology. 10th ed. Philadelphia, PA: Elsevier Saunders; 2012.
9. Hadidi AT. Classification of hypospadias. In: Hadidi AT, Azmy AF, editors. Hypospadias surgery: an illustrated guide. 1st ed. Berlin: Springer Verlag; 2004. p. 80.
10. Avellán L. Morphology of hypospadias. Scand J Plast Reconstr Surg. 1980;14(3):239–47.
11. Bush NC, DaJusta D, Snodgrass WT. Glans penis width in patients with hypospadias compared to healthy controls. J Pediatr Urol. 2013;9(6 Pt B):1188–91.
12. Abbas TO, Vallasciani S, Elawad A, Elifranji M, Leslie B, Elkadhi A, et al. Plate objective scoring tool (POST); an objective methodology for the assessment of urethral plate in distal hypospadias. J Pediatr Urol. 2020;5(1):e1–8.
13. Bhat A, Sabharwal K, Bhat M, Saran R, Singla M, Kumar V. Outcome of tubularized incised plate urethroplasty with spongioplasty alone as additional tissue cover: a prospective study. Indian J Urol. 2014;30(4):392–7.
14. Jordan G, Schlossberg S. Surgery of the penis and urethra. In: Wein A, Kavoussi L, Novick A, Partin A, Peters C, editors. Campbell-Walsh urology, vol. 2. Philadelphia: Saunders-Elsevier; 2007.
15. Groat WC, Steers WD. Neuroanatomy and neurophysiology of penile erection. In: Tanagho E, Lue TF, McClure RD, editors. Contemporary Management of Impotence and Infertility. Baltimore, MD: Williams & Wilkins; 1988. p. 3–27.
16. Dodat H, Landry J-L, Szwarc C, Culem S, Murat F-J, Dubois R. Spongioplasty and separation of the corpora cavernosa for hypospadias repair. BJU Int. 2003;91(6):528–31.

17. Hayashi Y, Mizuno K, Moritoki Y, Nakane A, Kato T, Kurokawa S, et al. Can Spongioplasty prevent fistula formation and correct penile curvature in TIP urethroplasty for hypospadias? Urology. 2013;81(6):1330–5.
18. Yerkes EB, Adams MC, Miller DA, Pope JC, Rink RC, Brock JW. Y-to-I wrap: use of the distal spongiosum for hypospadias repair. J Urol. 2000;163(5):1536–9.
19. Nesbit RM. Congenital curvature of the phallus. J Urol. 1965;93:230–2.
20. Baskin L. What is hypospadias? Clin Pediatr. 2017;56(5):409–18.
21. Cunha GR, Sinclair A, Cao M, Baskin LS. Development of the human prepuce and its innervation. Differentiation. 2020;111:22–40.
22. Brooks JD. Anatomy of the lower urinary tract and male genitalia. In: Wein A, Kavoussi L, Novick A, Partin A, Peters C, editors. Campbell-Walsh urology, vol. 1. Philadelphia: Saunders-Elsevier; 2007.
23. Radojicic ZI, Perovic SV. Classification of the prepuce in hypospadias according to morphological abnormalities and their impact on hypospadias repair. J Urol. 2004;172(1):301–4.
24. Juskiewenski S, Vaysse P, Moscovici J. A study of the arterial blood supply to the penis. Anat Clin. 1982;4:101–7.
25. Perovic SV, Radojicic ZI. Vascularization of the hypospadiac prepuce and its impact on hypospadias repair. J Urol. 2003;169(3):1098–101.
26. Yucel S, Guntekin E, Kukul E, et al. Comparison of hypospadiac and normal preputial vascular anatomy. J Urol. 2004;172:1973–6.
27. Hinman F Jr. The blood supply to preputial island flaps. J Urol. 1991;145(6):1232–5.
28. Zhao Z, Sun N, Mao X. Vascularization of vessel pedicle in hypospadias and its relationship to near-period complications. Exp Ther Med. 2018;16(3):2408–12.
29. Redman J. Anatomy of the genitourinary system. In: Gillenwater J, Grayhack J, Howards S, Duckett J, editors. Adult and Pediatric urology, vol. 1. St. Louis: Mosby; 1991.
30. Baskin LS, Erol A, Li YW, Liu WH. Anatomy of the neurovascular bundle: is safe mobilization possible? J Urol. 2000;164(3 Pt 2):977–80.
31. Baskin LS, Duckett JW, Lue TF. Penile curvature. Urology. 1996;48(3):347–56.
32. Baskin LS, Duckett JW. Dorsal tunica albuginea plication for hypospadias curvature. J Urol. 1994;151(6):1668–71.
33. Hsu GL, Brock G, Martínez-Piñeiro L, von Heyden B, Lue TF, Tanagho EA. Anatomy and strength of the tunica albuginea: its relevance to penile prosthesis extrusion. J Urol. 1994;151(5):1205–8.
34. Baskin LS, Lue TF. The correction of congenital penile curvature in young men. Br J Urol. 1998;81(6):895–9.
35. Baskin LS, Erol A, Li YW, Cunha GR. Anatomical studies of hypospadias. J Urol. 1998;160(3 Pt 2):1108–15. discussion 1137
36. Hayashi Y, Mizuno K, Kojima Y, Moritoki Y, Nishio H, Kato T, et al. Characterization of the urethral plate and the underlying tissue defined by expression of collagen subtypes and microarchitecture in hypospadias. Int J Urol. 2011;18(4):317–22.
37. Snodgrass W, Patterson K, Plaire JC, Grady R, Mitchell ME. Histology of the urethral plate: implications for hypospadias repair. J Urol. 2000;164(3 Pt 2):988–9. discussion 989–990
38. Erol A, Baskin LS, Li YW, Liu WH. Anatomical studies of the urethral plate: why preservation of the urethral plate is important in hypospadias repair. BJU Int. 2000;85(6):728–34.
39. Werner S, Smola H, Liao X, Longaker MT, Krieg T, Hofschneider PH, et al. The function of KGF in morphogenesis of epithelium and reepithelialization of wounds. Science. 1994;266(5186):819–22.
40. Snodgrass W. Tubularized, incised plate urethroplasty for distal hypospadias. J Urol. 1994;151(2):464–5.
41. Zeid A, Soliman H. Penile torsion: an overlooked anomaly with distal hypospadias. Ann Pediatr Surg. 2010;6(2):93–7.
42. Bhat A, Bhat MP, Saxena G. Correction of penile torsion by mobilization of urethral plate and urethra. J Pediatr Urol. 2009;5(6):451–7.
43. Bhat A, Sabharwal K, Bhat M, Singla M, Upadhaya R, Kumar V. Correlation of the severity of penile torsion with the type of hypospadias & ventral penile curvature and their management. Afr J Urol. 2015;21(2):111–8.
44. Cox K, Kyriakou A, Amjad B, O'Toole S, Flett ME, Welsh M, et al. Shorter anogenital and anoscrotal distances correlate with the severity of hypospadias: a prospective study. J Pediatr Urol. 2017;13(1):57.e1–5.

Penile Anthropometry

Mahakshit Bhat and Amilal Bhat

4.1 Introduction

Penile size reflects the exposure of the male fetus to androgens, starting from hypothalamic/pituitary gonadotropins down to testicular androgens. An abnormal growth pattern of the penis may be a cause of physiological illnesses in the child and may lead to psychosocial diseases, especially in adolescents [1]. The appearance of male external genitalia has a vital role to play in the psychological health of children and adolescents. Penile size is a common concern of parents and patients. Hypospadiologists, Pediatric Urologists, and Pediatricians frequently come across questions regarding the size of penis of their child. Parents/patients visiting the pediatric urology outpatient department might have numerous misconceptions regarding penile size. Therefore, nomograms are needed to define the average penile dimensions. With a defined penile nomogram, the patients and parents can be counseled regarding the penile size. However, as the physical stature differs across racial and ethnical spectrums, it stands to reason that penile size may vary too. A separate penile dimensions chart may be necessary to define the standard penile dimensions among various population groups. A micropenis is defined as a penis >2.5 SD below the mean penile size. If a discrepancy is present between the penile size of the patients' population group and the population as a whole, the case may be misdiagnosed with a micropenis. Penile dimensions in hypospadiacs are necessary to plan the surgery as the size of the penis may affect the outcome of hypospadias surgery and also in post hypospadias repair to schedule surgery, if any penile lengthening measures are required. Glans size is also an important variable in the outcome of hypospadias repair. Patients with small glans and small size of penis require hormonal treatment before and after surgery.

M. Bhat
Department of Urology, National Institute of Medical Sciences Medical College, Jaipur, Rajasthan, India

A. Bhat (✉)
Bhat's Hypospadias and Reconstructive Urology Hospital and Research Centre,
Jaipur, Rajasthan, India

Department of Urology, Jaipur National University Institute for Medical Sciences and Research Centre, Jaipur, Rajasthan, India

Department of Urology, Dr. S.N. Medical College, Jodhpur, Rajasthan, India

Department of Urology, S.P. Medical College, Bikaner, Rajasthan, India

P.G. Committee Medical Council of India, New Delhi, India

Academic and Research Council of RUHS, Jaipur, Rajasthan, India

4.2 Methods of Measuring the Penile Dimensions

Measuring the penile dimensions is more difficult in infants and children as compared to adults. Commonly used instruments are rigid tape, ruler, spatula, measuring with thread and Vernier Calipers. A disposable syringe may also be used for measurement of penile length (Fig. 4.1a–b). The main limitation in measuring the exact penile length is pubis fat. An adapted methodology for measurements may also influence the results. The stretched penile length is measured with a rigid tape from the pubo-penile skin junction to the tip of the penis, excluding the prepuce under maximal but not painful extension. Circumference of the penis is measured at the base of the penis (close to the pubis) with a measuring tape. For obese males, the abdominal adipose tissue is shifted manually to one side to measure penile length and circumference. We use Vernier calipers as it achieves the highest accuracy in comparison with rigid tape, measuring ruler, and others have used a spatula. Accuracy of Vernier calipers measurement makes it the method of choice despite a theoretical risk of trauma to the child (Fig. 4.2a–c).

We conducted a cross-sectional study on 1800 subjects with age ranging from birth to 18 years. One hundred participants were included in each age group with 1-year intervals between October 2012 and December 2014. The participants did not suffer from any genital, endocrinological, nutritional, or psychosocial disease. These were the relatives of other patients, boys admitted for conditions unrelated to genitalia, and healthy children, visiting for routine immunization.

A Vernier caliper was used to measure

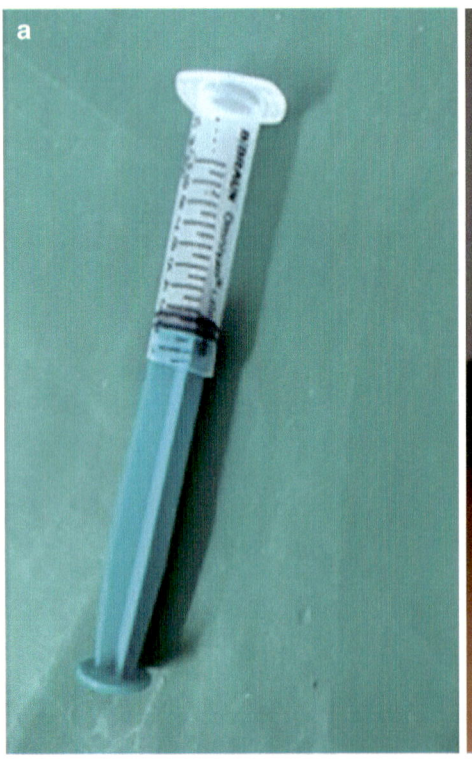
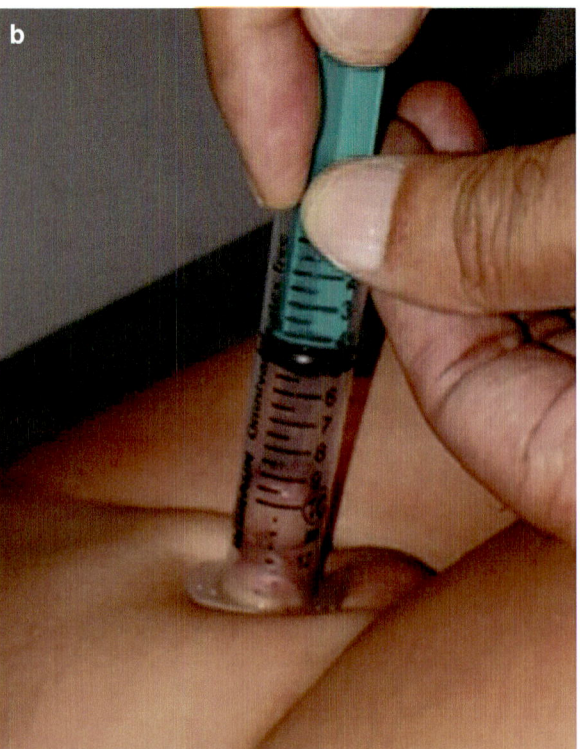

Fig. 4.1a–b Measuring the penile length with the disposal syringe

4 Penile Anthropometry

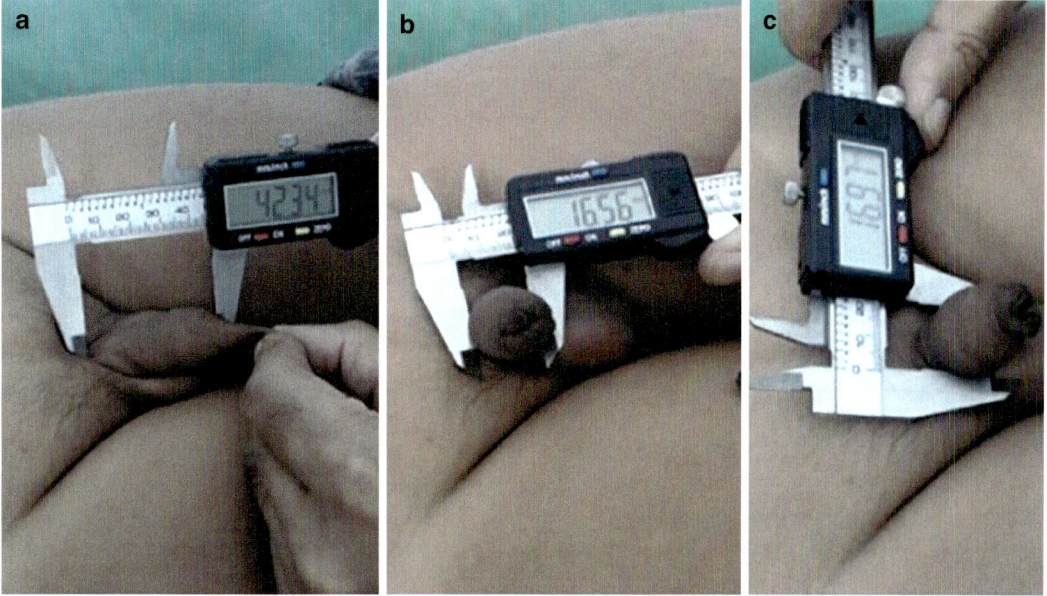

Fig. 4.2a–c Measuring the penile length and mid penile circumference with the Vernier calipers

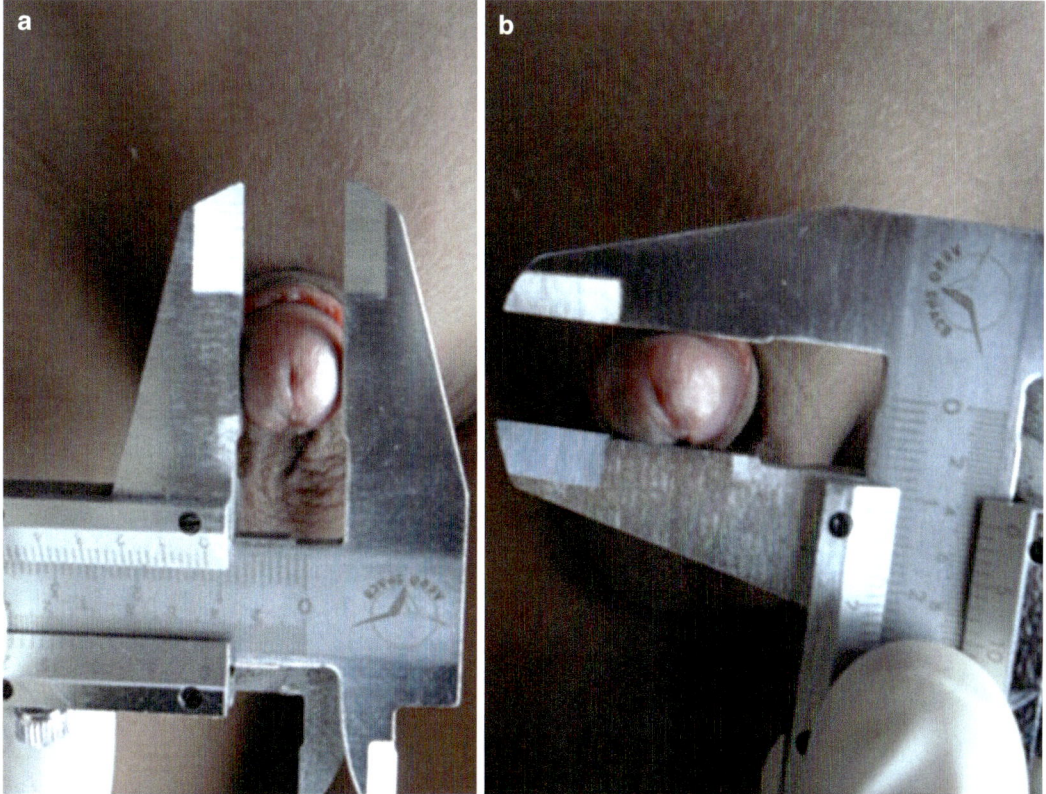

Fig. 4.3a–b Measuring the coronal circumference

- Stretched penile length (Fig. 4.2a).
- Penile shaft diameter.
- Penile circumference at the mid-shaft level (Fig. 4.2b & c).
- Coronal diameter.
- Coronal circumference (Fig. 4.3a & b).

We also measured the height, weight, and BMI of all subjects. Data were accumulated for the mean stretched penile length and the mean circumferences at the corona and mid-shaft in all the age groups. A Pearson coefficient was calculated for the correlation of penile length with weight, height, and BMI. Statistical analysis was also conducted to rule out the confounding factor of age, and different Pearson correlation coefficient values were obtained for each age group. The r values reaching statistical significance were derived for the study data. Nomograms were generated using graphical representations of the data collected for the penile dimensions with age. The data was compared with the similar studies, and the differences in the results were analyzed individually with each study using Student's t-test.

4.3 Results

As expected, with an increase in age, height, and weight of the child, all the penile dimensions increased. The curve of penile length with age was gradual up to the age of 11 years, after which the curve became steep up to the age of 18 years (Fig. 4.4). The mid-shaft circumference had a growth curve similar to penile length with a sharp rise in growth rate in the 11–16 year age group. (Fig. 4.5). A similar pattern of growth was observed in the measurement of the coronal circumference.

The height, weight, and BMI of all the participants were in the normal range as defined by the Indian Academy of Pediatrics using the growth charts from the Indian population. The Pearson correlation coefficient values followed a regular trend for neither weight, height, nor BMI. The inconsistent pattern in the Pearson correlation coefficient values in the various age groups is suggestive of the fact that the penile length does not have a direct correlation with weight, height, or BMI of the subjects.

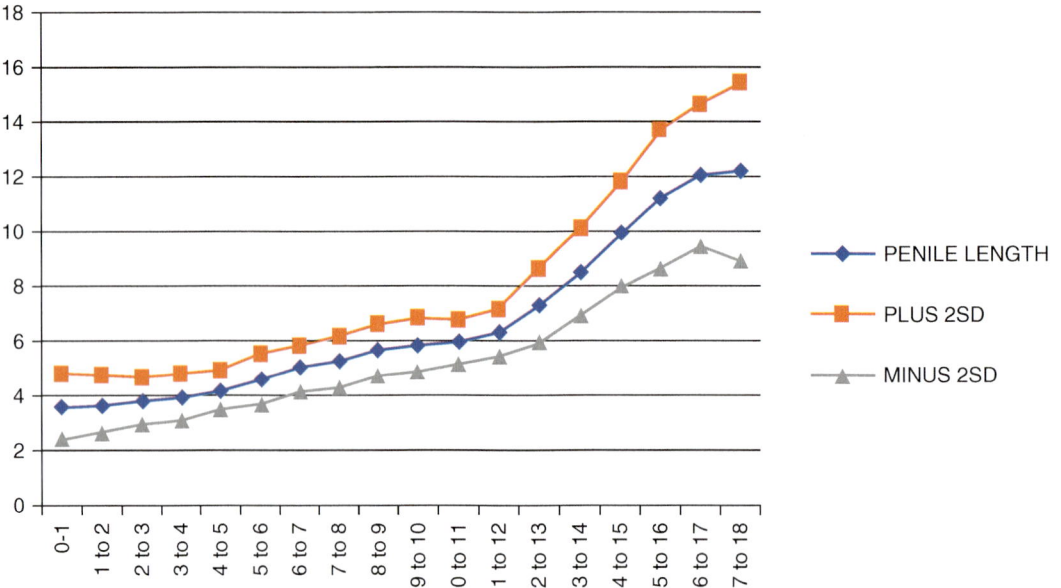

Fig. 4.4 Variation in penile length with age

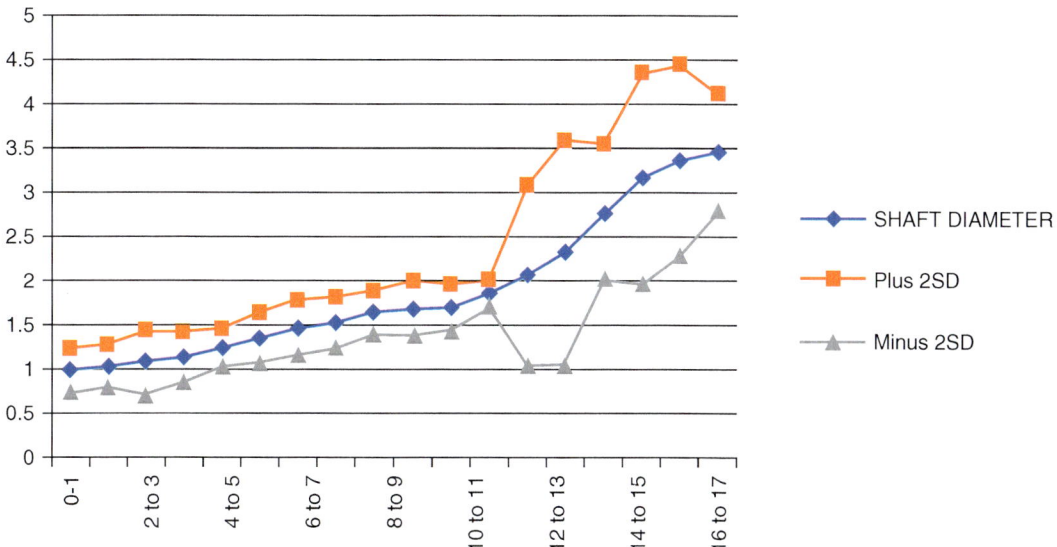

Fig. 4.5 Variation in penile shaft diameter with age

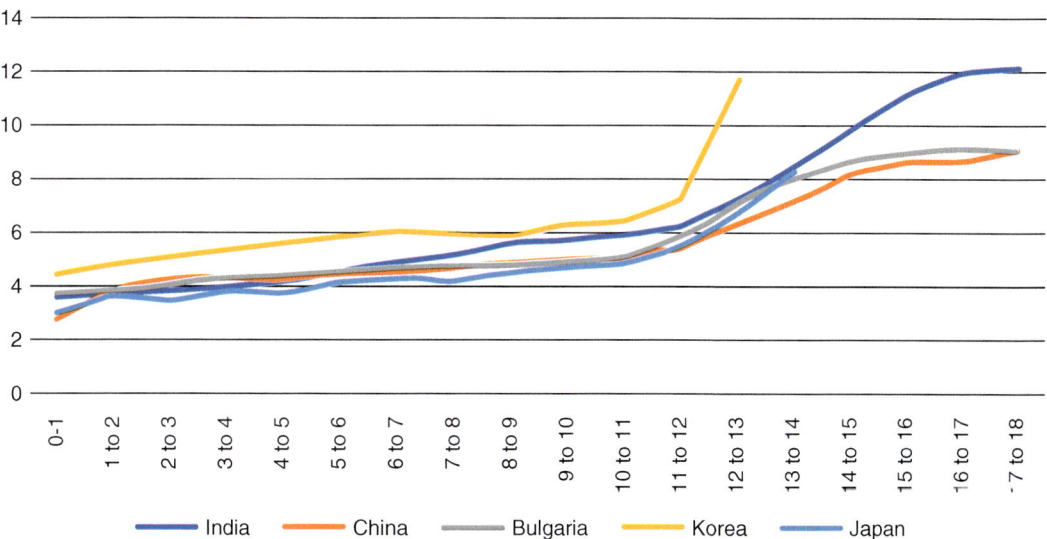

Fig. 4.6 Comparison of data of studies from different countries

Comparison of data from a variety of countries like China, Bulgaria, Korea, and Japan revealed data similar to our study. The graphs were parallel suggesting that the penile growth patterns are identical between the countries (Fig. 4.6).

4.4 Discussion

The typical age-related range of penile dimensions must be known to identify clinically abnormal penile size. Penile length increases gradually during childhood [2]. We observed that while the trend of slow penile growth was observed up to the age of 11 years, the rate of growth in penile dimensions at age 11 to 16 increased significantly. Differences in ethnicity, geographical location, genetics, and nutritional factors may lead to variation in penile anthropometry of several populations. A study conducted by Bhat et al. [3] tabulated data of 250 patients in age groups of 1-year intervals. It concluded that the penile length increases with advancing age, but observed no statistically significant relationship with body weight, height, or BMI. Our findings and data corroborate the results of the previous research and extend these findings up to the age of 18 years of age. We also found that the rate in increase in penile dimensions is higher from the age of 11 to 16 years as compared to the rest of the age groups (Table 4.1). The sharp rise in the rate of penile growth coincides with the onset of puberty in the Indian population [4]. We found no significant correlation in penile dimensions with age in any of the age groups. In all the age groups, height, weight, and BMI had a strong positive relationship with penile length during infancy, which suggests that birth weight and height may bear some influence on the penile length of the child. So, there are more chances of having a high incidence of hypospadias with a small phallus in the premature child.

The only other study in literature for Indian children was conducted by Vasudevan et al. [5]. These values are marginally higher than the values we obtained and may have been because of differences in growth parameters between the children of the North and South Indian population.

In our experience, penile size is a significant concern for parents after surgical repair of disorders such as hypospadias and DSD. This study provides a penile size nomogram using which the penile growth of such patients can be monitored on follow-up visits. This will reassure the parents as well as indicate to the clinician whether or not to intervene. If the penile length is found lesser than 2.5 SD from the mean, according to the nomogram, the patient can be diagnosed as a case of micropenis at an early age. Micropenis may result from a heterogeneous group of disorders, and the most common being fetal testosterone deficiency. In the male fetus, testosterone synthesis by the fetal Leydig cell during 8–12 weeks, the period of male differentiation is under the influence of placental human chorionic gonadotrophin. The fetal pituitary Luteinizing hormone modulates fetal testosterone synthesis by the Leydig cell and, consequently, affects the growth of the differentiated penis after mid-gestation. Growth hormone and insulin-like growth factors acting together are also modulated by androgen action. Thus, males with congenital hypopituitarism as well as isolated gonadotropin or growth hormone deficiency need to be further evaluated for hypogonadotropic hypogonadism, primary hypogonadism, testosterone activation defects, or androgen insensitivity syndrome and appropriate treatment is to be initiated according to the findings. The therapy includes intramuscular administration of testosterone, topical application of testosterone and LH-FSH administration. If testosterone administration does not result in an improvement in penile length, surgical intervention should be considered [6]. Similarly, post hypospadias repair patients with small (Fig. 4.7) penis should also be evaluated and treated with local testosterone and other endocrinological management.

Similar to our findings, Adriansyah et al. [7] in a study on 64 primary school students and 44 junior high school students in Indonesia found no significant variation in penile length with BMI. Wang et al. [8] in a study conducted in Taiwan formulated growth curves for boys aged 0 to 17 years and found growth curves similar to our research. They also made growth charts for penile dimensions form the data and found that the penile growth rates were on a gradual curve up to the age of 10 years. Similar to our study, they also found that the penile growth rate was increased from the age of 11–16 years.

Tomova et al. [9] conducted a study on 6200 boys aged 0–19 in Bulgaria and found that penile growth was gradual after birth. However, peak growth was observed from 12 to 16 years of age, which coincided with the maximal male pubertal growth spurt. They also reported the height and weight of the subjects enrolled in the study but did not perform any statistical analysis to evalu-

4 Penile Anthropometry

Table 4.1 Data of penile dimensions across all age groups

Age	Penile length	Coronal diameter	Coronal circumference	Shaft diameter	Shaft circumference	Height (Cm)	Weight (Kg)	BMI
0–1	3.557	1.0448	3.541682	0.972	3.27816	57.08	4.7695	13.82848
1 to 2	3.6522	1.1327	3.556678	1.0167	3.192438	80.247	10.3108	16.09062
2 to 3	3.7793	1.1594	3.640516	1.059	3.32526	91.1261	12.547	15.1565
3 to 4	3.9174	1.2235	3.842746	1.1254	3.533756	98.084	14.67	15.01702
4 to 5	4.1592	1.2981	4.075351	1.2229	3.839906	104.678	15.805	14.40422
5 to 6	4.5347	1.4149	4.277646	1.3455	4.22487	111.556	17.944	14.42327
6 to 7	4.9325	1.5203	4.693688	1.454	4.56556	118.026	21.197	15.22842
7 to 8	5.2033	1.59	4.991331	1.5095	4.73983	123.037	23.085	15.2667
8 to 9	5.6094	1.7202	5.389287	1.6293	5.116002	128.107	27.175	16.5647
9 to 10	5.7723	1.7809	5.592026	1.6689	5.240346	134.1	29.998	16.54269
10 to 11	5.9042	1.8012	5.61198	1.6895	5.30503	139.054	33.163	17.16101
11 to 12	6.212	1.9107	5.999598	1.8459	5.796126	144.121	37.075	17.85494
12 to 13	7.2202	2.2251	6.78949	2.052	6.44328	151.782	41.462	18.01596
13 to 14	8.4513	2.5958	7.199716	2.3044	7.312623	158.436	47.101	18.78035
14 to15	9.8483	3.1104	9.766656	2.7638	8.678332	163.123	50.666	19.05982
15 to 16	11.1223	3.5442	11.20806	3.1499	9.890686	166.137	55.12	19.98557
16 to 17	11.9706	3.787	11.86252	3.3578	10.54349	168.495	60.219	21.22025
17 to 18	12.1326	3.8171	11.98569	3.4521	10.83959	170.225	62.092	21.61512

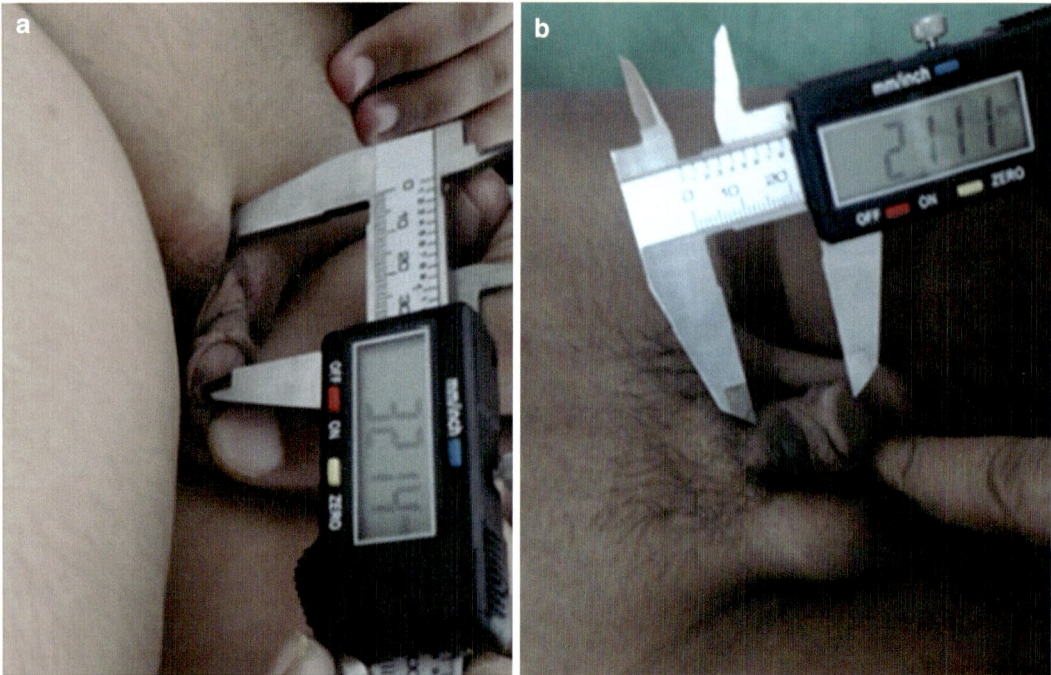

Fig. 4.7 Measuring the penile length postoperatively smaller for the age

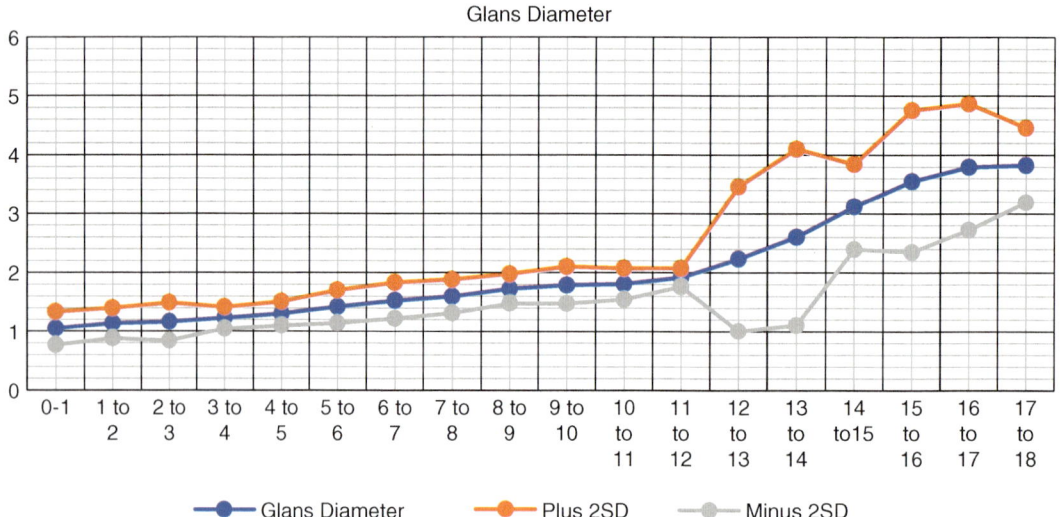

Fig. 4.8 Correlation of glans diameter with age

ate the correlation between penile dimensions and height and weight. Park et al. [10] measured the penile length in boys from the age of 0–14 years and found a peak penile growth rate at the age of thirteen years. On comparison, graphs from various studies were parallel suggesting that the penile growth patterns are similar between the countries (Fig. 4.6).

The glans circumference and glans diameter follow a similar relationship to age as the penile shaft and penile length (Figs. 4.8 & 4.9). It increases gradually till the age of 12 years with a

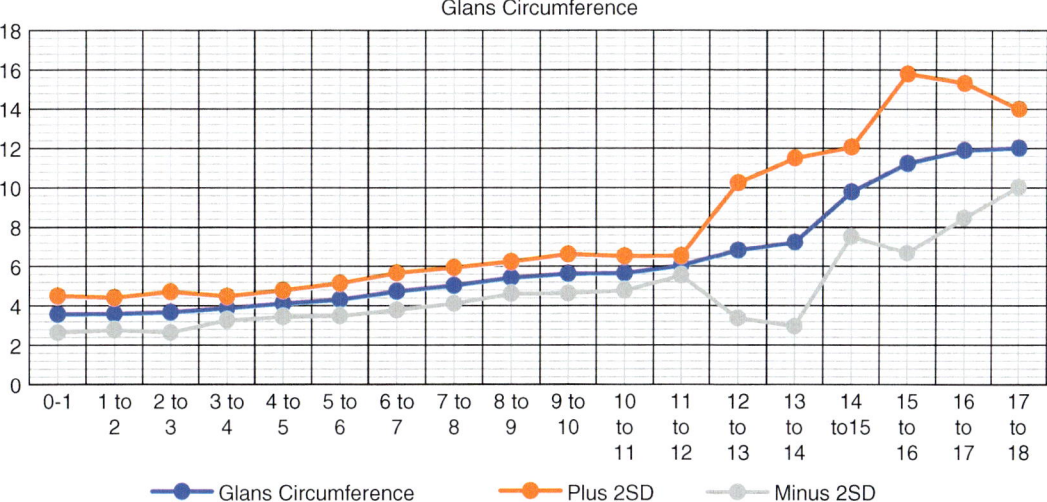

Fig. 4.9 Correlation of glans circumference with age

significant increment in the rate of increase in size from the ages 12–16 (Table 4.1). This change in the rate of growth can be attributed to puberty as with penile length and shaft diameter. The significance of glans size was described by Nicol C. Bush et al. who measured the glans diameter of 490 boys who underwent hypospadias repair and found that the glans size of <14 mm was an independent predictor of worse outcomes of hypospadias repair. In the same paper they commented that increasing age between 3 months and 10 years did not correlate with increasing glans size [11]. The p value of this statement was not significant and it contradicts with our findings. While the glans diameter and circumference increased in healthy individuals with age, an anomaly such as hypospadias may interfere with the penile growth and may be the reason of the discrepancy. These data can be charted on the graph shown in to compare the coronal dimensions of the selected patient with the population. On comparing the data on glans dimensions of normal patients, we can predict the outcome of hypospadias repair. This graph can also be used to decide on the technique to be used for hypospadias repair. A nomogram is necessary as the changes in biologic, environment, and feeding patterns are likely to affect the growth and development of specific organs. In a study from Korea (2012), they found a significant increase in penile (0.7 to 1.1 CMP<0.05) size in all age group and these anthropometric measurements such as height, body weight, and testicular size have also increased compared with those from 1987 study. So, a more extensive community-based population study is required to diagnose and treat size-related penile disorders. In cases of hypospadias, the role of testosterone deficiency has been documented as a causative factor in many studies [12]. Since the authors did not record androgen levels in the patients involved in the study, the penile growth retardation due to androgen deficiency may have confounded the correlation between age and size of the glans.

4.5 Conclusion

The penile length increases uniformly at a low rate up to the age of 11 years, but the penile growth rate increases from the age of 11–16 years corresponding to puberty. Penile dimensions did not correlate with body weight, height, or BMI. There was a sharp increase in penile size corresponding to puberty. Penile dimensions of the children were found to be statistically similar to previous studies conducted in other countries. The data of the study can be used to create a penile anthropometry chart which can be used for both pre- and post-operative assessment of hypospadiac penis and glans size. Pre-operatively the glans dimensions can be used to decide the technique to be used and to prognosticate the surgery. Penile length measurement is essential to rule out the micropenis as well as predict surgical outcome. Postoperatively the charts can be used to reassure parents regarding the size of the penis.

References

1. Schonfeld W. Adolescence: inappropriate sexual development and body image. J Am Med Womens Assoc. 1967;22(11):847–55.
2. Schonfeld WA, Beebe GW. Normal growth and variation in the male genitalia from birth to maturity. J Urol. 1942;48(6):759–77.
3. Bhat A, Upadhyay R, Bhat M, Sabharwal K, Singla M, Kumar V. Penile anthropometry in north Indian children. Indian J Urol. 2015;31(2):106.
4. Khadilkar V, Stanhope R, Khadilkar V. Secular trends in puberty. Indian Pediatr. 2006;43(6):475.
5. Vasudevan G, Bhat BV, Bhatia B, Kumar S. Genital standards for south Indian male newborns. Indian J Pediatr. 1995;62(5):593–6.
6. Hatipoğlu N, Kurtoğlu S. Micropenis: etiology, diagnosis and treatment approaches. J Clin Res Pediatr Endocrinol. 2013;5(4):217–23. https://doi.org/10.4274/Jcrpe.1135.
7. Adriansyah R, Ali M, Hakimi H, Deliana M, Lubis SM. The relationship of body mass index to penile length and testicular volume in adolescent boys. Paediatr Indones. 2012;52(5):267–71.
8. Wang Y-N, Zeng Q, Xiong F, Zeng Y. Male external genitalia growth curves and charts for children and adolescents aged 0 to 17 years in Chongqing, China. Asian J Androl. 2018;20(6):567.
9. Tomova A, Deepinder F, Robeva R, Lalabonova H, Kumanov P, Agarwal A. Growth and development of male external genitalia: a cross-sectional study of 6200 males aged 0 to 19 years. Arch Pediatr Adolesc Med. 2010;164(12):1152–7.
10. Park S, Chung JM, Kang DI, Ryu DS, Cho WY, Lee SD. The change of stretched penile length and anthropometric data in Korean children aged 0–14 years: comparative study of last 25 years. J Korean Med Sci. 2016;31(10):1631–4.
11. Bush NC, Villanueva C, Snodgrass W. Glans size is an independent risk factor for urethroplasty complications after hypospadias repair. J Pediatr Urol. 2015;11(6):355.e351–5.
12. Baskin LS. Hypospadias and urethral development. J Urol. 2000;163(3):951–6.

General Considerations in Hypospadias Surgery

5

Amilal Bhat and Nikhil Khandelwal

Abbreviations

TIP   Tubularized Incised Urethral Plate Urethroplasty
TUPU Tubularized Urethral Plate Urethroplasty

5.1 Introduction

Incidence of hypospadias is 1:300, and it is the second most common congenital anomaly. Diagnosis of the anomaly is made in the newborn by locating the ventral urethral opening/altered urinary stream and dorsal hood. The terminology "hypospadiologist" was coined by John Duckett's enduring legacies in hypospadias surgery. Hypospadiology is a well-recognized and evolving speciality. The surgeon dedicated to excellence, develops and maintains the high standards of specialist expertise, with sufficient case load in hypospadias surgery is called Hypospadiologist. John Duckett stated, "many successful methods for hypospadias surgery, no single technique works for all cases, so a suitable technique required to be chosen for the individual case". The outcomes of hypospadias surgery have improved significantly in the last three decades by sincerely following the quotes of Davis "I believe the time has arrived to state that the surgical repair of hypospadias is no longer dubious, unreliable, or extremely difficult. If tried and proven methods are carefully followed, a good result should be obtained in every case. Anything less than this suggests that the surgeon is not temperamentally fit for this kind of surgery" [1]. Now the "occasional" hypospadias surgeon is disappearing fast; the commitment and skill of the surgeon matter most in "Hypospadiology". The hypospadias surgery is technically demanding; so, anyone of the Urologist, Paediatric Surgeon, Paediatric Urologist, Plastic Surgeon, and general surgeon having the temperament for hypospadias surgery can perform the repair. The surgeon has to master at least six standard techniques in hypospadias with at least 40 to 50 cases load per year. The learning curve in hypospadias repair is lon-

A. Bhat
Bhat's Hypospadias and Reconstructive Urology Hospital and Research Centre, Jaipur, Rajasthan, India

Department of Urology, Jaipur National University Institute for Medical Sciences and Research Centre, Jaipur, Rajasthan, India

Department of Urology, Dr. S.N. Medical College, Jodhpur, Rajasthan, India

Department of Urology, S.P. Medical College, Bikaner, Rajasthan, India

P.G. Committee Medical Council of India, New Delhi, India

Academic and Research Council of RUHS, Jaipur, Rajasthan, India

N. Khandelwal (✉)
Department of Urology, Vijayanagar Institute of Medical Sciences, Bellary, Karnataka, India

ger and experience in hypospadias surgery co-relates with better results. The difference in results of hypospadias surgery done by the Hypospadiologists and Paediatric Surgeons versus other surgical specialists is significant [2, 3].

5.2 Epidemiological Trends

True worldwide prevalence of hypospadias is not known. Recently reported total international prevalence of hypospadias was 20.9 per 10,000 births. A rising trend in the prevalence in the past three decades has been reported, but it is localized to specific regions or periods. The prevalence of hypospadias is variable region-wise; Asia 0.6–69, Europe 18.6, North America 34.2 (6–129.8) per 10,000 births.

5.3 Should Hypospadias Be Operated?

Initially, the focus was mainly on proximal hypospadias repair with more on the creation of urethral passage, that too only up to corona. The proximal defect is most challenging to repair and has higher morbidity. With advancements in hypospadiology, the MAGPI technique came into practice and was described in the 1980s; it became the routine in distal hypospadias. But now, tubularized incised urethral plate urethroplasty is the most commonly done technique in distal hypospadias because of its better functional and cosmetic results. Hypospadias surgery is indicated because of ventral ectopic/stenotic meatus, ventral curvature, cleft/tilted glans, deformed hooded prepuce, penile torque, and penoscrotal transposition. The ideal outcome of the surgery includes the straight and adequate sized penis, right calibre urethra with meatus at the tip of the conical glans for normal voiding in a good stream, and unimpaired sexual activity. The development of the hypospadiac boys should be with self-confidence and a standard body image for young men after hypospadias surgery. Severe hypospadias with poor surgical results negatively impacts those with minor hypospadias and satisfactory surgical outcomes. Results, both functional and cosmetic, in modern-day hypospadias surgery have improved significantly; so, all types of hypospadias with or without chordee or torsion should be considered for surgery.

5.4 Preoperative Workup

The preoperative workup includes history, a medical checkup, and investigation of the child and counselling of the parents. The goals of the surgery must be discussed with the parents, and they should be told about the surgical plan, possible modifications during surgery, the period of hospitalization, peri and postoperative catheter care, dressings and medications, and expected outcome of the surgery and complication. The perineum should be inspected for any infection or diaper rashes, and surgery should be done only after its treatment. Genitalia should be examined to note the size of the penis, site and size of the meatus, width, length and development of the urethral plate, length of the hypoplastic urethra, chordee/torsion and their severity, shape and size of the dorsal hood, penoscrotal transposition and its severity and other associated anomalies like undescended testis, inguinal hernia. Multiple pinpoint dimples can be seen in the urethral plate along the side of the meatus. The location of the meatus should be confirmed by a probe in these cases [4]. Passing a probe is likely to diagnose the partial duplication of the urethra (Fig. 5.1a, b), which is laid open to convert it to one urethra during the repair. Careful examination and evaluation will diagnose the other associated congenital anomalies like undescended testis, inguinal hernia, hydrocele, the disorder of the sexual differentiation, renal agenesis, pelvic ureteric junction obstruction, and vesicoureteral reflux [5].

Careful inspection and examination of the median raphe depict much information about the embryological events. The degree of deviation of median raphe is directly proportional to the degree of torsion (Fig. 5.2a) and is an excellent method of measuring torque in cases of torsion with phimosis (Fig. 5.2b). Site of bifurcation of

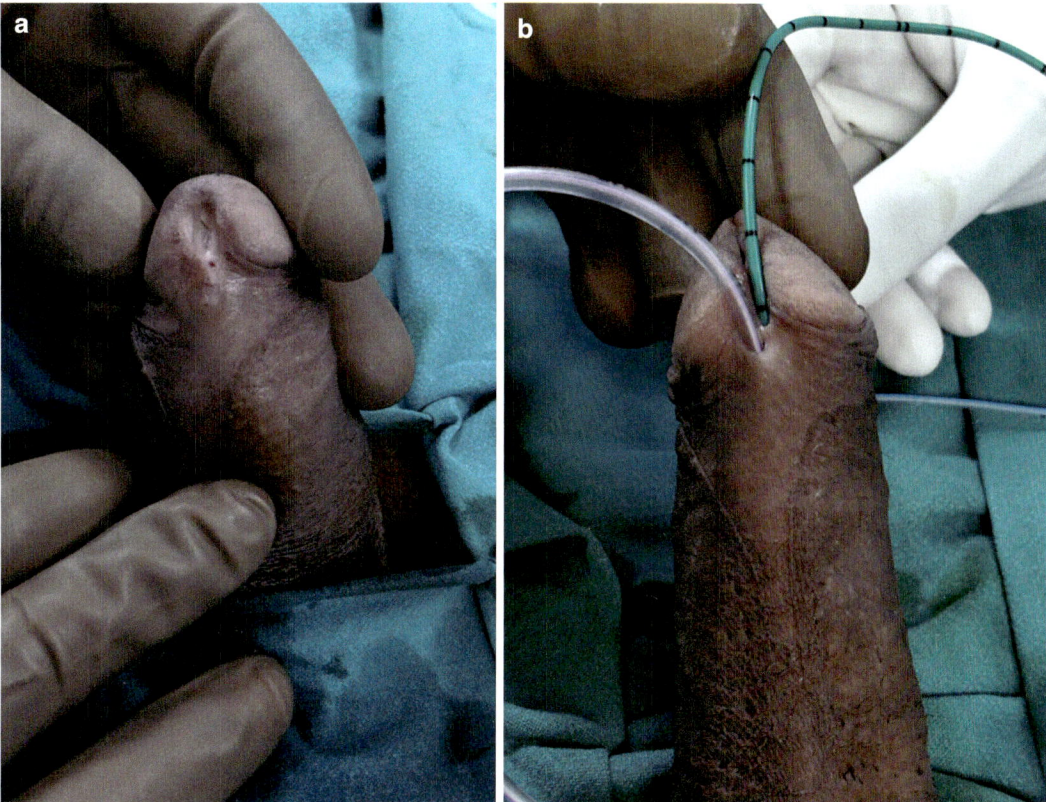

Fig. 5.1 Partial duplication of urethra (**a**) showing two openings. (**b**) Probing with ureteric catheter shows partial duplication of the urethra

median raphe and place of the dorsal Bull's eye indicate bifurcation of spongiosum and degree of chordee (Fig. 5.3a, b). Patients with severe hypospadias with or without penoscrotal transposition (Fig. 5.4a, b) are evaluated for internal sex organs, karyotyping, and USG for upper tract anomalies [6, 7]. Urethrogram and endoscopy are proper investigations to diagnose prostatic utricle. Large prostatic utricle makes catheterization difficult and can be a source of infection after surgery. Severe hypospadias with unilateral or bilateral undescended testis, a dimple in the perineum, or bifurcation of median raphe should be evaluated for disorders of sexual differentiation (Fig. 5.5a, b). Radiological imaging with ultrasonography and/or MRI for other urinary tract anomalies and internal genital organs and karyotyping should also be done in such patients [6]. Examination under anaesthesia helps better assess the type and severity of the hypospadias, degree of the chordee, and urethral plate quality. Therefore, the surgical plan is likely to be changed on the table [7].

5.5 Timing of Surgery

Hypospadias is usually diagnosed during the routine examination of the external genitalia just after the birth or during an inspection at the time of newborn circumcision. There is a delay in diagnosis of hypospadias with intact foreskin (Mega-meatus intact prepuce), and it is seen only with retraction of the foreskin or after circumcision later in life. The first milestone in the treatment is at the birth of the child. Parents must be informed and counselled about the anomaly, when the surgery is done, and the results. This is the proper time to establish a trust bond and confidence between parents and the surgeon to help remove the unknown fear, guilt, worry, better

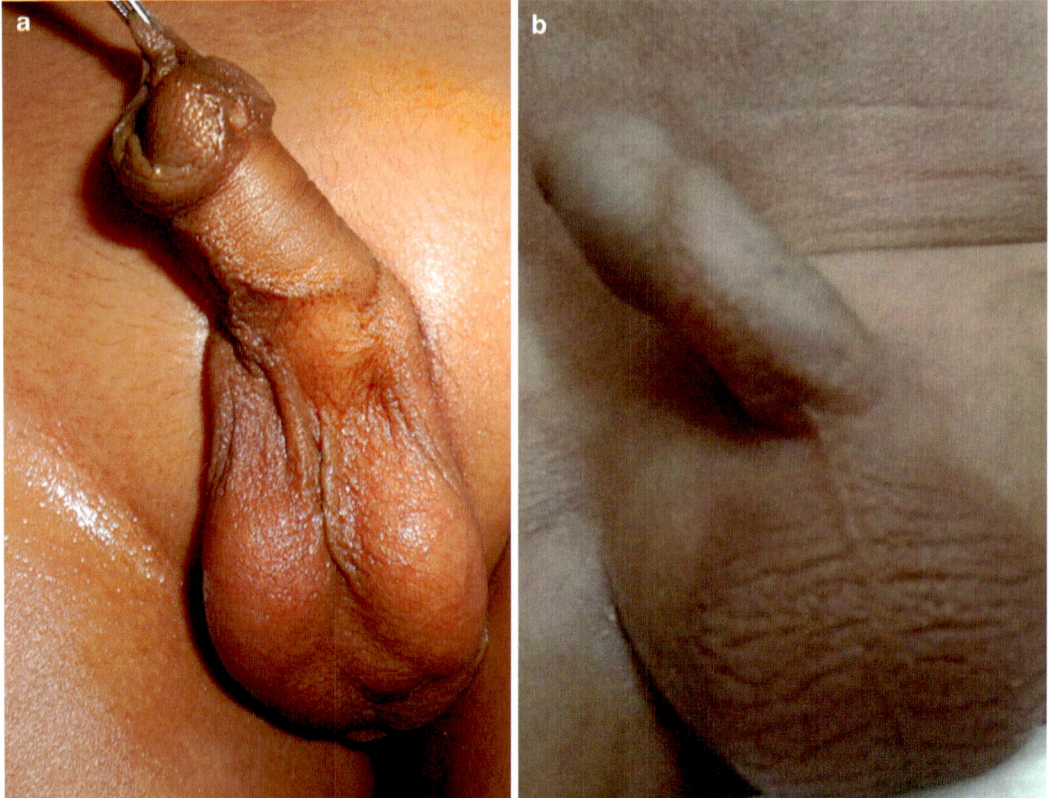

Fig. 5.2 (**a**) Torsion and deviation of median raphe in hypospadias. (**b**) Torsion and deviation of median raphe in isolated penile torsion

planning of surgical treatment, and co-operation of the family. Sometimes hypospadias may be associated with meatal stenosis. The meatal dilatation is required to prevent infection and back-pressure damage of the urinary tract during the first examination itself. The choice of surgery depends on the developmental milestones, penile length, size of glans, child's response to surgery, toilet training, and anaesthesia risk. The ideal age for hypospadias and genital surgery is 6 to 12 months, as per American Academy of Pediatrics guidelines [8]. The child develops good tolerance to surgery and anaesthesia by six months and becomes aware of his genitalia and toilet trained at 18 months. And even maybe operated at the age of 4 months if the baby is healthy and have adequate penile length [4]. The child who presents later after 18 months to a hospital, especially in developing countries, may be operated on at any age [9]. The general belief is that complications are lower in early repair. Though we had higher complications in adults (16.67%) than paediatric patients (6.67%) in tubularized and TIPU repairs, there is inconsistency in the literature. The issue of aesthetical genital surgeries without a functional impairment in minor hypospadias should be postponed to an age where he can give informed consent without a functional impairment of raising concern. Still, literature shows most of the surgeons are operating at an early age.

5.6 Hormonal Stimulation

Though the androgens increase the length of the penis, they improve the urethral plate tissue quality and have been used for a long time. But there is a lack of consensus on the type of androgen, whether local or systemic and the correct way of

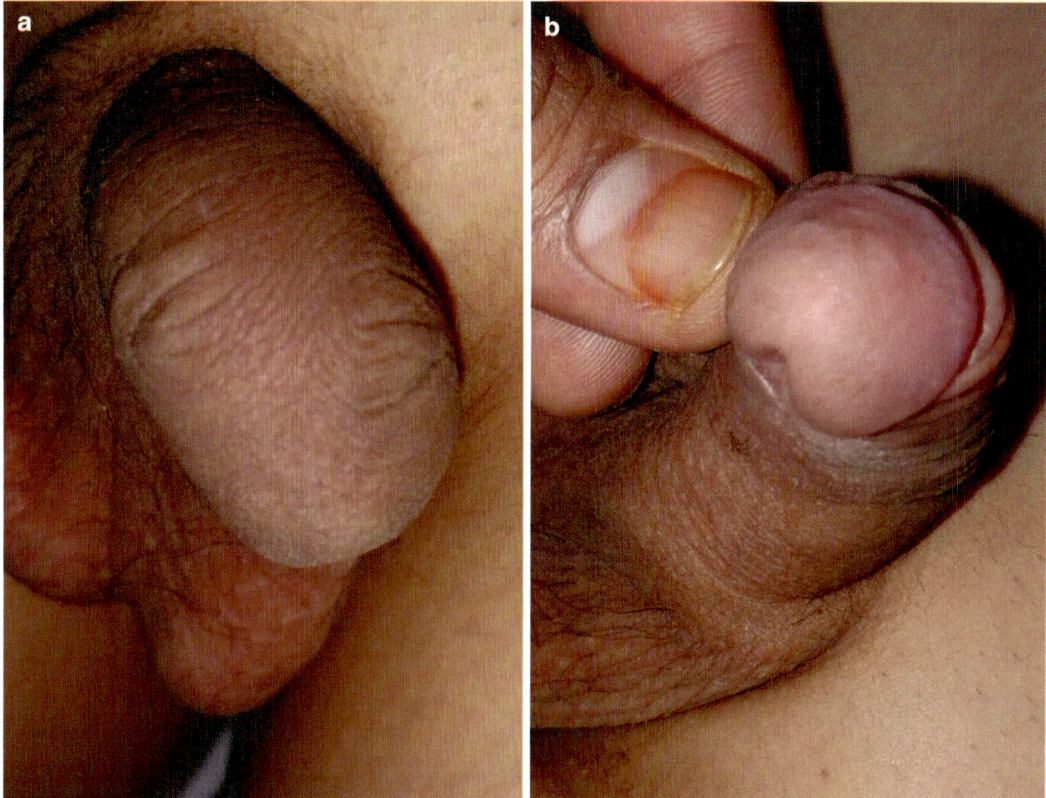

Fig. 5.3 (**a**). Site of dorsal Bull's eye. (**b**). Site of bifurcation of spongiosum ventrally

application. A thorough study of the potential side effects of androgens is needed. The real benefit of it in hypospadias surgery and the long-term effects of male sexual hormone application still needs to be defined [10]. The best-suited hormone for patients with undescended testis is HCG. Beta HCG, testosterone, and dihydrotestosterone are also used in the small penis or small penis after surgery. But it is unclear how safe these treatments are in the long term. HCG should be used cautiously as the experimental micropenis model supports delaying hormonal therapy until puberty [11]. Local 5% testosterone cream twice a day for five weeks or systemic testosterone two injections a week for five weeks (Koff's regimen) is preferred by most paediatric urologists. We use the local testosterone cream and found it effective in increasing the penile length, vascularity, and thickness of the corpus spongiosum significantly. Recently some studies have reported that androgen stimulation may impair wound healing and increases the risk of postoperative complications. Snodgrass (2014) compared the results of surgery in patients pre-treated with testosterone (to increase the glans size to 15 mm) and without hormones. He reported significantly higher complications and urethrocutaneous fistula in testosterone-treated patients [12].

5.7 Optical Magnification

Proper dissection and accurate approximation of tissues is the key to success in hypospadias surgery. The suture material should be very fine to prevent micro fistulae, and subcuticular sutures are preferred. Proper approximation of the tissue in hypospadias surgery is very important. So, magnification becomes an essential tool in these small children [10]. High powered glasses, magnification loupe, and operating microscope are used for magnification. Most hypospadias surgeons are using loupe, and a few prefer the operating microscope. Magnification minimizes complications

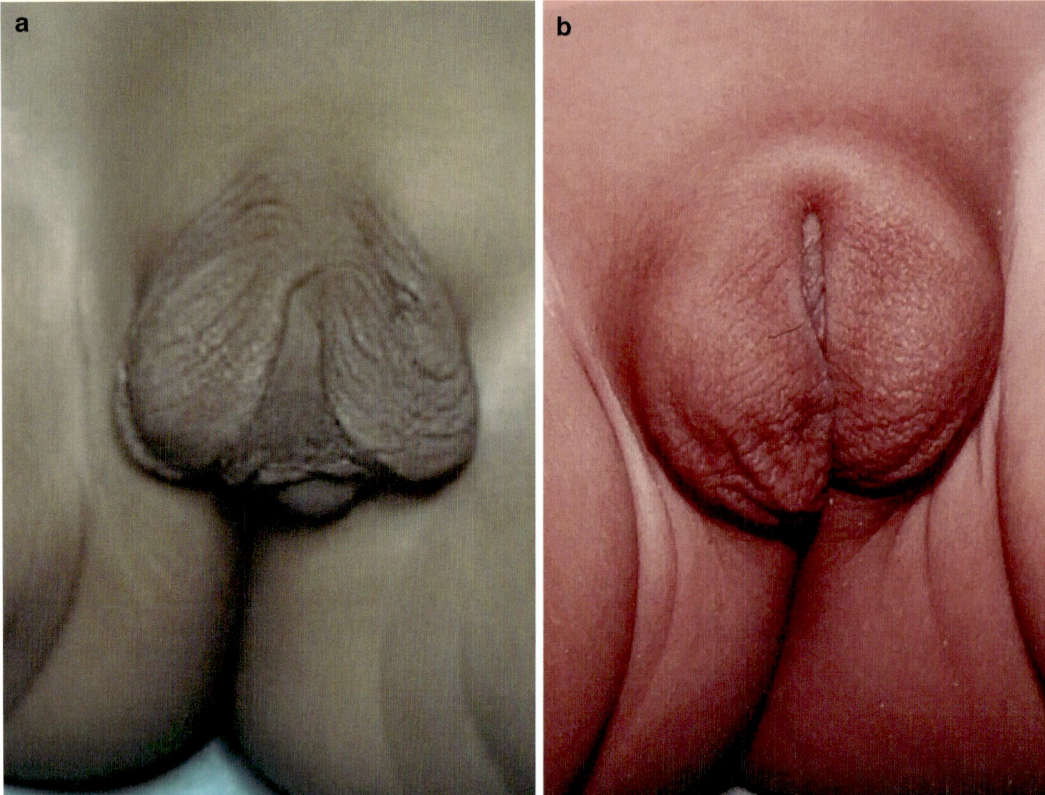

Fig. 5.4 (**a** & **b**). Severe hypospadias with penoscrotal transposition

and is indispensable in infants and toddlers' surgery. Gilbert et al. experienced fewer complications when using the microscope, and only 6.5% required reoperations in the microscope group while 24% in the non-microscope group [13]. A head-mounted microscope has been utilized in hypospadias surgery with a reported decrease in complications. Although this may provide magnification, there is no evidence to prove that it is more ergonomic than the surgical microscope. But authors prefer to use the magnification loupe rather than a head-mounted microscope or operating microscope for magnification.

5.8 Anaesthesia and Analgesia

After the preoperative assessment, a premedication is given to make the child comfortable. Midazolam 0.5 mg/kg IM/IV 30 minutes before surgery is commonly used. General anaesthesia is preferred with or without caudal or local penile block. The caudal block with bupivacaine, clonidine, ketamine, and midazolam is reported to have an increased duration of analgesia in the postoperative period. But there are divided opinions on the better efficacy over each other. In a recent meta-analysis (Goel et al. 2019 [14] and Tanseco et al. 2019 [15]), it was concluded that caudal analgesia might increase the risk of urethrocutaneous fistula and other complications of urethroplasty. The risk of urethrocutaneous fistula increased up to 14.6%, while overall urethroplasty-related complications up to 6.4% in the caudal analgesia patients. The explanation for the increase in complication given was a significant increase in penile volume after caudal block, which is likely to increase penile oedema and causing inadequate or delayed wound healing. But Braga et al. 2017 questioned the hypothesis of penile engorgement resulting in impaired postoperative healing and complications as they

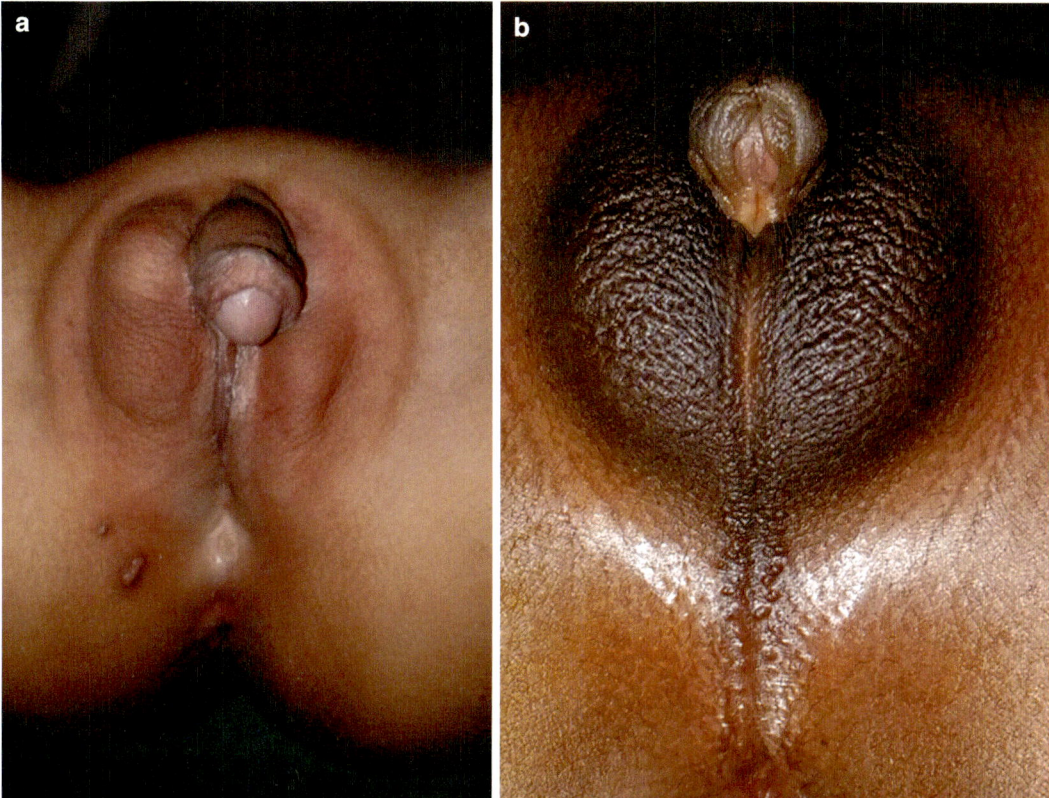

Fig. 5.5 (**a**) Perineal dimple and small left testis. (**b**) Bifurcation of median raphe

found no increased complications in hypospadias repair with caudal block analgesia [16]. Another study by the Philadelphia group 2018 found no association of the increased complications following caudal anaesthesia, including urethracutaneous fistula and glans dehiscence. The author is also of the same opinion.

5.9 Gentle Tissue Handling

Application of all the plastic and reconstructive surgical principles can yield better results in hypospadias repair. Minimal tissue trauma, pinpoint and minimal use of cautery, good haemostasis, tension-free closure in all layers, multiple layer well-vascularized tissue closure, and suturing with epithelial inversion [7]. The use of microsurgical instruments, magnification, proper handling of the tissues by using skin hooks, stay sutures minimize the tissue trauma. Using bipolar electro-cautery with fine tip forceps reduces tissue trauma. Needle holders and micro mosquito forceps should be reserved for hypospadias surgery, where a 6/o-7/o suture is used. Recently Riquelme et al. (2012) developed a new retractor for hypospadias surgery to minimize the tissue trauma, which has the following characteristics, can stabilize the penis in a position, easy to change the position of the penis, can be adjusted for the size of the penis, and maintains the bloodless field [17]. Dissection of the tissues in the right plane preserves the vascularity of the flap for neourethra and skin and helps prevent ischaemic complications. The plane of dissection is kept at Buck's fascia while penile de-gloving is done, and superficial and deep layers of the dartos fascia for raising the inner prepucial flap (Fig. 5.6a, b). A dissection plane is created to mobilize the urethral plate at the level of tunica albuginea, lifting Buck's fascia starting proximal to the meatus in the normal urethra and then dis-

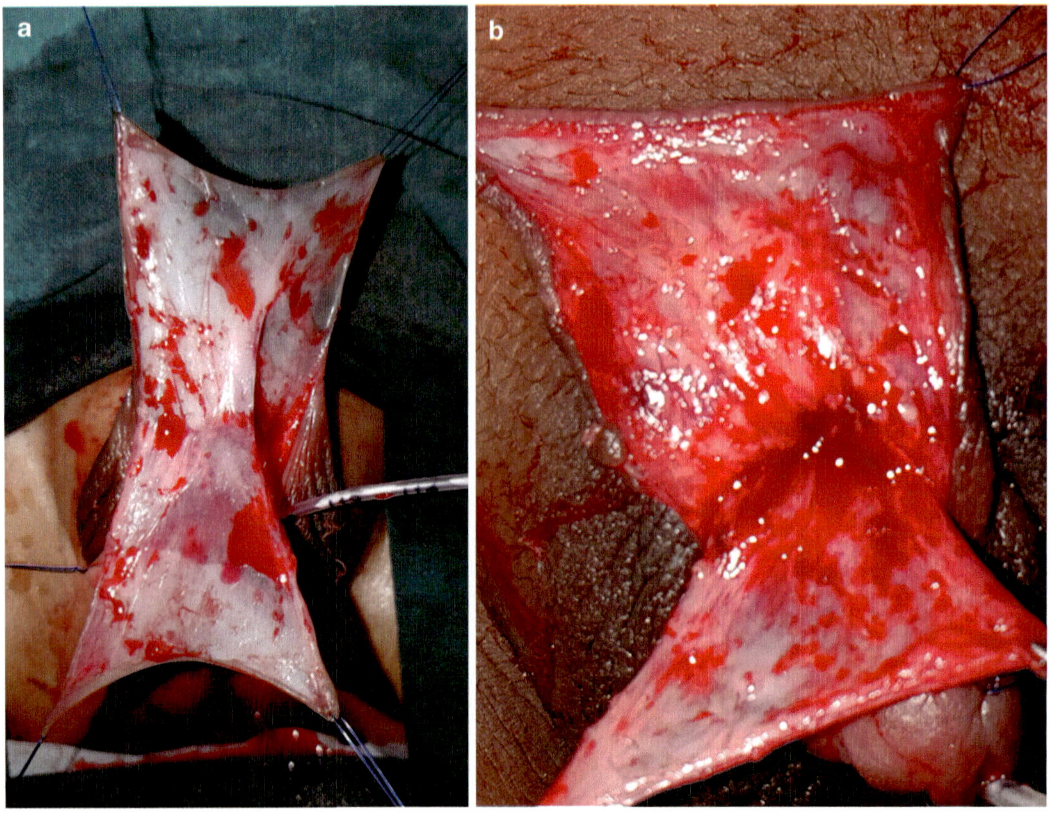

Fig. 5.6 (a & b) Dissection of dorsal dartos between the superficial and deep layer of dartos

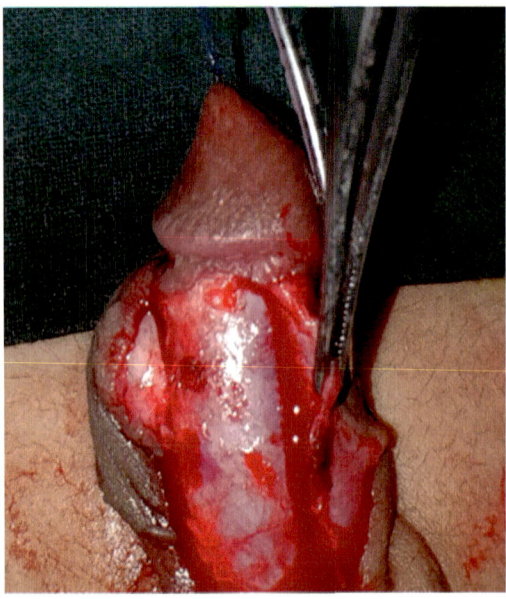

Fig. 5.7 Plane of dissection of spongiosum with urethral plate

sected in the same plane distally (Fig. 5.7). As the urethra is covered in two layers of Buck's fascia, it is easy to create the plane of dissection without damaging the corpus spongiosum and cavernosum. The glanular wings are incised in the same plane in continuity with corpus spongiosum into the glans (Fig. 5.8a, b).

5.10 Suture Material

Ideal suture material for urethroplasty in hypospadias repair should be absorbable and have good tensile strength for a period long enough to resist urinary flow after catheter removal till definitive healing occurs. Skin closure sutures should preferably be absorbable to prevent the anxiety and fear of the patients of suture removal. Though chromic catgut, the natural fibre suture, has been commonly used for urethroplasty in

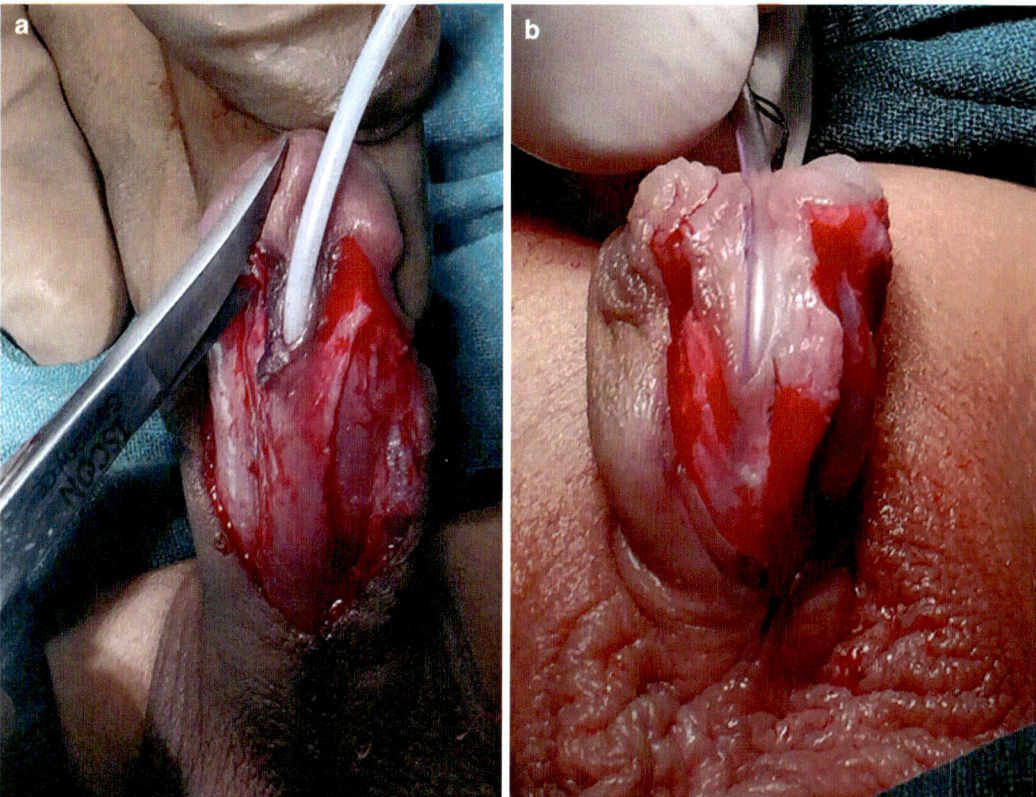

Fig. 5.8 (a & b). Dissection of spongiosum into the glans

hypospadias repair for many years, recent studies have shown a higher incidence of urethral fistula compared to polyglactin in tubularized urethral plate urethroplasty for mid-shaft to proximal hypospadias repair and a higher incidence of suture tracks when used for skin reconstruction. Snodgrass found a higher incidence of skin tracks (43%) in patients operated on using chromic catgut [18]. Recently, the monofilament Polydioxanone (PDS) and braided polyglactin (Vicryl), the late absorbable suture, are commonly used in either a continuous subcuticular and interrupted full-thickness fashion with 6/0–7/0 sutures. Larger and nonabsorbable sutures may leave behind the suture marks with comedo-like skin tracks. The size & the composition of suture material, and the type of sutures may affect the outcome of the hypospadias surgery. Ulman and co-workers reported a significantly low fistula rate (4.95%) in subcuticular repair than through and through technique (16.6%) [19]. While others believe subcuticular or through and through sutures does not affect the results provided, polyglactin suture is used [20]. The polyglactin absorbable sutures are useful for the innermost layer closure with epithelial inversion, while polyglyconate sutures are better for other layers. Shirazi et al., in an experimental study in the rats, compared the results Chromic, catgut, polydioxanone, poliglecaprone 25, polylactic acid, and polyglactin [21]. These were reported to have been associated with more vessel density and a wider urethral lumen with poliglecaprone 25, while the polydioxanone had more urethral epithelium. The authors believe that the key to success lies in the accurate approximation of the margin of the urethral plate or skin rather than the type of sutures and suture material. Suppose a surgeon wants to pass the suture through and through urethral plate epithelium or skin, then early absorbable suture like Vicryl rapid should be used, and for subcuticular suturing, any of the absorbable or late absorbable suture material can be used [22].

5.11 Urinary Diversion

Common practice in hypospadias surgery is to use a stent for urinary drainage for 5–7 days, but some use a suprapubic urinary diversion with a urethral stent. There are reports where no stents were utilized without compromising the results of hypospadias repair. Hakim et al., in a multicentric retroscopic review of Mathieu's repair, found no difference in urethrocutaneous fistula rate in stented versus non-stented repair and no urinary retention even in caudal anaesthesia group postoperatively [20]. Waterman et al. (2002) had used stent free repair successfully in modified incised plate tubularized urethroplasty, while Manzoni et al. reported a high fistula rate when the urethral stent was not used [7, 23]. Another issue that remains to be decided is whether the stent is placed in the bladder or urethra. In our opinion, placing the stent in the bladder is better to avoid extravasation of urine than urethral positioned stents. There is no clearly defined suitable size of the urethral stent in urethroplasty. Commonly 5 to 10 Fr size urethral stent according to the age and size of the urethra is used. Reconstructed neourethra is generally larger than or equal to the calibre of the urethral stent. We prefer a Silastic catheter of adequate size according to the child's age and keep it just inside the bladder for about 7–10 days [22]. Hypospadias surgery is usually done in a daycare centre at most places, and the child is sent home the same day after putting the stent in the diapers.

5.12 Dressing

There are different opinions about postoperative dressings like whether to go for dressing or not and whether to use the pressure dressing or not. An ideal dressing should be easily and quickly applied, dressing material must be non-allergenic and cheap, should not be adherent to the wound/incision, effectively absorb the leakages of the wound, put adequate pressure on the flaps and grafts effectively without damaging the blood circulation, protect against infections, and must be easily & painlessly removable. In a prospective trial, Van Savage et al. (2000) found no difference in surgery results, rate of adverse events and complications in patients with dressing and no dressing, and it was an easy postoperative ambulatory parent care at home [24]. Multi-layer fibrin glue has been used as an effective dressing as it is impervious to urine and stool and prevents oedema and haematoma. Many other techniques that have been found suitable in hypospadias surgery are SANAV polyurethane bio-occlusive foil, Peha-Haft and adhesive membrane dressings, Cavi care, and glove-finger Melolin. Silicon foam dressing effectively restricts oedema, haematoma formation and stabilization with easy removal [25]. A pressure dressing is a double-edged sword as excessive pressure may compromise the blood supply of skin flaps and skin, while no pressure is likely to lead to haematoma formation, oedema and infection, increasing the incidences of complications. The authors prefer postoperative dressing with optimum pressure to control postoperative oedema, prevent haematoma, and as a barrier to infection.

5.13 Surgical Treatment

The surgical goals of hypospadias surgery are a straight penis with adequate length, conical glans with a slit-like meatus at the tip, cosmetic symmetry of the glans and penile shaft, projectile stream, reconstructing a urethra of uniform calibre and adequate length, and normal erections; thereby imposing confidence in the child [22]. Orthoplasty, urethroplasty, meatoplasty and glanuloplasty, scrotoplasty and skin cover are needed to achieve the goals. A circumcoronal incision is given 5–7 mm away from the corona to raise para-glanular flaps. The approximation of the para-glanular flaps will reduce the incidence of subcoronal fistula. Orthoplasty is the most crucial milestone before proceeding to urethroplasty in 1-stage repair. The penis has to be straight for a successful repair. Therefore, the complete chordee's correction should be tested by Gittes test on the table before proceeding for the urethroplasty. The methods for correction of the chordee are penile skin de-gloving, mobilization of urethral plate and urethra, extended urethral mobilization, plication procedures, split and roll technique, dorsal plication, penile disassembly and corporoplasty with the graft. Gittes test is commonly used to assess the complete chordee correction. However, intra-corporeal injection of the Alprost and Prostaglandin E1 is very useful for both intra-operative and in follow-up visits to check for curvature correction. Glanuloplasty and meatoplasty are done to reconstruct a conical glans with wide meatus at the tip to produce a projectile stream. The meatoplasty is commonly done with V or W shaped flap. Raising an adequate length of the glanular wing is crucial in meatoplasty and glanuloplasty to prevent pressure on the neourethra and reduce ischaemic complications.

5.13.1 Urethroplasty

Penis and glans size, the severity of ventral curvature, type of hypospadias, the width of urethral plate width and spongiosal development, available ventral penile skin proximal to the meatus, hypoplastic urethral length, size, shape, and type of the dorsal hood, and penile shaft skin are important factors for choosing the type of urethroplasty. Urethral plate preservation procedures are preferred because of their better results. The type of urethroplasty can only be decided after chordee correction. TIPU with or without inlay graft and onlay flap urethroplasty can be done in most of the distal and middle hypospadias with minimal chordee or without chordee. An algorithm is proposed to choose the type of urethroplasty in hypospadias without curvature [22] (Fig. 5.9). Results of single-stage and two stages are comparable, and the choice depends on the training and experience of the surgeon in proximal hypospadias [2, 9, 26–29]. The urethral plate should be preserved and utilized to improve the results. Based on the rational approach taking into consideration all the factors influencing the repair, an algorithm is proposed [9, 22, 30] (Chap. 6, Fig. 6.8).

5.13.2 Healthy Vascular Tissue Cover

The critical factors for healing are adequate blood supply of the neourethra and waterproof suturing. Healthy vascularized tissue cover over neourethra helps in maintaining blood supply as well as waterproofing. Commonly used healthy and vascularized interposing tissues are corpus spongiosum, dorsal/ventral/lateral dartos flap, tunica vaginalis flaps, and denuded inner prepucial skin. The dorsal dartos vascular pedicle is mobilized up to the root of the penis to avoid penile torque. The tunica vaginalis flaps are very good vascularized tissue to cover the neourethra and yield better results than other tissues. Denuded skin flaps have also been used for results but need complete denudation to prevent buried skin inclusion dermoid. Spongiosum is a well-vascularized and healthy tissue available locally. Spongioplasty is an ideal healthy tissue cover for neourethra and also reconstructs a near-normal urethra [22]. Dartos flap may also be added with spongiosum for a better outcome.

5.14 Preputioplasty

Many parents and patients demand prepucial reconstruction for cosmetic appearance. As the circumcision is less acceptable, the prepuce can be saved and utilized to reconstruct the prepuce and have good cosmetic results [31]. Preputioplasty can be done in both distal and proximal hypospadias in tubularized urethral plate urethroplasty on parents' demand. The foreskin reconstruction adds about 20 minutes to the operating time without increasing the complication of urethroplasty. However, Kljin et al. reported increased urethroplasty complications with preputioplasty and discouraged prepucial

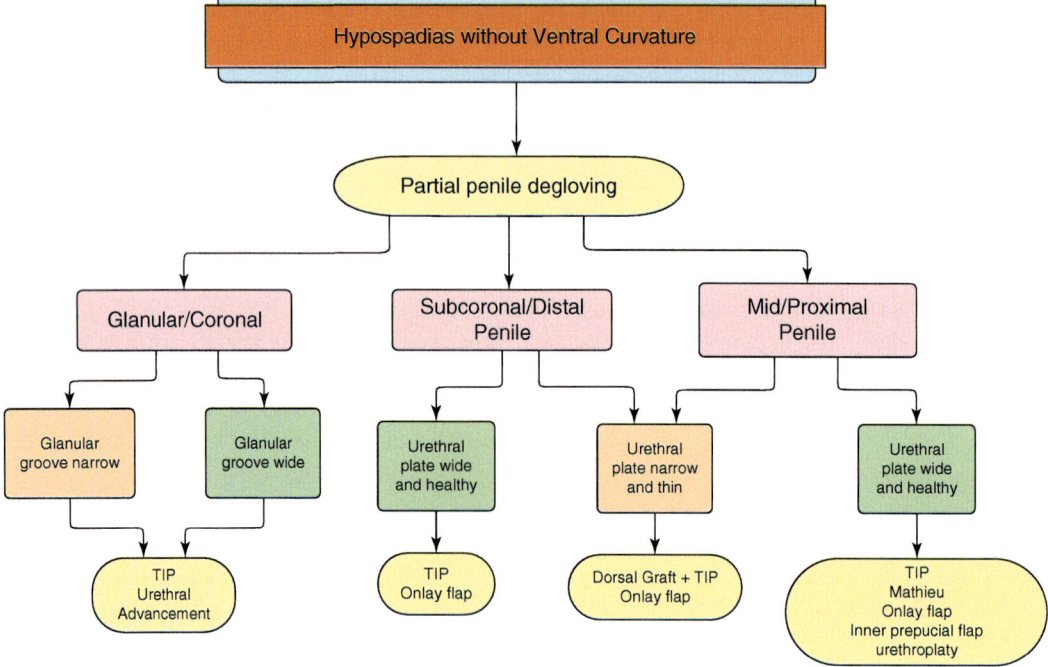

Fig. 5.9 Algorithm for hypospadias without ventral curvature

reconstruction [32]. But others recommended preputioplasty because they had no difference in urethroplasty results with preputioplasty [26, 31, 33]. Details of prepucioplasty are described in Chap. 25.

5.15 Postoperative Care

Dressing, catheter care, analgesics, and antibiotics are the essential points that require attention in the postoperative period. Local anaesthetic agents and acetaminophen or acetaminophen with codeine are needed to relieve the incisional pain. Bladder spasms and related problems can be treated acutely with Oxybutynin in the dose 0.2 mg/kg/dose six hourly. Prophylactic antibiotics should be continued till the per urethral catheter or stent is removed. The parents are counselled for postoperative care and asked to apply an antibiotic ointment to the glans penis and urethra tip every time the diapers are changed or after passing urine.

5.16 Postoperative Follow-Up Protocol

Daycare surgery is the routine in hypospadias surgery in most of the centres. Longer hospital and repeated visits of the clinician's may remind the child of his abnormality and have psychological implications. The child is called at 1,3,6 month and then yearly up to 2 years, and review follow-up adolescence to adulthood up to the genital maturity; when the patient can express his social and sexual problems. Any complications beyond two years period will automatically bring the patients to the surgeon. A previous asymptomatic fistula is likely to appear, and chordee may occur due to failure of growth of scarred urethra later. The patients are concerned about the size of the penis and cosmesis. So they should be followed up to adolescence & adulthood for the actual outcome of surgery and real incidence of chronic complications. The post-surgical outcome is evaluated in view of cosmesis, functional and psychosexual functions. Adult urologists may contribute positively in adolescence and adulthood follow-up and management of the complications.

5.17 Surgical Outcome

5.17.1 Cosmetic Function

Cosmesis is an important issue in postoperative follow-up. Hypospadiac patients are concerned about the size of the penis and penile appearance. A better cosmetic appearance with an adequate size of the penis yields a better sexual outcome. Hypospadias Objective Scoring Evaluation, Paediatric Penile Perception Score, Hypospadias Objective Penile Evaluation Score are used for objective evaluation of the hypospadiacs. An independent person done scoring, can be kept in the patients' notes for future progression (for details, see Chap. 28).

5.17.2 Functional Outcome

Function evaluation of the hypospadiac patients is recommended by the uroflow study after toilet training. Children with findings of borderline obstructed flow, postvoid residual urine, lower urinary tract symptoms, recurrent urinary tract infection, or other urinary signs are evaluated for obstruction & bladder functions. They should be followed until adulthood (for details, see Chap. 28).

5.17.3 Psychosexual Outcome

Psychosexual well-being is one of the long-term goals of hypospadias surgery and is a challenge to evaluate. Only a few studies are available for assessing long-term psychosexual adjustment and sexual function. Most hypospadiacs do well in adulthood in terms of sexual function, and the strength and duration of erection, ejaculation, and masturbation are unimpaired. However, in a few patients with severe hypospadias with chordee, long skin urethroplasty, and surgery burden, the sexual functions are affected and concern the patients. They need standardized assessment available for objective scores (for details, see Chap. 27).

5.18 Future

Despite innovations and concepts, the importance of the current techniques is unlikely to be obsolete. The innovation and the use of modern technology like laser soldering, tissue engineering, use of Robots and radiological evaluation for chordee tissue, and objective anatomical details will show the pathway to the future of hypospadiology. Tissue engineering may regenerate the urethra for urethral replacement. In experimental studies, the tubular cellular collagen matrices seeded with urothelial cells are used as a medium to grow the urethra and utilized successfully to repair created urethral defects in a rabbit model. Similarly, others have grown the corpus cavernosum [34, 35]. The complex anatomy of the urethral mucosa surrounded by spongiosum is the foremost hurdle to replace the urethra by tissue engineering and its routine use in hypospadias surgery. However, the regenerated urethra can be used in complex redo cases and hypospadias cripple. Robots may play an important role in hypospadias surgery by removing the effects of tremors for meticulous suturing with magnification but have not been used till date.

References

1. Davis DM. Surgical treatment of hypospadias, especially scrotal and perineal. J Urol. 1951;65(4):595–602.
2. Titley OG, Bracka A. A 5-year audit of trainees experience and outcomes with two-stage hypospadias surgery. Br J Plast Surg. 1998;51(5):370–5.
3. Snyder CL, Evangelidis A, Hansen G, Peter SDS, Ostlie DJ, Gatti JM, Gittes GK, Sharp RJ, Murphy JP. Management of complications after hypospadias repair. Urology. 2005;65(4):782–5.
4. Shukla AR, Patel RP, Canning DA. Hypospadias. Urol Clin. 2004;31(3):445–60.

5. Duckett J, Walsh P, Retik A, Vaughan E. Campbell's urology. Hypospadias. 1998;5:353–95.
6. Khuri F. Urological anomalies associated with hypospadias. Urol Clin North Am. 1981;8:565.
7. Manzoni G, Bracka A, Palminteri E, Marrocco G. Hypospadias surgery: when what and by whom? BJU Int. 2004;94(8):1188–95.
8. Kass EJ, Bolong D. Single-stage hypospadias reconstruction without fistula. J Urol. 1990;144(2 Part 2):520–2.
9. Bhat A. Extended urethral mobilization in incised plate urethroplasty for severe hypospadias: a variation in technique to improve chordee correction. J Urol. 2007;178(3):1031–5.
10. Mouriquand P, Mure PY. Current concepts in hypospadiology. BJU Int. 2004;93:26–34.
11. McMahon D, Kramer S, Husmann D. Micropenis: does early treatment with testosterone do more harm than good? J Urol. 1995;154(2):825–9.
12. Snodgrass W, Villanueva C, Bush NC. Duration of follow-up to diagnose hypospadias urethroplasty complications. J Pediatr Urol. 2014;10(2):208–11.
13. Gilbert DA, Devine CJ Jr, Winslow BH, Horton CE, Getz SE. Microsurgical hypospadias repair. Plast Reconstr Surg. 1986;77(3):460–5.
14. Goel P, Jain S, Bajpai M, Khanna P, Jain V, Yadav DK. Does caudal analgesia increase the rates of urethrocutaneous fistula formation after hypospadias repair? Systematic review and meta-analysis. Indian J Urol. 2019;35(3):222.
15. Tanseco PP, Randhawa H, Chua ME, Blankstein U, Kim JK, McGrath M, Lorenzo AJ, Braga LH. Postoperative complications of hypospadias repair in patients receiving caudal block vs noncaudal anaesthesia: a meta-analysis. Can Urol Assoc J. 2019;13(8):E249.
16. Braga LH, Jegatheeswaran K, McGrath M, Easterbrook B, Rickard M, DeMaria J, Lorenzo AJ. Cause and effect versus confounding—is there a true association between caudal blocks and tubularized incised plate repair complications? J Urol. 2017;197(3 Part 2):845–51.
17. Riquelme M, Aranda A, Rodarte-Shade M, Rodriguez-Gomez J, Torres-Riquelme J. A new surgical stabilizing instrument for hypospadias repair. Eur J Pediatr Surg. 2013;23(02):148–9.
18. Snodgrass W, Bush N. Recent advances in understanding/management of hypospadias. F1000Prime Rep. 2014;6:101. https://doi.org/10.12703/P6-101.
19. Ulman I, Erikci V, Avanoğlu A, Gökdemir A. The effect of suturing technique and material on complication rate following hypospadias repair. Eur J Pediatr Surg. 1997;7(03):156–7.
20. Hakim S, Merguerian PA, Rabinowitz R, Shortliffe LD, McKenna PH. Outcome analysis of the modified Mathieu hypospadias repair: comparison of stented and unstented repairs. J Urol. 1996;156(2):836–8.
21. Shirazi M, Noorafshan A, Serhan A. Effects of different suture materials used for the repair of hypospadias: a stereological study in a rat model. Urol Int. 2012;89(4):395–401.
22. Bhat A. General considerations in hypospadias surgery. Indian J Urol. 2008;24(2):188.
23. Waterman BJ, Renschler T, Cartwright PC, Snow BW, de Vries CR. Variables in successful repair of urethrocutaneous fistula after hypospadias surgery. J Urol. 2002;168(2):726–30.
24. Van Savage JG, Palanca LG, Slaughenhoupt BL. A prospective randomized trial of dressings versus no dressings for hypospadias repair. J Urol. 2000;164(3):981–3.
25. Gangopadhyay A, Sharma S. Brief report-Peha-haft bandage as a new dressing for pediatric hypospadias repair. Indian J Plast Surg. 2005;38(2):162–4.
26. Snodgrass W, Yucel S. Tubularized incised plate for mid-shaft and proximal hypospadias repair. J Urol. 2007;177(2):698–702.
27. Braga LH, Pippi Salle JL, Lorenzo AJ, Skeldon S, Dave S, Farhat WA, Khoury AE, Bagli DJ. Comparative analysis of tubularized incised plate versus onlay island flap urethroplasty for penoscrotal hypospadias. J Urol. 2007;178(4):1451–7.
28. Gershbaum MD, Stock JA, Hanna MK. A case for the 2-stage repair of perineoscrotal hypospadias with severe chordee. J Urol. 2002;168(4 Part 2):1727–9.
29. Ferro F, Zaccara A, Spagnoli A, Lucchetti M, Capitanucci M, Villa M. Skin graft for 2-stage treatment of severe hypospadias: back to the future? J Urol. 2002;168(4):1730–3.
30. Kajbafzadeh A-M, Arshadi H, Payabvash S, Salmasi AH, Najjaran-Tousi V, Sahebpor ARA. Proximal hypospadias with severe chordee: single-stage repair using corporeal tunica vaginalis free graft. J Urol. 2007;178(3):1036–42.
31. Gray J, Boston V. Glanular reconstruction and preputioplasty repair for distal hypospadias: a unique daycase method to avoid urethral stenting and preserve the prepuce. BJU Int. 2003;91(3):268–70.
32. Klijn AJ, Dik P, De Jong TP. Results of preputial reconstruction in 77 boys with distal hypospadias. J Urol. 2001;165(4):1255–7.
33. Erdenetsetseg G, Dewan P. Reconstruction of the hypospadiac hooded prepuce. J Urol. 2003;169(5):1822–4.
34. Kwon TG, Yoo JJ, Atala A. Autologous penile corpora cavernosa replacement using tissue engineering techniques. J Urol. 2002;168(4):1754–8.
35. Atala A. Recent developments in tissue engineering and regenerative medicine. Curr Opin Pediatr. 2006;18(2):167–71.

Chordee Correction in Hypospadias Repair

Amilal Bhat and Mahakshit Bhat

6.1 Introduction

Hypospadiology is still not well understood and is in the evolution phase. This is evident from the fact that more than 300 procedures and modifications are described in the literature. One must be aware that we operate upon the corpus spongiosum and cavernosum, responsible for erection. The surgical principle in correcting a congenital anomaly is reconstructing the organ to the normal or near-normal with the existing tissue or supplementing the tissue. Hypospadias surgery is one example of applying this principle. The most commonly used methods are penile de-gloving, dorsal plication and/or resection of the urethral plate, and corporotomies/corporoplasty in selected patients. Methods used for chordee correction in hypospadias seem to be away from the embryological basis of the cause and applied without looking into the etiological factors in the individual case. The rational approach is required to correct curvature as per anatomical principles of surgery and the step-by-step approach dealing with the all-etiological factors in modern Hypospadiology.

A. Bhat (✉)
Bhat's Hypospadias and Reconstructive Urology Hospital and Research Centre,
Jaipur, Rajasthan, India

Department of Urology, Jaipur National University Institute for Medical Sciences and Research Centre, Jaipur, Rajasthan, India

Department of Urology, Dr. S.N. Medical College, Jodhpur, Rajasthan, India

Department of Urology, S.P. Medical College, Bikaner, Rajasthan, India

P.G. Committee Medical Council of India, New Delhi, India

Academic and Research Council of RUHS, Jaipur, Rajasthan, India

M. Bhat
Department of Urology, National Institute of Medical Sciences Medical College, Jaipur, Rajasthan, India

6.2 Definition of Chordee

Chordee is a French word and is derived from the word cord or band. In hypospadias, it is used to describe scar-like tissue from meatus to corona, responsible for bending the penis. There is hardly any description of chordee in the literature of the late 1880s to 1920. Smith (1937) used the word chordee in his presentation at AUA Meeting. Von Hook, in 1950 used it for corporal maldevelopment and ventral bending. Then onwards, it seems to be commonplace in using the terminology. In the name of the "chordee," the fibrous bands of dysplastic mesenchymal tissues were resected to correct the ventral curvature. Unfortunately, the interchangeable use of the term "chordee" and "fibrous tissues" unnecessarily perpetuates confusion. The tissue is not fibrous tissue, but it is a hypoplastic corpus spongiosum [1]. Baskin et al. found the increased vascularity in the spongiosum during hypospadias evaluation of fetal penises [2].

Kaplan and Lamm found no histological evidence of fibrous scar in fetal specimens contributing to bending and suggested that the ventral curvature is a normal phase during the development of the penis [3]. The histology of the excised dartos and spongiosum tissues during hypospadias repair showed well-vascularized connective tissues without evidence of a fibrous scar which disapproves the concepts "dysplastic dartos, and corpus spongiosum forms the fibrous 'chordee' tissues and require resection to correct the chordee" [1]. The arrest in the development of urethra is the cause of hypospadias and often results in curvature with relatively shortened ventral structures.

6.3 Causes of Chordee

Ultimately the entrapment of the corporeal body in the coverings of the penis leads to the curvature, and the various factors leading to curvature are:

1. Short ventral skin
2. Short Dartos fascia
3. Short Bucks fascia
4. Short Corpus spongiosum
5. Dorso-ventral disproportion of Corpus cavernosum
6. Congenital short urethra

Either a single or a combination of the factors mentioned above may be responsible for the curvature.

6.4 Incidence of Chordee

Though the Chordee is defined and discussed, its exact incidence is unknown. Prevalence and severity of ventral curvature vary with the type of hypospadias. We reported 24.16 % chordee in a study of 120 cases, having distal 6 %, mid 29.5 %, and proximal having 100% in the cases chosen for tubularized plate urethroplasty [4]. But in 115 patients with all types of hypospadias and repair selected for hypospadias repair, chordee was present 80 (69.56 %). It was mild 29 (36.25%), Moderate 27 (33.75%) and Severe i24 (30%) respectively.

Stojanovic B (2011) et al. reported approximately 30% of all patients with hypospadias had a curvature, and the incidence of curvature was 23.5% in distal, 29.4% in the middle, and 68.3% in the proximal hypospadias. Snodgrass reported ventral curvature in 11% of primary distal cases, 30% mid-shaft repairs, and 81% proximal repairs. Ventral curvature in all mid-shaft and distal hypospadias patients was less than 30 degrees. Ventral curvature in the proximal penile to perineal hypospadias was found less than 30 degrees in 31% and more than 30 degrees in 50%. Fifty percent of proximal hypospadias patients after the penile degloving either had no chordee or had minor chordee, which was corrected by a single dorsal plication [5]. The incidence of residual curvature varies from 9.3% to 25 % of redo surgeries [6].

6.5 Classification of Chordee

Chordee may be classified into:

1. **Congenital:** Isolated or associated with hypospadias, chordee without hypospadias and epispadias.
2. **Acquired:** Secondary to stricture, trauma, post-surgery.

Hypospadias and its variants of chordee fall in the congenital group and are classified as shown in Figs. 6.1 and 6.2).

According to the severity of the curvature, it is graded in degrees as:
Mild <30 degrees
Moderate- 30–45 degrees
Severe- >45 degrees

6.6 Penile Chordee and Sexual Problem

Significant chordee is reported to impact sexual relationships, self-esteem and confidence, and sexual function. Adult men with more than 30 degrees seek medical advice more frequently for sexual dysfunction. Such patients with untreated chordee reported having more dissatisfaction with the appearance of the penis, increased difficulty with sexual intercourse, and more mental stress [7]. A straight, functional, and cosmetically

6 Chordee Correction in Hypospadias Repair

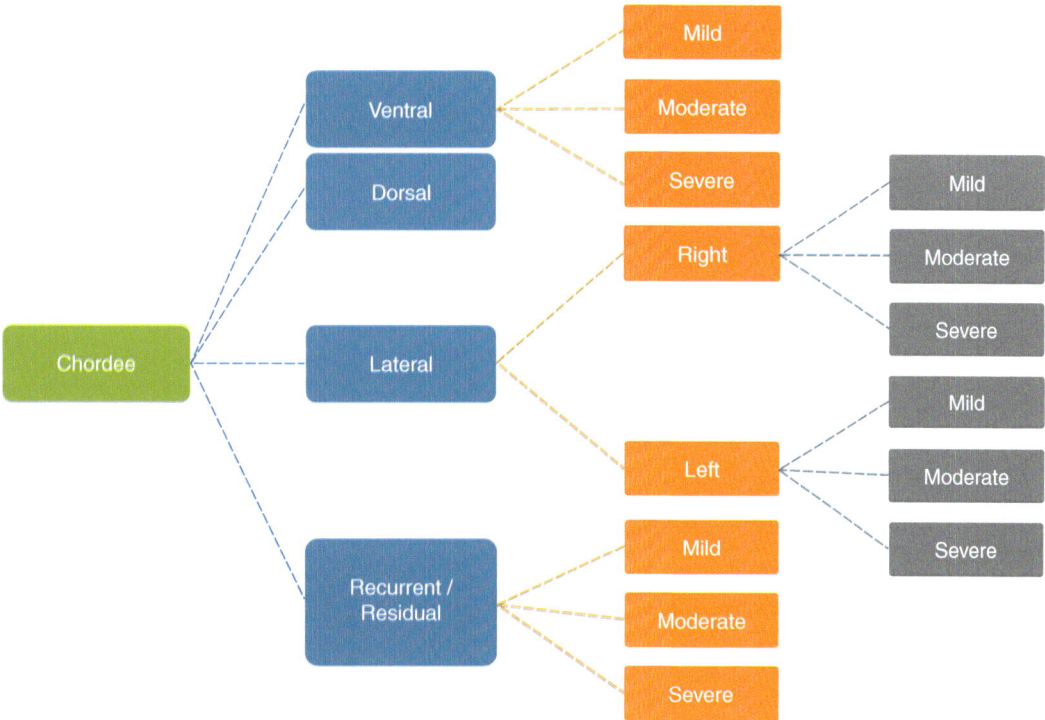

Fig. 6.1 Classification of chordee

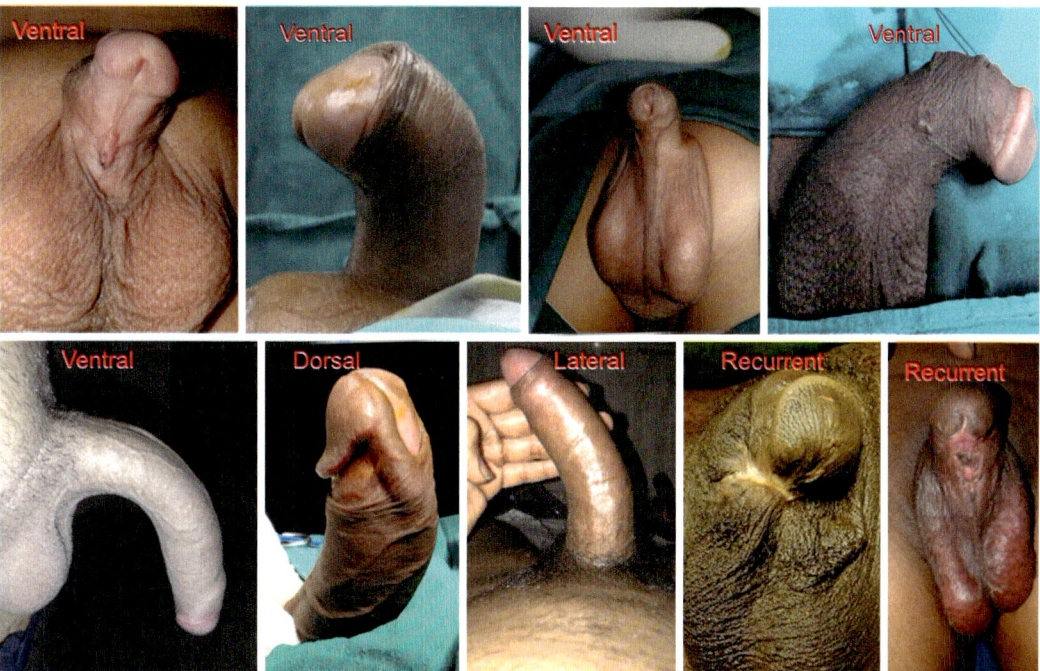

Fig. 6.2 Showing various types of chordee

normal penis to minimize the psychological effects on the child in the future can only be obtained by chordee correction.

6.7 Assessment of Chordee

A preoperative assessment alone cannot assess the degree of the chordee and the methods required for its correction. Apparent bending may improve or resolve after the penile de-gloving. The skin adjacent to the meatus may retract as far as the penoscrotal junction after de-gloving, and it is additional proof of short ventral skin contributing to chordee. A cephalad traction on the glans by stay suture makes the ventral surface taught and palpates the chordee tissue with fingers. Such observations formed the basis for determining ventral curvature until Gittes and McLaughlin described saline corporeal injection in 1974 [8].

6.7.1 Gittes and McLaughlin Test [8]

The saline injection induces penile erection to assess the severity of ventral curvature and document it for successful correction. Artificial erection of the penis by intracavernous saline injection is the most commonly used maneuver for the chordee evaluation and is widely known as Gitte's test. A Goniometer does the exact degree's measurement in a fully erect penis. The main criticisms of the technique is the potential for supra-physiologic or sub-physiologic intra-corporeal pressure at the time of saline injection distorting the findings. In addition, it is difficult to repeat the test after the corporoplasty due to the corporeal leak of saline. Still, this test is followed by most of the surgeons practicing hypospadias surgery.

6.7.2 Vasoactive Drugs

Another technique followed by some pediatric urologists are vasoactive drugs. The drug is injected to induce erection during hypospadias surgery. The main advantage is being a physiologic assessment than erection by saline injection. But the disadvantages are empirical dose regimens in children, long-lasting erection than with saline injection, the requirement of a reversal agent, and increased chances of bleeding due to the prolonged erection. It is observed that all curvature assessments are determined subjectively by visual impression only without direct measurement with a protractor. Kogan induced pharmacological erection by administering 14 micrograms of Alprost intracavernous in 56 boys of 6 months to 13 years of age, and Phenylephrine (40 micrograms.) was given for detumescence [9]. They concluded that the pharmacological erection is effective and reliable, without significant complications. Perovic et al. used the intracorporeal injection of Prostaglandin E1 in a study of 672 patients (a mean age of 5.7 years), in doses ranging from 0.5 to 15 micrograms according to the age, weight and penis size. They found it useful both intra-operative as well as in follow-up visits to check for correction of curvature [10]. The advantage of it is that the effect of PGE1 is based on the inhibition of alpha1-adrenergic activity in penile tissue and its relaxant effect, thus producing physiologic erection, but the disadvantage is the prolonged erection.

6.7.3 Elasto-Sonography

Sono-elastography is a useful imaging technique to evaluate tissue elasticity and is the emerging newer modality for documentation of inelastic tissue in hypospadias repair. The modality allows real-time assessment stiffness of the tissues in a focused area [11]. Standard is yet to be established, but penile ultrasound and strain elastography may become a part of evaluating the hypospadias patient in future research [details in Chap. 29 Role of Imaging in Hypospadias] (Fig. 6.3).

6.8 Correction of Ventral Curvature/Chordee [12–14]

The straight penis is the most important requirement for a successful hypospadias repair, mandating the complete chordee correction. Chordee

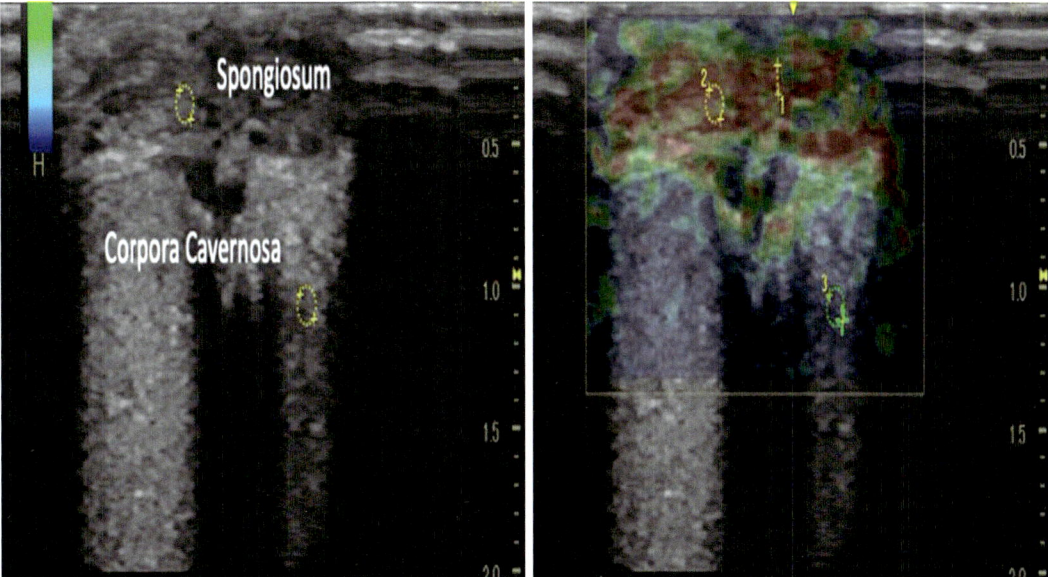

Fig. 6.3 Figure showing tissue stiffness in elasto-sonography

correction must always be checked during hypospadias surgery by doing an artificial erection test (Gitte's test) on the table before proceeding for the urethroplasty. Visual correction may mislead about complete correction. If chordee is not checked and left uncorrected or under corrected, then the residual chordee in adulthood may create sexual problems and needs surgery again, which may be more difficult in the majority. The common methods used to chordee correction are:

1. Penile De-gloving
2. Dorsal Midline Plication and Plication of the Tunica Albuginea
3. Nesbit's Plication, Multiple Parallel Suture Plication
4. Resection of chordee tissue / spongiosum and urethral plate
5. Corporotomies and Corporoplasty by Tunica Vaginalis Free Graft, Dermal Graft
6. Penile Disassembly/ Corporeal Rotation

Among these most commonly used methods are penile de-gloving with/without dorsal plication and transection of the urethral plate irrespective of the etiological factor. The commonest complaint of all hypospadiacs in adulthood is the shortening of the penis. The dorsal plication of the tunica may lead to the penis shortening in severe hypospadias. The chordee correction needs a step-by-step approach taking care of the above-mentioned etiological factors. The step-by-step technique differs in urethral plate preserving procedures, urethral plate transection procedures, and chordee without hypospadias.

6.9 Correction of Curvature Preserving the Urethral Plate [12, 15]

Upadhyay et al. recommended preserving the urethral plate in the modern approach of hypospadias repair [16]. So, the rational approach in hypospadias repair is to preserve the urethral plate, utilize it and add spongioplasty to create a near-normal urethra that is nearer to an ideal replacement of the urethra. The steps described for curvature correction preserving the urethral plate are:

1. De-gloving of penis
2. Urethral plate and corpus spongiosum mobilization up to the corona

3. Urethral plate with spongiosum mobilization into glans
4. Proximal urethral mobilization
5. Tethering tissue resection
6. Midline dissection of corporal bodies and Lateral mobilization of the Buck's fascia
7. Spongioplasty and Glanuloplasty
8. Single stitch Dorsal Plication
9. Superficial corporotomy and Corporoplasty
10. Penile disassembly with or without corporoplasty

6.9.1 Surgical Techniques [12–15]

A stay suture is applied in the glans penis, and the urethra is stented with an infant feeding tube. Assessment of chordee is done with the Gittes test (Fig. 6.4a). After subcutaneous injection of 1 in 1,00,000 solution of adrenaline into the corona, a circumcoronal circumferential incision is given, and de-gloving of the penile skin is done, keeping the level of dissection at the level of Buck's fascia (Fig. 6.4b). Care is taken not to injure the underlying corpora. The Gittes test is then repeated to see the degree of correction achieved (Fig. 6.4c). A plane of dissection created proximal to the divergence of the corpus spongiosum at the level of tunica albuginea and urethral plate with corpus spongiosum is mobilized up to corona (Fig. 6.4d), and Gittes test is repeated to see the chordee correction. If chordee persist, the urethral plate with spongiosum is mobilized into the glans (Fig. 6.4e), and the Gittes test re-assesses the correction (Fig. 6.4f). At this stage, if the visual impression shows the shortening of the spongiosum segment, then the urethra is further mobilized proximally up to the bulbar urethra according to the shortness of the spongiosum segment, and the Gittes test is repeated to confirm the chordee correction. Still, ventral curvature remains uncorrected because of

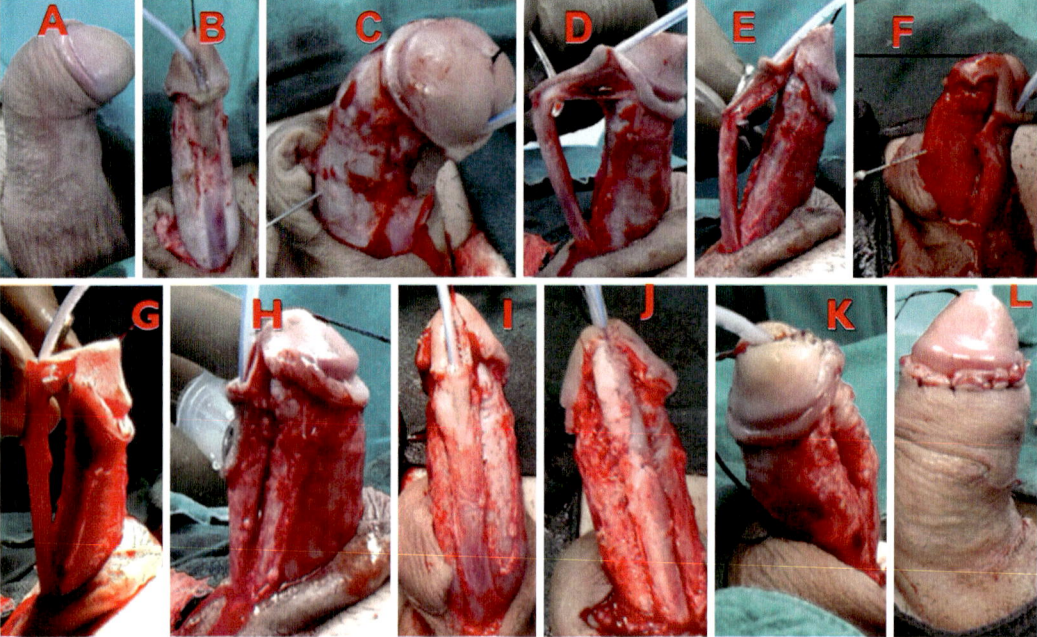

Fig. 6.4 Showing the chordee correction, preserving the urethral plate. (**a**) Coronal hypospadias, Gittes test showing severe curvature. (**b**) De-gloving of the Penile skin. (**c**) Gittes test showing curvature persisting after penile de-gloving. (**d**) Mobilization of the urethral plate with spongiosum up to corona and urethra up to the penoscrotal junction proximally. (**e**) Mobilization of the urethra with spongiosum into glans. (**f**) Gittes test showing minimal chordee. (**g**) Midline dissection of Bucks fascia and lateral mobilization of Buck's Fascia. (**h**) Gittes test showing correction of chordee. (**i**) Showing resection of skin from Hypoplastic urethra. (**j**) Tubularization of urethral plate and Spongioplasty. (**k**) Showing Glanuloplasty and correction of chordee. (**l**) Showing final skin closure

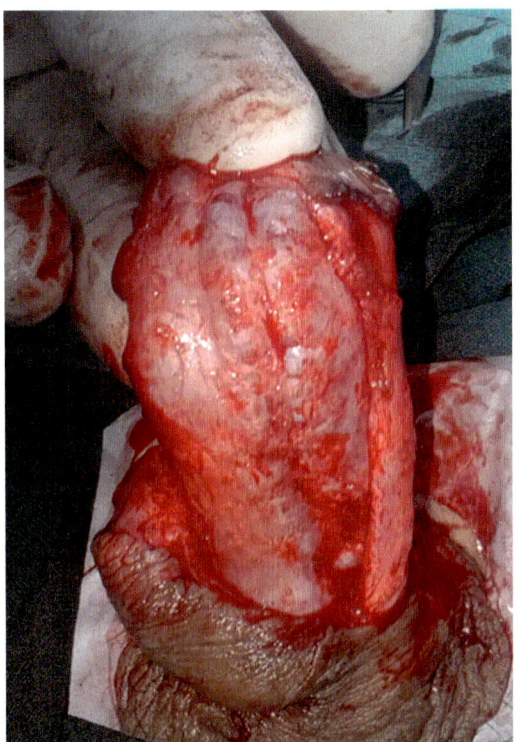

Fig. 6.5 Resection of tethering tissue and midline dissection

tethering tissue attached to the ventral surface, causing the entrapment of ventral corpora. In that case, this tissue is resected to correct the curvature (Fig. 6.5) and midline dissection of the corporal bodies and lateral dissection of Buck's fascia if required (Fig.6.4g). In the next step, a single stitch dorsal midline plication is done at 12 o'clock if chordee persisted of less than 30 degrees and ventral transverse superficial corporotomies / corporoplasty is done if chordee more than 30 degrees. Final chordee correction is confirmed before proceeding for urethroplasty (Fig. 6.4h).

After confirmation of chordee correction, the skin adjacent to the mobilized urethral plate is excised (Fig. 6.4i), and the urethral plate's tubularization is done. Next, Spongioplasty is done by suturing the mobilized divergent (Y-shaped) corpus spongiosum from the normal urethra to the tip of the glans. Suturing the Y-shaped corpus spongiosum to an "I" shape adds length to the spongiosum segment, which helps chordee correction and reconstructs near the normal urethra (Fig. 6.4j). Glansplasty is done by suturing the glanular flaps, reshaping the glans to conical, and bringing the meatus to the tip. Glanuloplasty pushes the urethra distally towards the tip, which eventually helps to correct the glanular chordee (Fig. 6.4k). After that, finally, skin closure is done (Fig. 6.4l). The step-by-step procedure may preserve the urethral plate even in scrotal or perineal hypospadias, and TIPU is feasible in such cases.

6.10 Correction of Curvature in Severe Hypospadias Transecting Urethral Plate [17]

Proximal hypospadias with severe curvature, the poor urethral plate and spongiosum requires transection of urethral plate to correct the curvature. Traditionally, the urethral plate and spongiosum in these patients are resected. However, even in such cases where the urethral plate and spongiosum are responsible for tethering the corporal bodies, the urethral plate and spongiosum are transected at corona and mobilized, and should be preserved & utilized.

The steps for curvature correction preserving the urethral plate are:

1. Penile skin De-gloving.
2. Mobilization of urethral plate and spongiosum just proximal to the meatus after transecting coronal level.
3. Resection of Tethering tissue.
4. Midline Dissection of Corporal bodies.
5. Mobilization of Buck's fascia laterally.
6. Proximal mobilization of urethra.
7. Ventral lengthening procedures.
    a. Superficial Corporotomies.
    b. Corporoplasty by Tunica Vaginalis Free Graft, Dermal Graft.
8. Corporeal rotation/ dorsal plication.
9. Penile disassembly.

6.10.1 Surgical Technique [17]

Though the type of urethroplasty is decided on the table whether to transect the urethral plate or preserve it, but many cases, either the urethral plate are very poorly developed, or the chordee is so severe and looks likely because of short spongiosum segment, (Fig. 6.6a–f) in such cases urethral plate is transected at the corona.

A stay suture is applied into the glans penis, and the urethra is stented with an infant feeding tube. Assessment of chordee is done with the Gittes test. After subcutaneous injection of 1 in 1,00,000 solution of adrenaline, a circumferential circum-coronal incision is given at the corona. And the penile de-gloving is done, keeping the plane of dissection at the level of tunica albuginea, and the urethral plate is transected at corona. Urethral plate and spongiosum are mobilized along with penile de-gloving up to the penoscrotal junction (Fig. 6.7a–c), and Gittes test is done to confirm the chordee correction (Fig. 6.7d). Resection of Buck's fascia and any remained part of the adherent spongiosum is resected to release the corporal bodies (Fig. 6.7e) and Gittes test is repeated to confirm chordee correction (Fig. 6.7f).

This simple maneuver of penile de-gloving along with mobilization of urethral plate and spongiosum corrects chordee many a time (Fig. 6.8a and b). The mobilized urethral plate and spongiosum are preserved for tubularization to add a length to the urethra to go for one-stage repair. Midline dissection of Buck's fascia releases the entrapped corporal bodies to correct the chordee and lateral mobilization of Buck's fascia in the next step if curvature persists and is confirmed with the Gittes test (Figs. 6.7g and h and 6.9a and b).

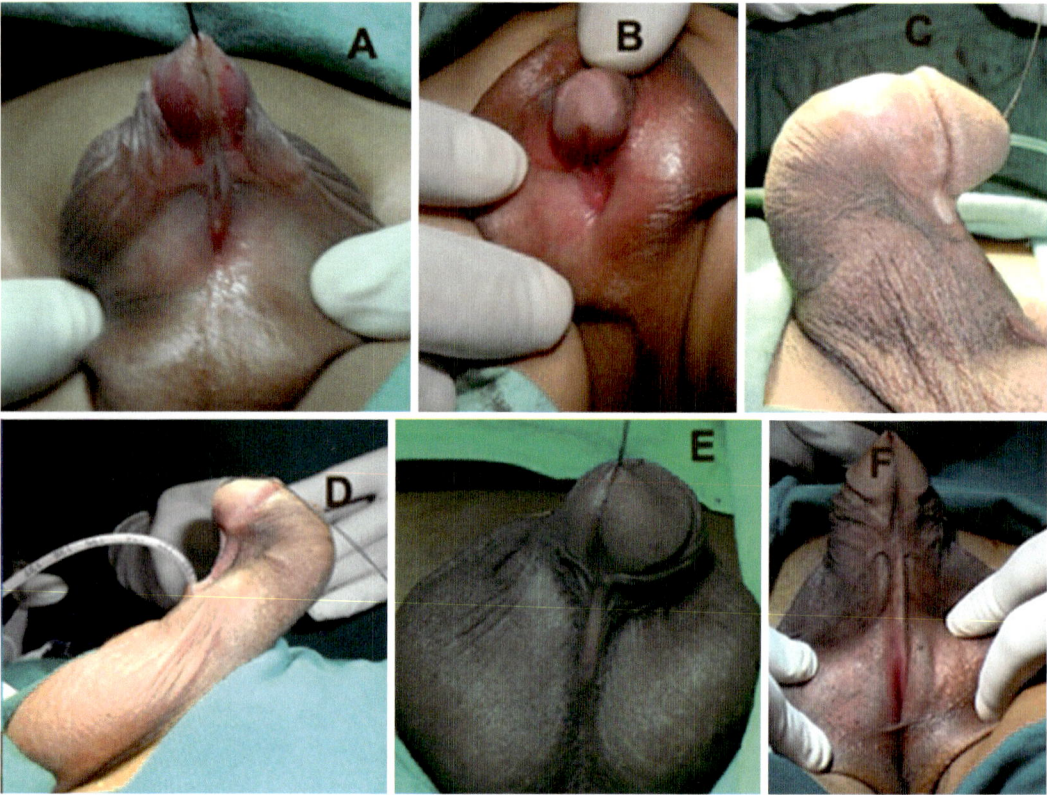

Fig. 6.6 Proximal hypospadias with severe curvature and very narrow urethral plate A&B Scrotal hypospadias with severe chordee in Children C&D Proximal penile hypospadias with severe chordee Adult E&F Scrotal hypospadias with severe chordee adult

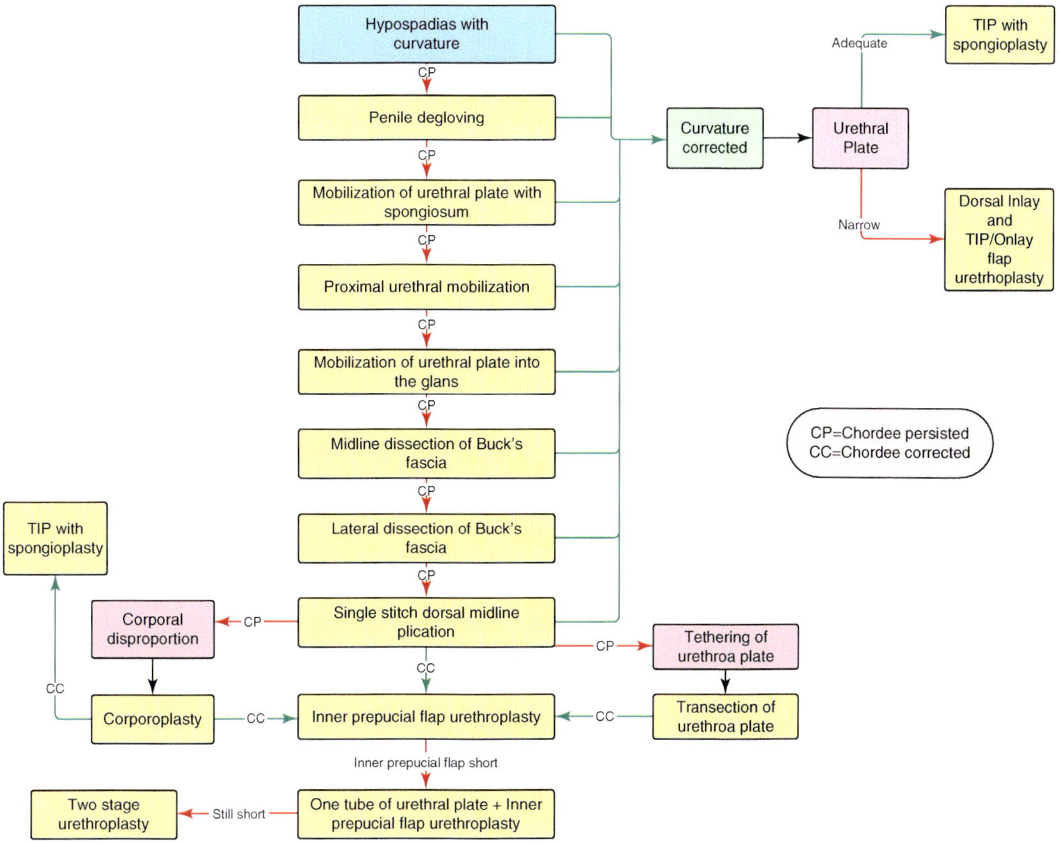

6 Chordee Correction in Hypospadias Repair

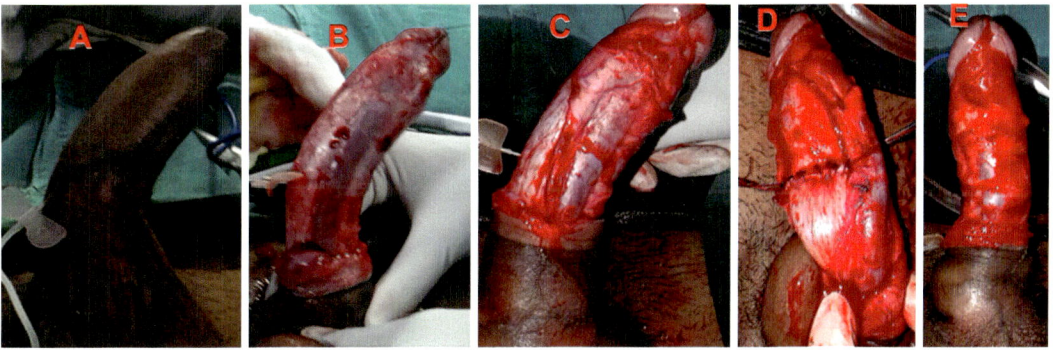

Fig. 6.11 Algorithm for correction of chordee in hypospadias with curvature

Fig 6.12 Correction of lateral chordee without hypospadias. (**a**) Gittes test showing Moderate Lateral Chordee in an adult without hypospadias. (**b**) Penile skin degloving lateral chordee persisting. (**c**) Mobilization of Buck's fascia lateral chordee persisting but reduced. (**d**) Tunica Albuginea Plication. (**e**) Gittes test complete correction of Chordee

the underlying urethra [19]. King (1970) named it "cutaneous chordee" and incorporated it into tubularized urethroplasty [20]. Smith (1955) and others have utilized pedicled preputial skin as an aid to the correction of penile curvature in the two-stage correction of severe hypospadias [21]. Allen and Roehrborn (1993) utilized the same technique for correcting minor penile curvature

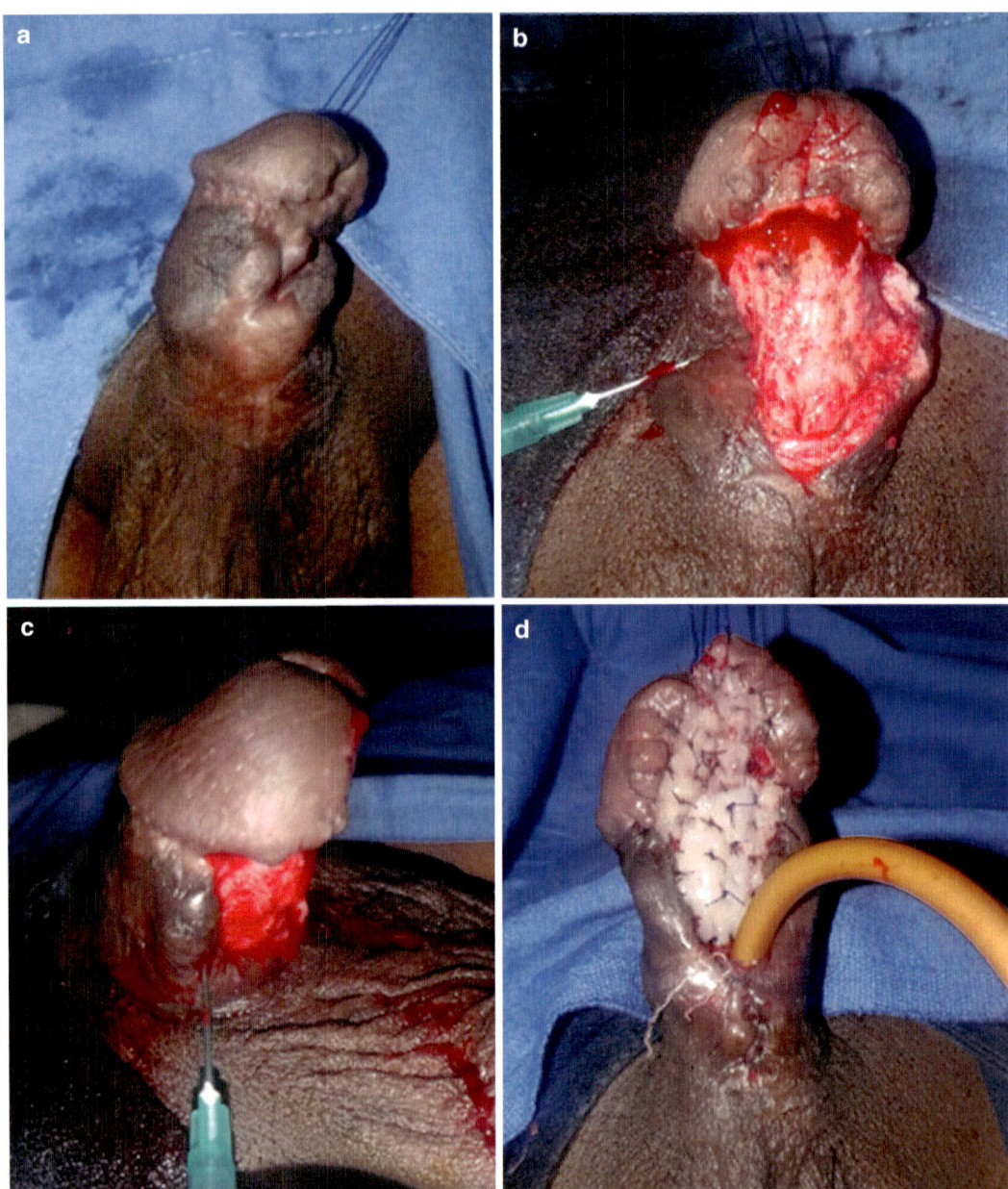

Fig. 6.13 Correction of secondary chordee in reoperative case. (**a**) Fistula with chordee. (**b** and **c**). Gittes test showing chordee correction after Partial penile degloving and resection of chordee tissue. (**d**) Buccal Mucosal graft

in Chordee without hypospadias [22]. Penile degloving itself releases the ventral shortening in more than 50% of cases. Weber (2014) et al. reported a satisfactory correction of ventral curvature with complete penile de-gloving in 77%, 29.5%, and 2% ($p < 0.001$) with mild, moderate, and severe chordee with hypospadias, respectively [23].

6.13.2 Urethral Plate and Spongiosum Mobilization

Urethral plate and spongiosum mobilization is done along with penile de-gloving to correct the curvature. If the dissection level is kept at the tunica albuginea level, the curvature of the skin and hypoplastic spongiosum will be corrected

6 Chordee Correction in Hypospadias Repair

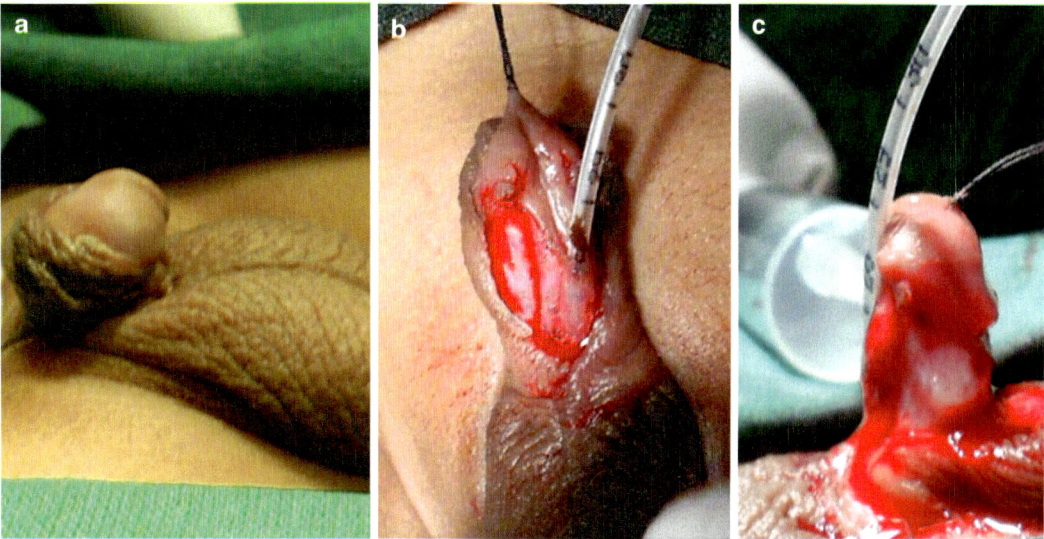

Fig. 6.14 Correction of curvature by mobilization technique. (**a**) Penoscrotal hypospadias with curvature, (**b**) Partial Penile de-gloving and Mobilization of urethral plate, (**c**) Gittes test showing chordee correction

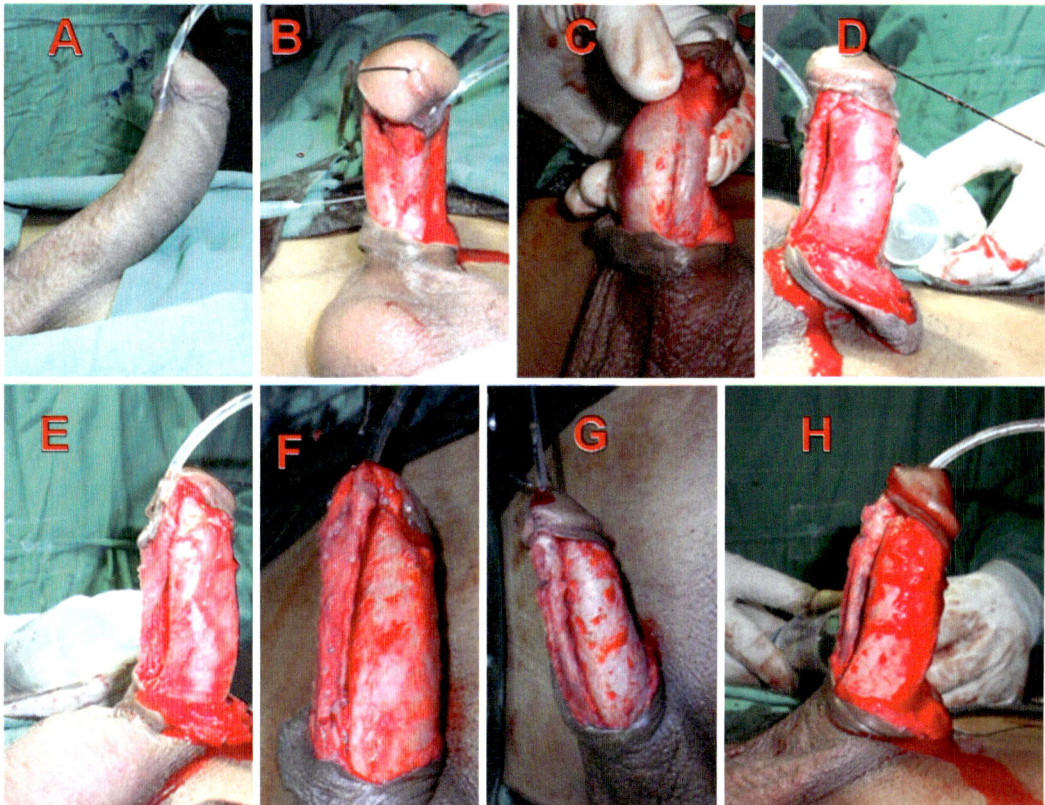

Fig. 6.15 Steps of the mobilization technique in distal hypospadias with severe chordee. (**a**) Distal penile hypospadias with severe chordee. (**b**) Chordee persisting after Penile skin de-gloving. (**c**) Mobilization of urethral plate and spongiosum. D. Gittes test showing partial chordee correction. (**e**) Gittes' test showing the chordee correction after mobilization of urethral plate and spongiosum into glans. (**f**) Tubularization of urethral plate. (**g**) Spongioplasty and Glanuloplasty. (**h**) Gittes test confirms chordee correction after spongioplasty and glanuloplasty

Table 6.1 The steps of chordee correction and etiological factor corrected

Surgical step	Factor corrected
Penile de-gloving	Skin, Dartos and Buck's Fascia
Mobilization of spongiosum	Spongiosum
Resection of chordee tissue, Midline dissection, and lateral dissection	Buck's fascia
Spongioplasty and Glansplasty	Spongiosum
Dorsal plication/ Superficial corporotomy/ Corporoplasty	Dorsoventral corporeal disproportion

[12, 18]. Mollard and Costagnola used the urethral plate's mobilization for chordee correction, and they mobilized it from meatus to corona. They added dorsal plication to fix the chordee and preserve the urethral plate as the urethral plate mobilization alone did not correct the chordee [24]. According to patient age, the urethral plate and corpus spongiosum mobilization add the urethral length of 2 to 3.5 cm, which helps in chordee correction in the short corpus spongiosum segment. Adequate mobilization of glanular flaps and the urethral plate and corpus spongiosum mobilization into the glans corrects the glanular chordee. The bulbar artery blood supply to the urethral plate and urethra is preserved since the urethral plate is mobilized with corpus spongiosum. Both proximal and distal ends remain intact, maintaining the continuity of the corpus spongiosum. Care is taken not to damage the corpus spongiosum or cavernosum, which may hamper the blood supply. The urethral plate and the corpus spongiosum mobilization facilitates the urethral plate tubularization without incision, provided the width of the urethral plate is adequate [25]. Bhat A (2007) could correct the chordee in 88% of the cases by the urethral plate with the corpus spongiosum and the proximal urethral mobilization preserving the urethral plate, and tubularization urethral plate was done. It was feasible to tubularize without incising the urethral plate in 35% of cases [9]. The urethral plate with spongiosum and proximal urethral mobilization up to the bulbar region corrects the curvature in STAG repair. The same principle is used by Snodgrass and Bush during the first stage for chordee correction in proximal hypospadias with severe curvature. Snodgrass et al. reported in 50% of patients with proximal hypospadias, chordee correction was possible by degloving, and dartos dissection and a chordee of less than 30 degrees were easily corrected single midline dorsal plication. The other 50% had a chordee greater than 30 degrees. Still, with mobilization of the corpus spongiosum wings, the urethral plate and, as needed, the normal proximal urethra, combined with ventral corpora incisions described above, it was possible to correct the chordee and preserve the urethral plate in 50% of these. Thus, in 75% of patients with proximal hypospadias with chordee, the urethral plate could be preserved for tubularization to perform the TIPU. The plate transaction was done to correct the chordee followed by a two-stage graft procedure in the remaining 25 % of cases [6].

6.13.3 Spongioplasty and Glanuloplasty

Fanning out spongiosum on the ventral surface and its attachment on corpora's ventral surface may cause shortening of the ventral surface. Mobilization of the spongiosum makes the ventral surface of corpora free, which corrects the curvature. Spongioplasty with Y to I technique increases the length of the spongiosum segment, which helps in the correction of chordee (Fig. 6.16a). Glansplasty, after well mobilized glanular wing, reconstructs the normal-looking glans and corrects the glanular chordee (Figs. 6.16b, 6.15g and h, and 6.17a and b). Modifications of Dodat et al. and Bhat et al. in spongioplasty have the added advantages; help improve the chordee correction, more rounded appearance of the glans, and reduce fistula chances [26, 27].

6.13.4 Separation of Corporal Bodies

Urethral is encircled in the two Buck's Fascia layers, superficial and deep. The deep layer is attached to the midline septum, and its shortening is responsible for the ventral chordee. So, midline dissection of corporal bodies in the avascular

6 Chordee Correction in Hypospadias Repair

Table 6.2 Incidence of chordee & the steps of chordee correction

Type of hypospadias	No of cases (%)	No of cases with curvature (%)	Penile degloving	Urethral plate & spongiosum mobilization	Proximal urethral mobilization	Dorsal plication	Transection of urethral plate	Superficial corporotomies	Mobilization Back's fascia in midline &/laterally
Anterior	41 (35.65%)	21 (51.22%)							
Coronal Distal penile	11 30	12 (57.14%); Moderate 07 (33.33%); Severe 02 (09.52%)	8 (39%)	9 (42%)	4 (19%)	Nil	Nil		
Middle	42 (36.52%)	27 (64.29%); Mild 15 (55.55%); Moderate 07 (25.93%); Severe 05 (18.52%)	7 (25.92%)	12 (44.44%)	6 (22.22%)	2 (7.40%)	Nil		2 (7.40%)
Proximal	32 (27.83%)	32 (100%)							
Proximal penile	19	Mild 02 (06.25%); Moderate 13 (40.63%); Severe 17 (53.13%)	2 (6.25%)	5 (15.625%)	2 (6.25%)	16 (50%)	2 (6.25%)	3 + 2 (15.625%)	
Penoscrotal	6								
Scrotal	4								
Perineo-Scrotal	3								
	Total 115	Total 80 (69.56%); Mild 29 (36.25%); Moderate 27 (33.75%); Severe 24 (30%)	17 (21.75%)	21 (26.25%)	15 (18.75%)	4 (5%)	16 (20%)	2 (2.5%)	7 (8.75%)

Fig. 6.16 (**a**) Y-I Spongioplasty, (**b**) Glanuloplasty

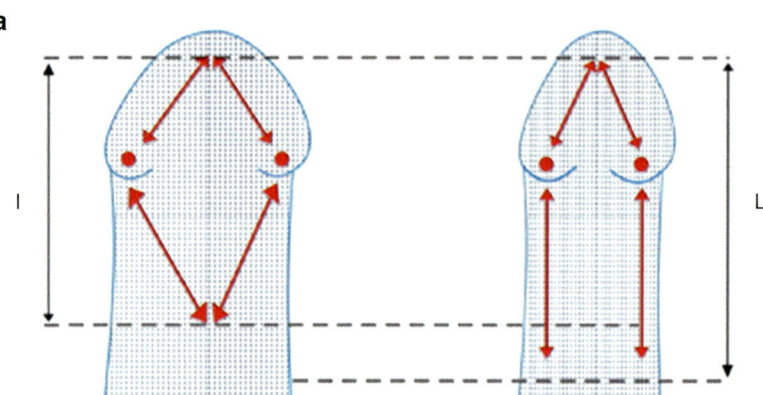

Y – I Spongioplasty I-L Increased length

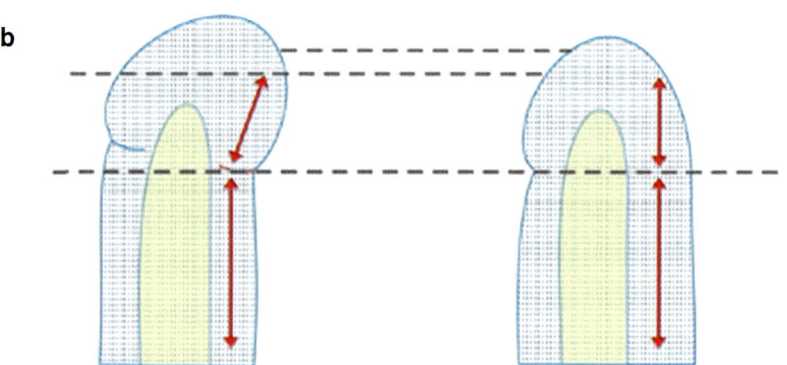

Glanuloplasty correcting glanular Chordee

plane and lateral mobilization of Buck's fascia will release the ventral entrapment and correct the ventral curvature (Fig. 6.18a–f). The same principle was applied in corporal separation and split and roll techniques to fix chordee with minimal complication without shortening the penis. The Shaeer used the same principle to free the corporal bodies by midline dissection as a corporal rotation technique to correct severe curvature without shortening the penis [28].

6.13.5 Lateral Mobilization of Buck's Fascia

Attachment of Bucks fascia to midline and shortening on the ventral surface. Lateral mobilization will release the ventral surface of the corporal bodies and helps in the correction of curvature. This step, along with the penile de-gloving, mobilization of the spongiosum with the urethral plate and proximal urethra, corrects the curvature (Fig. 6.19a–c). The same principle is used to release the ventral corporal entrapment by incision or corporal separation and split and roll technique to correct chordee with minimal complication without shortening the penis [29].

6.14 Other Methods Used for Chordee Correction

6.14.1 Heineke-Mikulicz Principle

Heineke-Mikulicz principle of transverse incision and suturing the same longitudinally increases the length and is used in gut, corpora, and skin. Lengthening of the tunica albuginea

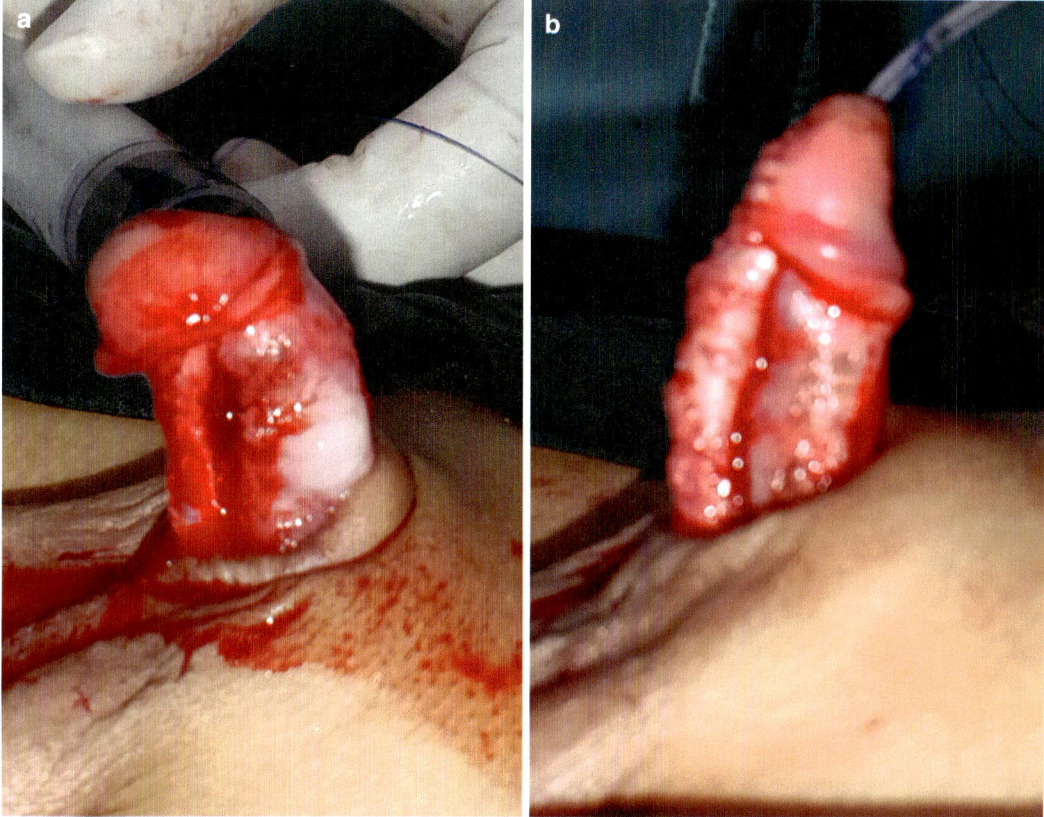

Fig. 6.17 (a) Gittes test showing chordee persisting after penile gloving and mobilization of the urethral plate. (b) Chordee corrected after glansplasty and spongioplasty

the shorter concave surface was done by Udall (1980) using the Heineke-Mikulicz principle to correct the chordee [30]. Saalfeld et al. (1973) used a similar technique of incising the tunica transversely at multiple places and sutured them longitudinally to increase the shorter concave surface of the penis [31]. Perovic et al. (1998) used the principle by multiple parallel plicating sutures in the midline opposite the maximal curvature site to correct the chordee. This technique does not require neurovascular bundle mobilization and is the preferred technique for treating penile curvature [32, 33].

6.14.2 Dorsal Plicating Techniques

Dorsal plication to shorten the convex surface is commonly used after penile de-gloving without evaluating the etiological factor. Various procedures are Nesbit's technique, Plication of Tunica Albuginea, Midline Plication dorsally, and Parallel Multiple Plications [34–36].

Nesbit (1965) described the shortening of the longer dorsal surface by excising the elliptical segments of tunica albuginea and then suturing it on the dorsal aspect of the penis to correct curvature [34]. Baskin and Duckett (1994) reported plication of Tunica albuginea for correction of ventral curvature. The neurovascular bundle is dissected from the surface of both corpora cavernosa after penile de-gloving. Two parallel incisions are given approximately 1.0 cm long at the distance of 0.5 to 1.0 cm on the tunica albuginea's anterior-lateral surface, directly opposite the point of maximal penile curvature bilaterally. Application of the tourniquet helps to decrease bleeding and optimizes visualization. The outer edges of incised tunica are sutured with interrupted suture and inverting the knots burring the intervening strip of tunica albuginea [36].

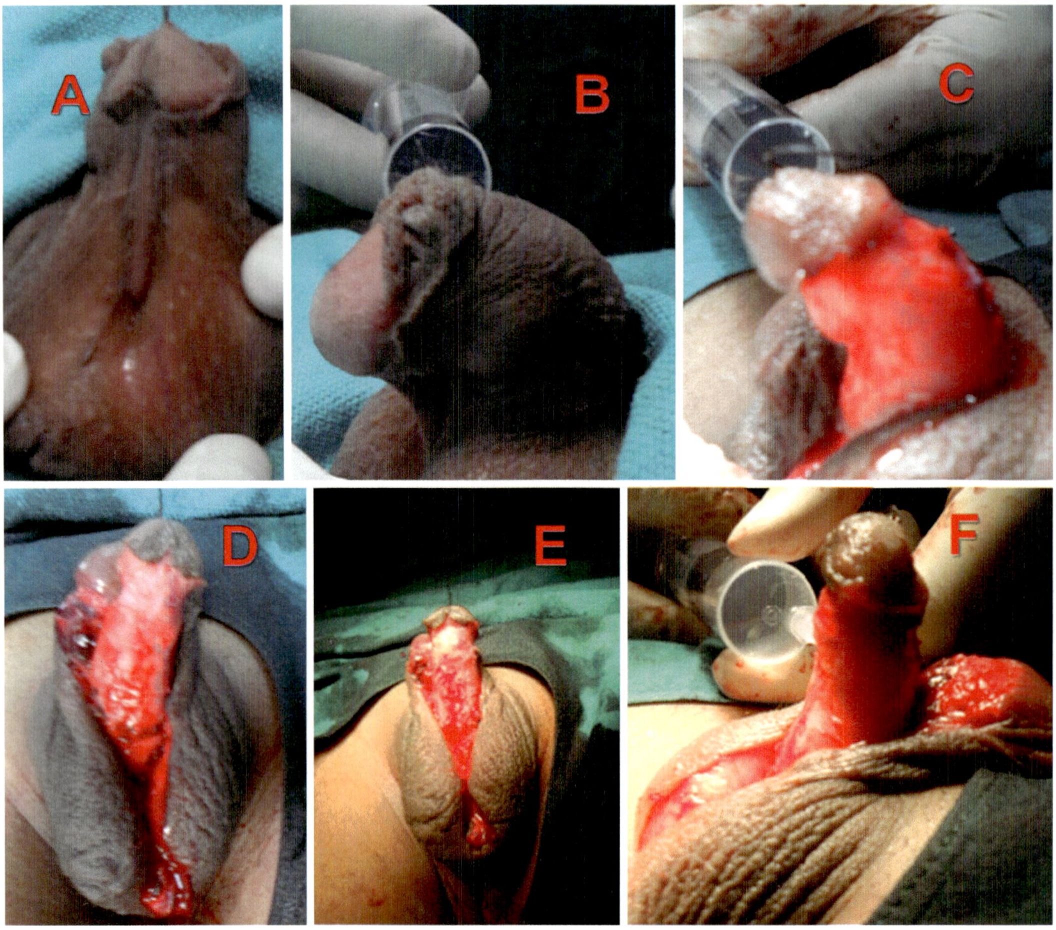

Fig. 6.18 The correction of curvature in severe hypospadias. (**a**) Scrotal hypospadias with poor urethral plate, (**b**) Gittes test showing severe chordee, (**c**) Penile skin degloving and Gittes test showing persistence of Chordee, (**d** and **e**). Resection of tethering tissue and midline dissection of corpora, (**f**) Gittes test showing correction of chordee

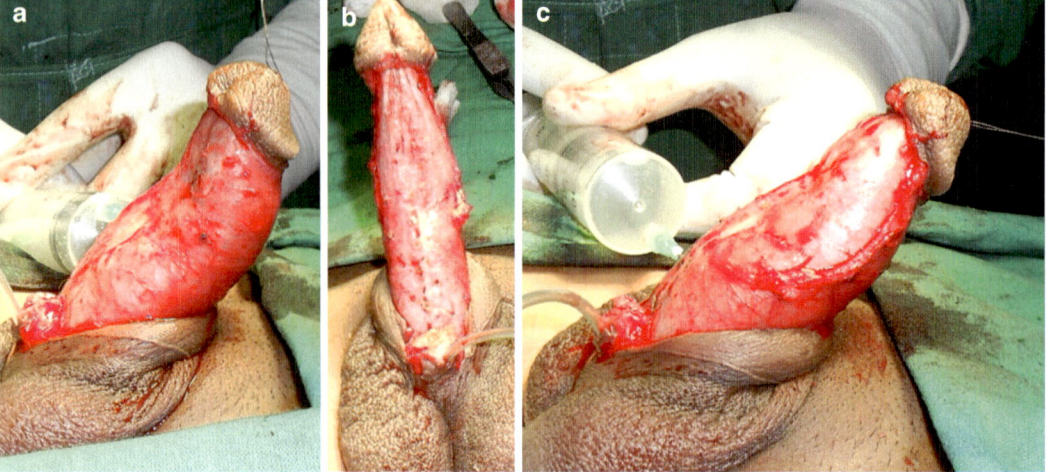

Fig. 6.19 Correction of chordee with midline and lateral dissection of Buck's fascia. (**a**) Gittes test showing persistence of chordee after penile de-gloving and resection of tethering tissue. (**b**) Lateral dissection of the Buck's fascia. (**c**) Gittes test showing complete correction of chordee

Dorsal midline plication is done by giving a 5–10 mm long longitudinal incision in the tunica albuginea in the dorsal midline and approximating the edges transversely to correct the ventral curvature. Chertin et al. (2004) reported long-term satisfactory results of dorsal plication without penile shortening/recurrence of chordee in a median follow-up of 6 years [37], and dorsal plication is the most commonly used technique for chordee correction of minor degree.

6.14.2.1 Dorsal Multiple Plications

The multiple dorsal plications have also been used by many who advocate the plication procedure as the first line for chordee correction. Wang X (2018) reported 16-64-dot plication multiple dorsal plications in correcting Donnahoo type III chordee in a post-pubertal patient with good and long-standing arthroplasty [38].

The commonest complaint of hypospadiac patients is the short penis. The plication procedures are applicable only in mild chordee as correction of moderate to severe chordee will lead to penile shortening. Another critical factor in dorsal plication procedures is that this approach is against the anatomical principles of surgery. The technique deals with the normal dorsal surface incising it, leading to fibrosis, making that pathological. Rather than dealing with the embryological abnormal ventral surface, the normal dorsal surface goes against the anatomical principles of surgery. Besides, there are chances of nerve injury leading to penile pain, numbness to the penile shaft and glans, and sometimes impotence and recurrent curvature. So, preference in mild curvature (up to 30 degrees) persist after mobilization should be the single stitch dorsal plication.

6.14.3 Corporal Rotation

Koff and Eakins (1984) first described in 1984 ventral penile curvature correction by midline longitudinal incision and corporal rotation in hypospadias. Midline corporal incision releases the midline entrapment of the corporal bodies. The medial rotation and fixing the dorsal aspect of the corpora cavernosa change the corporal bodies' direction and correct the ventral curvature [39]. Snow (1989) and Kass (1993) added sutures into the dorsal lateral corpus cavernosum and ventral midline incision in the corpora cavernosa to rotate the corpora. Placing the sutures without mobilization of a neurovascular bundle is subject to the risk of compression injury caused by these sutures [40, 41]. Decter (1999) used the same principle to release corporal bodies by a midline incision and corporal rotation with neurovascular mobilization for chordee correction in severe hypospadias. The midline incision and freeing of the neurovascular bundles on the dorsal aspect of the corpora cavernosa facilitate medial rotation of the dorsal part of the corpora. Nonabsorbable sutures are placed at the maximal convex curvature area from the dorsolateral aspect of one corpus cavernosum across the midline to the other side in such a way that the corpora are rotated toward the dorsal midline [29]. The separation of corpora and split and roll technique can be used to correct chordee with minimal complication without shortening the penis and increases the performing single-stage hypospadias reconstruction with plate preservation procedures. Shaeer has used the corporal rotation technique to correct severe curvature up to 90 degrees without shortening the penis [28].

6.14.4 Superficial Corporotomy

The most significant disadvantage of the dorsal shortening procedures is the shortening of the penis, the commonest complaint of the hypospadiacs. So, the ventral lengthening procedures should be preferred, and the method used is superficial corporotomies and corporoplasty stepwise. Due to dorsoventral corporal disproportion, mild to moderate curvature is amenable to superficial corporotomies by incising tunica albuginea's superficial layer at the maximum curvature. Multiple superficial corporotomy (fairy cuts) can be made into the tunica albuginea from 4 to 8 O'clock, exposing erectile spongy tissue. It is technically easy without the need for grafts. These corporotomies are covered by mobilized urethral plate and spongiosum in the first stage of STAG repair. The disadvantages are mild bleeding, and sometimes there may be fibrosis on healing the corporotomies, causing the recurrence of chordee [42, 43].

6.14.5 Corporoplasty:

6.14.5.1 Small Intestinal Submucosa

Severe curvature may require corporoplasty. Various tissues used are skin graft, tunica albuginea flaps, and grafts and single layer SIS graft. Small intestinal submucosa (SIS) is an acellular collagen-based material derived from the porcine small intestine used as an interposition graft for severe penile curvature. Though the three- and single-layer results are similar, single-layer SIS appears to have an advantage over multilayer SIS, most likely secondary to one-layer SIS's ability to regenerate and revascularize. Leslie et al. in 2008 used corporoplasty with dermal graft, tunica albuginea, and 1ply SIS for correction of curvature in severe cases of hypospadias with promising results [44]. Miguel et al. in 2011 used SIS for corporoplasty in hypospadias. They found that corporal body grafting with 1 ply SIS is viable for correcting severe chordee associated with penoscrotal/ perineal hypospadias and penile corporal body disproportion without compromising penile length. Single-layer SIS is a material with reliable results, easy availability, no donor site-associated morbidity, and no reported graft-related complications [45].

The single-layer material is used by most of the proponent's small intestine mucosa, and a few use the four-layer small intestine submucosa. This can be used in both urethral preservation and urethral plate transection procedures.

6.14.5.2 Dermal Graft [46]

Ventral lengthening is the preferred procedure for the short phallus with severe ventral penile curvature preventing further shortening. The dermal graft is commonly used for corporoplasty, and the dermal graft is harvested from the groin, a non-hair-bearing area. After the Gittes test, the corporotomy incision is given on the ventral surface at the maximal curvature (concavity) identified site to straighten the penis and required graft length is measured. The donor site is marked in the elliptical shape slightly longer than the required length after transverse linear corporotomy. The graft is prepared by sharp dissection, defatted, and preserved in saline. The dermal graft is the suture to the margins of the incised corpora with a simple running suture of 5-6/0 polyglactin. Penile erection is done to see the major leak and apply suture to seal it if any [46].

6.14.5.3 Tunica Vaginalis Graft

Perlmutter and colleagues (1985) described the utility of the tunica vaginalis free graft for corporoplasty to repair severe curvature. On follow-up, only one patient had "some degree" of ventral angulation ranging from 2 to 37 months [47]. Kajbafzadeh et al. (2007) used tunica vaginalis-free graft for correction chordee in 18 proximal hypospadias patients with severe chordee. The urethral plate could be preserved in thirteen patients for single-stage urethroplasty [48]. Braga et al. (2007) reported a success rate of up to 95% following the tunica vaginalis graft in the short term. They had a higher recurrence of curvature with Dural graft than the Tunica vaginalis graft and opined that tunica vaginalis graft repair is a better option for correcting the ventral curvature [49].

6.14.6 Penile Disassembly with or Without Corporoplasty

Ventral curvature is due to the entrapment of corporal bodies. Penile disassembly will separate both corporal bodies and spongiosum segment. This will free all the three components (two corporal and one spongiosum) from the coverings and attachments and correct the chordee if it is due to the penis' coverings. But if there is the dorsoventral disproportion of corporal bodies, then corporoplasty will be required. Perovic (1998) described the penile disassembly technique and concluded that this is the most effective procedure for selecting severe hypospadias with severe chordee, severe glans tilt, and a small penis chordee as corporoplasty adds length to the penis. Penile disassembly with extensive urethral mobilization restored the hypospadiac meatus to normal without the need for urethroplasty to reconstruct neo-urethra and increased the penile length [31]. This technique is rarely used. Most chordee cases can be corrected with penile de-gloving, urethral plate with spongiosal mobilization, proximal urethral mobilization, midline and lateral mobilization of Buck's fascia, and dorsal plication tunica without shortening the penis.

6.15 Conclusions

The step-by-step approach of chordee correction deals with the chordee's causative factor preserving spongiosum as per surgery's anatomical principles. The spongiosum can be utilized as a healthy tissue cover to prevent the fistula. Mobilization helps in the ventral lengthening of the penis. Even if dorsal tunica plication is required after mobilization, the length needed will be less, again preserving the length of the penis. Thus, it helps in preventing penile shortening, which is the commonest complaint post hypospadias surgery. Ventral lengthening procedures, corporotomy and corporoplasty, are better than dorsal shortening procedures. The common grafts used are skin, tunica vaginalis, and intestinal mucosa. Penile disassembly is rarely required.

References

1. Snodgrass W. A farewell to chordee. J Urol. 2007;178(3):753–4.
2. Baskin LS, Duckett JW, Lue TF. Penile curvature. Urology. 1996;48:347–56.
3. Kaplan GW, Lamm DL. Embryogenesis of chordee. J Urol. 1980;114:769–72.
4. Bhat A, Bhat M, Kumar V, Kumar R, Mittal R, Saksena G. Comparison of variables affecting the surgical outcomes of tubularized incised plate urethroplasty in adult and pediatric hypospadias. J Pediatr Urol. 2016;12(108):101–8.
5. Snodgrass W, Macedo A, Hoebeke P, Mouriquand PDE. Hypospadias dilemmas: a round table discussion. J Paed Urol. 2011;7:145–57.
6. Stojanovic B, Bizic M, Majstorovic M, Kjovic V, Djordjevic M. Penile curvature incidence in hypospadias: can it be determined? Adv Urol. 2011:813205. https://doi.org/10.1155/2011/813205.
7. Menon V, Breyer B, Copp HL, Baskin L, Disandro M, Schlomer BJ. Do adult men with untreated ventral penile curvature have adverse outcomes? J Pediatr Urol. 2016;12:31.e31–31.e317. https://doi.org/10.1016/j.jpurol.2015.09.009.
8. Gittes R. Injection technique to induce penile erection. Urology. 1974;4:473–4.
9. Kogan BA. Intraoperative pharmacological erection as an aid to pediatric hypospadias repair. J Urol. 2000;164:2058–61.
10. Perovic S, Djordjevic M, Djakovic N. Natural erection induced by prostaglandin-E1 in the diagnosis and treatment of congenital penile anomalies. Brit J Urol. 1997;79(1):43–6.
11. Camoglio FS, Bruno C, Zambaldo S, Zampieri N. Hypospadias anatomy: elastosonographic evaluation of the normal and hypospadic penis. J Pediatr Urol. 2016 Aug 1;12(4):199–e1.
12. Bhat A. Extended urethral mobilization in incised plate urethroplasty for severe hypospadias: a variation in technique to improve chordee correction. J Urol. 2007;178(3):1031–5.
13. Bhat A, Sabharwal K, Bhat M, Singla M, Kumar V, Upadhyay R. Correction of penile torsion and chordee by mobilization of the urethra with spongiosum in chordee without hypospadias. J Pediatr Urol. 2014;10:1238–43.
14. Bhat A, Bhat MP, Saxena G. Correction of penile torsion by mobilization of urethral plate and urethra. J Pediatr Urol. 2009;5(6):451–7.
15. Bhat A, Gandhi A, Saxena G, Choudhary GR. Preputial reconstruction and tubularized incised plate urethroplasty in proximal hypospadias with ventral penile curvature. Indian J Urol. 2010;26(4):507.
16. Upadhyay J, Shekarriz B, Khoury AE. Midshaft hypospadias. Urol Clin. 2002;29:299–310.
17. Bhat A, Bhat M, Sabharwal K, Kumar R. Bhat's modifications of Glassberg–Duckett repair to reduce complications in management severe hypospadias with curvature. Afr J Urol. 2017;23(2):94–9.
18. Bhat A, Saxena G, Abrol N. A new algorithm for management of chordee without hypospadias based on the mobilization of the urethra. J Pediatr Urol. 2008;4:43–50.
19. Allen TD, Spence HM. The surgical treatment of coronal hypospadias and related problems. J. Urol. 1968;100(4):504–8.
20. King L. Cutaneous chordee and its implications in hypospadias repair. Urol Clin North Am. 198(8):397–402.
21. Smith DR. Surgical treatment of hypospadias. J Urol. 1955;73(2):329–34.
22. Allen TD, Roehrborn CG. Pedicled preputial patch in the repair of minor penile chordee with or without hypospadias. Urology. 1993;42(1):63–5.
23. Weber BA, Braga LH, Patel P, Salle JL, Bägli DJ, Khoury AE, Lorenzo AJ. Impact of penile degloving and proximal ventral dissection on curvature correction in children with proximal hypospadias. Can Urol Assoc J. 2014;8:424.

24. Mollard P, Castagnola C. Hypospadias: the release of chordee without dividing the urethral plate and onlay island flap (92 cases). J Urol. 1994;152:1238–40.
25. Bhat A, Singla M, Bhat M, Sabharwal K, Upadhaya R, Kumara V. Incised plate urethroplasty in perineal and perineo-scrotal hypospadias. Afric J Urol. 2015;21:105–10.
26. Dodat H, Landry JL, Szwarc C, Culem S, Murat FJ, Dubois R. Spongioplasty and separation of the corpora cavernosa for hypospadias repair. Brit J Urol Int. 2003;91(6):528–31.
27. Bhat A, Singla M, Bhat M, Sabharwal K, Kumar V, Upadhayay R, Saran RK. Comparison of results of TIPU repair for hypospadias with "spongioplasty alone" and "spongioplasty with dorsal dartos flap". Open J Urol. 2014;2014
28. Shaeer O. Shaeer's corporal rotation for length-preserving correction of penile curvature: modifications and 3-year experience. J Sex Med. 2008 Nov;5(11):2716–24.
29. Decter RM. Chordee correction by corporal rotation: the split and roll technique. J Urol. 1999;162:1152–15.
30. Udall DA. Correction of 3 types of congenital curvatures of the penis, including the first reported dorsal curvature case. J Urol. 1980;124(1):50–2.
31. Saalfeld J, Ehrlich RM, Gross JM, Kaufman JJ. Congenital curvature of the penis: successful results with variations in corporoplasty. J Urol. 1973;109:64–5.
32. Perovic SV, Djordjevic ML, Djakovic NG. A new approach to the treatment of penile curvature. J Urol. 1998;160:1123–7.
33. Baskin LS, Erol A, Li YW, Cunha GR. Anatomical studies of hypospadias. J Urol. 1998;160:1108–15.
34. Nesbit RM. Congenital curvature of the phallus: report of three cases with description of corrective operation. J Urol. 1965;93(2):230–2.
35. Baskin LS, Duckett JW. Dorsal tunica albuginea plication for hypospadias curvature. J Urol. 1994;151(6):1668–71.
36. Mingin G, Baskin LS. Management of chordee in children and young adults. Urol Clin. 2002;29(2):277–84.
37. Cheritin B, Koulikov D, Fridman A, Farkas A. Dorsal tunica albuginea plication to correct congenital and acquired penile curvature: a long-term follow-up. BJU Int. 2004;93:379–81.
38. Wang X, Mao Y, Chen S, Tang Y, Quin D, Liu M, Chen Y. Multiple dorsal midline plication (MDMP) for correction of Donnahoo type III chordee in post-pubertal patient. Chinese J Urol. 2018;12:42–4.
39. Koff SA, Eakins M. The treatment of penile chordee using corporeal rotation. J Urol. 1984;131(5):931.
40. Snow BW. Transverse corporeal plication for persistent chordee. Urology. 1989;34:360–1.
41. Kass EJ. Dorsal corporeal rotation: an alternative technique for the management of severe chordee. J Urol. 1993;150:635–6.
42. Snodgrass W, Bush N. Tubularized incised plate proximal hypospadias repair: continued evolution and extended applications. J Pediatr Urol. 2011;7(1):2–9. https://doi.org/10.1016/j.jpurol.2010.05.011.
43. Snodgrass W, Bush N. Staged tubularized autograft repair for primary proximal hypospadias with 30-degree or greater ventral curvature. J Urol. 2017;198:680–6.
44. Leslie JA, Cain MP, Kaefer M, Meldrum KK, Misseri R, Rink RC. Corporeal grafting for severe hypospadias: a single institution experience with 3 techniques. J Urol. 2008;180(4):1749–52.
45. Miguel C, Rafael G, Joshi D, Yuval B-Y, Andrew L. Ventral corporal body grafting for correcting severe penile curvature associated with single or two-stage hypospadias repair. J Pediatr Urol. 2011;7:289–93.
46. Devine CJ, Horton CE. Use of the dermal graft to correct chordee. J Urol. 1975;113:56–8.
47. Perlmutter AD, Montgomery BT, Steinhardt GF. Tunica vaginalis free graft for the correction of chordee. J Urol. 1985;134(2):311–3.
48. Kajbafzadeh A-M, Arshadi H, Payabvash S, Salmasi AH, Najjaran-Tousi V, ARA S. Proximal hypospadias with severe chordee: single-stage repair using corporeal tunica vaginalis free graft. J Urol. 2007;178(3):1036–42.
49. Braga LP, Sallae JLP, Dave S, Bagli DJ, Lorenz AJ, Khoury AE. Outcome analysis of severe chordee correction using tunica vaginalis as a flap in boys with proximal hypospadias. J Urol. 2007;178:1693–7.

Management of Distal and Mid-Penile Hypospadias

Ujwal Kumar, Vikash Singh, and Amilal Bhat

7.1 Introduction

Hypospadias is the most common congenital anomalies of male external genitalia where urethra opens on the ventral aspect of the penis with or without penile curvature [1]. Based on the external urethral meatus location has been classified as distal, mid and proximal hypospadias. Distal variants are found in the majority (70%-85%) and are usually associated with no or mild ventral curvature [2–4]. Deviation of urinary stream and poor cosmetic appearances are usually the only problem with these variants. Proximal hypospadias is less common (10%–25%) still, surgically challenging [5]. But this classification system does not consider the severity of ventral curvature, glans size and quality of the urethral plate and penile skin proximal to external meatus are important for surgical planning. A new scoring system considering the quality of glans and urethral plate, location of the meatus and penile curvature (GMS score) has been proposed to define the severity of hypospadias and hence, surgical complexity as chances of complications [6, 7]. Hundreds of surgical techniques had been described in the literature to manage hypospadias, but the appropriate selection of a surgical procedure in a particular case is important. Most of the surgical techniques are described for distal and proximal variants. Mid-penile hypospadias is managed by one of these techniques.

7.2 Preoperative Assessment

A thorough history and physical examination are of utmost importance [8, 9]. Detailed family history, including hypospadias in father or sibling, should be documented. History of previous hypospadias surgery or circumcision must be ascertained, as it plays a crucial role in surgical planning.

In an examination, the patient should be examined for penile length, location and size of the external urethral meatus, hooded prepuce, quality of glans and urethral plate, the severity of ventral

U. Kumar
Department of Urology, IMS, BHU,
Varanasi, Uttar Pradesh, India

V. Singh
Maa Rajwati Hospital Pvt Ltd,
Varanasi, Uttar Pradesh, India

A. Bhat (✉)
Bhat's Hypospadias and Reconstructive Urology Hospital and Research Centre,
Jaipur, Rajasthan, India

Department of Urology, Jaipur National University Institute for Medical Sciences and Research Centre,
Jaipur, Rajasthan, India

Department of Urology, Dr. S.N. Medical College,
Jodhpur, Rajasthan, India

Department of Urology, S.P. Medical College,
Bikaner, Rajasthan, India

P.G. Committee Medical Council of India,
New Delhi, India

Academic and Research Council of RUHS,
Jaipur, Rajasthan, India

curvature or glans tilt, quality of skin proximal to the meatus, degree of associated spongiosal hypoplasia, penile deviation (rotation) and scrotal transposition. Chordee is best assessed intra-operatively. Testicular descend should be documented as undescended testis may be associated with the disorder of sexual dysfunction.

7.3 Timing of Surgery

Six to 18 months is the ideal age, as advised by the American Academy of Physicians to avoid behavioural problem and psychological stress [5, 10]. If this milestone is missed, the patient can be operated on whenever they come to the hospital.

7.4 Preoperative Androgen Therapy

At present, there is not much evidence to support preoperative androgen use (Testosterone, HCG) [11, 12]. Several reports suggest negative impacts of testosterone on wound healing and have found increased intraoperative bleeding [13, 14]. Significant variations in terms of the androgen used, dosage and evaluation of results or hypospadias outcomes have been reported [15]. Details of it are described in Chap. 5 General considerations.

7.5 Aim of Surgical Correction

Hypospadias repair aims to make the penis normal or near-normal for voiding and sexual activities. Penile cosmesis is also an important aspect. The external urethral meatus should be vertically slit-shaped and at the tip of the conical glans and a straight penis.

7.6 Principles of Surgery

Out of so many surgical techniques, selecting a surgical procedure for a particular case is very important. The principle of surgery is almost similar for all patients regardless of the surgical technique, and these are:

1. Orthoplasty (correction of ventral curvature)
2. Urethroplasty including glanuloplasty and meatoplasty
3. Vascularized coverage over neo-urethra
4. Circumcision or prepucioplasty

7.6.1 Correction of Ventral Curvature (Orthoplasty)

Ventral curvature is better assessed intraoperatively after penile degloving. Artificial erection test described by Gittes and McLaughlin in 1974 revolutionized the assessment, hence, correction of penile curvature [16]. The severity of penile curvature has traditionally been divided into mild (<30 degrees), moderate (30–45 degrees) and severe (45 degrees).

A step-by-step approach is preferred, the steps are penile degloving, mobilization of urethral plate, spongiosum and urethra, single stitch dorsal plication, superficial corporotomy and corporoplasty [17, 18]. Details of chordee correction are described in Chap. 6 chordee correction. Ventral lengthening procedures are preferred in severe chordee to avoid shortening of the penis. Various options available are mobilization of the urethral plate and urethra, multiple superficial incisions into the ventral aspect of corpora cavernosa, Multiple full-thickness corporotomies through the ventral corpora from 4 to 8 o'clock without grafting and single full-thickness ventral corporotomy from 3 to 9 o'clock followed by grafting [19, 20]. Usually, dermal grafts are used from non-hair-bearing areas of the body. Multiple studies showed good long-term results with ventral lengthening procedures [21, 22].

7.6.2 Urethroplasty Techniques

Advancement Procedures
- Meatal Advancement and Glanuloplasty Procedure (MAGPI)
- Urethral mobilization and Advancement Procedure (UAP)
- Meatal Mobilization technique (MEMO)
- GUD (Glandar Urethral Disassembly)

Tubularization of the Urethral Plate
- Thiersch-Duplay technique
- Glanular Approximation Procedure (GAP)
- Glanular-Frenular Collar (GFC) technique
- TIP procedure (Tubularized Incised Plate)
- Augmented Urethral plate tubularization G-TIP
- Tubularized Reconstructed Plate Urethroplasty (TRPU)

Augmentation of the Urethral Plate
- Meatal-based flap techniques
- Slit-Like Adjusted Mathieu (SLAM)
- Transverse preputial island flap

Replacement of the Urethral Plate
- Tubularization of TPIF (Asopa I, II, and Duckett tube).
- Koyanagi repair and its modifications.
- Double-faced tubularized inner prepucial flap urethroplasty.
- Two-stage urethroplasty with an initial preputial graft placement/ Buccal mucosa, Byars flap followed by a second-stage tubularization after six months.

7.7 Meatal Advancement and Glanuloplasty Procedure (MAGPI)

MAGPI repair was first described by Duckett et al. in 1981 for distal hypospadias repair [23]. Before introducing Duckett's MAGPI procedure, distal hypospadias was usually not repaired due to fear of surgical complications. The variants that decide the appropriateness of MAGPI are based upon the meatus' location and size, quality of parameatal skin and glans configuration [24]. This procedure was mainly used for glandular, coronal and mildly sub-coronal hypospadias with minimal or no ventral curvature or glans tilt. Meatus proximal to this usually gives poor results. Meatus size should not be very wide, which hampers adequate lateral mobilization and glanuloplasty. Narrow meatus is not a problem with MAGPI as Heineke-Mikulicz closure makes the meatus wide. If there is stenotic meatus, extend the vertical incision well into the meatus.

Parameatal tissue should be thick and pliable to be easily elevated off the overlying urethra to advance distally. This elevation will make the conical glans. The glans should be wide enough to allow wrapping of elevated urethra ventrally. This will prevent fistula and meatal retraction.

Duckett et al. and other proponents reported excellent results of this surgery in properly selected patients [24–26]. They gave the reason for poor results by opponents [27–29] because of an appropriate case selection rather than the original description. Duckett in his original series of 1111 cases, reported 5 fistulas (0.45%), 7 meatal retraction (0.6%), 1 residual chordee (0.09%) and overall, 1.2% patients needed re-surgery [24]. No meatal stenosis was recorded. Since the introduction of this technique in 1981, various modifications have been proposed to minimize the complications [24, 30–32]. Duckett modified the glans closure from single layer to two-layer to minimize gland dehiscence and meatal retraction [24]. Somoza et al. removed a triangular segment of glanular tissue distal to the meatus. Dorsal and lateral urethral sides were dissected leads to urethral advancement without any tension. Glans was approximated above this ventral urethral wall. They reported no complications in a series of 20 patients by this modification [30]. Arap proposed the MAGPI procedure for more proximal cases. The ventral meatal edge held at two places about 7–10 mm apart makes 'M' configuration. The middle 'V' of the 'M' was closed to make a urethral extension, and this was covered by glandular approximation [32]. Though the MAGPI procedure is an outpatient & simple technique but is not very widely used due to its relatively poor cosmetic results and meatal retrusion [33].

7.8 Urethral Mobilization and Advancement

Beck first described urethral advancement for hypospadias repair in 1898, but his technique was not consistently successful [34]. Belman (1977) presented his experience of urethral mobilization and advancement technique for distal hypospadias with good results [35]. This technique is used for glanular, coronal and subcoronal hypospadias with or without chordee. Atala described this procedure for mid-penile hypospadias with acceptable complications and excellent cosmetic outcomes [36]. Advantage of this technique over MAGPI is the glans' excellent cosmetic appearance. Here, meatus, along with distal urethra, is mobilized proximally off the underlying corpora. The proximal extent of urethral mobilization depends on hypospadiac meatus's distance to glans tip or future meatus. The ratio of urethral mobilization length and hypospadiac meatus to future meatus length is usually 3-5:1 in different series (Fig. 7.1a–c) [36–38]. Adequate urethral mobilization avoids meatal retraction and ventral curvature.

This Technique's basic principle is to use the urethral elasticity and excellent/extensive urethral blood supply. After penile degloving, external urethral meatus is circumscribed and mobilized proximally. Glans wings should be dissected widely to avoid meatal stenosis (Fig. 7.2a, b). The mobilized urethra is then anastomosed dorsally at glans tip with interrupted 7/0 PDS, and ventrally glans wings are closed over urethra in two layers (Fig. 7.2c). Since the urethra is already intact, there is no need for any vascularized coverage and chances of urethrocutaneous fistula is nil [37]. Use of magnification and meticulous urethral mobilization is necessary to decrease the urethral injury, spongiosclerosis and stricture. In conclusion, this mobilization and advancement procedure is an excellent option for distal variants with excellent cosmetic outcomes and minimal complications.

7.9 Meatal Mobilization Technique (MEMO)

A modification of UAP is published with minimal mobilization called meatal mobilization(MEMO) technique. The technique is feasible only in cases with an appropriately mobile urethra. The meatus is incised circumferentially starting laterally on both sides of the meatus. Dorsally it is dissected up to the corporal bodies. Along with this plane dissection, the meatus is dissected 1 to 1.5 cm proximally. The length of mobilization depends upon the mobility of the urethra, but dissection should not be done too far proximally to avoid the curvature and fistula. Glanular wings are mobilized adequately for tension-free closure, and glanuloplasty is done (Fig. 7.3a, b). Seibold J et al. (2010) reported the results in 46 boys of the MEMO technique with a success rate of 97% No urethral stricture or urethrocutaneous

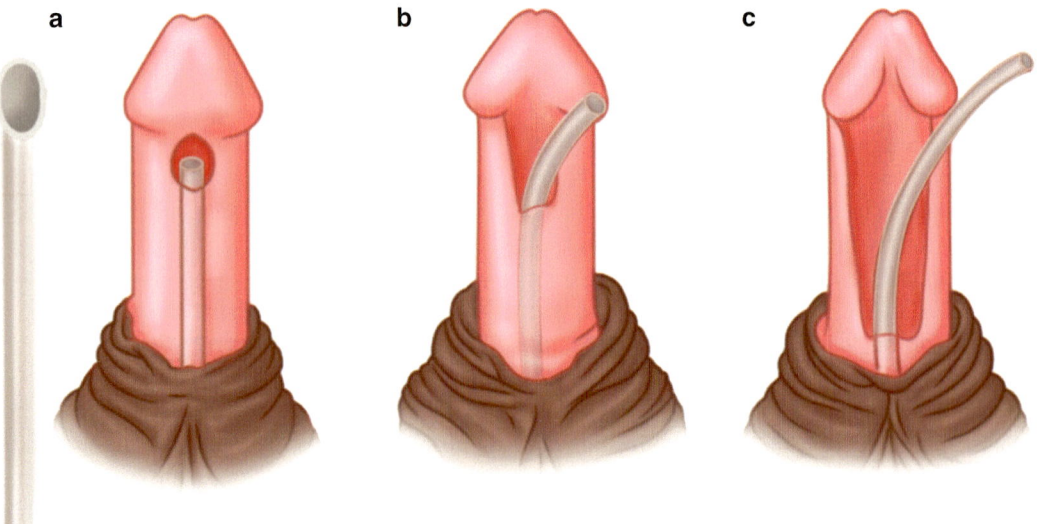

Fig. 7.1 Urethral mobilization. (**a**) Distal penile hypospadias. (**b**) Partial mobilization of urethra. (**c**) Proximal urethral mobilization

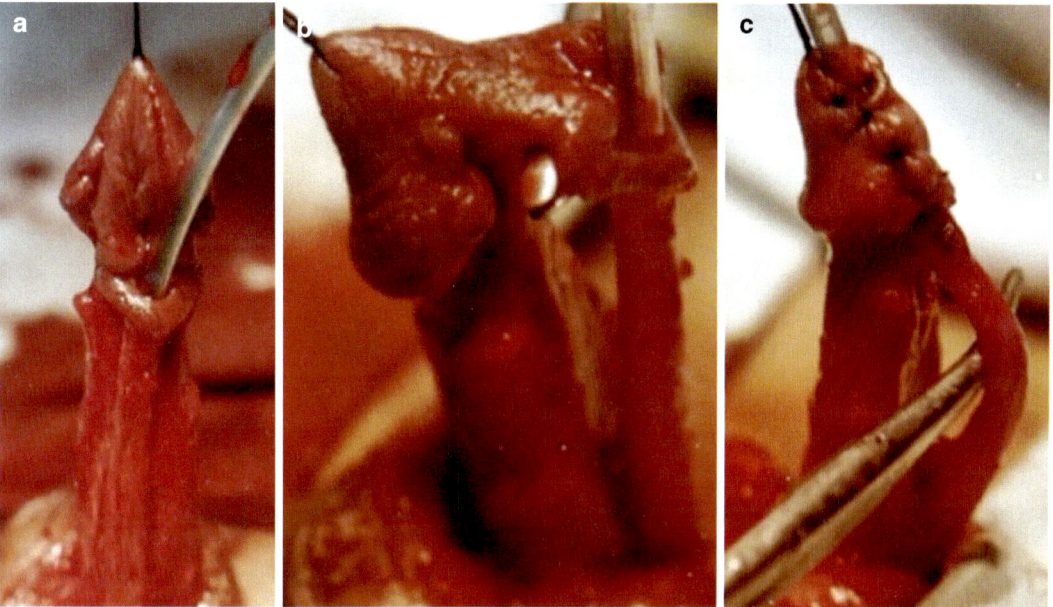

Fig. 7.2 Urethral mobilization. (**a**) Penile de-gloving in distal penile hypospadias. (**b**) Partial mobilization of the urethra and urethral plate. (**c**) Urethroplasty and glanuloplasty

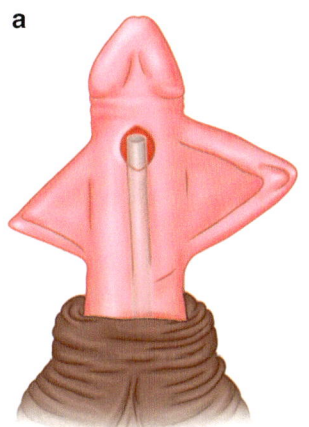 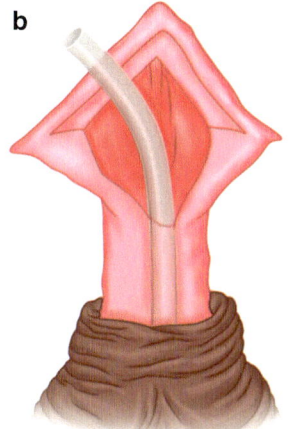

Fig. 7.3 Meatal mobilization technique. (**a**) Sub-coronal hypospadias. (**b**) Meatal mobilization and raising the glanular wing

fistula was seen. Only one meatal retraction (3%) occurred in the short term. The final decision of the MEMO technique's feasibility can only be made after degloving of the penile skin. The ventral aspect of the urethra should not be too flimsy, and the urethra should be mobile enough [33].

7.10 GUD (Glandar Urethral Disassembly) [39]

The technique combines urethral mobilization technique and penile disassembly. The extensive mobilization of glanular wing for partial glanular disassembly allows the mobilized distal urethra to bring at the tip and cosmetically better glans after glansplasty.

Technique A sub-coronal circumferential incision is given, and penile degloving is done. This exposes the Y-shaped spongiosum and distal urethra. A tourniquet is applied to prevent the bleeding during mobilization of glans wings and spongiosum The Buck's fascia is incised lateral to the spongiosal pillar on both sides of the urethra spongiosum is released from the corpora and mobilized. The spongiosum is mobilized in the same plane of dissection up to the tip of the glans. The glanular wing is mobilized extensively to do the partial glanular disassembly keeping the urethral plate attached to the glans. After partial disassembly of the glans, the urethra can be easily lifted cranially and can be repositioned distally by two interrupted anchors 5.0 vicryl sutures, one on each side. Both glandular wings can embrace the distal repositioned urethra, and the glans will show a conical conformation. The urethra is sutured to the glans by 6.0 PDS sutures. The mobilized spongiosal pillar is sutured over the urethral in the midline to complete the spongioplasty. A dorsal dartos flap designed from inner foreskin is rotated to cover the entire urethra whenever necessary. Finally, the glans' lateral borders are brought together over the urethra with subcutaneous/ subepithelial 5.0 PDS sutures to complete the glans reconstruction. A urethral stent is positioned to be kept for 5–7 days. Macedo et al. reported 7.01% complications, consisting of fistulas (5.3%) and glans dehiscence (5.3%) since two patients had both complications in a mean in a mean follow up of 7 months [39]. Though the technique aimed to prevent the fistula without urethroplasty, the authors had the fistula in 5.3%. The causes of the fistula may be damage of hypoplastic urethra during mobilization or compromise to the blood supply of the distal urethra.

7.11 Thiersch-Duplay Technique

Professor C. Thiersch in 1869, reported tubularization of the urethral plate in a child with an epispadias [40]. He designed the flaps and the lateral incisions so that the urethral suture lines are unopposed. Duplay in 1874, described tubularization of the urethral plate distal to the urethral orifice [41]. He was able to provide the first successful hypospadias repair with this technique in five cases. Stock and Hanna reported the largest series of Thiersch-Duplay repair [42]. They combined the Heineke-Mikulicz meatoplasty to widen the meatus along with tubularization of the urethra. Earlier this technique was used for hypospadias with meatus at or just proximal to coronal sulcus. Later on, it was extended for more proximal cases with mild (<30°) or no chordee. Patients with moderate to severe chordee (>30°) are not fit for this technique.

The surgery starts with 5/0 silk stay suture at the glans dorsal the future meatus. Heineke-Mikulicz closure is done at 12 o' clock for stenotic meatus with interrupted 7-0 polyglycolic suture over 8-F feeding tube in the urethra. For thin and hypoplastic perimeatal skin, an incision is made ventrally until healthy skin is seen and the skin edges are then approximated with interrupted 7-0 polyglycolic sutures. Dorsally, laterally and ventrally around the meatus, a sub-coronal incision is given followed by penile degloving with a width of the urethral plate being 12 mm, leaving 2 mm of skin around the meatus. Subcuticular 7-0 polydioxanone suture (PDS) continuously is used to tubularize the urethral plate over the catheter. The skin over the glans is approximated with horizontal mattress interrupted 7-0 polyglycolic sutures. Among 512 children operated by Stock and Hanna [42] reported the complication rate of only 2.1%. Urethrocutaneous fistula and stricture were the most common complications. Vascularized coverage over neo-urethra by dartos flap from the dorsal penile skin reduces the incidence of urethrocutaneous fistula.

7.12 Glans Approximation Procedure (GAP)

Zaontz described a modified glanuloplasty, glans approximation procedure (GAP) to repair glanular and coronal hypospadias with a wide and deep glans groove. This repair was based on the Thiersch-Duplay technique. Functional and cosmetic results were excellent and among 24 children operated only one case developed a distal fistula [43]. Details of the technique are described in Chap. 17 Management of Mega Meatus Intact Prepuce. We prefer tubularized urethral plate urethroplasty in cases of distal hypospadias with wide urethral meatus.

7.13 Tubularized Incised Plate (TIP) Procedure

Tubularization of the urethral plate is the most commonly utilized repair for distal hypospadias without curvature. TIPU is the modification of the Thiersch Duplay technique; the addition of the dimension of relaxing incision in the urethral plate by Snodgrass (1994). Tubularized incised plate urethroplasty warrants a wide and healthy urethral plate and a minimal ventral curvature. Almost all distal hypospadias cases can be dealt with TIP repair [44–46], middle hypospadias with mild curvature and curvature can be corrected with step-by-step procedures preserving the urethral plate.

Surgical Technique After determining the glans width, the dorsal prepuce corners are held, and the incision line is marked. The incision is about 2 mm below the meatus or more proximal on the ventral side depending on the availability of underlying dartos and corpus spongiosum

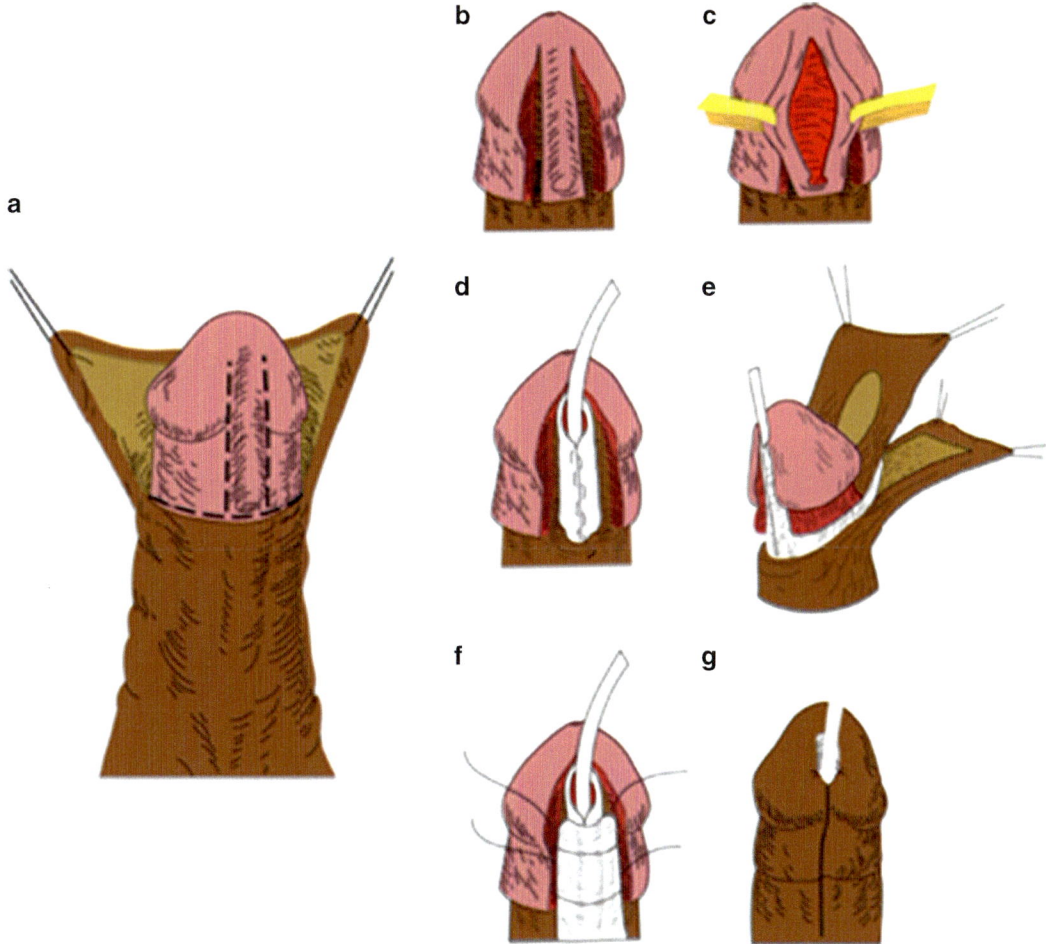

Fig. 7.4 Tubularized urethral plate urethroplasty. (**a**) Marking the incision. (**b**) Dissection of urethral plate. (**c**) Incising the urethral plate. (**d**) Tubularization of the urethral plate. (**e**) Raising the Dartos flap. (**f**) Dartos cover over neo-urethra. (**g**) Glansplasty and Skin closure

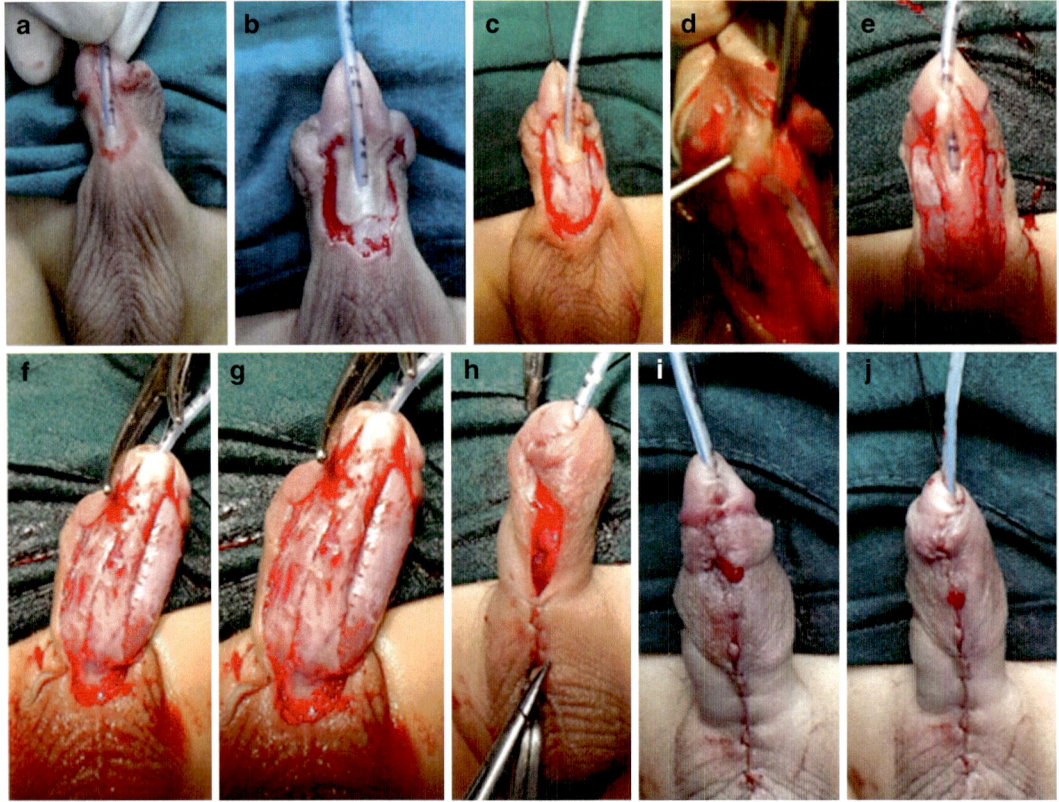

Fig. 7.5 Incised urethral plate urethroplasty in mid hypospadias with preputioplasty. (**a**) Mid-penile hypospadias; (**b**) U-shaped incision; (**c**) Partial penile degloving; (**d**) Mobilization of urethral plate and spongiosum and Incising the urethral plate; (**e**) First suture to create the meatus; (**f**) Tubularization of urethral plate; (**g**) Spongioplasty (**h**, **i**, and **j**) Glansplasty and prepucioplasty

(Figs. 7.4a, 7.5a and 7.6d). Penile de-gloving is done in two different planes, ventrally under the shaft skin and dorsally along the Buck fascia up to the penopubic and penoscrotal junctions. After applying a tourniquet at the base of the penis, the junctions of the glans wings to the urethral plate are marked, and 1:100,000 epinephrine is injected along the marking and an incision is given. Dissection is continued down to the corpora's surface and then laterally on each side to approximately 3 and 9 o'clock (Figs. 7.4b and 7.5b, c). For tension on glans wings approximation or if glans width is less than 14 mm, additional extended dissection is done at 3 and 9 o'clock, further releasing the wings for a distance of approximately 4 mm distally. The incision is given in midline within the meatus down to the surface of the underlying corpora (Figs. 7.4c and 7.5d). A 6-Fr urethral stent is passed into the bladder and is tied to the glans traction suture. Tubularization of the urethral plate is done in two subepithelial layers using 7-0 polyglactin (Fig. 7.4d). The stitch starts distally approximately 3 mm below the plate's end to create an oval neo-meatal opening to avoid iatrogenic meatal stenosis (Fig. 7.5e). Continuous suturing is done proximally to the meatus, and then the same suture is continued distally for the second layer (Fig. 7.5f, g). After raising a ventral dartos flap Fig. 7.4e and splitting it into two longitudinal segments whenever possible, it is crossed over the neo-urethra to provide double-layered coverage. Neo-urethra is covered by dorsal dartos Fig. 7.4f. Glansplasty is completed using 6-0 polyglactin.

Subepithelial interrupted stitches. The remaining ventral shaft skin attached to the inner prepuce is then excised, and the collar is sutured using 7-0 polyglactin interrupted sub-epithelial

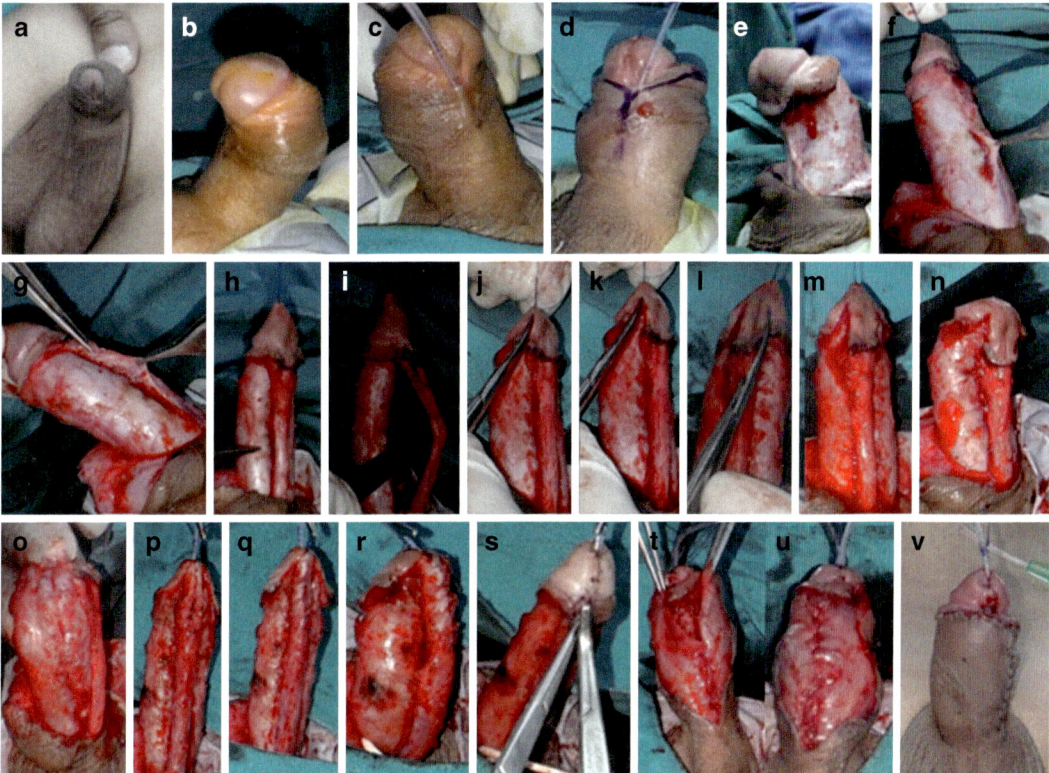

Fig. 7.6 Incised urethral plate urethroplasty in distal hypospadias with Moderate curvature. (**a**) Distal penile hypospadias; (**b**) Gittes test showing moderate chordee; (**c**) Hypoplastic urethra up to mid-penis; (**d**) Marking the incision; (**e**) Penile degloving and chordee persist; (**f**) Creation of Dissection plane proximal to hypoplastic urethra; (**g, h, i**) Mobilization of the urethral plate with spongiosum; (**j, k, l, m**). Mobilization of a urethral plate into glans; (**n**) Gittes test sowing persistence of chordee; (**o**) Resection of tethering tissue and midline dissection of corpora; (**p**) Tubularization of urethral plate; (**q**) Spongioplasty; (**r**) Gittes test Chordee corrected; (**s**) Glauloplasty; (**t, u**). Dartosorraphy (**v**) Skin closure

stitches Fig. 7.4g. The median raphe is made by closure of the ventral midline skin and the skin laterally on either side is excised. Prepucioplasty is added if parents want a reconstruction of the foreskin (Fig. 7.5h–j).

In cases with curvature, the curvature is corrected by mobilization of the urethral plate, and spongiosum Fig. 7.6e–o or with dorsal plication and TIPU is done Fig. 7.6p–v.

Post-operative cosmesis following TIP repair was found superior (Fig. 7.7a, b) to other procedures including Mathieu and onlay flap repairs [47]. TIP repair complications are more in proximal (4-33%) cases than in distal cases (2.5%). Most common complications are urethrocutaneous fistula and meatal stenosis while neo-urethral strictures are rare [44].

7.14 G-TIP Urethroplasty

The patients with narrow urethral plate simple tubularization may not always be suitable. The principle relied on is that there is the epithelization/granulation of the raw dorsal urethra, but the mechanism of healing the incised plate still remains to be decided. A school of thought favours a complete re-epithelization with urothelium while others think that the healing is by granulation tissue and fibrosis later on in that area. Worse outcomes in narrow urethral plates have been reported. The healing of a larger incised raw area of neo-urethra is unpredictable and may exert tension on the ventral suture line affecting its primary healing. To overcome this shortcoming and to improve healing of the neo-

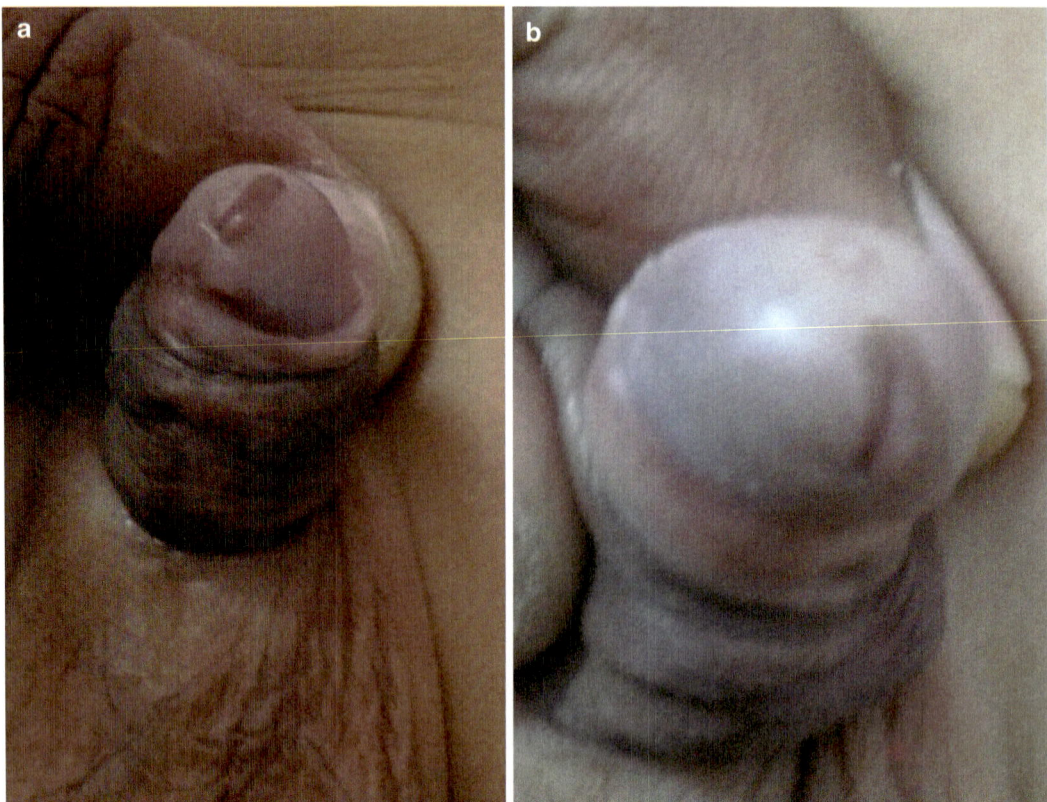

Fig. 7.7 (**a** and **b**) Post-operative after TIPU repair almost normal looking meatus and glans with the well-retracted prepuce

urethra grafting of the dorsal incised (GTIP) area using the inner prepuce (Fig. 7.8a, b) has been described by several authors. We put dorsal inlay when the deep incision is required to tubularize the urethral plate and cover with single or dorsal double dartos cover (Fig. 7.9a–h). Objective criteria to decide about the narrow urethral plate and dorsal inlay graft were suggested by Abbass & Pippi Salle (2018). They measured the ratio of the urethra before and after an incision to help decide to graft or not the incised plate. The urethral plate should be maximally stretched and measured at its widest point. It is then deeply incised to the corpora. The same measurements are repeated, therefore producing a urethral plate ratio before and after incision. If the ratio is less than 0.5, these cases should be grafted (Fig. 7.10) [Urethral plate ratio = width of urethral / width of urethral plate after incision = < 0.5] [48].

Limit of grafting first was considered to fill the defect up to mid-glans and ensure healing without stenosis. More recently, proponents report incising into glans just beyond the urethral plate and then grafting to better position the meatus at the tip. G-TIP is an option for most patients with distal hypospadias narrow urethral plate, but the disadvantage being it is not possible to do prepucioplasty. No comparative study has demonstrated a significant difference in urethroplasty outcomes between TIP and G-TIP. Similarly, there is no report comparing the appearance of the meatus between these techniques [49].

7.15 Tubularized Reconstructed Plate Urethroplasty (TRPU) Technique [50]

Tanelli C et al. (2020) published tubularized reconstructed urethral plate urethroplasty in 29 patients with shallow groove and flat glans and a well-vascularized, thick, compliant, elastic

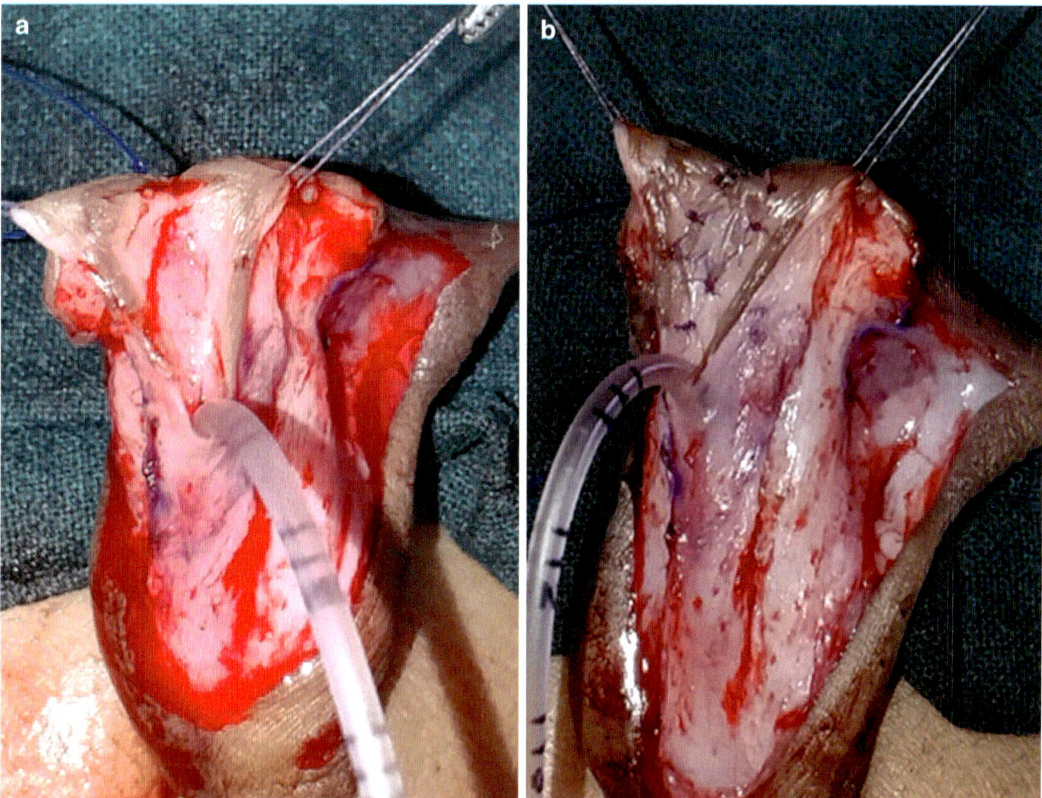

Fig. 7.8 The Dorsal inlay graft. (**a**) Incised the urethral plate. (**b**) Graft fixed

plates, with urethral defect not longer than 2–3 cm. A vertical incision is given from the tip of glans to mid-glans after applying the tourniquet (Fig. 7.11a). The incision is deepened to create a diamond-shaped defect. Subsequently, longitudinal wedges of the spongiosum tissue from the urethral plate base extending to the hypospadiac meatus are excised, and a wedge-shaped groove is carved out from the posterior of the native urethral plate (Fig. 7.11b). The tissue's subepithelial excision is done from the native urethral plate base to thin out it and increase the epithelialized surface area (Fig. 7.11c). The plate's enlargement resembles like the stretched graft by cleaning the fat tissue under the skin. A vertical incision is closed horizontally by Heineke-Mikulicz principle, which also widens the narrow plate's diameter (Fig. 7.11d). Thinned, stretched and finally enlarged native urethral plate is re-secured into its bed using quilting stitches to reduce the risk of mobilization (Fig. 7.11e). Reconstructed urethral plate ensures the required width to allow the tubularization of neo-urethra of the adequate circumference. A U-shaped incision is done along the lateral margins of the urethral plate (Fig. 7.11f) and the urethral plate is tubularized. Though the authors.

Claim that the procedure simulates created fossa navicularis and solves the problem of meatal stenosis, with an overall complication rate was 3.4% only [50]. Still, the long-term follows up will decide the real advantages of the modification.

7.16 Glanular-Frenular Collar (GFC) Technique [51]

Ozbey H and Etker S did a modification to create the frenulum to produce near-normal anatomy of the penis in the study of 121 patients with varying degrees of hypospadias. The glans penis' split

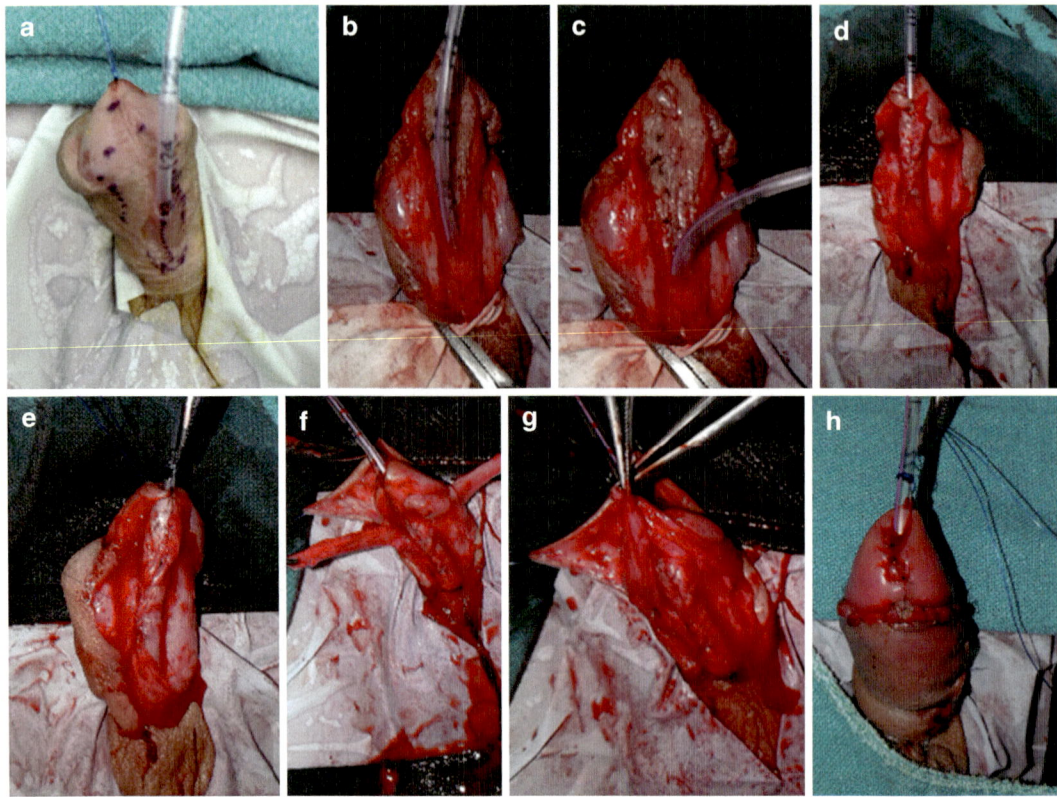

Fig. 7.9 The Dorsal inlay graft in and double dartos cover in mid-penile hypospadias (**a**) Mid-penile hypospadias. (**b**) Partial penile degloving and mobilization of urethral plate. (**c**) Dorsal inlay graft (**d**) Tubularization of urethral plate. (**e**) Spongioplasty (**f** and **g**) double dorsal dartos cover. (**h**) Skin Closure and final picture

wings or so-called ventral cleft between the glans wings that accommodate the frenulum are part of normal anatomy. Hence, in hypospadias surgery, the approximated glans wings should allow for ventral support of the glanular and sub-coronal urethra through a reconstructed neo-frenulum. A V-shaped incision is given to dissecting the inner foreskin, in a fashion that allowed for its ventral mobilization as a frenular mucosal collar for Y-shaped closure. After tubularization of the proximal urethra, a partial spongioplasty is performed up to the sub-coronal level. Well mobilized glans wings are approximated only at their outermost convexities creating a wide slit-like meatus. The cleft-like area between the split wings of the glans penis is filled with the terminal ends of the spongiosum and the dartos of the mucosal collar, which converged to form a septum and a neo-frenulum. The midline skin closure of the ventral collar and the circumferential foreskin closure is completed as usual. Prepucioplasty can also be done on the desire of the parents.

7.17 Meatal-Based Flap Techniques

Mathieu described this meatal-based flap technique in 1932 for distal hypospadias variants [52]. This procedure is mainly suited for meatus cases at the distal penile shaft, at the sub-coronal level and at the corona with mild or no chordee. Glanular groove should be wide, and skin proxi-

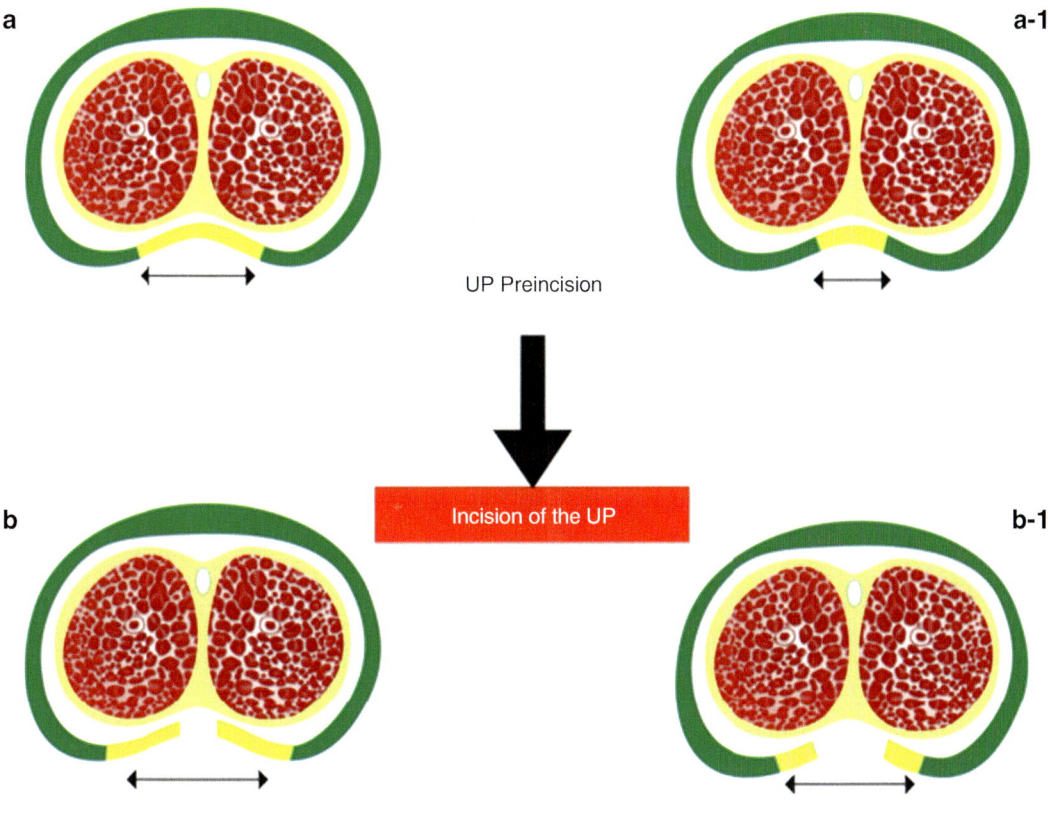

Fig. 7.10 Measuring urethral plate for G-Tip [a / b = > 0.5, a1 / b1 = < 0.5]. (**a** and **a1**) Urethral plate width prior to incising. (**b** and **b1**) Urethral Plate width after to incising

mal to meatus should be thick and well vascularized. Since the Mathieu technique description, others have presented their modified meatal-based flap techniques that offered good results [53, 54].

In this technique, first, a 5/0 monofilament suture with a round body needle is applied for traction at the tip of gland just dorsal to the future meatus. Then flap outline is marked proximal to the meatus. The distance between hypospadiac meatus and glans tip is the proximal flap length which should be marked. The width of the proximal flap (7-8 mm) should be 2-3 mm more than that of the glanular flap (5-6 mm) to maintain distal vascularity (Fig. 7.12a, b). Flap dissection started proximally, and maximum possible vascularized subcutaneous tissue should be dissected along with skin flap. An incision made along with the glanular tissue and lateral glans wings is mobilized. The proximal flap is then flipped to the glanular flap and anastomosed with 7/0 PDS or vicryl in subcuticular fashion over 8 Fr infant feeding tube (Fig. 7.12c). The anastomotic line can be covered with vascularized subcutaneous tissue with proximal flap, if available. Other options are dorsal dartos subcutaneous flap and tunica vaginalis [55–57]. Glanular wings are then closed with 6/0 PDS or vicryl in an interrupted fashion (Fig. 7.12d).

Urethrocutaneous fistula, urethral stricture, meatal stenosis, glans dehiscence and meatal retraction are common complications [58–60]. Unsightly appearance of external urethral meatus was another concern. Several modifications have been proposed to reduce these complications. MAVIS technique described by Boddy and

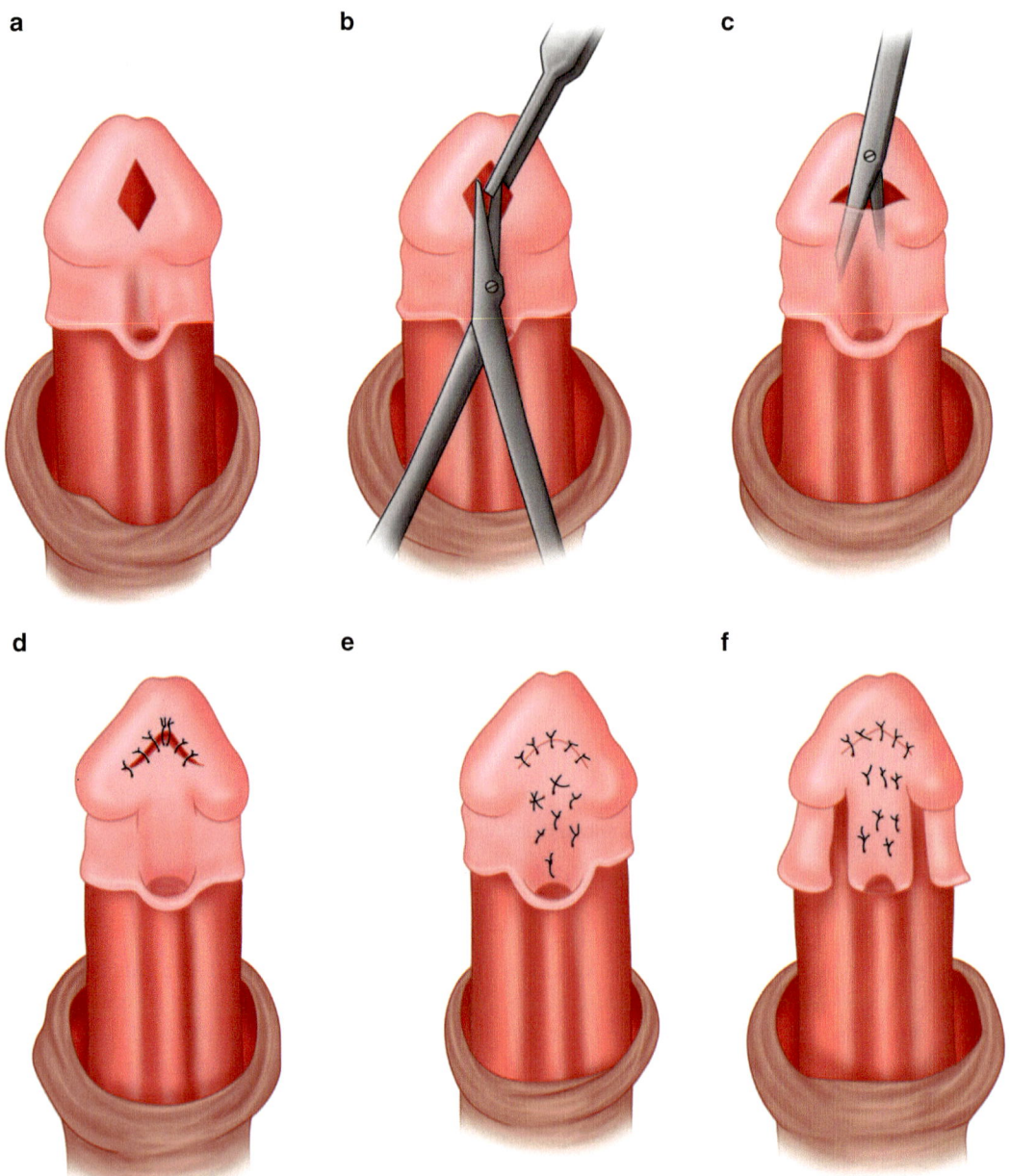

Fig. 7.11 The TRPU technique. (**a**) A vertical incision tip of glans to mid-glans. (**b**) Excision of glanular spongiosum to deepen the urethral plate. (**c**) Releasing the urethral plate from underlying to widen it. (**d**) Vertical incision and horizontal closure (Heineke-Mikulicz). (**e**) Quilting of the thinned, stretched and enlarged urethral plate. (**f**) U-shaped incision on the urethral plate's lateral margins

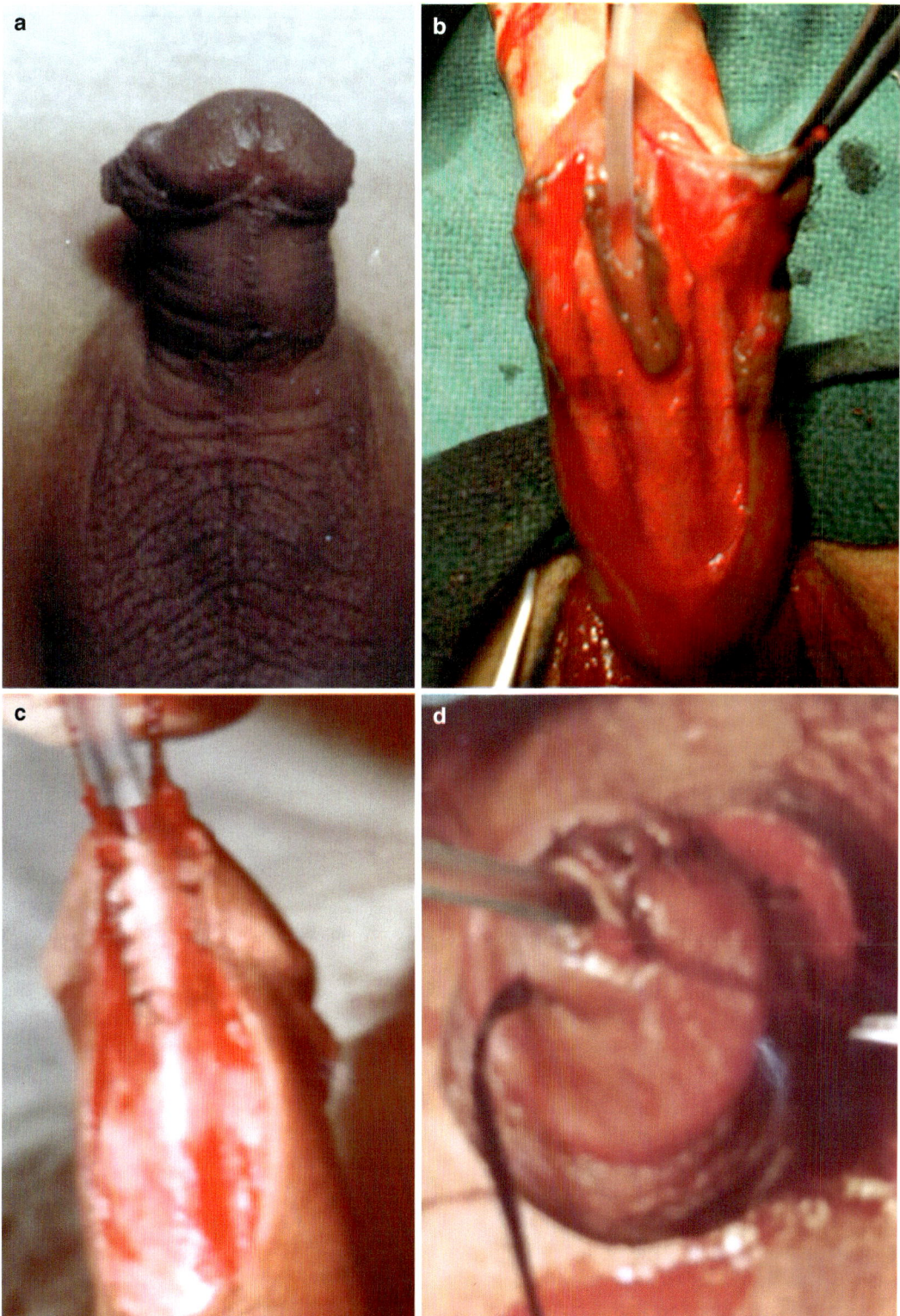

Fig. 7.12 Mathieu repair. (**a**) Coronal hypospadias. (**b**) Raised flap sutured. (**c**) Closure of the flap over the urethral plate. (**d**) Glansplasty

Samuel was proposed to make meatus slit-like by excising a V-shaped tissue from the tip of the anterior lip of meatus [61].

7.18 SLAM Technique (Slit-Like Adjusted Mathieu Technique) [62]

The technique is modifying Mathieu's parameatal-based technique to create a slit-like opening. The principal drawback of the Mathieu technique was the shape of meatus not being slit-like. Hadidi modified V-Y meatoplasty and sutures the flap little proximal to the neo-meatus and creates a slit-like a meatus.

The distance is measured from the meatus to the flap and an inverted u shaped is given in the glans and penile shaft proximal to the meatus slightly larger than required. If the flap length falls short, an oblique flap is raised preventing the inclusion of hair-bearing scrotal skin. The width of the skin flap is taken larger in cases of the narrow urethral plate. The wide glanular wings are created by dissecting the glans deep in the parallel incision. At the distal end, the two incisions converge to have a slit-like meatus and to avoid having sutures at the meatus.

The flap is mobilized by using sharp scissors, the incision is deepened starting near the coronal sulcus and then mobilized proximally including the dartos fascia and corpus spongiosum with the flap as much as possible to maintain the blood supply of the flap. The angle epithelium is excised to trim the dog-earing at the flap's proximal two angles, keeping the fascia to reduce fistula chances. The urethroplasty's first step is to suture the flap's distal end to the end of the glans 2 mm from the tip. This helps to have a slit-like meatus and place one stitch only at the meatus at the 6-o'clock position. The flap suturing starts 3 mm proximal to the flap's angle and is carried out using 6/0 Vicryl in a continuous subcuticular fashion. A sealing second suture layer with continuous sutures is carried out. A V triangle is removed from the tip of the flap to help to have a slit-like meatus. The Glans wings are approximated around the new urethra with 6 0 Vicryl to complete the glanuloplasty, and the penile skin closure is done.

The important points to prevent the complications in the technique are the urethroplasty's suturing should start a few millimetres proximal to the original meatus to have the knot proximal and away from the neo-meatus. Care must be taken to elevate Buck fascia and part of the corpus spongiosum with the flap because this constitutes the main blood supply to the flap. Size of the urethra is designed to be the same size or slightly larger than the normal proximal urethra. Epithelium from margins at meatus is excised.

Hadidi reported satisfactory results (97%) in 848 patients. Fourteen patients (1.65%) developed a fistulae, 7(0.82%) had wound dehiscence and 4 (0.48%) patients developed meatal stenosis [62].

7.19 Transverse Preputial Island Flap

Preputial island flap was first introduced by Hook in the nineteenth century [63]. Asopa and Duckett used the island flap in severe cases by tubularizing it [64, 65]. This technique can be used for cases where the urethral plate's width is not sufficient to undergo Theirsch-Duplay or TIP. Distal and mid-hypospadias cases with poor proximal skin are also a candidate for this procedure. Ventral curvature should be of a mild degree, and the patient should not be circumcised. Since the results of on lay flap urethroplasty are better than the tubularized flap; it should be tried when moderate curvature can be corrected while preserving the urethral plate. Moderate chordee can be rectified by mobilizing urethral plate and spongiosum with/ without single stitch dorsal plication or incising the urethral plate with or without a single stitch dorsal plication and Z-plasty of the urethral plate to increase the length urethral.

After penile degloving ventral chordee is assessed and corrected either by the urethral plate's mobilization with spongiosum and urethra with or without dorsal plication. A transverse flap

7 Management of Distal and Mid-Penile Hypospadias

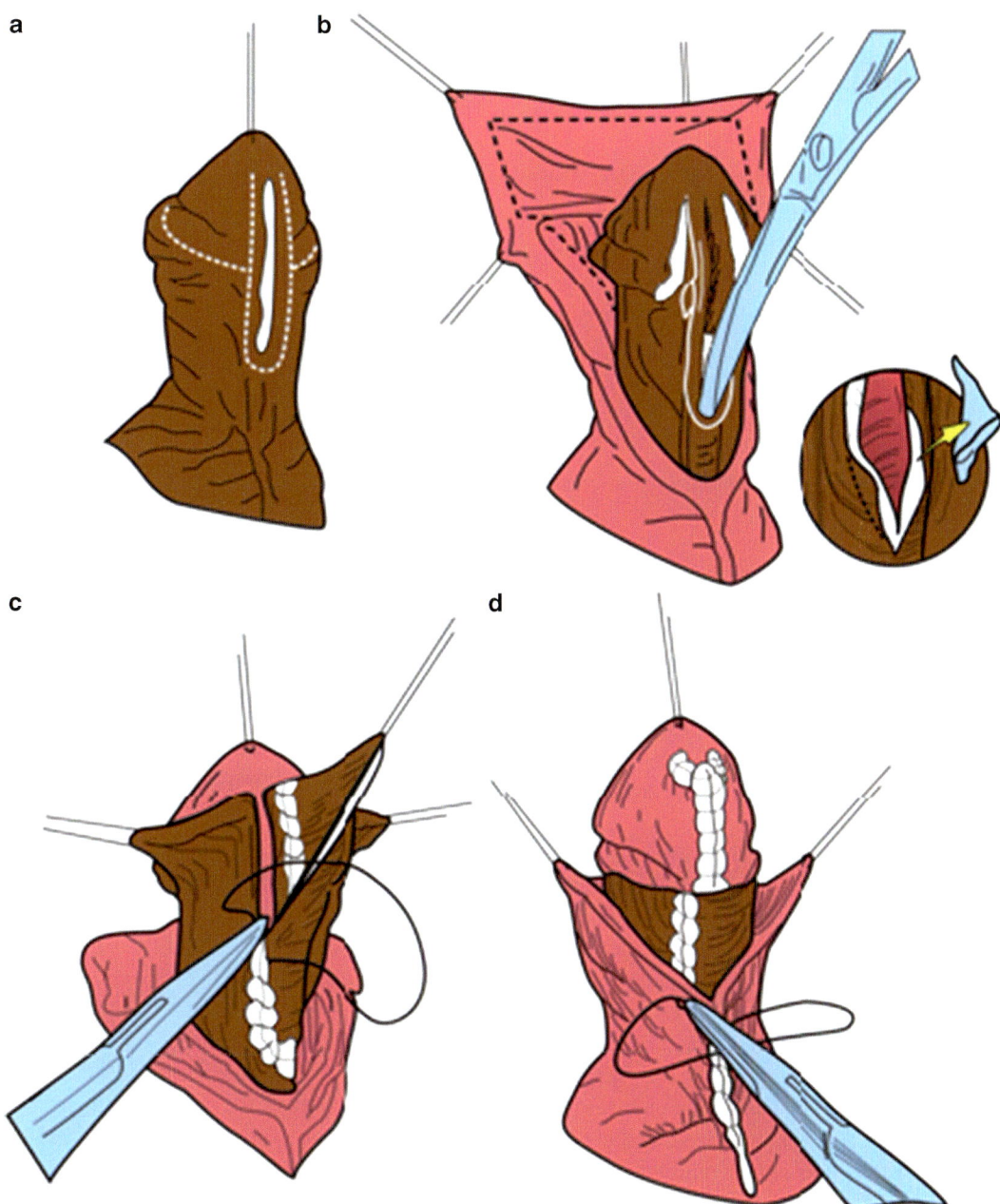

Fig. 7.13 (a) Mid-penile hypospadias. (b) Penile de-gloving, incising the hypoplastic urethra and raising the transverse island flap. (c) Bringing the transverse flap ventrally and suturing it to urethral plate. (d) Glansplasty and skin closure

of width 1.5–2 cm and length as per meatus location is measured and marked Fig. 7.13a. The flap is dissected in a plane between penile skin dorsally and dartos flap ventrally. Dissection continued till the base of the penis. The flap is then rotated ventrally and anastomosed with native urethral plate with 7/0 PDS or vicryl subcuticular sutures (Fig. 7.13b, c). The anastomosis is covered with dartos flap or tunica vaginalis. Glanuloplasty followed by penile skin closure after dorsal splitting completes the procedure (Fig. 7.13d).

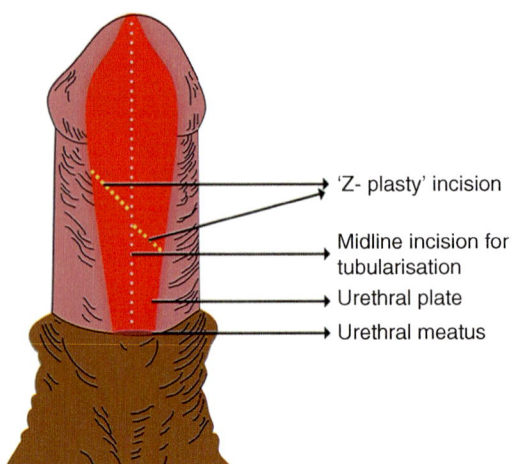

Fig. 7.14 Z-plasty of the urethral plate to correct the curvature

Urethrocutaneous fistula, urethral stricture, meatal stenosis and penile skin necrosis are common complications associated with this procedure [66]. Fistula can be reduced by covering the anastomoses with well-vascularized tissue, and the closure should not be in tension. Flap dissection in the right plane reduces flap necrosis and the incidence of urethral stricture and the chances of penile skin necrosis.

Mild curvature can be corrected by penile degloving, mobilization of the urethral plate or dorsal plication. Sarma et al. used the Z-plasty of the urethral plate to augment the urethral plate and used onlay flap urethroplasty. A single Z-plasty incision is given on the urethral plate at the maximum chordee site, to divide the short urethral plate, pre-serving the vascular plexus/spongiosum deep to the urethral plate (Fig. 7.14). The urethral plate can be tubularized if adequate width can be gained with a midline incision [67]. Double-faced on the lay flap is utilized to reduce the complications and better ventral skin closure. El dahshpury et al. (2013) reported functional and cosmetic success in 96.6% and complications reported were 0.5% glanular disruption, 1.09% fistula, 0.5% urethral diverticulum and 1.09% lateral penile torsion [68].

In patients with moderate to severe chordee where urethral plate transection is needed, single-stage repair with tubularization of island flap (Fig. 7.15a–f) or modified tubularized island urethroplasty (Fig 7.16a–h) and two-stage urethroplasty remains the option. Commonly used one-stage tubularized techniques are Asopa I, II Duckett Hodgson X, XX. Though Asopa started the technique earlier but Duckett deserves the credit to popularize it. In the Asopa modification of the procedure, the inner prepuce is also used as a pedicle flap. Still, the neo-urethra is left attached to the underneath surface of the foreskin.

Therefore, the skin and the neo-urethra share a common blood supply. Double-faced tubularized preputial flap technique seems a superior choice, which provides better vascular supply with better results than standard ventral preputial tubularized flap in one-stage penoscrotal hypospadias repair, with reported fewer complications, better urinary function and good cosmetic results [69]. The tubularized flap and graft details are described in Chap. 9 single-stage repair in proximal hypospadias, Chap. 14 modified flap repair and Chap. 12 flaps and grafts in hypospadias repair.

7.20 Conclusion

Hypospadias surgery is technically complex with long-term results on the child's physical, mental and aesthetic well-being. Mid and distal hypospadias management's success depends on the appropriate preoperative assessment of the degree of chordee, quality of the urethral plate, location of the meatus and proper surgical technique surgeon experience. Most distal hypospadias can be managed by TIP, G-TIP and Gap procedures. The choice in middle hypospadias remains TIP, G, TIP, Urethral mobilization, Mathieu procedure and onlay flap urethroplasty. Mid-hypospadias with severe curvature may require transection of urethral plate and can be managed by tubularized flap or graft urethroplasty or two-stage repairs.

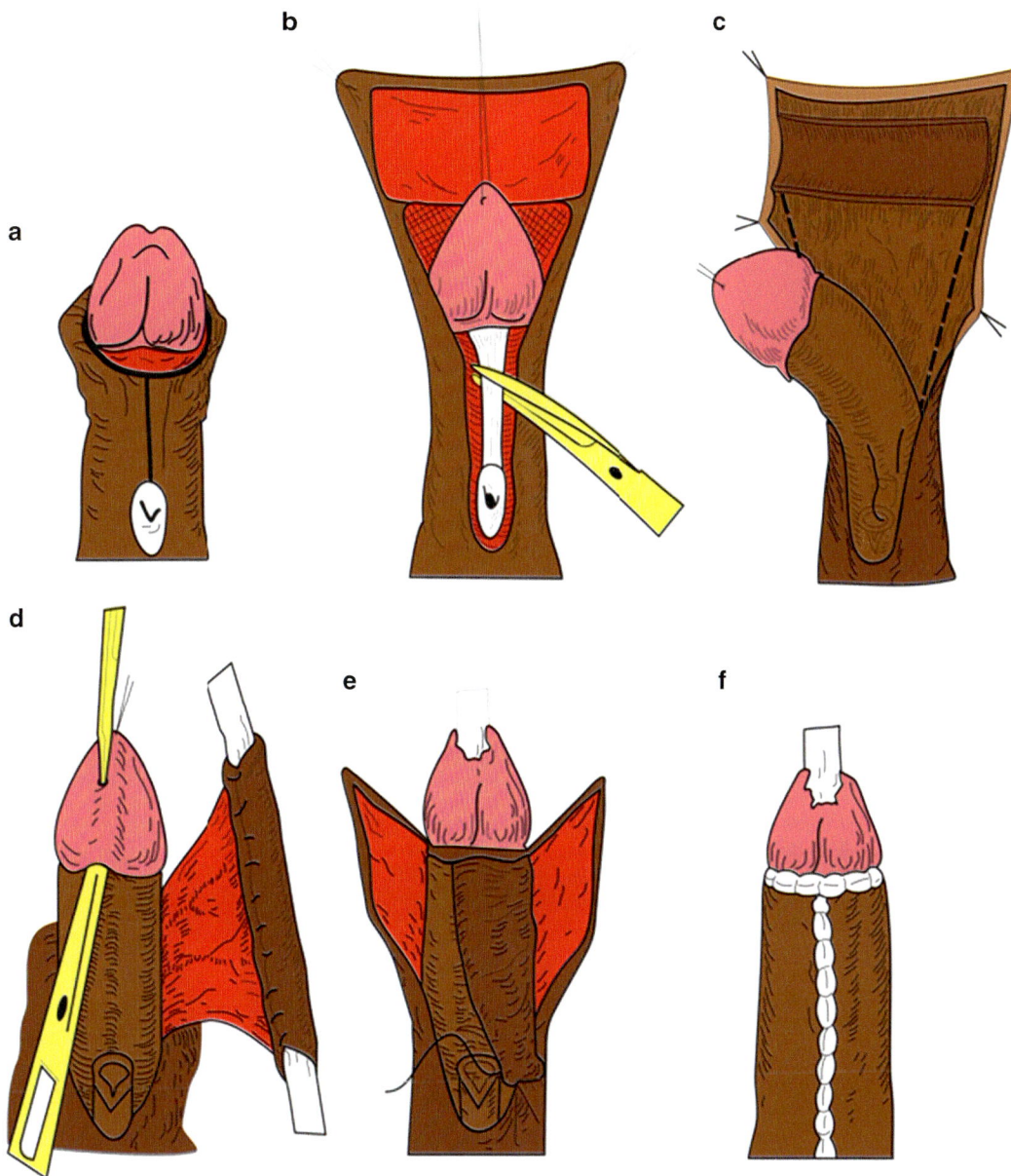

Fig. 7.15 (a) Proximal hypospadias. (b) Transaction of the urethral plate to correct the chordee. (c) Raising the inner prepucial flap. (d) Tubularization of the flap and crating the glans tunnel. (e) Suturing the skin tube to the native urethra taking out through glans tunnel. (f) Skin closure

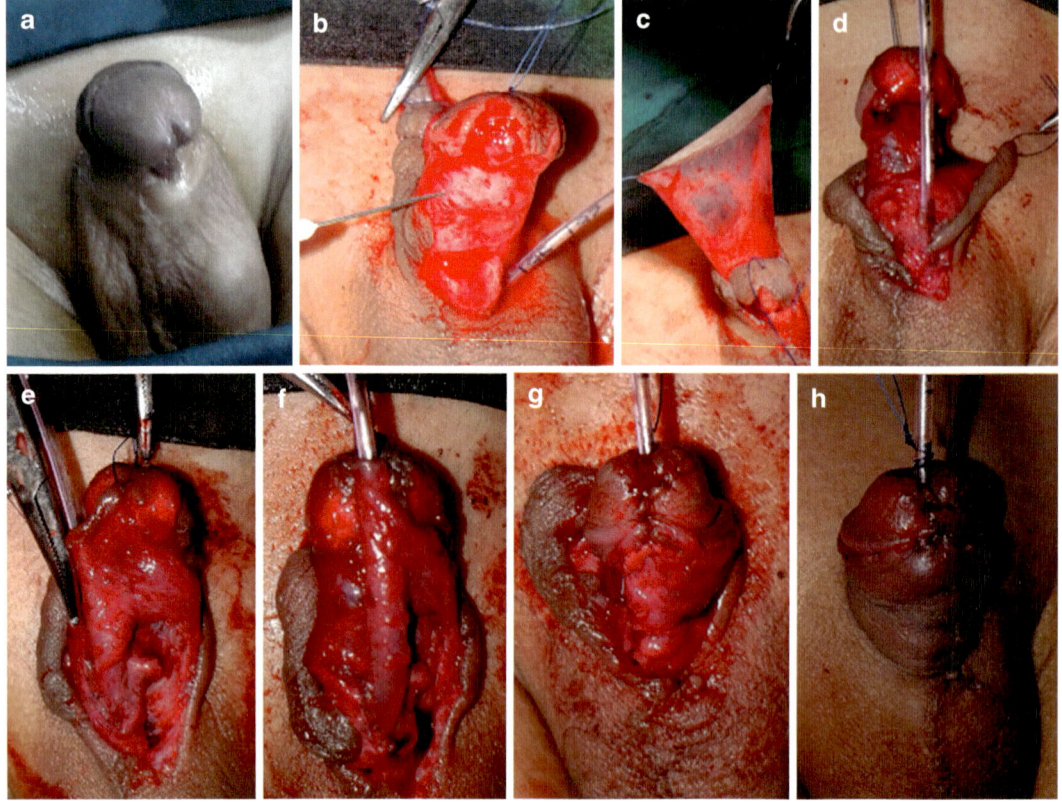

Fig. 7.16 Modified transverse Island flap urethroplasty. (**a**) Mid-penile hypospadias with severe curvature. (**b**) Gittes test after penile degloving and resection of Chordee tissue. (**c**) Dissecting inner prepucial flap. (**d**) Anastomosis of flap with urethral with healthy spongiosum. (**e**) tubularization of the flap. (**f**) Anastomosis of the tube to glans. (**g**) Glansplasty. (**h**) Skin closure

References

1. Kraft KH, Shukla AR, Canning DA. Hypospadias. Urol Clin North Am. 2010;37(2):167–81.
2. Duckett JW Jr. Hypospadias. Pediatr Rev. 1989;11(2):37–42.
3. Borer JG, Bauer SB, Peters CA, et al. Tubularized incised plate urethroplasty: expanded use in primary and repeat surgery for hypospadias. J Urol. 2001;165(2):581–5.
4. Pfistermuller KL, McArdle AJ, Cuckow PM. Meta-analysis of complication rates of the tubularized incised plate (TIP) repair. J Pediatr Urol. 2015;11(2):54–9.
5. Manzoni G, Bracka A, Palminteri E, et al. Hypospadias surgery: when what and by whom? BJU Int. 2004;94(8):1188–95.
6. Merriman LS, Arlen AM, Broecker BH, et al. The GMS hypospadias score: assessment of inter-observer reliability and correlation with post-operative complications. J Pediatr Urol. 2013;9(6 Pt A):707–12.
7. Arlen AM, Kirsch AJ, Leong T, et al. Further analysis of the Glans-Urethral Meatus-Shaft (GMS) hypospadias score: correlation with postoperative complications. J Pediatr Urol. 2015;11(2):71.e1–71.e75.
8. Cimador M, Vallasciani S, Manzoni G, et al. Failed hypospadias in pediatric patients. Nat Rev. 2013;10:657–65.
9. Snodgrass W, Macedo A, Hoebeke P, et al. Hypospadias dilemmas: a round table. J Pediatr Urol. 2011;7:145–57.
10. American Academy of Pediatrics. Timing of elective surgery on the genitalia of male children with particular reference to the risks, benefits, and psychological effects of surgery and anaesthesia. Paediatrics. 1996;97:590–4.
11. Steven L, Cherian A, Yankovic F, et al. Current practice in pediatric hypospadias surgery: A specialist survey. J Pediatr Urol. 2013;9:1126–30.
12. Springer A, Krois W, Horcher E. Trends in hypospadias surgery: Results of a worldwide survey. Eur Urol. 2011;60:9.

13. Gilliver SC, Ashworth J, Ashcroft GS. The hormonal regulation of cutaneous wound healing. Clin Dermatol. 2007;25:56–62.
14. Gorduza DB, Gay CL, de Mattos E, et al. Does androgen stimulation prior to hypospadias surgery increase the rate of healing complications? A preliminary report. J Pediatr Urol. 2011;7:158–61.
15. Netto JMB, Ferrarez CEPF, Leal AAS, et al. Hormone therapy in hypospadias surgery: A systematic review. J Pediatr Urol. 2013;9:971–9.
16. Gittes RF, McLaughlin AP III. Injection technique to produce penile erection. Urology. 1974;4:473–5.
17. Bhat A. Extended urethral mobilization in incised plate urethroplasty for severe hypospadias: a variation in technique to improve chordee correction. J Urol. 2007;178(3):1031–5.
18. Bhat A, Sabharwal K, Bhat M, Singla M, Kumar V, Upadhyay R. Correction of penile torsion and chordee by mobilization of the urethra with spongiosum in chordee without hypospadias. J Pediatr Urol. 2014;10(6):1238–43.
19. Pippi Salle JL, Sayed S, Salle A, et al. Proximal hypospadias: a persistent challenge. Single institution outcome analysis of three surgical techniques over 10 years. J Pediatr Urol. 2016;12(1):28.e1–7.
20. Devine CJ Jr, Horton CE. Use of the dermal graft to correct chordee. J Urol. 1975;113(1):56–8.
21. Lindgren BW, Reda EF, Levitt SB, et al. Single and multiple dorsal grafts for the management of severe penile curvature. J Urol. 1998;160:1128–30.
22. Pope JC 4th, Kropp BP, McLaughlin KP, et al. Penile orthoplasty using dermal grafts in the outpatient setting. Urology. 1996;48:124–7.
23. Duckett JW. MAGPI (Meatoplasty and Glanuloplasty): a procedure for subcoronal hypospadias. Urol Clin No Am. 1981;8:513–9.
24. Duckett JW, Snyder HM. The MAGPI hypospadias repair in 1111 patients. Ann Surg. 1991;213(6):620–5.
25. Livine PM, Gibbons MD, Gonzales E. Meatal advancement and glanuloplasty: an operation for distal hypospadias. J Urol. 1984;131:95.
26. Mc Millan RDH, Churchill BM, Gilmore RF. Assessment of urinary stream after repair of anterior hypospadias by meatoplasty and glanuloplasty. J Urol. 1985;134:100–2.
27. Hastie KJ, Deshpande SS, Moisey CN. Long-term follow-up of the MAGPI operations for distal hypospadias. Br J Urol. 1989;63:320.
28. Isa MM, Gearhart JP. The failed MAGPI: management and prevention. Br J Urol. 1989;64:169–71.
29. Ozen HA, Whitaker RH. Scope and limitations of the MAGPI hypospadias repair. Br J Urol. 1987;59:81.
30. Somoza I, Liras J, Abuin AS, Mendez R, Tellado MG, Rios J, et al. N Modern Magpi Cir Pediatr. 2004;17:76–9.
31. Shukla AK, Singh AP, Sharma P, Shukla J. MAGPI technique for distal penile hypospadias; modifications to improve outcome at a single centre. Arch Int Surg. 2016;6:201–5.
32. Arap S, Mitre AI, De Goes GM. Modified meatal advancement and glanuloplasty repair of distal hypospadias. J Urol. 1984;131:1140.
33. Seibold OG, Amend B, Alloussi SH, Colleselli D, Todenhoef T, et al. Meatal mobilization (MEMO) technique for distal hypospadias repair: technique, results AND long-term follow-UP Central European. J Urol. 2010;63(3):125–8.
34. Beck C. A new operation for balanic hypospadias. NY Med J. 1898;67:147.
35. Belman AB. Urethroplasty. Soc Pediatr Urol Newslett. 1977;12:1–2.
36. Atala A. Urethral mobilization and advancement for midshaft to distal hypospadias. J Urol. 2002;168(Pt 2):1738–41. discussion of 1741
37. Hassan HS, Almetaher HA, Negm M, Elhalaby EA. Urethral mobilization and advancement for distal hypospadias. Ann Pediatr Surg. 2015;11:239–43.
38. Elemen L, Tugay M. Limited Urethral Mobilization Technique in Distal Hypospadias Repair with Satisfactory Results. Balkan Med J. 2012;29:21–5.
39. Macedo A Jr, Ottoni SL, Garrone G, Liguori R, Mattos RM, da Cruz ML. The GUD technique: glandar urethral disassembly. An alternative for distal hypospadias repair. Int Braz J Urol. 2020;46(6):1072–4.
40. Thiersch C. über die Entstehungweise und operative Be- handlung des Epispadie. Arch Heilkd. 1869;10:20.
41. Duplay S. De l'hypospadias perineo-scrotal et de son traite- ment ehirugieal. Areh Gen Med. 1874;1(613):657.
42. Stock JA, Hanna MK. Distal urethroplasty and glanuloplasty procedures: Results of 512 repairs. Urology. 1997;49:449.
43. Zaontz MR, The GAP. (glans approximation procedure) for glanular/coronal hypospadias. J Urol. 1989;141(2):359–61.
44. Snodgrass WT. Utilization of urethral plate in hypospadias surgery. Indian J Urol. 2008;24:195–9.
45. Snodgrass WT, Bush N, Cost N. Tubularized incised plate hypospadias repair tor distal hypospadias. J Pediatr Urol. 2010;6:408–13.
46. Snodgrass W, Bush N. Primary hypospadias repair techniques: A review of the evidence. Urol Ann. 2016;8:403–8.
47. Ververidis M, Dickson AP, Gough DC. An objective assessment of the results of hypospadias surgery. BJU Int. 2005;96:135–9.
48. Abbas TO, Pippi Salle JL. When to graft the incised plate during TIP repair? A suggested algorithm that may help in the decision- making process. Front Pediatr. 2018;6:326–8.
49. Snodgrass W, Bush N. Primary hypospadias repair techniques: A review of the evidence. Urol Ann. 2016;2016(8):403–8.
50. Taneli C, Tanriverdi HI, Genc A, Sencan A, Gunsar C, Yilmaz O. Tubularized reconstructed plate urethroplasty: an alternative technique for distal hypospadias repair. Urology. 2021;148:243–9.

51. Ozbey H. Etker Sharif Hypospadias repair with glanular Frenular technique. J Ped Urol. 2017 Feb;13(1):34–6.
52. Mathieu P. Traitment en un temps de l'hypospadias balani- que et juxta balanique. J Chir. 1932;39:481–4.
53. Mustarde JC. One-stage correction of distal hypospadias and other people's fistulae. Br J Plast Surg. 1965;18:413–22.
54. Ir DCI, Horton CE. Hypospadias repair. J Urol. 1977;118:188–93.
55. Retik AB, Mandell J, Bauer SB, al. Meatal based hypospadias repair with the use of the dorsal subcutaneous flap to prevent urethrocutaneous fistula. J Urol. 1994;152:1229–31.
56. Churchill BM, van Savage JG, Khoury AE, et al. The dartos flaps as an adjuant in preventing urethrocutaneous fistulas in repeat hypospadias surgery. J Urol. 1996;156:2047–9.
57. Snow BW, Cartwright PC, Unger K. Tunica vaginalis blanket wrap to prevent urethrocutaneous fistulas. An 8-year - experience. J Urol. 1995;153:472–3.
58. Delong TP, Boomers TM. Improved Mathieu repair for coronal and distal shaft hypospadias with moderate chordee. Br J Urol. 1993;72:972–4.
59. Minevieh E, Pecha BR, Ackman J, Sheldon CA. Mathieu hypospadias repair: An experience in 202 patients. J Urol. 1999;162:2141–3.
60. Murphy JP. Hypospadias. In: Ashcraft KW, Murphy JP, Sharp RJ, Sigalet DL, Snyder CL, editors. Pediatric surgery. 3rd ed. Philadelphia: Saunders; 2000. p. 763–82.
61. Boddy SA, Samuel M. A natural glanular meatus after "Mathieu and V incision sutured" MAVIS. BJU Int. 2000;86:394–7.
62. Hadidi AT. The slit-like adjusted Mathieu technique for distal hypospadias. J Pediatr Surg. 2012;47:617–23.
63. Horton CE. Devine CI Ir, Barcat N: Pietorial history of hypospadias repair techniques. In: Horton CE, editor. Plastie and reconstructive surgery of the genital area. Boston: Little Brown; 1973. p. 237–48.
64. Asopa HS, Elhence IP, Atri SP, Bansal NK. One-stage correction of penile hypospadias using a foreskin tube. Int Surg. 1971;55:435.
65. Duckett JW. Transverse preputial island flap technique for repair of severe hypospadias. Urol Chn North Am. 1980;7:423.
66. Eider JS, Duckett JW, Snyder HM. Onlay island flap in the repair of mid and distal penile hypospadias without chordee. J Urol. 1987;138:376–9.
67. Sarma VP. The feasibility of urethral plate preservation in proximal and mid hypospadias: Sequential and anatomical approach. Ann Pediatr Surg. 2020;16:26. 4 of 9
68. El dahshoury ZM, Gamal W, Hammady A, Hussein M, Salem E. Modified double-faced onlay island preputial skin flap with augmented glanuloplasty for hypospadias repair. J Pediatr Urol. 2013;9:745–9.
69. Daboos M, Helal AA. Salama A Five years' experience of double-faced tubularized preputial flap for penoscrotal hypospadias repair in paediatrics. J Pediatr Urol. 2020;16:673–7.

Modified Tubularized Incised Urethral Plate Urethroplasty

Amilal Bhat

8.1 Introduction

Most of the innovations claimed today are described in the history of hypospadias. The principle of tubularization was described by Professor C. Thiersch (1869) in a child of epispadias. Later, the same was used for hypospadias & is known as the Thiersch-Duplay urethroplasty [1]. King (1981) tubularized the urethral plate for distal hypospadias [2]. The glanular approximation procedure described by Zaontz (1989) is based on the same principle and is suitable for coronal and glanular hypospadias with a deep glans groove [3]. Snodgrass (1994) added the dimension of relaxing incision in the urethral plate and deserved the credit of making it the most popular and commonly used technique world over [4]. There have been many modifications to the original description of TIP described by Snodgrass to improve the results. These modifications have led to significant improvement in the outcome and a few reports appearing in the literature with nil fistula rate. The technique described here is with few modifications to improve the results of TIPU.

8.2 Modified TIPU Surgical Technique

The important steps of our modified TIPU are:

1. Partial/Total penile degloving
2. Mobilization of spongiosum and urethral plate
3. Incising the urethral plate
4. Tubularization of the urethral plate
5. Spongioplasty
6. Glanuloplasty
7. Frenuloplasty
8. Dartosorraphy
9. Prepucioplasty

8.2.1 Penile Degloving

Surgical technique I:1,000,000 solution adrenaline solution injected at the planned site of the incision after taking a stay suture on the glans and inserting the urethral stent. A Y-shaped incision is given by the side of the urethral plate

---

A. Bhat (✉)
Bhat's Hypospadias and Reconstructive Urology Hospital and Research Centre,
Jaipur, Rajasthan, India

Department of Urology, Jaipur National University Institute for Medical Sciences and Research Centre,
Jaipur, Rajasthan, India

Department of Urology, Dr. S.N. Medical College,
Jodhpur, Rajasthan, India

Department of Urology, S.P. Medical College,
Bikaner, Rajasthan, India

P.G. Committee Medical Council of India,
New Delhi, India

Academic and Research Council of RUHS,
Jaipur, Rajasthan, India

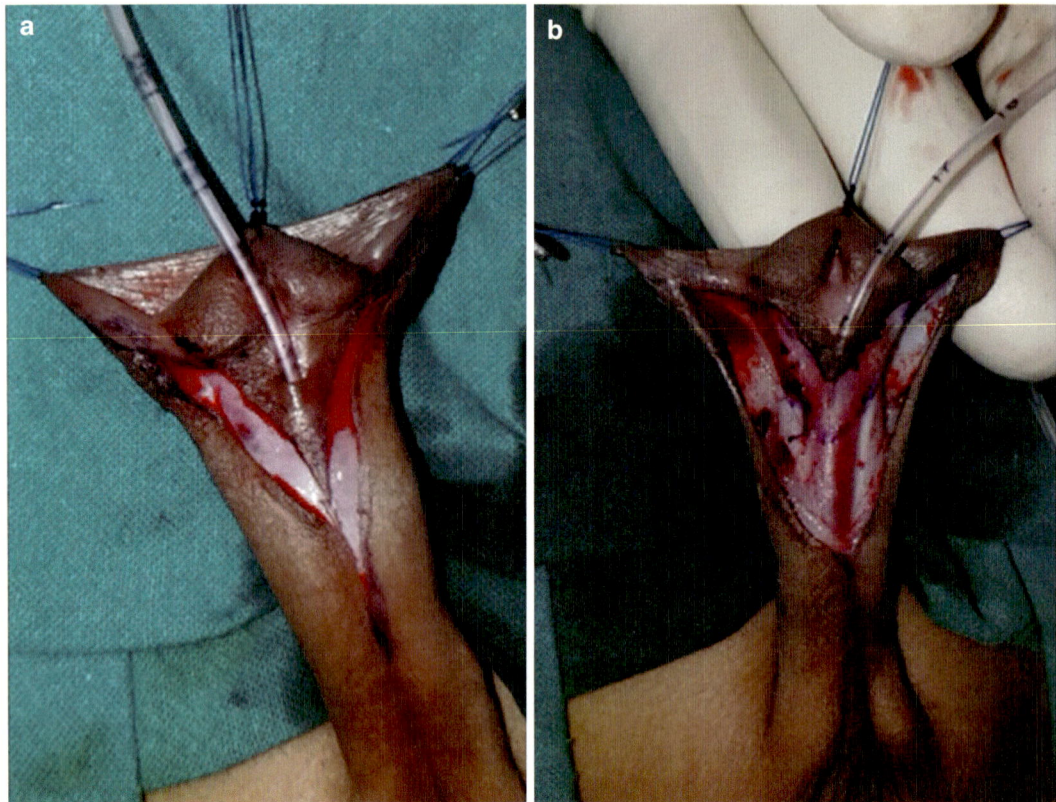

Fig. 8.1 Partial Penile degloving. (**a**) Distal penile hypospadias Y-shaped incision. (**b**) Partial Penile degloving

encircling the meatus midline extension on the penis' shaft (Fig. 8.1a). The wings are extended into the dorsal hood in patients having no chordee and circumferential circum-coronal incision in cases with chordee. Skin and dartos are incised, and partial penile degloving is done (Figs. 8.1b and 8.11a–c). A complete penile degloving is done down up to the root of the penis to correct chordee in cases with chordee. The level of dissection is kept at Buck's fascia. Then, the chordee correction is evaluated by Gitte's test.

8.2.2 Mobilization of Urethral Plate and Spongiosum

After creating a dissection plane at the tunica albuginea level proximal to the meatus, the urethral plate and corpus spongiosum are mobilized starting just proximal to the meatus up to corona (Figs. 8.2a, b and 8.11c–d). Partial mobilization is done for the patients without chordee. This mobilization helps in tubularization of urethral plate and spongioplasty with tension-free sutures. The spongiosum is then dissected into the glans in the same plane of dissection beyond mid-glans (Figs. 8.3a, b and 8.11e–f), and the glanular wings are raised. Glanular wings are dissected adequately on both sides and deep up to the tip of corporal bodies. This will help get done the spongioplasty up to neo-meatus covering the sub-coronal area with spongiosum to prevent sub-coronal fistula. Deep and adequate mobilization of the glanular wings allows tension free glanuloplasty even in cases of small glans.

8.2.3 Incising the Urethral Plate

The urethral plate is incised with the knife starting just inside the meatus to glans (Figs. 8.4a and 8.11g). The incision's depth is done according to

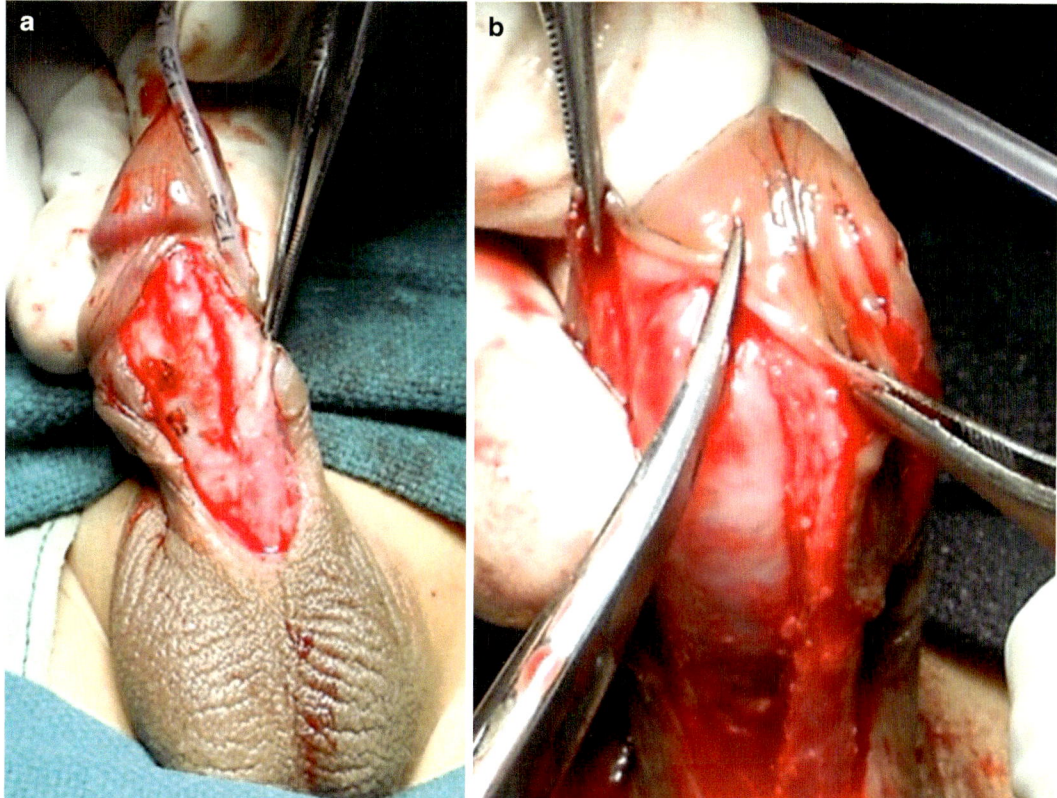

Fig. 8.2 (**a** and **b**) Mobilization of urethral plate and spongiosum up to the corona

the urethral plate's width to tubularize the urethral plate with tension-free suturing. In case of the deep incisions, we prefer to place the dorsal inlay graft in the urethral plate (Fig. 8.11g, h). The care is taken not to extend the incision beyond mid-glans, but in cases of the narrow urethral plate with small glans incision may be extended up to the tip of glans and an inlay graft is placed to prevent the meatal stenosis (Fig. 8.4b).

8.2.4 Tubularization of Urethral Plate and Spongioplasty

Skin around the meatus and adherent to the hypoplastic urethra is excised. A suture is taken at the distal end of the urethral plate to create a wide meatus. Tubularization of the urethral plate is started proximal to meatus at the bifurcation of spongiosum and then continued distally with 6/0-7/0 PDS inverting continuous sub-epithelial sutures. Care is taken to avoid the sutures' passing through the epithelium, and there should not be buckling of the neo-urethra. Distal tubularization is done up to mid-glans to reconstruct a wide meatus. Then spongioplasty is done starting proximal to the urethral plate's tubularization, distally up to the tip of neourethra. Depending upon the development of the spongiosum, spongioplasty (Figs. 8.5a, b and 8.11j) or double breasting spongioplasty is done (Fig. 8.6a–c). Mobilization of the urethral plate and spongiosum allow the tension-free suturing of the spongiosum. The spongiosum is a vascular healthy tissue cover supporting the urethral plate and maintains the urethral plate's blood supply and reconstructs a near-normal urethra.

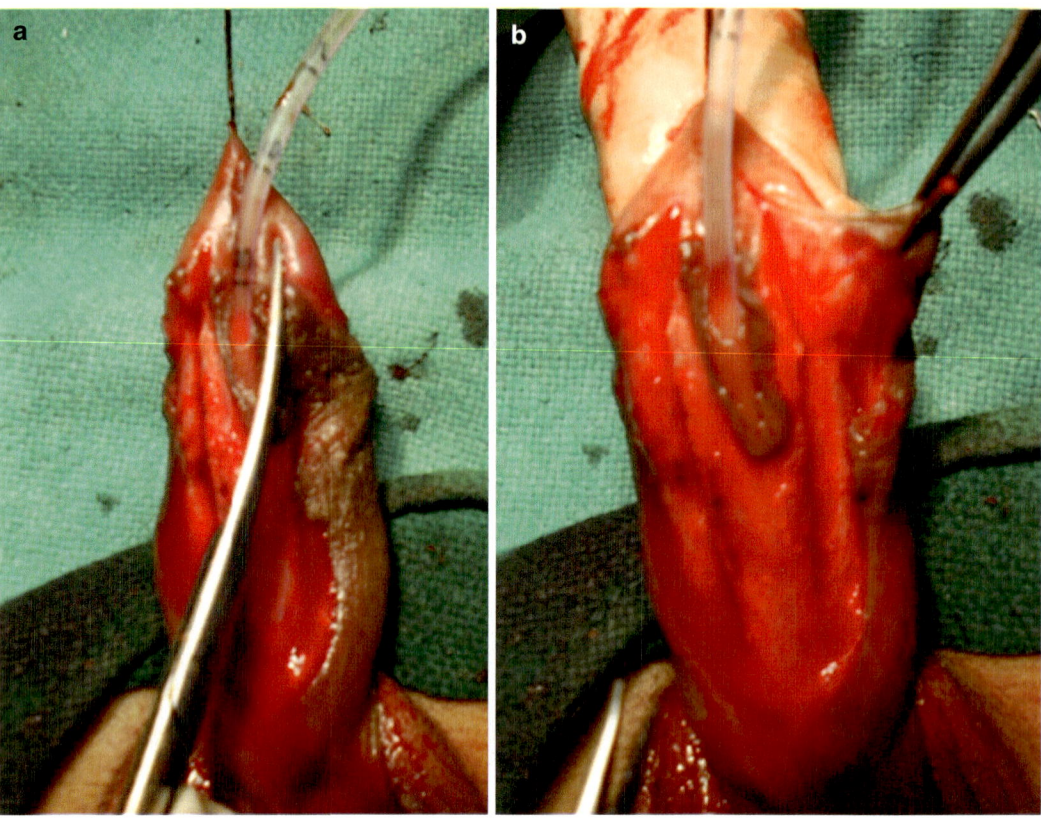

Fig. 8.3 (**a** and **b**) Mobilization of urethral plate and spongiosum into glans

8.2.5 Glanuloplasty and Frenuloplasty

The first suture is taken at the meatus, creating a wide meatus (Fig. 8.11k). Adequate space is left between the neo-urethra and glans wings. Suturing is continued up to the corona to complete the first layer of glanuloplasty (Fig. 8.11l). Then the second layer is completed starting from meatus to corona. Sutures may be taken subepithelial or through the epithelium (Fig. 8.7a, b). The suture is taken in the inner prepucial skin, and traction is applied towards meatus. Two to three sutures are taken to reconstruct the fraenulum of an adequate length, (Figs. 8.8a, b and 8.11m), and the inner layer of the prepucioplasty is completed keeping a wide prepucial opening. The last suture is kept as a stay suture to apply traction (Fig. 8.11n).

8.2.6 Dartosorraphy and Prepucioplasty

The ventral dartos covers the neo-urethra. Approximation of the dartos is started from the proximal end of the incision keeping the traction on the prepucial stay suture. A thick layer of dartos is available if partial penile degloving is done by dissecting at Buck's fascia This thick layer of the dartos is sutured over the neourethra as a healthy interposing tissue layer and dartosorraphy is completed starting from the proximal to distal up to the end of prepuce keeping traction on the preputial suture. The closure of the dartos in prepuce completes the second layer of the prepucioplasty (Figs. 8.9a, b and 8.11o, p). The prepuce's outer layer is sutured to complete the prepucioplasty and skin closure done by sub-cuticular or through & through sutures (Figs. 8.9c and 8.11q, r, and s).

8 Modified Tubularized Incised Urethral Plate Urethroplasty

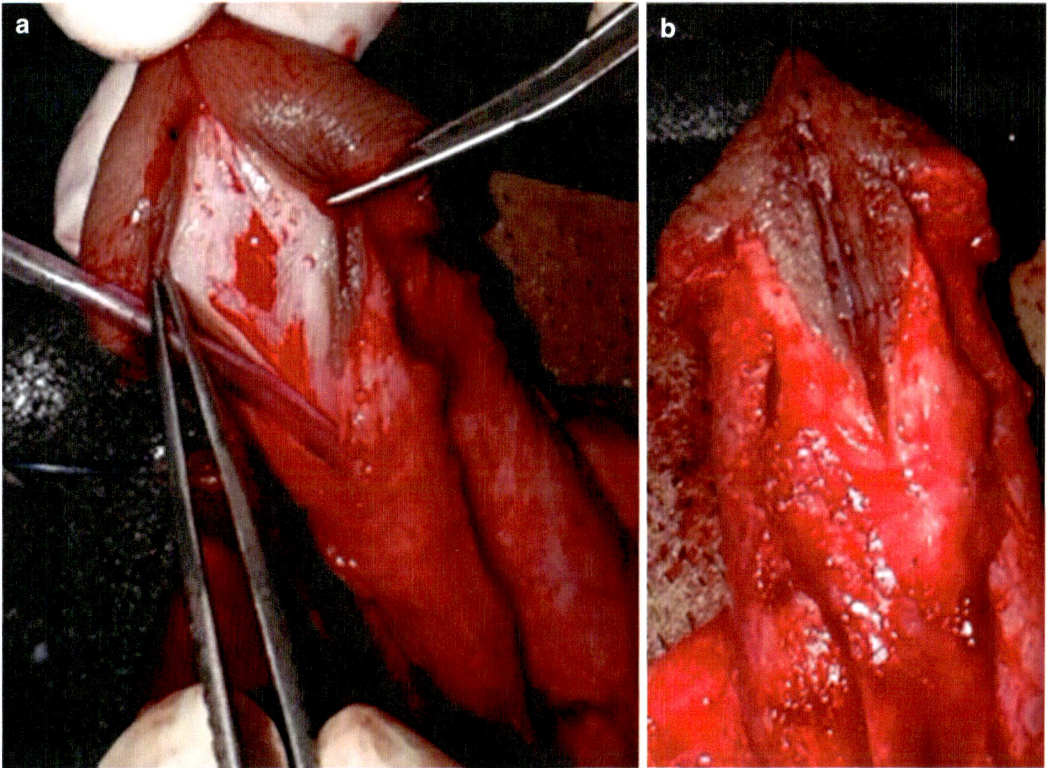

Fig. 8.4 Incision up to the tip of glans. (**a**) Incising urethral plate up to the tip of glans. (**b**) Dorsal inlay graft

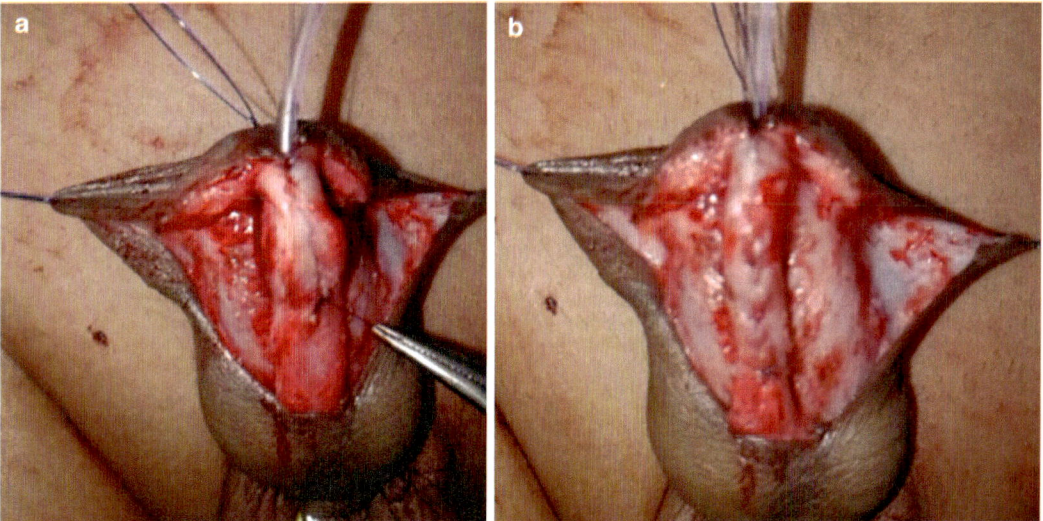

Fig. 8.5 (**a**) Tubularization of the urethral plate and (**b**) Spongioplasty

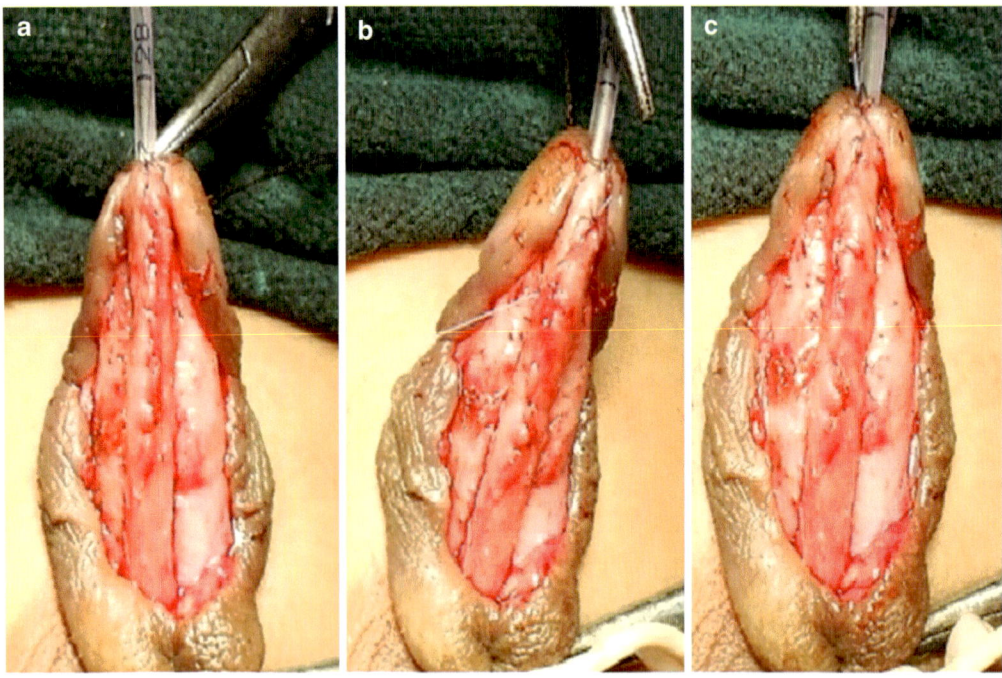

Fig. 8.6 Double breasting Spongioplasty. (**a**) One side of spongiosum sutures to side of the suture line. (**b**) Measuring the flap for double breasting. (**c**) Spongiosum sutured to the other side

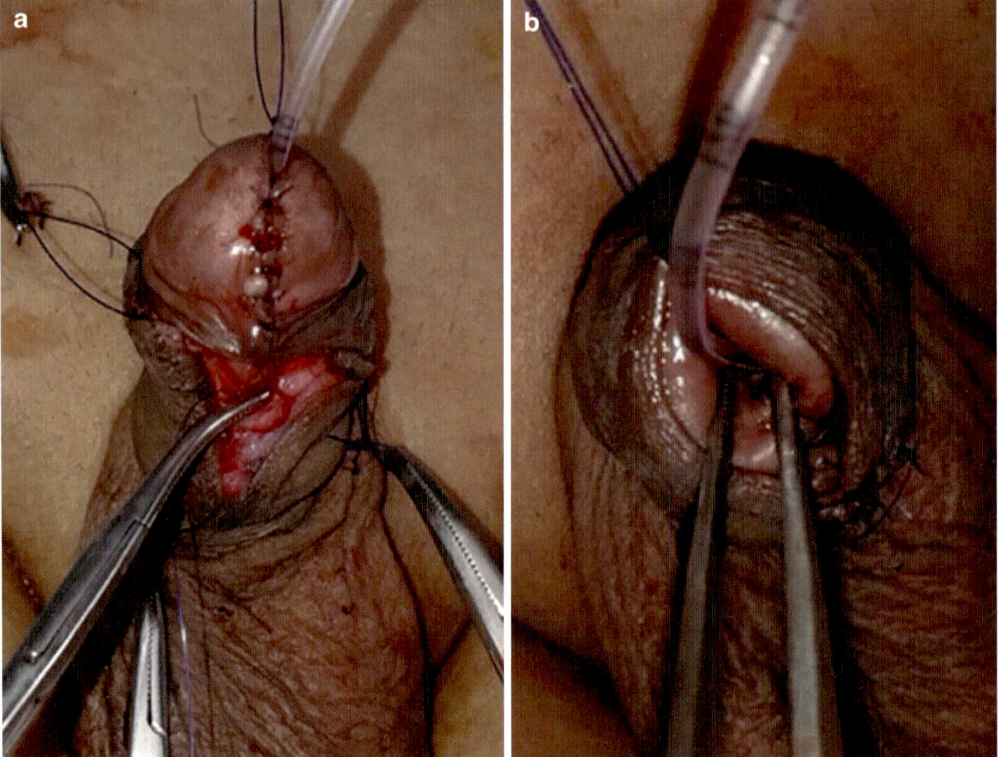

Fig. 8.7 Glanuloplasty. (**a**) Glanuloplasty. (**b**) Wide meatus

8 Modified Tubularized Incised Urethral Plate Urethroplasty

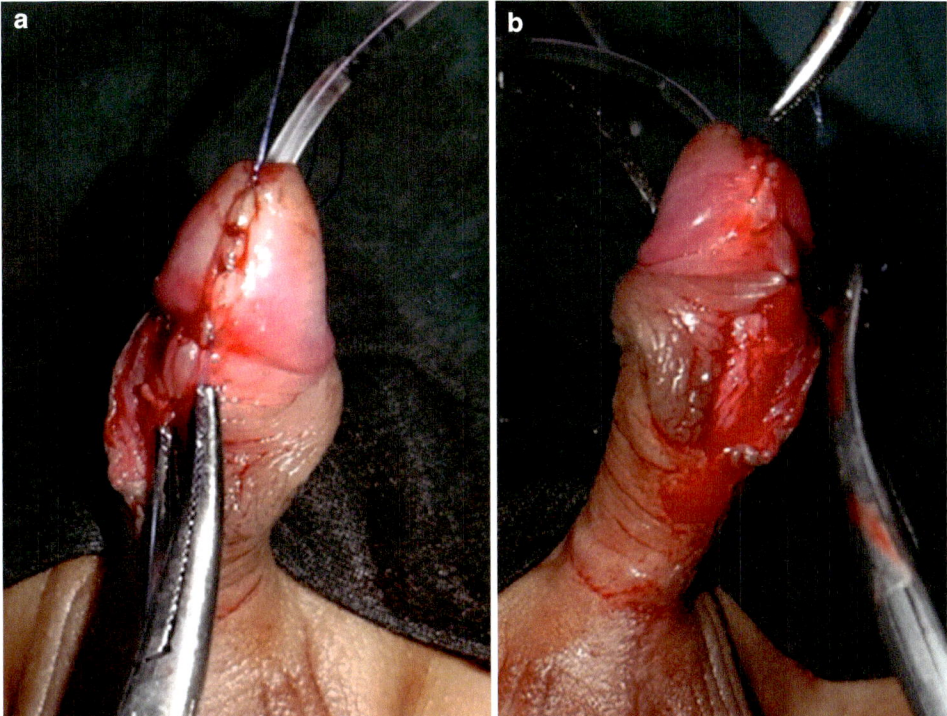

Fig. 8.8 (**a** and **b**) Frenuloplasty

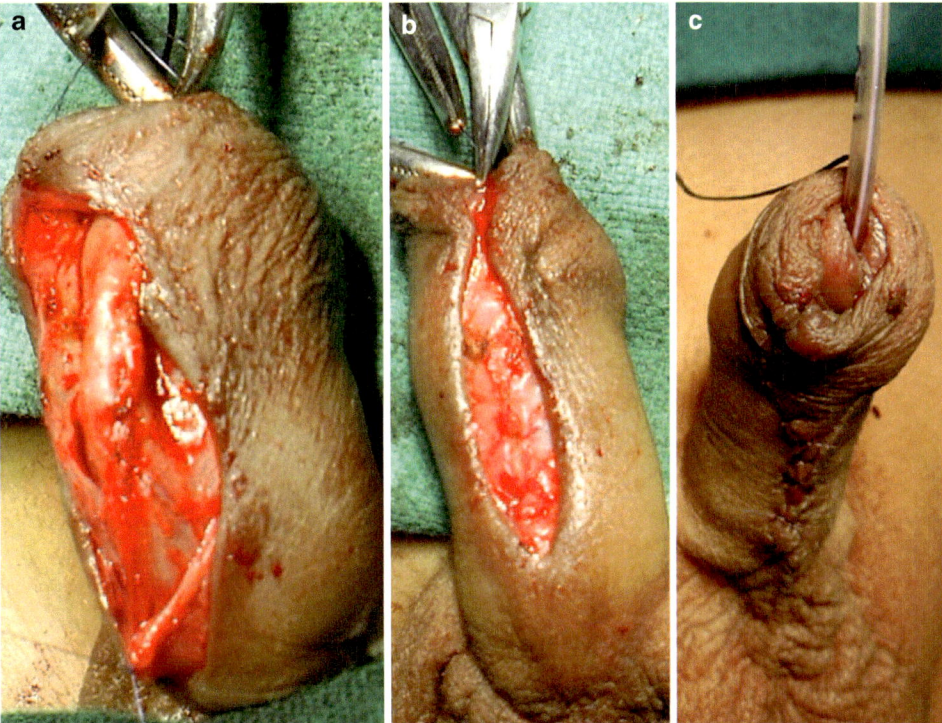

Fig. 8.9 Reconstitution of dartos "Dartosorraphy". (**a**) Dartos suturing started. (**b**) Dartos suturing completed. (**c**) Prepucioplasty and skin closure

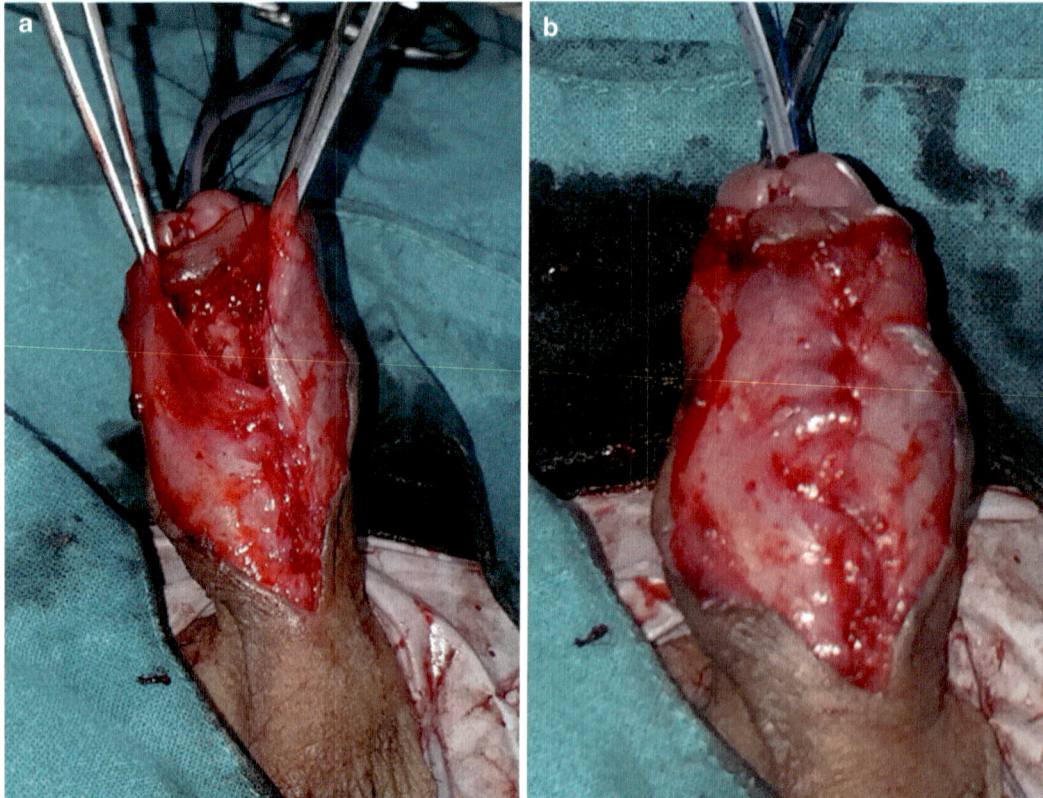

Fig. 8.10 Reconstitution of dartos "Dartosorraphy". (**a**) Dartos suturing halfway down. (**b**) Dartos suturing completed

Even in cases of complete penile degloving, the thick dartos is available, and dartosorraphy is feasible (Fig. 8.10a, b). Then urethral stent is fixed, and a pressure dressing is done. All the steps mentioned above are depicted in Fig. 8.11a–s.

8.3 Modifications

Our Modifications to the original TIPU described by Snodgrass in 1994:

1. Partial penile degloving.
2. Mobilization of spongiosum and urethral plate from bifurcation of spongiosum to mid-glans.
3. Spongioplasty/Double Breasting spongioplasty.
4. Frenuloplasty.
5. Interposing healthy tissue ventral dartos-Dartosorraphy.
6. Prepucioplasty.

Among our TIPU modifications, the mobilization of urethral plate and spongiosum and spongioplasty are the most important ones. The mobilization of urethral plate and spongiosum has the advantages of easy tubularization with or without incising the urethral plate, correcting mild chordee and spongioplasty without any tensions in the suture line. We could tubularize the urethral plate without an incision in 35% of cases [5]. Snodgrass incises the urethral plate deep up to tunica albuginea, but we modified its depth up to superficial spongiosum only, and deeper incisions are supplemented with inner prepucial inlay graft. The incision in these patients of the narrow urethral plate is extended to the glans' tip and covered

8 Modified Tubularized Incised Urethral Plate Urethroplasty

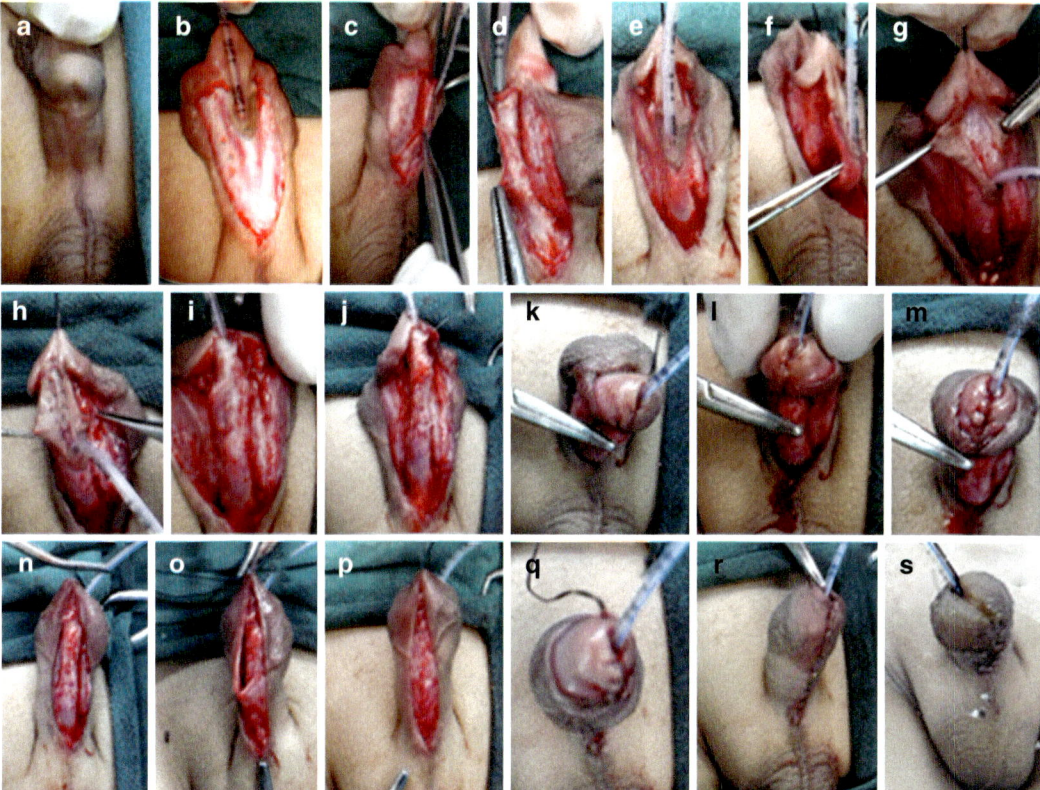

Fig. 8.11 Modified TIPU with inner prepucial dorsal inlay graft. (**a**) Distal penile hypospadias. (**b**) Partial penile degloving. (**c** and **d**) Mobilization of urethral plate and spongiosum up to corona. (**e** and **f**) Mobilization of urethral plate and spongiosum up to mid-glans. (**g**) Incising the urethral plate. (**h**) inner prepucial dorsal inlay graft. (**i**) Tubularization of urethral plate. (**j**) Spongioplasty. (**k** and **l**) Glanuloplasty. (**m**) Frenuloplasty. (**n**) Inner prepucial layer closed for the first layer of Prepucioplasty. (**o** and **p**) Dartosorraphy. (**q** and **r**) Completion of Prepucioplasty. (**s**) Oedema of prepuce on the fifth-day dressing. Post-operative normal looking penis

with a graft to have a wide meatus. This Modification of incising up to the tip of glans is similar to that described by Rama Jayanti. The spongioplasty reconstructs a near-normal urethra, and that is the objective in the hypospadias repair. We mobilize the urethral plate and spongiosum up to mid-glans and spongioplasty is done up to neo-meatus which covers the neo-urethra with spongiosum at corona and helps in prevention of fistula at corona, which is the commonest site of the fistula. We used the concept of mobilization of the urethral plate with spongiosum and proximal urethra and Spongioplasty. Our results of spongioplasty in 2007 in 34 cases of proximal hypospadias were very good and had an acceptable fistula rate of 9% [5]. Later (in 2010 and 2014) we published our results of spongioplasty in all types of hypospadias with an overall fistula rate of 7.40% and 7.96%, respectively, and nil in distal hypospadias with well-developed spongiosum [6, 7]. Recently, we have added the double breasting spongioplasty that almost eliminates the chances of fistula, and the fistula rate was 1.66% only [8]. Snodgrass also added spongioplasty to his original description in 2013 [9]. The addition of frenuloplasty and prepucioplasty reconstructs near-normal penis and operated child may not appreciate whether he has been operated or not and satisfy the parents and the patient (Fig. 8.12a–d). We do penile degloving keeping the plane of dissection at Buck's fascia, So both layers of dartos are available for reconstituting the dartos "dartosorraphy".

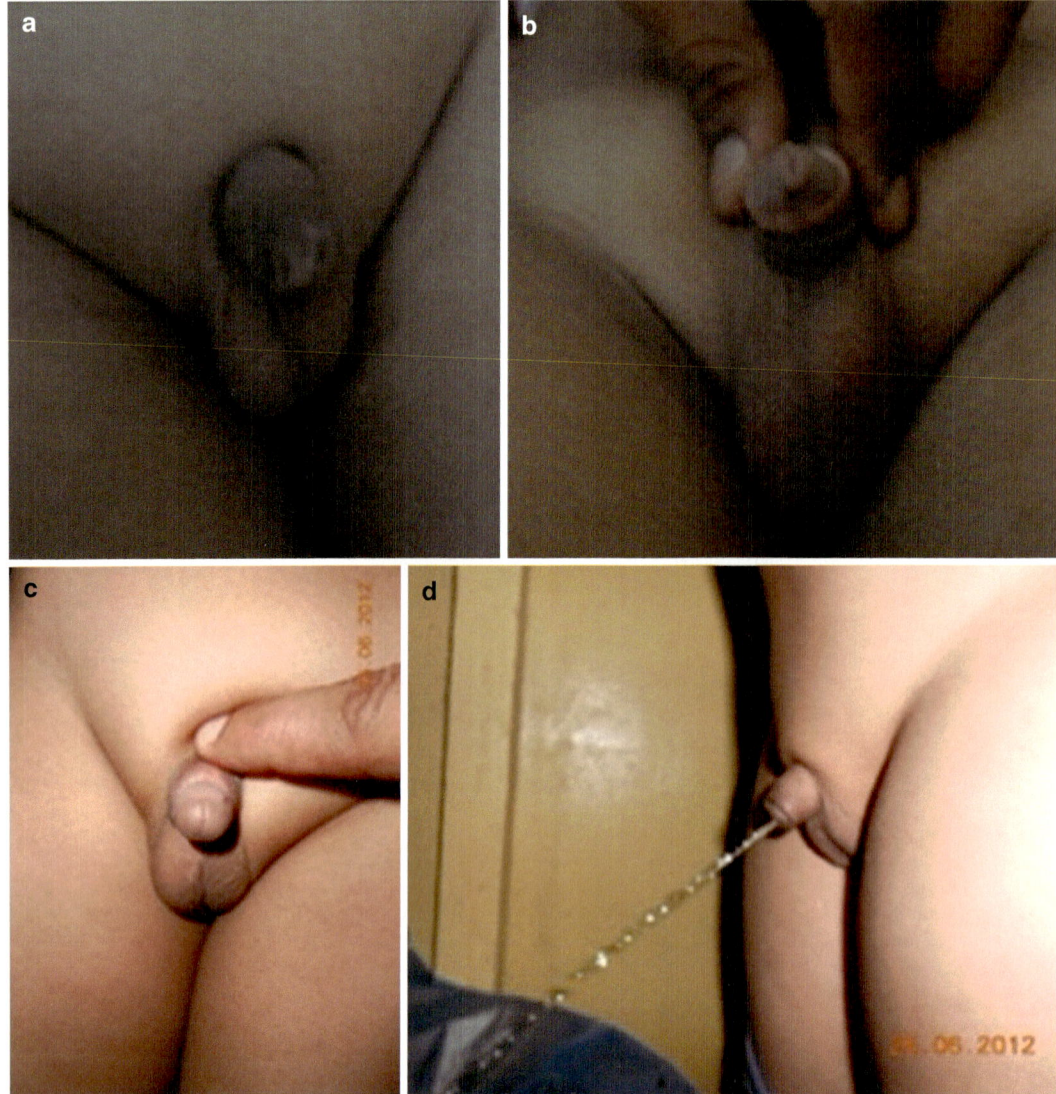

Fig. 8.12 Post-operative picture normal looking penis and projectile stream. (**a**) Penis with prepuce. (**b**) Conical glans with normal-looking meatus at the tip. (**c**) Easily Retractable Prepuce. (**d**) Projectile stream

Which is the second layer of healthy tissue cover over neo-urethra. Using ventral dartos as interposing tissue, we can spare the prepuce for prepucioplasty and avoid the vascular compromise of skin due to dorsal dartos mobilization. We reported our results of prepucioplasty in proximal hypospadias 2010 without increasing the complications of urethroplasty [6] and later on in 2013. Snodgrass also reported similar results after adding prepucioplasty with TIPU in distal hypospadias [9].

8.4 Technical Modification by Snodgrass and Bush [9]

1. Changing from chromic to polyglactin sutures and epithelial to subepithelial suturing.
2. Two-layer subepithelial urethroplasty using interrupted polyglactin and continuous polydioxanone sutures, and adding spongioplasty. A dartos flap again covered the entire repair.

Subsequent outcomes review showed a reduction to 10% fistulas in the next series of patients.
3. In the last published series, a tunica vaginalis flap replaced dartos as the barrier layer, and no fistulas occurred during a mean follow-up of 12 months.
4. Extended dissection of the glans wings, not only at 3 and 9 o'clock but also distally from the corpora for approximately 4 mm diminishes tension subsequent approximation. This Modification reduced glans dehiscence in all primary and re-operative patients from 8% before the Modification to 4% after (p Z 0.039, data not published). Technical modifications to improve outcomes have rarely been reported with other hypospadias repairs.
5. Snodgrass in 2013 added foreskin reconstruction without any change in urethroplasty complications.

8.5 Rama Jayanti Modification

These three modifications improved the results of TIPU [10]

1. The urethral plate is incised from the meatus to the tip of the glans.
2. The urethral plate is tubularized starting at the meatus and working proximally.
3. The meatus is calibrated larger to accept a 10 to 12 Fr Bougie, even before tubularization.

8.6 Discussion

Most of the TIPU modifications had been on covering the neo-urethra with various interposing healthy tissue. The described variations are a local de-epithelialized skin flap, a lateral skin flap, a ventral-based dartos flap, & a double dartos flap. Fistula rate reported was 0 to 26% in various studies. Though a few studies reported reducing fistula rate the double-dartos flaps, Still, a statistically significant difference was only reported by Appignani et al. [11]. Maarouf A M et al. (2012) [12] reported that the fistula rate was higher with a single layer dartos cover (8%) than with a double layer (none) However, the difference was not statistically significant (P = 0.1). Elsayed et al. reported no considerable difference in subsequent urethrocutaneous fistula between a double-layered and single layer dorsal dartos flap cover of the neo-urethra in TIP urethroplasty for repairing hypospadias [13]. We use well mobilized ventral dartos as dartosorraphy. Belman (1988) used the de-epithelialized preputial skin flap as a vascular cover for hypospadias repairs. Belman reported a fistula rate of 3.5% after the wrapping of the neo-urethra with a de-epithelialized preputial skin flap brought ventrally by rotating to the ventrum from the dorsal aspect [14]. Canning and his group recommended antegrade dissection of the dartos pedicle to preserve the dartos fascia's vasculature for covering the TIP repair and the better vascular supply of the attached preputial flap for on lay hypospadias repair. The predominant arteries can be identified by transillumination and followed distally to preserve their fine branches; therefore, the maximum fascial vascularity is preserved [15]. Unification of all these factors in a well-designed prospective randomized and controlled study on sufficient patients followed for an optimal period could give a solid and evidence-based answer to whether multi-layered dartos interposition is superior to a single layer or not.

The most crucial modification has been the addition of dorsal inlay grafts for covering the raw surface of the incised plate with a preputial or buccal mucosal graft. Dorsal inlay graft urethroplasty was first described in redo cases by Kolon and Gonzales in 1998 [16]. Asanuma et al. in 2007 reported the results of dorsal inlay graft urethroplasty for primary hypospadias and achieved good results with a fistula rate of 3.6% [17]. Gundeti et al. 2005 reported good results with augmentation of the narrow urethral plate with dorsal inlay graft in primary cases [18]. Mouravas et al. in 2014 reported a lower rate of meatal stenosis and fistula rate in G-TIP on comparative analysis of TIP and G-TIP in 47 patients. They recommended it as the procedure of choice in patients in primary hypospadias [19]. Gupta et al. (2016) in a prospective study of 263 cases of primary hypospadias incised at the tip of glans was reconstructed successfully in 96% of patients. Irrespective of glans size and degree of hypospadias and the urethral fistula was reported in 3.7% only [20].

8.7 Conclusions

Objective in congenital anomalies is to reconstruct the organ with the existing tissue or supplementation of tissue. The Modification of mobilization of the urethral plate with spongiosum helps in tension-free tubularization. Tubularization of urethral plate and spongiosum reconstructs a near-normal urethra with minimal complication. Long-term complications in middle and posterior hypospadias such as postvoid dribble and retained ejaculate are because of the urethra devoid of spongiosum. Spongioplasty will help to reduce these complications. Adding Frenuloplasty and Prepucioplasty reconstructs prepuce giving the penis a normal appearance. Spongioplasty with dartosorraphy is a perfect healthy interposing tissue layer based on sound surgical principles.

References

1. Rogers B. History of external genital surgery. Plast Reconstruct Surg Genital Area. 1973:3–47.
2. King LR. Hypospadias—a one-stage repair without skin graft based on a new principle: chordee is sometimes produced by the skin alone. J Urol. 1970;103(5):660–2.
3. Zaontz MR. The GAP (glans approximation procedure) for glanular/coronal hypospadias. J Urol. 1989;141(2):359–61.
4. Snodgrass W. Tubularized, incised plate urethroplasty for distal hypospadias. J Urol. 1994;151(2):464–5.
5. Bhat A. Extended urethral mobilization in incised plate urethroplasty for severe hypospadias: a variation in technique to improve chordee correction. J Urol. 2007;178(3):1031–5.
6. Bhat A, Gandhi A, Saxena G, Choudhary GR. Preputial reconstruction and tubularized incised plate urethroplasty in proximal hypospadias with ventral penile curvature. Indian J Urol. 2010;26(4):507.
7. Bhat A, Sabharwal K, Bhat M, Saran R, Singla M, Kumar V. Outcome of tubularized incised plate urethroplasty with spongioplasty alone as additional tissue cover: A prospective study. Indian J Urol. 2014;30(4):392.
8. Bhat A, Bhat M, Kumar R, Bhat A. Double breasting spongioplasty in tubularized/tubularized incise plate urethroplasty: A new technique. Indian J Urol. 2017;33(1):58.
9. Snodgrass W, Dajusta D, Villanueva C, Bush N. Foreskin reconstruction does not increase urethroplasty or skin complications after distal TIP hypospadias repair. J Pediatr Urol. 2013;9(4):401–6.
10. Jayanthi VR. The modified Snodgrass hypospadias repair: reducing the risk of fistula and meatal stenosis. J Urol. 2003;170(4 Part 2):1603–5.
11. Yıldız A, Bertozzi M, Akın M, Appignani A, Prestipino M, Dokucu Aİ. Feasibility of a tubularised incised-plate urethroplasty with double de-epithelised dartos flaps in a failed hypospadias repair: A preliminary report. Afr J Paediatr Surg. 2012;9(1)
12. Maarouf AM, Shalaby EA, Khalil SA, Shahin AM. Single vs double dartos layers for preventing fistula in a tubularised incised-plate repair of distal hypospadias. Arab J Urol. 2012;10(4):408–13.
13. Elsayed ER, Zayed AM, El Sayed D, El Adl M. Interposition of dartos flaps to prevent fistula after tubularized incised-plate repair of hypospadias. Arab J Urol. 2011;9(2):123–6.
14. Belman AB. De-epithelialized skin flap coverage in hypospadias repair. J Urol. 1988;140(5):1273–6.
15. Elbakry A. Tissue interposition in hypospadias repair: a mechanical barrier or healing promoter? Arab J Urol. 2011;9(2):127.
16. Kolon TF, Gonzales ET. The dorsal inlay graft for hypospadias repair. J Urol. 2000;163(6):1941–3.
17. Asanuma H, Satoh H, Shishido S. Dorsal inlay graft urethroplasty for primary hypospadiac repair. Int J Urol. 2007;14(1):43–7.
18. Gundeti M, Queteishat A, Desai D, Cuckow P. Use of an inner preputial free graft to extend the indications of Snodgrass hypospadias repair (Snodgraft). J Pediatr Urol. 2005;1(6):395–6.
19. Mouravas V, Filippopoulos A, Sfoungaris D. Urethral plate grafting improves the results of tubularized incised plate urethroplasty in primary hypospadias. J Pediatr Urol. 2014;10(3):463–8.
20. Gupta V, Yadav SK, Alanzi T, Amer I, Salah M, Ahmed M. Grafted tubularised incised-plate urethroplasty: an objective assessment of outcome with lessons learnt from surgical experience with 263 cases. Arab J Urol. 2016;14(4):299–304.

Single Stage Repair in Proximal Hypospadias

Pramod P. Reddy and Mahakshit Bhat

9.1 Introduction

Hypospadias is a diverse condition with a wide spectrum of clinical phenotypes ranging from a glanular meatus to a perineal meatus with varying degrees of chordee, glanular configurations, and penile skin coverage. It is estimated that approximately 25% of all hypospadias cases will have a proximal meatus and its associated findings, i.e. significant ventral curvature +/− penile torsion, with ventrally deficient shaft skin, a flattened hypoplastic glans, and penoscrotal transposition.

The management of proximal hypospadias has undergone significant evolution over the past few decades based on understanding the results, complications, and long-term clinical outcomes. The treatment strategies evolved based on data and information from expert opinions and retrospective case reports to incorporating more evidence-based medicine into the care algorithms that determine surgical management. From 1960 through the 1970s, there was a preference for two-stage repairs, and then Dr. Duckett popularized urethral substitution with a single-stage repair using a preputial flap tube urethroplasty. Procedures also evolved from urethral substitution (tube urethroplasty) to urethral augmentation (onlay flap urethroplasty), with improved clinical outcomes.

The goals of surgery in the management of a patient with proximal hypospadias include addressing the various components of the clinical phenotype and achieving sustainable optimal functional and cosmetic outcomes; this includes:

- Normalization of penile anatomy.
  - Correction of penile chordee and any associated penile torsion.
  - Address the location of the meatus to enable proper voiding.
  - Achieve normal glans configuration.
    Achieve proper skin coverage of the penis—with either circumcision or preservation of the foreskin if possible, in accordance with the parental request.
  - Address penoscrotal relationship with correction of any transposition.
- Enable the proper function of the reconstructed urethra.
- Anticipate and prepare for changes related to physiological growth and erectile function from infancy to adulthood. There is, on

P. P. Reddy (✉)
Division of Pediatric Urology, Cincinnati Children's, Univ. of Cincinnati College of Medicine, Cincinnati Children's Hospital Medical Center, Cincinnati, OH, USA
e-mail: Pramod.Reddy@cchmc.org

M. Bhat
Department of Urology, National Institute of Medical Sciences Medical College, Jaipur, Rajasthan, India

average, a 320% change in flaccid penile length during this period [1].
- Ensure optimal sexual function to permit painless, penetrative intercourse.
- Allow for optimal body image perception by the patient.

The preference for managing proximal hypospadias has swung from a choice for single-stage repair to most pediatric urologists (76.6%) preferring the two-stage repair over the past decade [2, 3].

There are certainly some significant benefits of a single-stage hypospadias repair as they decrease the burden of care, reduce the cost of treatment, diminished anesthetic risk and therapy duration. However, these benefits may come at the cost of a higher complication rate than two-stage repairs.

A review published in 2010 demonstrated that the complication rates for proximal hypospadias repairs were:

- Single-stage repairs that involved urethral substitution—32-46%.
- Single-stage repairs that involved urethral augmentation or reconfiguration—24.2%.
- Two-stage procedures—22.2%.

9.2 General Principles of Repair

There is no age beyond which it is not safe to undertake the hypospadias repair. However, there is a minimum age at which it is safe to proceed with the repair, and most surgeons would recommend waiting till the child is at least six months old.

The minimal age for undertaking surgery is based on the following patient factors:

- Anesthetic risk [4, 5].
- Anatomy—vascularity improves after mini-puberty [6–8].
- The psychological impact of surgery on the parents of infants [9].

When undertaking the repair of a proximal penile shaft hypospadias, the surgeon has to consider the following:

- Degree of chordee.
- Whether to perform urethral reconstruction, augmentation, or substitution.
- Glansplasty.
- Penoscrotal transposition.
- Skin coverage.

9.3 Proper Assessment of the Chordee

The assessment of penile curvature/chordee is critically important as this is a crucial determinant in the decision to proceed with either a single-stage procedure or a multi-staged procedure.

The intra-operative artificial erection test with injectable saline is the preferred test used to assess the chordee's degree, originally described by Gittes and McLaughlin [10].

There is a consensus among pediatric urologists that chordee greater than 20 degrees is clinically significant and warrants repair [11]. In cases when the proximal hypospadias is associated with greater than 30 degrees of ventral chordee, and the degree of chordee is unchanged after degloving, it is the opinion of this author that these patients should be diverted into a staged repair pathway [12, 13].

I would direct the reader to the chapter dedicated to issues related to Chordee in this textbook for a more comprehensive review of this very important aspect of caring for a child with hypospadias.

9.4 Urethroplasty

The urethroplasty can be achieved with one of the three techniques:

- Tubularization of the existing urethral plate with or without need for incision of the back wall of the urethral plate.
- Augmentation of the existing urethral plate:
  - Grafting the existing urethral plate to permit tension-free tubularization.
  - Transverse island onlay preputial flap (TIOF).
  - Double onlay preputial flap (DOPF).
- Substitution of the existing urethral plate:

- Duckett Procedure (TVIF).
- Asopa-I urethroplasty.
- Koyanagi-Nonomura urethroplasty.

The source of tissue for urethral augmentation or substitution for single-stage repairs of proximal hypospadias includes the following:

- Urethral mobilization, by dissecting and elevating the existing urethra and distal advancement to permit a glanular meatus. The main disadvantage of this option is a bias towards the inadequate treatment of chordee. If the chordee does recur, it will cause the urethroplasty to fail [14].
- Penile shaft skin distal to the existing meatus.
- Skin proximal to the existing meatus.
- Preputial skin.

  - Skin graft to form neourethra [15].
  - Skin flap to form neourethra [14, 16–27].

Surveys of practicing Pediatric Urologists and Pediatric Surgeons indicate that when caring for a patient with less than 30 degrees of ventral chordee, 51% prefer a single-stage procedure to preserve the urethral plate. Among the single-stage procedures, 43% would perform a TIP procedure, and 10–30% of them would use the TVIF procedure to correct a proximal hypospadias [2, 3].

9.5 Urethral Tubularization Procedures

9.5.1 TIP Procedure (Figs 9.1a–i)

In a few cases of proximal hypospadias where there is minimal chordee (<30 degrees) and a healthy urethral plate that extends into the glans, an extended TIP procedure can be considered [28]. After an initial enthusiasm for this procedure as a single-stage repair for such cases, this was tempered by the long-term results that showed recurrent chordee and fistulas [29].

In the instance where the anatomy is conducive, one may perform a TIP repair following the distal TIP repair principles.

- Degloving of the penis using a circumcising incision and preservation of the dorsal blood supply. The incision may be modified in those cases where the family has requested foreskin preservation (Fig. 9.1a–c).
- Mobilization of the divergent spongiosal tissue along the length of the urethral plate for later use in the spongioplasty to cover the tubularized urethral plate (Fig. 9.1d, e).
- Assessment of ventral chordee with artificial erection test and if less than 30 degrees, proceed with single-stage repair and correction of the chordee with dorsal plication(s). If more than two plications are required to achieve an orthotopic penis—the surgeon may have to reconsider the choice of a single-stage repair.
- Creation of glans wings—the spongiosal flaps should be mobilized so that they create a 90-degree angle with the urethral plate; this will permit tension-free closure of the glans (Fig. 9.1e).
- Deep midline incision of the urethral plate to permit two-layer tubularization of the urethra in a tension free manner. It is important to stop the tubularization approximately 2–3 mm from the distal end of the urethral plate to reduce risk of meatal stenosis (Fig. 9.1f).
- The urethral plate's tubularization is performed with interrupted sutures for the initial layer and running sutures for the second layer. This should be performed around a stent (caliber depends on the age of the patient at the time of surgery - I typically use a 6 Fr stent in infants).
- Spongioplasty, reconfiguration of the divergent spongiosum ventral to the reconstructed urethra—Y to I reconfiguration [30–34] (Fig. 9.1g).
- Glanuloplasty: Suturing the glans wings to reapproximate them in the ventral midline with adequate space between the neourethra and glans wings (Fig. 9.1h).
- Harvesting of a tunica vaginalis flap from one of the testis and reinforcement of the urethroplasty as a vascularized barrier flap. It is important to mobilize the tunica vaginalis along the spermatic cord adequately, otherwise, it can cause penile torsion.

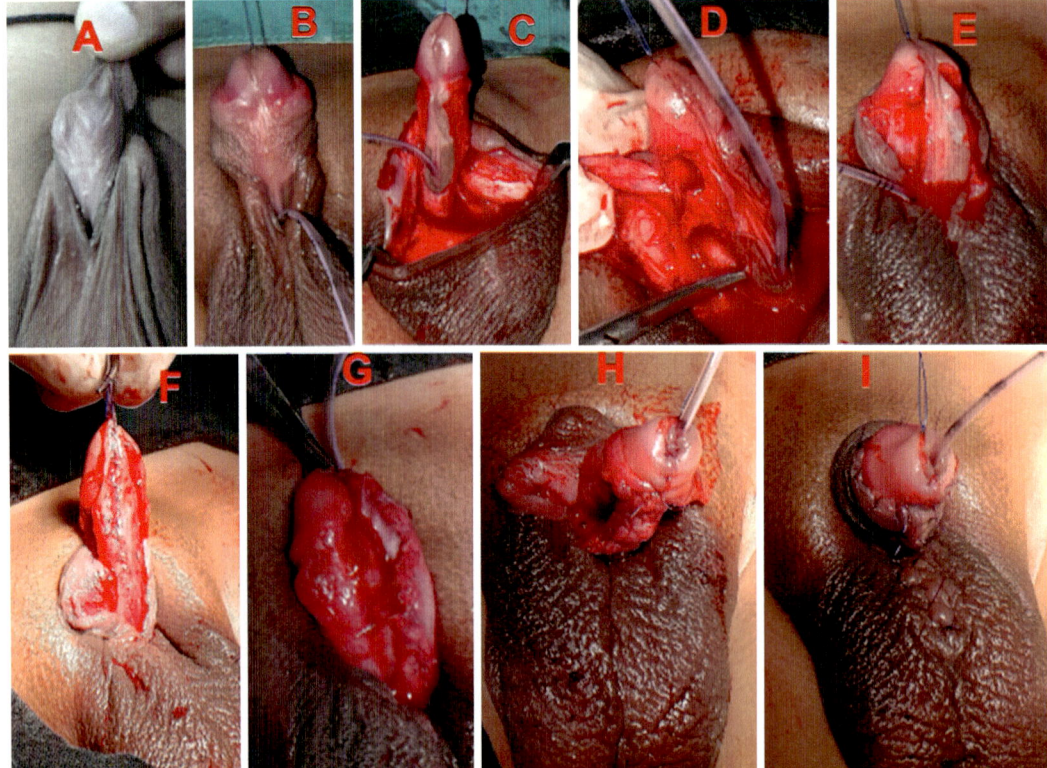

Fig. 9.1 Demonstrates the TIP urethroplasty technique for treating proximal hypospadias. (**a** & **b**). Penoscrotal hypospadias. (**c**). Penile degloving. (**d**). Incising the urethral plate. (**e**). Mobilization of urethral plate into glans. (**f**). Tubularization of urethral plate. (**g**). Spongioplasty. (**h**). Glansplasty. (**i**). Skin closure

- Skin coverage, this is an often over looked aspect of hypospadias surgery, it is important to bear in mind that attention to detail and ensuring an aesthetically pleasing skin coverage of the reconstructed penis will result in high patient and parental satisfaction as the child grows (Fig. 9.1i).

- The use of intermediate protective barrier layers between the urethra and the skin has been shown to reduce the risk of complications, in particular the occurrence of fistulae. The principles to be followed with respect to this layer, whether it be spongiosal tissue, local dartos tissue, or a tunica vaginalis flap are that it: (1) provides mechanical support to the reconstructed urethra, (2) brings neovascularity that aids in healing and (3) prevents directly overlapping suture lines. Snodgrass has shown that by incorporating a tunica vaginalis barrier flap, spongioplasty, and a two-layer closure for the urethroplasty, he has significantly reduced his fistula rate for proximal TIP procedures [28]. The initial reports of outcomes after the TIP procedure for proximal hypospadias demonstrated a complication rate of approximately 24.2%; this included a 20% incidence of fistula/dehiscence and a 3% rate of stricture/meatal stenosis.

9.6 Urethral Augmentation Procedures

9.6.1 Grafted-Tubularized Incised Plate (G-TIP) [35] Also Known as Single Primary Stage Dorsal Inlay Urethroplasty (Fig. 9.2a–h)

This procedure is performed in the same manner as a regular Tubularized Incised Plate (TIP) repair, with one additional step, using either a prepucial or buccal mucosa graft to augment the existing urethral plate after incising it dorsally [35]. This modification of the TIP procedure has expanded the indications for a TIP repair in proximal hypospadias cases, to even include cases where previously the existing urethral plate may have been deemed to be too narrow to permit a tension-free tubularization <8 mm [36].

Steps of the procedure:

- Degloving of the penis using a circumcising incision and preservation of the dorsal blood supply. The incision may be modified in those cases where the family has requested foreskin preservation and prepucial reconstruction (Fig. 9.2a, b).
- Mobilization of the divergent spongiosal tissue along the length of the urethral plate for later use in the spongioplasty to cover the tubularized urethral plate.
- Assessment of ventral chordee with artificial erection test and if less than 30 degrees, proceed with single-stage repair and correction of the chordee with dorsal plication(s). If more than two plications are required to achieve an orthotopic penis—the surgeon may have to reconsider the choice of a single-stage repair (Fig. 9.2b).
- Creation of glans wings—the spongiosal flaps should be mobilized so that they create a 90-degree angle with the urethral plate; this will permit tension-free closure of the glans.
- Deep dorsal midline incision of the entire urethral plate, that stops approximately 3 mm from the distal end to reduce the risk of meatal stenosis. As shown in Fig. 9.2c, it is important to make a deep incision in the urethra plate such that the two halves of the ure-

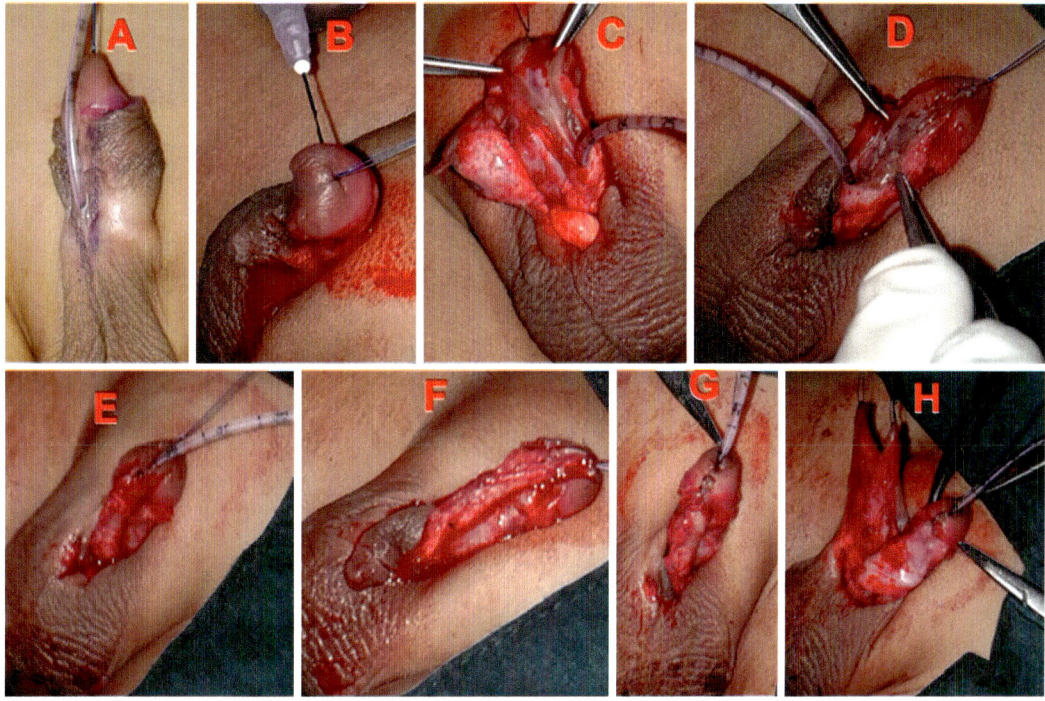

Fig. 9.2 Demonstrates the dorsal inlay graft technique. (**a**). Proximal penile hypospadias. (**b**). Checking the degree of chordee after penile degloving and mobilization of the existing urethra. (**c**). Incising the urethral plate. (**d**). Dorsal inlay graft. (**e**). Tubularization of the augmented urethral plate. (**f**). Spongioplasty. (**g**). Glanuloplasty. (**h**). Covering the tubularized urethra with dorsal dartos flaps

thral plate can be easily drawn apart—this dissection and the gap are dependent on the width of the existing urethral plate, need at least 14–16 mm total width (urethral plate + graft) to permit an adequate tension-free urethroplasty.
- Measure the length of the defect in the urethral plate and harvest an adequate sized graft from either the inner layer of the prepuce or from the inner aspect of the lip in cases where the child has been circumcised, or the family has requested a foreskin preserving procedure.
- The graft is laid into the defect in the urethral plate, the lateral edges of the graft are secured to the urethral plate with monofilament interrupted sutures, and the graft is quilted to the underlying corporal tissue (Fig. 9.2d).
- The grafted urethral plate is then tubularized with interrupted sutures for the initial layer and running sutures of the 2nd layer. This should be performed around a stent (caliber depends on the age of the patient at the time of surgery, in infants, I usually will perform this portion of the procedure around a 8 Fr feeding tube, but replace it with a 6 Fr stent that will remain during the post-operative healing) (Fig. 9.2e).
- Spongioplasty, reconfiguration of the divergent spongiosum ventral to the reconstructed urethra—Y to I reconfiguration (Fig. 9.2f) [30–34].
- Glanuloplasty: Suturing the glans wings with adequate space between the neourethra and glans wings (Fig. 9.2g).
- Harvesting dorsal dartos flap to cover the neourethra (Fig. 9.2h) or harvesting of a tunica vaginalis flap from one of the testis and using this to reinforce the urethroplasty as a vascularized barrier flap. It is important to mobilize the tunica vaginalis along the spermatic cord adequately, failure to do so can cause penile torsion.
- Skin coverage.

9.6.2 Onlay Transverse Island Preputial Flap (TVIF)

In instances where there is favorable anatomy for a single-stage repair, i.e. healthy skin, less than 30-degree ventral chordee, and an intact urethral plate, one can consider the onlay transverse island flap (TVIF) [17, 37] using prepucial skin to augment the existing urethral plate. This is a useful technique where the urethral plate is not wide enough or healthy enough (i.e., elastic) to permit a TIP procedure. The technique evolved as a modification of the tubularized transverse island flap described by Duckett.

Steps of the procedure:

- Degloving of the penis with a circumcising incision—preserve the dorsal blood supply and also the urethral plate—allow for a minimum of 8 mm of the urethral plate to be left intact.
- Intra-operative artificial erection test, if less than 30 degrees ventral chordee, correct with dorsal plication (if greater than 30 degrees, optimal results may be achieved with a staged procedure).
- Apply the tourniquet at the base of the shaft and create glans wings.
- In patients that have a prominent lip at the distal end of the glanular groove, this can be addressed with a Heineke-Mikulicz maneuver that eliminates the lip, deepens the glans groove, and extends the neourethra to the tip of the glans.
- Cut back on the existing urethra till a healthy urethra with healthy supporting corpus spongiosum is encountered. This ensures a wide proximal anastomosis and reduces the risk of an anastomotic stricture.
- Harvest a rectangular flap from the inner prepucial tissue along with its vascular pedicle. The length of the longer side is determined by the length of the urethra to be reconstructed.
- The flap is rotated to the ventrum and anastomosed to the urethral plate. The rethrocutaneous suture line is covered with a second layer

that incorporates the vascular pedicle of the flap (Fig. 9.3a–c).
- Closure of the glans wings and glansplasty, as shown in Fig. 9.3d, e.
- Skin coverage (Fig. 9.3f).

9.6.3 Double Onlay Preputial Flap (DOPF)

Holland and Smith reported that when the urethral plate is less than 8 mm in width, there is a higher complication rate when such a plate is tubularized, i.e. fistulae and wound dehiscence [36]. The Double Onlay Preputial Flap (DOPF) [38] technique of hypospadias repair can be utilized in cases of proximal hypospadias that meet the following criteria:

- Have minimal chordee.
- Have healthy penile skin and have not been circumcised.
- Urethral plate is <8 mm in width.
- Conical or flat glans penis.

Steps of the procedure:

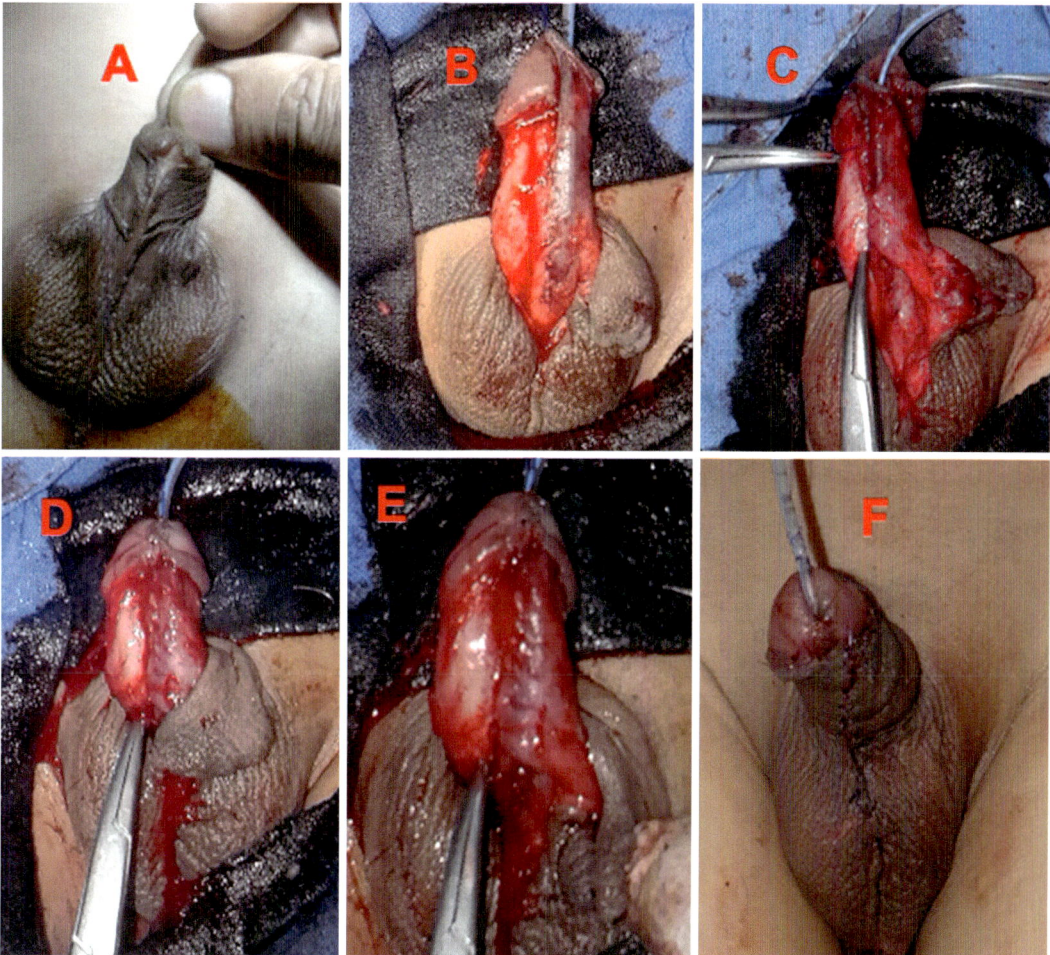

Fig. 9.3 Demonstrates the dorsal transverse island onlay flap technique. (**a**). Proximal penile hypospadias Narrow urethral plate. (**b**). Penile degloving and partial sutured island flap. (**c**). Onlay flap sutured up to meatus. (**d**). Glansplasty. (**e**). Covering the neourethra with dorsal dartos flap taking few sutures in the pedicle. (**f**). skin closure and final intra-operative result

- Place a traction suture through the glans penis.
- Make a "U" shaped incision around the existing urethral plate and the current meatus.
- Circumcising incision is performed, leaving a 5 mm glans cuff.
- The penis is then degloved down to the penopubic and penoscrotal junctions.
- Artificial erection test (Gittes test) is performed, and if any significant chordee present (between 10–30 degrees), this is corrected with dorsal plications or Nesbit procedure, (if the chordee is greater than 30 degrees, optimal results may be achieved with a staged procedure).
- A tourniquet is then applied, and glans wings are then created, ensuring a urethral plate of uniform width from the original meatus to the location of the neomeatus in the glans penis.
- The prepuce is then divided vertically into two transverse segments (one being 2/3rd the width of the prepuce and the other being 1/3rd the width).
- The larger prepucial segment (2/3rd of the prepuce) is rotated around the right side of the penile shaft to the ventral aspect and oriented vertically. It is then trimmed to the desired dimensions, and a two-layer anastomosis of the flap to the urethral plate is performed around a urethral catheter.
- The glans wings are then approximated over the neourethra distally, leaving a 2–3 mm gap at the proximal aspect of the glans.
- The 1/3rd segment of the prepucial flap is now rotated around the left side of the penile shaft and trimmed to a triangle-shaped flap that is sutured to the glans over the neourethra.
- Skin coverage.

9.7 Urethral Substitution Procedures

9.7.1 The Duckett, Transverse Preputial Island Flap Technique [Figs. 9.4a–g and 9.5a–i, 9.6a–g]

In 1980, Duckett published his technique for a single-stage procedure intended to treat those patients in whom 2–6 cm of urethra needed to be created after the release of chordee and excision of the original urethral plate [17–19, 39].

Steps of the procedure:

- Circumcising incision is performed leaving a 5 mm glans cuff and circumscribes the existing urethral meatus on the ventral aspect of the penis.
- The penis is then degloved down to the penopubic and penoscrotal junctions (Figs. 9.4a, b, 9.5a, b).
- The native urethral tissue and any ventral chordee tissue are sharply excised (Fig. 9.4b, 9.5c).
- Artificial erection test (Gittes test) is performed (Fig. 9.6a, b) and if any significant chordee present (between 10 and 30 degrees), this is corrected with dorsal plications or Nesbit procedure.
- Required length of urethra and inner prepucial flap length are measured (Figs. 9.5d, e, 9.6c).
- The creation of a vascularized neourethra is undertaken. Holding sutures are placed in the dorsal prepuce's skin, and tension maintained on the ventral aspect of the prepuce. The neourethral flap is marked out to be 15 mm wide, and as long as the defect from the existing meatus to the tip of the glans.
- The outlined flap is dissected, maintaining the blood supply intact, and then rolled into a urethra over a 10 or 12 Fr catheter (depending on the age of the patient), a combination of running sutures in the middle of the flap and interrupted sutures on the ends to permit trimming of the tube as needed (Figs. 9.4c, 9.5f).
- Dissection between the dorsal prepucial skin and the tubularized flap ensuring a generous vascularized pedicle to the flap is carried about 2/3rd of the way down the penile shaft to enable transposition of the flap to the ventrum of the penile shaft (Fig. 9.4d).
- The flap is then transposed to the ventrum by wrapping around one side of the penile shaft (usually on the right side, based on surgeon preference) (Figs. 9.5h, 9.6c) Alternatively, this can be achieved by carefully creating a buttonhole in the vascular pedicle and passing the glans penis and shaft through this opening

9 Single Stage Repair in Proximal Hypospadias

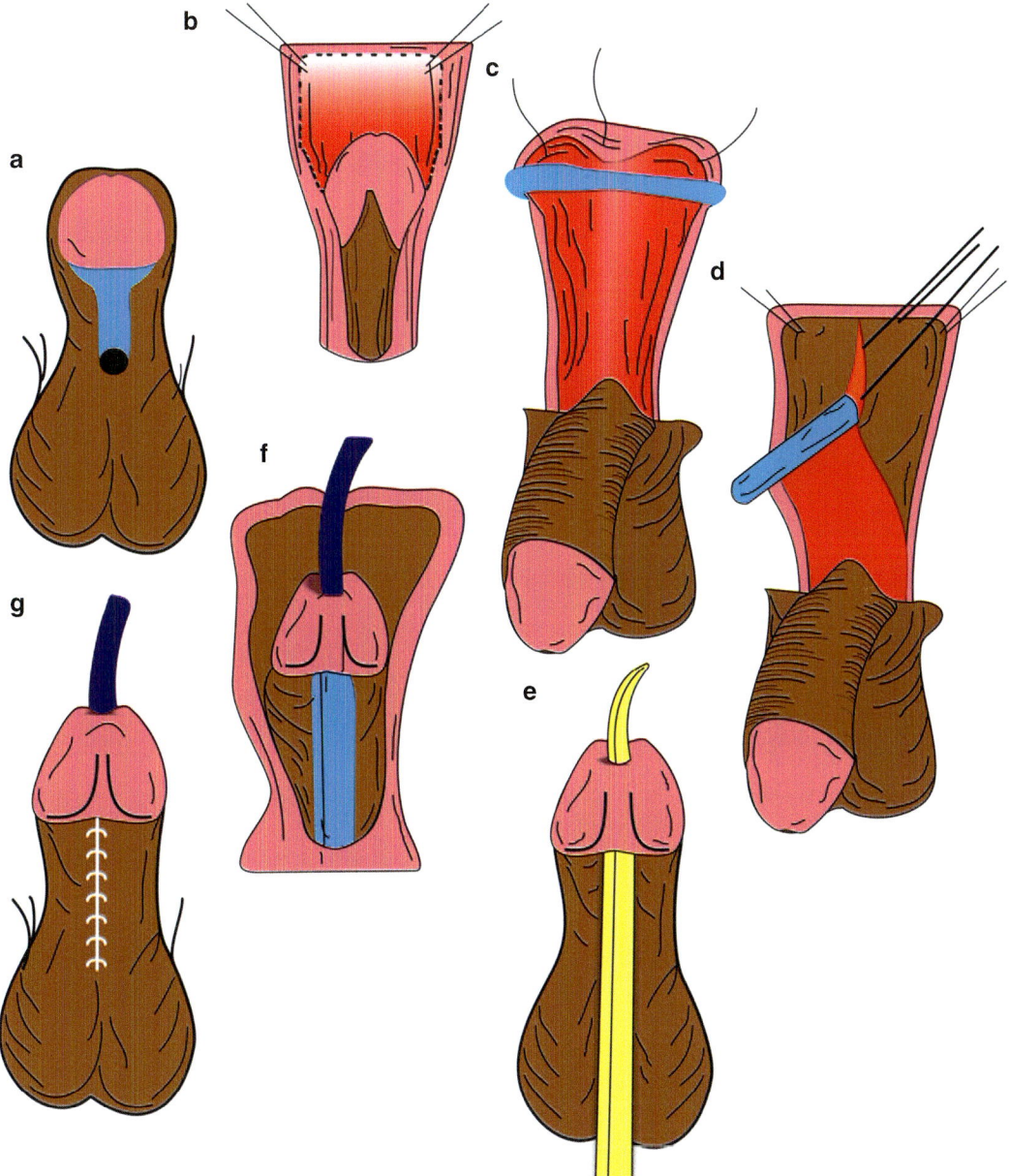

Fig. 9.4 Demonstrates the inner prepucial flap repair for severe hypospadias. (**a**). Proximal hypospadias. (**b**). Penile degloving and correction of chordee. (**c**). Mobilization of inner prepucial flap. (**d**). Tubularization of prepucial flap. (**e**). Creating a Tunnel in the glans. (**f**). Proximal and distal anastomosis of skin tube with stent in situ. (**g**) Skin closure

to allow for ventral transposition of the tubularized neourethra.
- The flap is then anastomosed to the proximal urethral meatus, ensuring that the spongiosum is included in the anastomosis (Figs. 9.5g, 9.6e).
- A glans penis channel is then created by sharply dissecting into the glans, such that the

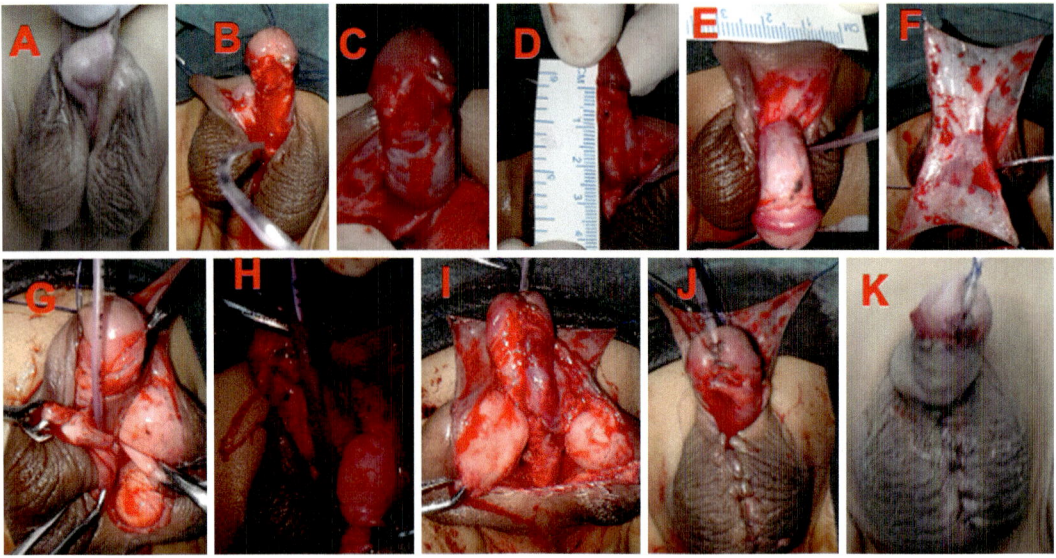

Fig. 9.5 Demonstrates the inner prepucial flap repair in scrotal hypospadias. (**a**). Scrotal hypospadias. (**b**). Penile degloving. (**c**). Correction of chordee. (**d**). Measuring the required urethral length. (**e**). Measuring the length of inner prepucial flap. (**f**). Mobilization of inner prepucial flap. (**g**). Anastomosis of skin flap with the urethra. (**h**). Tubularization of inner prepucial skin flap. (**i**). Anastomosis of skin tube to glans, covering the skin tube with dartos. (**j**). Glansplasty. (**k**). Skin closure

neomeatus is just superior to the level of the blind-ending glanular pit. A button of glanular tissue is then sharply excised (Fig. 9.4e).
- The glanular channel is calibrated with a 14 Fr urethral sound.
- The tubularized neourethra is pulled through the glans channel and gently pulled taut to avoid any kinking in the neourethra (avoid pulling too hard as this can result in secondary chordee). The excess tube is then excised, and the tube is anastomosed to the glans with interrupted sutures (Fig. 9.3f). Alternatively glans wing are raised and skin tube is sutured to the margins of the glans and then glansplasty is done (Figs. 9.4i, 9.5e, f).
- Skin coverage, in the majority of cases, adequate skin is available for penile resurfacing (Figs. 9.4g, 9.5k & 9.6g) but in patients where there is a paucity of penile shaft skin, the Cecil–Culp maneuver has been utilized with satisfactory results.

9.7.2 The Asopa-I Repair

Asopa initially described the Asopa technique in 1971 [16, 40]. Similar to results with other techniques that deployed vascularized pedicle tube repairs, long-term follow-ups of patients managed with this procedure were noted to have diverticula formation. The tubularized preputial repairs do not provide a stable foundation for the neourethra on the underlying tunica albuginea. During voiding, there is some mobility of the entire neourethra, resulting in turbulent flow of urine within the neourethra, the eddy currents created result in varying degrees of tension being exerted on the wall of the neourethra and result in diverticula formation. In 2010, the modified Asopa-I repair was proposed [41]. The modifications included fixation of the neourethral edges to the underlying tunica albuginea, to reduce the risk of diverticula formation.

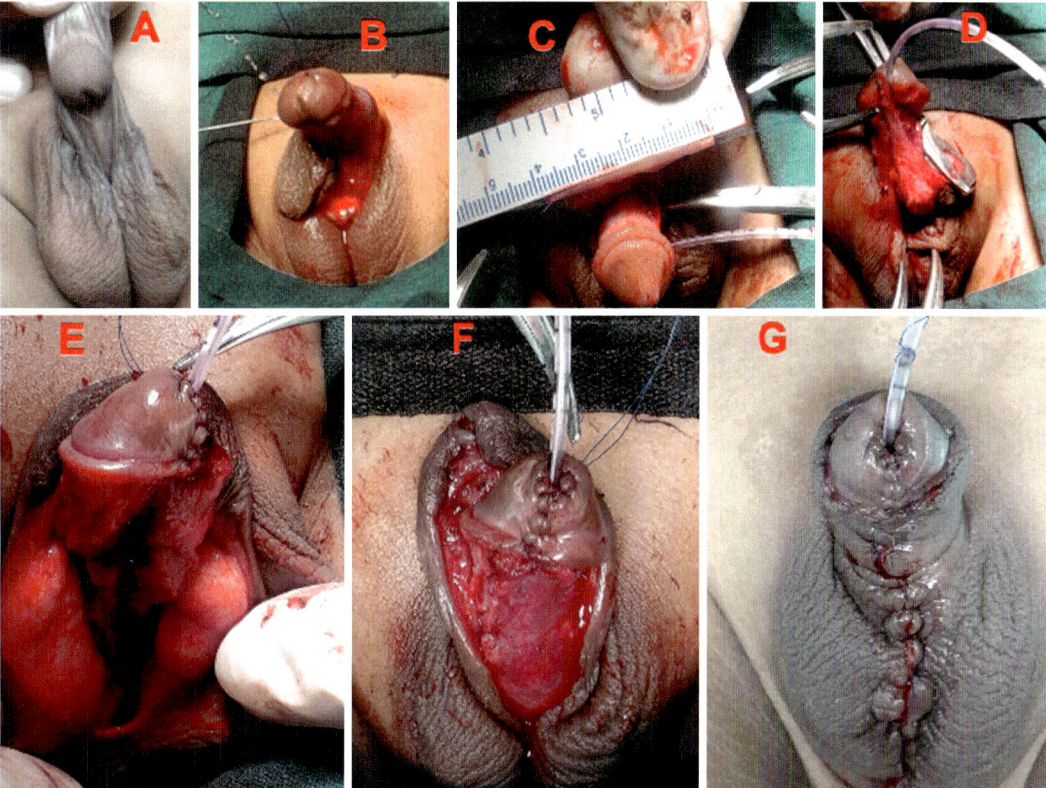

Fig. 9.6 Demonstrates the inner prepucial flap repair in penoscrotal hypospadias. (**a**). Penoscrotal hypospadias. (**b**). Gittes test after penile degloving and resection of chordee tissue. (**c**). Measuring the length of inner prepucial flap. (**d**). Anastomosis of skin flap with the urethra. (**e**). Anastomosis of skin tube to glans and glansplasty. (**f**). Covering the skin tube with dartos; Tubularized inner prepucial skin tube brought ventrally from left side. (**g**). Skin closure

Steps of the procedure:

- A subcoronal, racquet-shaped incision down the ventral aspect of the penis is created incorporating the existing meatus.
- The penis is then degloved down to the penopubic and penoscrotal junctions.
- Artificial erection test (Gittes test) is performed, and if any significant chordee present (between 10 and 30 degrees), this is corrected with dorsal plications or Nesbit procedure.
- A tourniquet is then applied, and glans wings are then created.
- An inner prepucial flap based on the superficial dorsal penile vessels is marked out and then separated from the outer preputial skin by sharp dissection.
- An oblique cut at the junction of the right-sided (2/3rd) and left (1/3rd) segments of the penile shaft skin, being careful to preserve the blood supply.
- The cranial margin of the inner prepucial flap is dissected from the vascular pedicle—this margin will function as a free graft.
- The caudal margin of the inner prepucial flap is circumferentially anastomosed to the proximal urethra, and then the flap is anchored to the penile shaft using absorbable sutures along the entire length of the neourethra into the glans.
- The flap is then tubularized over a stent.
- An additional row of sutures between the dartos of tubularized preputial flap and the tunica is now placed to ensure secure attachment of

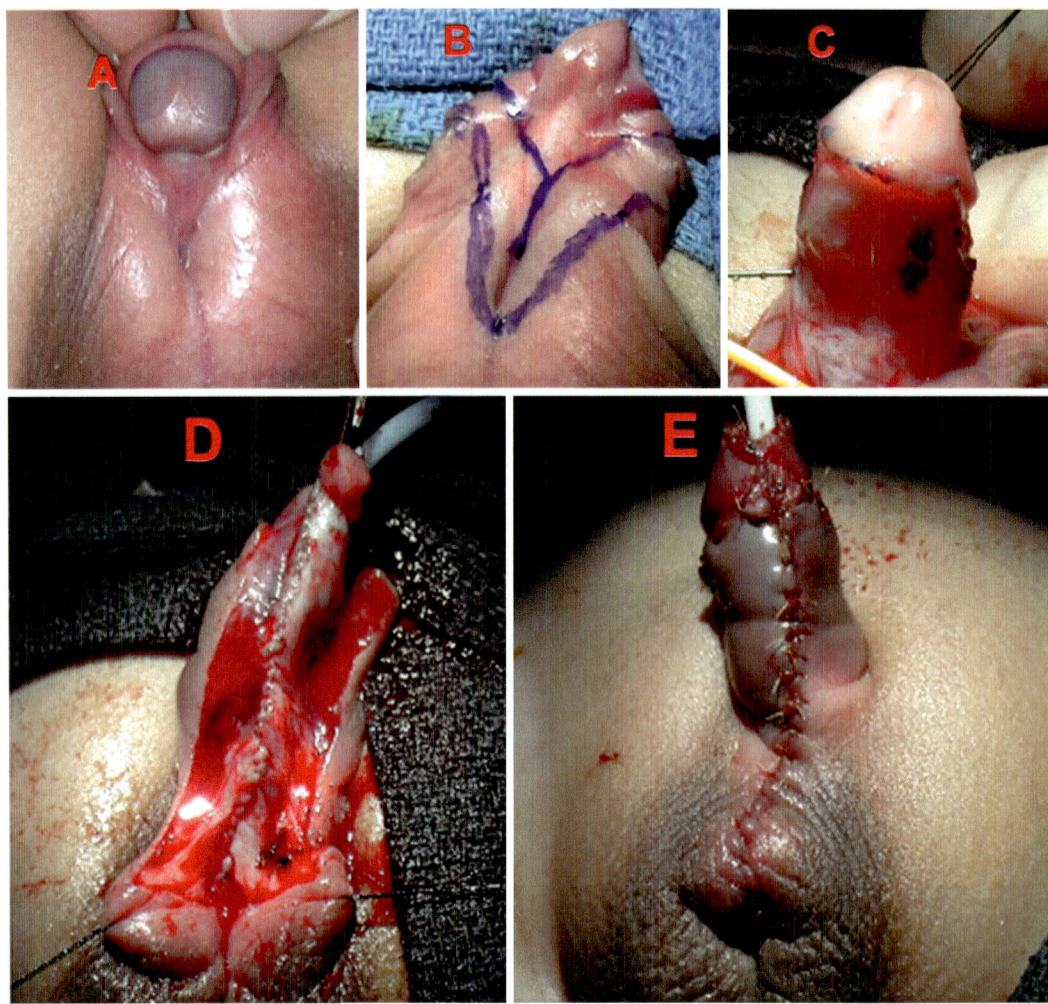

Fig. 9.7 Demonstrating the Koyanagi–Nonomura urethroplasty in proximal hypospadias. (**a**). Scrotal hypospadias and chordee. (**b**). Skin markings for Koyanagi–Nonomura urethroplasty. (**c**). Correction of chordee by excision of urethral plate and chordee tissue on ventrum of the penis. (**d**). Urethroplasty completed. (**e**). Completed Koyanagi–Nonomura hypospadias repair with orthotopic penis and distal glanular meatus

the neourethra to the underlying penile shaft (this is to reduce the risk of sacculation and diverticula formation).
- The glans wings are then approximated over the neourethra.
- Skin coverage.

9.7.3 The Koyanagi–Nonomura 1 Stage Bucket Repair

The repair initially described by Koyanagi and Nonomura has been modified to optimize the clinical outcomes [24, 42–44]. The steps of the modified procedure include the following:

- Create a circumferential incision around the glans, approximately 0.8 cm from the coronal sulcus (Fig. 9.7a, b).
- The existing urethral plate is proximally circumscribed in a "U" shaped manner.
- The incision around the urethral plate is carried parallel to the initial circumcising incision; when the flap of skin is freed up, it has the appearance of a bucket handle.
- The penile shaft skin is now degloved.

- Create glans wings.
- Correct the chordee (Fig. 9.7c).
- The medial aspects of the two limbs that make up the bucket handle are sewn together (7–0 PDS) and create a neourethra (Fig. 9.7d).
- The neourethra is formed by the skin tube.
- The glans wings are closed around the neourethra (Fig. 9.7e).
- Correct any penoscrotal transposition (Glenn and Anderson technique).
- Skin closure using Byar's flaps (Fig. 9.7e).

9.7.4 Skin Coverage

Planning for and ensuring adequate skin coverage at the culmination of the repair is important and has to be something that is proactively considered when making the initial incisions. In cases of proximal hypospadias, there is typically redundant dorsal hooded foreskin and ventral deficiency of skin. When achieving penile shaft skin coverage at the end of the procedure, ensuring a tension-free closure with the symmetric distribution of skin will reduce the risk of acquired penile curvature from skin tethering as the repair heals. In most cases, ventral midline skin closure can be achieved; however, if this cannot be accomplished, Byar's skin flaps can be used.

Preserving the foreskin as part of the hypospadias repair can be either due to parental preference or cultural practice. In single-stage repairs for proximal hypospadias, the foreskin can be preserved; however, this has to be determined at the onset of the procedure as foreskin preserving incisions are different to an incision that accounts for a circumcision to be performed as part of the procedure [Fig. 9.8a–e]. The actual parental satisfaction and complication rate of preserving the foreskin in these cases remains unknown due to infrequent reports in the literature.

9.7.5 Penoscrotal Transposition

The penoscrotal transposition associated with proximal penile shaft hypospadias is almost always partial but can be extensive in some cases. This can be corrected at the time of the single-stage repair or undertaken as a separate procedure after healing the hypospadias repair. The repair consists of creating rotational skin flaps encompassing the scrotal skin and rotating them inferior to the penile shaft. The technique described by Glenn and Anderson provides an excellent cosmetic result [45]. The Koyanagi–Nonomura single-stage bucket repair is also an option as it permits the correction of the penoscrotal transposition at the hypospadias repair time [46]. Postoperative results show meatus at the tip and good cosmetic results (Fig. 9.9a–c).

9.7.6 Stents/Dressings

Urinary diversion after a single-stage repair is the norm. When performing this procedure in children who are not yet toilet trained, we place a fenestrated urethral stent into the bladder and secure it to the glans with stay stitches. One can choose to cut the stent short as a drip stent, have it drip into the diaper, or leave it longer and teach the parents the double diaper technique. I recommend that the parents apply Vaseline as a barrier cream to protect the skin from an infection resulting in dehiscence.

For those children who are already toilet trained, we prefer to place a suprapubic tube at the time of the repair and continuously drain the bladder. We do leave a stent across the repair but do not place it proximal to the sphincter, thereby avoiding the need to place the older child in a diaper. The catheter is left in place for 10–14 days and is usually removed in the clinic after assessing the wound.

The nature of dressings after hypospadias is as varied as the number of operations. I have been using Cyanoacrylate dressing (Dermabond) for the past ten years and reinforcing this with a Coban wrap [47, 48]. The wrap is removed after 24 hrs, and the Dermabond is allowed to dissolve and separate (usually 4–7 days).

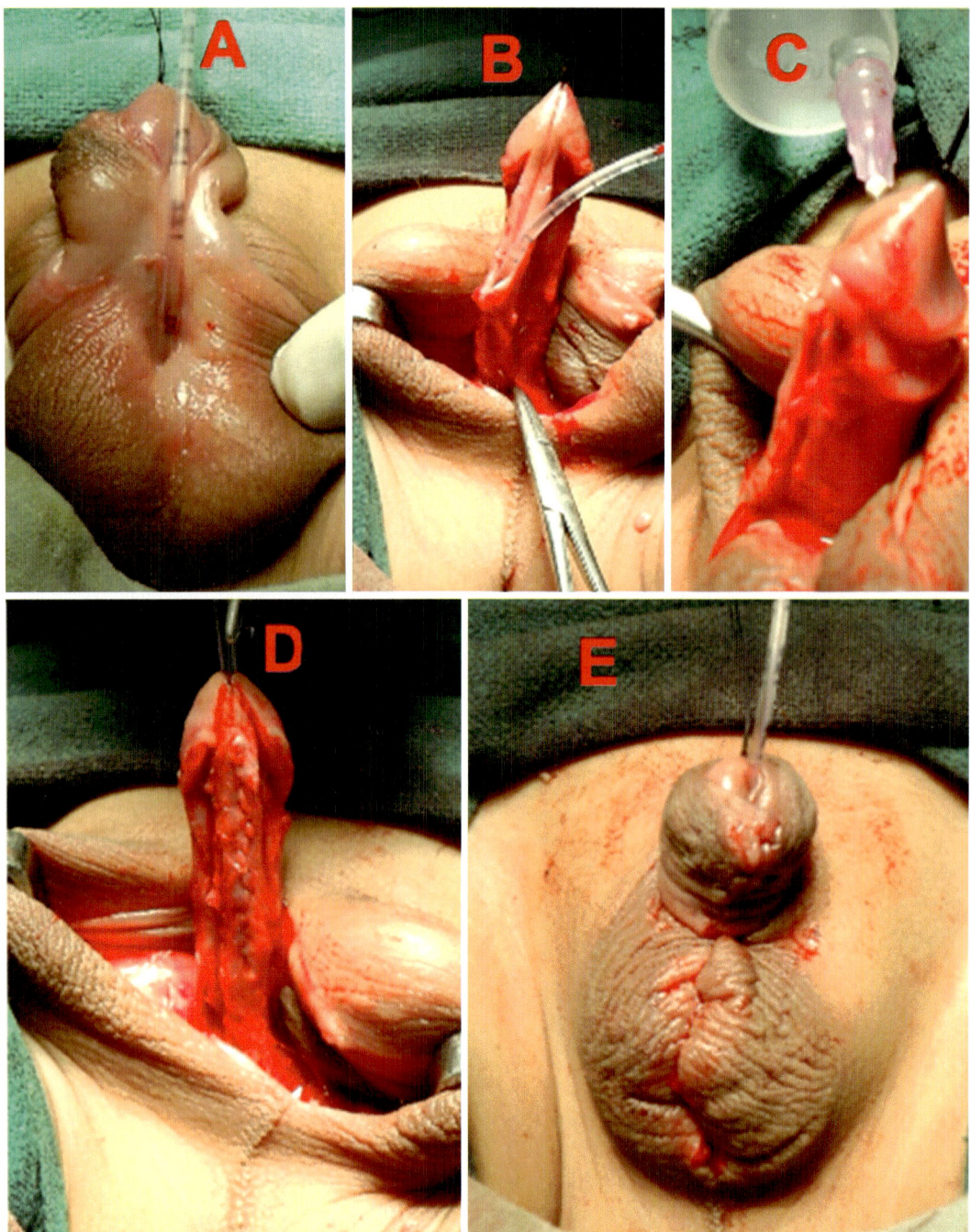

Fig. 9.8 Techniques for preservation of prepucial skin and preputioplasty. (**a**). Scrotal hypospadias. (**b**). Penile degloving and mobilization of the urethral plate and spongiosum. (**c**). Gittes test to assess for any residual chordee that might need to be corrected. (**d**). Tubularization of urethral plate. (**e**). Glanuloplasty and Prepucioplasty.

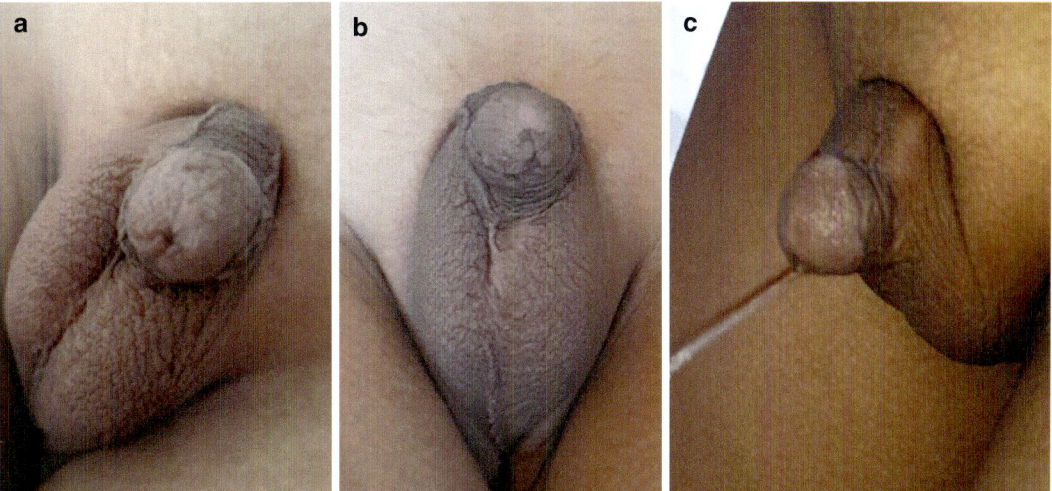

Fig. 9.9 Postoperative photograph of scrotal hypospadias after inner prepucial flap repair. Meatus at tip with conical glans, well-formed scrotum, and a single laminar urinary stream

9.7.7 Perioperative Care

Intra-operative antibiotics are administered. Typically Cefazolin (Clindamycin for those with Penicillin allergy).

Post-operatively they are sent home on Bactrim BID (if they have a Sulfa allergy, consider Keflex TID) until the urethral catheter is removed.

Oxybutynin (Ditropan—0.6 mg/kg in three divided doses) is prescribed as needed for bladder spasms.

9.7.8 Why Consider a One-Stage Procedure

Management of distal hypospadias is well established and uniformly agreed upon, but the dilemma still continues whether to perform a one-stage repair or multi-stage repair in cases of proximal hypospadias. One-stage repair is an attractive option because of reduced cost, hospital stay, anesthetic risks, and time to the final result.

Badawy and Fahmy (2013) reported similar complication rates in single-stage and two-stage techniques including mostly minor complications in the form of fistula, meatal stenosis, partial glans dehiscence, and urethral diverticulum, with their surgical technique. The 2-stage repair is versatile and has satisfactory outcomes, but necessitates a second procedure. There is a paucity of high-quality evidence supporting the superiority of one approach over the other [49–51]. Gonzalez R et al. in 2018 published their results of *one*-stage repair in mid and proximal hypospadias preserving the urethral plate and using a TPF for the urethroplasty and coverage of the ventral penis with a success rate of 77.5%. Compared to a planned two-stage approach, the technique described in this report resulted in significantly fewer procedures till complete resolution of the problem [52].

The results of the single-stage repair can be improved with modifications of the double faced flap. In a recent report, Daboos et al. present their five year experience using the double faced tubularized preputial flap for penoscrotal hypospadias repair in a prospective randomized study. 152 of 160 children (95%) had good clinical urinary functional outcomes (short micturition time, good urinary stream without straining or post voiding dribbling, and satisfactory cosmetic results) obtained by parents' interview at follow-up visits. They proposed the double faced tubularized preputial flap technique as a superior option compared to two-stage repairs with reported fewer complications (15% VS 25%),

Table 9.1 Showing complications of single-stage repair in proximal hypospadias

Complication rates of single-stage repair

Author	Year	Technique	No. of cases	Complication No	Complication rate
Castagnetti [59]	2013	Transverse preputial island flap	31	5	16%
		TIPU	26	7	27%
		OIFA	18	4	22%
Bhat et al. [60]	2015	TIPU	14	3	21.42%
Singhal et al. [61]	2015	Transverse preputial island flap	92	16	17%
Huang et al. [62]	2017	Preputial onlay flap	32	6	18.7%
Elemam et al. [63]	2017	Transverse preputial island flap	40	10	25%
		Double face	40	6	15%
Bhat A et al. [55]	2017	TIPU+ TOIF	21	4	19.04%
Gonzalez et al. [52]	2018	Preputial onlay flap	49	11	22.5%
Patil et al. [64]	2018	Transverse preputial island flap	30	6	20%
Badaway et al. [51]	2018	Inner prepucial flap	40	18	45%
Daboos et al. [53]	2020	Double face	80	12	15%
		Duckett	80	20	25%
Cui et al. [65]	2020	Transverse preputial island flap	155	92	59.35%
Total			748	220	29.41%

Table 9.2 Complications of two-stage repair in proximal hypospadias

Complication rates of two-staged repair

Author	Year	Technique	Total cases	Complications No	Complication rate
McNamara et al. [66]	2015	Inner prepucial flap	134	71	53%
Stanasel I et al. [67]	2015	Inner prepucial flap	56	38	68%
Manasherova [68]	2020	PSG (Free Graft)	108	33	31%
		BMG	112	23	20%
Misra et al. [69]	2020	BMG/prepucial grafts	36	11	30.6%
Castagnetti [59]	2013	Prepucial graft	18	5	28%
Pippi Salle [70]	2015	Prepucial graft	60	19	32%
Snodgrass [13]	2017	Prepucial graft or labial mucosa	43	10	23%
Total			567	210	37%

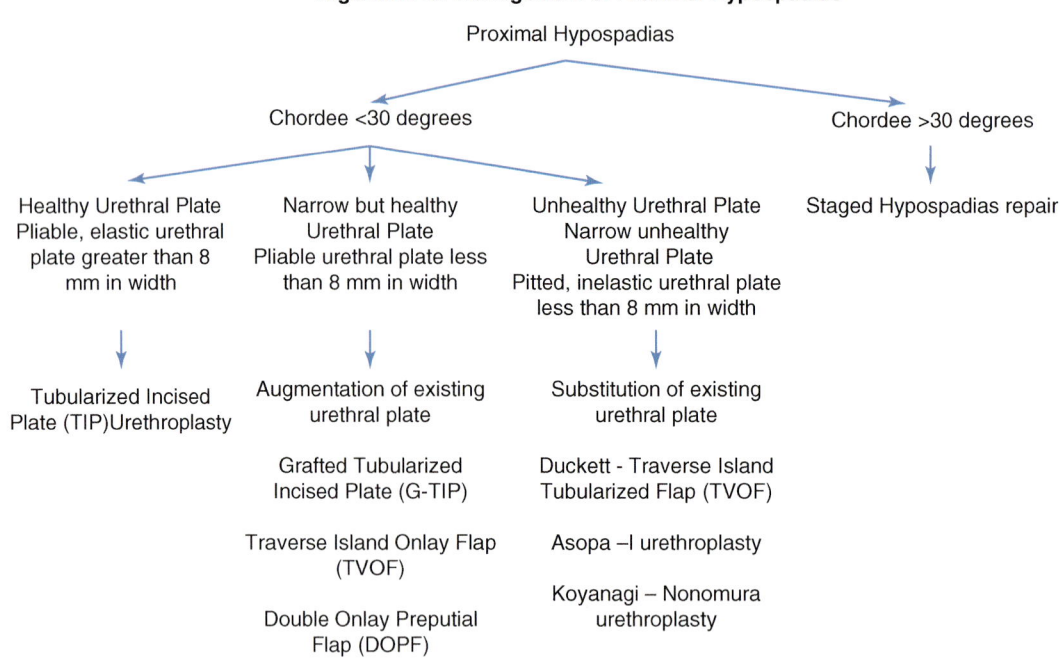

Fig. 9.10 Algorithm in proximal hypospadias repair

better urinary function, and good cosmetic results [53]. In cases where inner prepucial skin flap fails to cover the required urethral defect, midline nonhair bearing skin may be used to cover the remaining length with the technique proposed by Glassberg-Duckett. Tiryaki (2010) reported the success rate of 74% in cases where they utilized a combination of Duckett's preputial tube and the Thiersch–Duplay procedure in 34 patients with a mean follow-up of 4.1 years in severe hypospadias [54]. Similar results were reported by Bhat et al. 2017 where they tubularized the mobilized & preserved urethral plate as a proximal segment of urethra with a success rate of 80.06% [55].

Hensle et al. reported 32% long-term complications after a two-stage repair. Graft contracture and slough was noted in 46% and 54% had meatal stenosis and fistula. They reported that their complications in first 3 years of their experience were 60%. This decreased to 19% in last 7 years of the reporting period indicative of a definitive learning curve in two-stage repairs [56]. Hueber et al. (2016) reported that the obstructive urinary flow pattern observed in patients early on is a frequent finding after proximal hypospadias surgery, and that the flow rates become comparable with those of normal unoperated males on follow-up to adulthood. They advocated that because of the remarkable improvement observed at puberty a watchful waiting approach is proposed in order to avoid unnecessary intervention [57]. Similarly Rynja SP (2018) published long-term results of proximal and distal hypospadias as compared to control with a mean age of 20.6 years and found that in their cohort of TPIF patients, long-term urinary, sexual, and cosmetic outcomes were similar to those in patients with distal hypospadias repairs and controls [58].

We reviewed the recent published literature reporting on the clinical outcomes of one-stage and two-stage repairs for proximal hypospadias. The data are presented in Table 9.1 (single-stage repair) and Table 9.2 (two-stage repair). The literature would suggest that the clinical outcomes are comparable whether one chooses a single-stage repair or a staged option. Longer-term follow-up is going to be very important to demonstrate if this remains true or if one strategy is better than the other, especially since the data for the long-term outcomes for the contemporary two-stage repairs are not yet available for review.

We strongly recommend that each surgeon who undertakes hypospadias repairs should develop their own personal approach based on their training, experience, and clinical outcomes. In order to ensure best practice, they should track their own clinical outcomes with frequent and periodic reviews, and make evidence-based adjustments to their treatment algorithm.

It is the personal preference of the authors to undertake a two-stage repair in cases of proximal hypospadias with ventral chordee that is greater than 30 degrees, we propose the following algorithm to be considered (Fig. 9.10).

9.8 Conclusion

Proximal hypospadias continues to be a challenging clinical phenotype to repair. Choosing between a single-stage versus a staged hypospadias repair depends on the degree of chordee (< 30 degrees will permit a single-stage procedure) and the surgeon's experience. There are a number of surgical techniques to choose from, and it is advisable to master a technique from each of the various strategies in managing a child with proximal hypospadias, i.e. tubularization of the urethral plate, augmentation of the urethral plate, and substitution of the urethral plate. It is critical as a surgeon to track your personal clinical outcomes and complications proactively to assess your own performance objectively.

When assessing the outcome of hypospadias repair, it is vitally important to keep in mind that the patient and his family's reporting may be very different from what is noted and reported by the surgeon [71]. While as a surgeon, one might be willing to accept a complication rate of >30%, please remember for our patients that we are so privileged to be caring for, it is either "All or None," they either have a complication or do not. For patients who develop complications, the burden of care and cost of ongoing care can significantly impact the family and the mental well-being of the affected patient.

References

1. Wang YN, et al. Male external genitalia growth curves and charts for children and adolescents aged 0 to 17 years in Chongqing, China. Asian J Androl. 2018;20(6):567–71.
2. Steven L, et al. Current practice in paediatric hypospadias surgery; a specialist survey. J Pediatr Urol. 2013;9(6 Pt B):1126–30.
3. Springer A, Krois W, Horcher E. Trends in hypospadias surgery: results of a worldwide survey. Eur Urol. 2011;60(6):1184–9.
4. Brockel MA, Polaner DM, Vemulakonda VM. Anesthesia in the Pediatric patient. Urol Clin North Am. 2018;45(4):551–60.
5. Paterson N, Waterhouse P. Risk in pediatric anesthesia. Paediatr Anaesth. 2011;21(8):848–57.
6. Kurtoglu S, Bastug O. Mini puberty and its interpretation. Turk Pediatri Ars. 2014;49(3):186–91.
7. Copeland KC, Chernausek S. Mini-puberty and growth. Pediatrics. 2016;138(1):37.
8. Pasterski V, et al. Postnatal penile growth concurrent with mini-puberty predicts later sex-typed play behavior: evidence for neurobehavioral effects of the postnatal androgen surge in typically developing boys. Horm Behav. 2015;69:98–105.
9. Schultz JR, Klykylo WM, Wacksman J. Timing of elective hypospadias repair in children. Pediatrics. 1983;71(3):342–51.
10. Gittes RF, McLaughlin AP 3rd. Injection technique to induce penile erection. Urology. 1974;4(4):473–4.
11. Bologna RA, et al. Chordee: varied opinions and treatments as documented in a survey of the American Academy of Pediatrics, Section of Urology. Urology. 1999;53(3):608–12.
12. Gong EM, Cheng EY. Current challenges with proximal hypospadias: we have a long way to go. J Pediatr Urol. 2017;13(5):457–67.
13. Snodgrass W, Bush N. Staged tubularized autograft repair for primary proximal hypospadias with 30-degree or greater ventral curvature. J Urol. 2017;198(3):680–6.
14. Waterhouse K, Glassberg KI. Mobilization of the anterior urethra as an aid in the one-stage repair of hypospadias. Urol Clin North Am. 1981;8(3):521–5.
15. Devine CJ Jr, Horton CE. A one stage hypospadias repair. J Urol. 1961;85:166–72.
16. Asopa HS, et al. One stage correction of penile hypospadias using a foreskin tube. . A preliminary report. Int Surg. 1971;55(6):435–40.
17. Duckett JW Jr. Transverse preputial island flap technique for repair of severe hypospadias. Urol Clin North Am. 1980;7(2):423–30.
18. Duckett JW. The island flap technique for hypospadias repair. Urol Clin North Am. 1981;8(3):503–11.
19. Duckett JW. The island flap technique for hypospadias repair. 1981. J Urol. 2002;167(5):2148–52. discussion 2157-8

20. Duckett JW Jr. Transverse preputial island flap technique for repair of severe hypospadias. 1980. J Urol. 2002;167(2 Pt 2):1179–82. discussion 1183
21. Filmer RB, Duckett JW, Sowden R. One-stage correction of hypospadias/chordee. Birth Defects Orig Artic Ser. 1977;13(5):267–70.
22. Hodgson NB. A one-stage hypospadias repair. J Urol. 1970;104(2):281–3.
23. Hodgson NB. A one-stage hypospadias repair. 1970. J Urol. 2002;167(2 Pt 2):1176–8.
24. Koyanagi T, et al. Complete repair of severe penoscrotal hypospadias in 1 stage: experience with urethral mobilization, wing flap-flipping urethroplasty and "glanulomeatoplasty". J Urol. 1983;130(6):1150–4.
25. Koyanagi T, et al. One-stage repair of perineal hypospadias and scrotal transposition. Eur Urol. 1984;10(6):364–7.
26. Koyanagi T, et al. Experience with one-stage repair of severe proximal hypospadias: operative technique and results. Eur Urol. 1993;24(1):106–10.
27. Nonomura K, et al. One-stage total repair of severe hypospadias with scrotal transposition: experience in 18 cases. J Pediatr Surg. 1988;23(2):177–80.
28. Snodgrass W, Bush N. Tubularized incised plate proximal hypospadias repair: continued evolution and extended applications. J Pediatr Urol. 2011;7(1):2–9.
29. Snodgrass W, Bush N. Recurrent ventral curvature after proximal TIP hypospadias repair. J Pediatr Urol. 2020;17(2):222.e1–5.
30. Bhat A. General considerations in hypospadias surgery. Indian J Urol. 2008;24(2):188–94.
31. Bhat A, et al. Double breasting spongioplasty in tubularized/tubularized incise plate urethroplasty: a new technique. Indian J Urol. 2017;33(1):58–63.
32. Bhat A, et al. Outcome of tubularized incised plate urethroplasty with spongioplasty alone as additional tissue cover: a prospective study. Indian J Urol. 2014;30(4):392–7.
33. Delaage PH, Bargy F, Beaudoin S. Spongioplasty in the treatment of hypospadias. Prog Urol. 2005;15(6):1120–3.
34. Hayashi Y, et al. Can spongioplasty prevent fistula formation and correct penile curvature in TIP urethroplasty for hypospadias? Urology. 2013;81(6):1330–5.
35. Gundeti M, et al. Use of an inner preputial free graft to extend the indications of Snodgrass hypospadias repair (Snodgraft). J Pediatr Urol. 2005;1(6):395–6.
36. Holland AJ, Smith GH. Effect of the depth and width of the urethral plate on tubularized incised plate urethroplasty. J Urol. 2000;164(2):489–91.
37. Hollowell JG, et al. Preservation of the urethral plate in hypospadias repair: extended applications and further experience with the onlay island flap urethroplasty. J Urol. 1990;143(1):98–100. discussion 100-1
38. Eldahshoury ZM, et al. Modified double face onlay island preputial skin flap with augmented glanuloplasty for hypospadias repair. J Pediatr Urol. 2013;9(6 Pt A):745–9.
39. Duckett JW. Hypospadias. Clin Plast Surg. 1980;7(2):149–60.
40. Asopa HS. Newer concepts in the management of hypospadias and its complications. Ann R Coll Surg Engl. 1998;80(3):161–8.
41. Dahiphale AM, Chawada J, Asopa HS. Retrospective and prospective study of modified Asopa-I repair in hypospadias patients. New Indian J Surg. 2018;9(5):567–73.
42. Koyanagi T. Repair of severe proximal hypospadias associated with bifid scrotum. Int Urol Nephrol. 1984;16(2):115–21.
43. Koyanagi T, et al. Further experience with one-stage repair of severe hypospadias and scrotal transposition. Modifications in the technique and its result in eight cases. Int Urol Nephrol. 1988;20(2):167–77.
44. Koyanagi T, et al. One-stage repair of severe penoscrotal hypospadias. Nihon Hinyokika Gakkai Zasshi. 1983;74(8):1440–6.
45. Glenn JF, Anderson EE. Surgical correction of incomplete penoscrotal transposition. J Urol. 1973;110(5):603–5.
46. Glassberg KI, Hansbrough F, Horowitz M. The Koyanagi-Nonomura 1-stage bucket repair of severe hypospadias with and without penoscrotal transposition. J Urol. 1998;160(3 Pt 2):1104–7. discussion 1137
47. Hosseini SM, et al. Cyanoacrylate glue dressing for hypospadias surgery. N Am J Med Sci. 2012;4(7):320–2.
48. Tan HL, et al. The use of octyl cyanoacrylate (superglue) in hypospadias repair including its use as a fixator for urethral stents. J Pediatr Surg. 2012;47(12):2294–7.
49. Dason S, Wong N, Braga LH. The contemporary role of 1 vs. 2-stage repair for proximal hypospadias. Transl Androl Urol. 2014;3(4):347–58.
50. Badawy H, Fahmy A. Single- vs. multi-stage repair of proximal hypospadias: the dilemma continues. Arab J Urol. 2013;11(2):174–81.
51. Badawy H, et al. Posterior hypospadias: evaluation of a paradigm shift from single to staged repair. J Pediatr Urol. 2018;14(1):28 e1–8.
52. Gonzalez R, Lingnau A, Ludwikowski BM. Results of Onlay preputial flap urethroplasty for the single-stage repair of mid- and proximal hypospadias. Front Pediatr. 2018;6:19.
53. Daboos M, Helal AA, Salama A. Five years' experience of double faced tubularized preputial flap for penoscrotal hypospadias repair in pediatrics. J Pediatr Urol. 2020;16(5):673 e1–7.
54. Tiryaki T. Combination of tubularized island flap and ventral skin flap techniques in single-stage correction of severe proximal hypospadias. Urol Int. 2010;84(3):269–74.
55. Bhat A, Bhat M, Sabharwal K, Kumar R. Bhat's modification of Glassberg-Duckett repair to reduce complications in management of severe hypospadias with curvature. Afr J Urol. 2017;7(23):94–9.

56. Hensle TW, Kearney MC, Bingham JB. Buccal mucosa grafts for hypospadias surgery: long-term results. J Urol. 2002;168(4 Pt 2):1734–6. discussion 1736-7
57. Hueber PA, et al. Long-term functional outcomes after penoscrotal hypospadias repair: a retrospective comparative study of proximal TIP, Onlay, and Duckett. J Pediatr Urol. 2016;12(4):198 e1–6.
58. Rynja SP, et al. Proximal hypospadias treated with a transverse preputial island tube: long-term functional, sexual, and cosmetic outcomes. BJU Int. 2018;122(3):463–71.
59. Castagnetti M, Zhapa E, Rigamonti W. Primary severe hypospadias: comparison of reoperation rates and parental perception of urinary symptoms and cosmetic outcomes among 4 repairs. J Urol. 2013;189(4):1508–13.
60. Bhat A, Sabharwal K, Bhat M, Singla M, Upadhayaa R, Kumara V. Correlation of severity of penile torsion with type of hypospadias and ventral penile curvature and their management. Afr J Urol. 2015;17(21):111–8.
61. Singal AK, Dubey M, Jain V. Transverse preputial onlay island flap urethroplasty for single-stage correction of proximal hypospadias. World J Urol. 2016;34(7):1019–24.
62. Guo L, et al. Utilities of scrotal flap for reconstruction of penile skin defects after severe burn injury. Int Urol Nephrol. 2017;49(9):1593–603.
63. Elemam A, Taha SM, Gismalla M. Transverse ventral island preputial tube versus double face preputial tube in the repair of penoscrotal hypospadias: does the dissection of the tube from dorsal preputial skin affect the outcome of repair? Glob J Med Res. 2017;17(1):1.
64. Patil A, Sharma A, Mane N, Parab S, Andankar M, Pathak H. Hypospadias repair using Tranverse Preputial Island flap (modified Asopa procedure). J Pediatr Nephrol. 2018;6(3):1–7.
65. Cui X, et al. Clinical efficacy of transverse preputial island flap urethroplasty for single-stage correction of proximal hypospadias: a single-centre experience in Chinese patients. BMC Urol. 2020;20(1):118.
66. McNamara ER, et al. Management of Proximal Hypospadias with 2-stage repair: 20-year experience. J Urol. 2015;194(4):1080–5.
67. Stanasel I, et al. Complications following staged hypospadias repair using transposed preputial skin flaps. J Urol. 2015;194(2):512–6.
68. Manasherova D, et al. Bracka's method of proximal hypospadias repair: preputial skin or buccal mucosa? Urology. 2020;138:138–43.
69. Misra D, et al. Urethral fistulae following surgery for scrotal or perineal hypospadias: a 20-year review. J Pediatr Urol. 2020;16(4):447 e1–6.
70. Pippi Salle JL, et al. Proximal hypospadias: a persistent challenge. Single institution outcome analysis of three surgical techniques over a 10-year period. J Pediatr Urol. 2016;12(1):28 e1–7.
71. Braga LH, et al. Ventral penile lengthening versus dorsal plication for severe ventral curvature in children with proximal hypospadias. J Urol. 2008;180(4 Suppl):1743–7. discussion 1747-8

10

Tubularized Incised Urethral Plate Urethroplasty in Severe Hypospadias

Amilal Bhat

10.1 Introduction

Tubularized incised urethral plate urethroplasty is the choice of procedure in distal and middle hypospadias [1]. But there is significant variability in preference of the procedures to proximal hypospadias with chordee. The available techniques for proximal hypospadias repair are TIPU, with or without dorsal inlay and on lay flap urethroplasty and urethral plate transection procedures and replacement urethroplasty are Duckett's repair, Asopa's I & II, Double island urethroplasty, Koyanagi, Hodgson's X, Hodgson's XX, Glassberg–Duckett technique, Bhat's modification of Glassberg–Dukette technique and two-stage procedures [2]. Among these transverse island procedures, Duckett and Asopa are commonly practised. Complications are more in these replacement urethroplasties than in on lay flaps urethroplasty and TIPU. In the modern approach of hypospadias repair, the urethral plate is to be preserved as far as possible [3]. Results of two-stage procedures and single-stage have been reported similar [4]. The choice, whether to go for a single stage or two, depends on the training and experience of the surgeon. But single-stage repair with excellent results will be preferred by the parents or patients because of the greater convenience to the patient, decreased cost, anaesthesia risk, decreased separation anxiety and psychological impact. This will give better results because of the availability of healthy and unscarred urethral plate and skin [4]. Long-term complications like spraying of urine, post-void dribble, the dribble of the ejaculate, milking of the ejaculate and retained ejaculate with two-stage are very high (33–42.5%) [5, 6]. Neourethra devoid of with spongiosum is the leading cause of these complications. Tubularized urethral plate urethroplasty with spongioplasty reconstructs near-normal urethra and is likely to reduce these complications. Complications of TIPU in proximal hypospadias are comparable to other procedures of hypospadias repair in severe hypospadias [7]. The main limitation in the application of TIPU repair is presence of chordee. Mild to moderate curvature correction is feasible by the mobilization technique preserving the urethral plate making these cases suitable for TIPU.

A. Bhat (✉)
Bhat's Hypospadias and Reconstructive Urology Hospital and Research Centre,
Jaipur, Rajasthan, India

Department of Urology, Jaipur National University Institute for Medical Sciences and Research Centre,
Jaipur, Rajasthan, India

Department of Urology, Dr. S.N. Medical College,
Jodhpur, Rajasthan, India

Department of Urology, S.P. Medical College,
Bikaner, Rajasthan, India

P.G. Committee Medical Council of India,
New Delhi, India

Academic and Research Council of RUHS,
Jaipur, Rajasthan, India

10.2 Surgical Technique

Main steps of the technique are

1. Penile de-gloving and chordee correction.
2. Incising the urethral plate and its tubularization with or without the dorsal inlay.
3. Spongioplasty and glanuloplasty.
4. Scrotoplasty.
5. Skin closure.

10.2.1 Penile De-gloving and Chordee Correction

A stay suture is placed on glans, and 1:100000 adrenaline solution is injected at the planned site of the incision. A circumferential circumcoronal incision is given and is extended down on the shaft as an inverted U-shape at the margins of the urethral plate encircling the meatus and then extended in the midline in the scrotum. Penile skin de-gloving is done at Buck's fascia up to the root of the penis (Fig. 10.1a) for chordee correction. Then, the Gittes test is done to assess the chordee correction (Fig. 10.1b). Dissection plane is created just proximal to the meatus at tunica albuginea, the urethral plate and corpus spongiosum is mobilized (Fig. 10.1c) distally into the glans. The spongiosum is mobilized lateral to the medial. If there is no curvature and parents demand prepucioplasty, partial ventral penile de-gloving is done (Fig. 10.2a, b). The mobilization of the urethral plate is done medially just inside

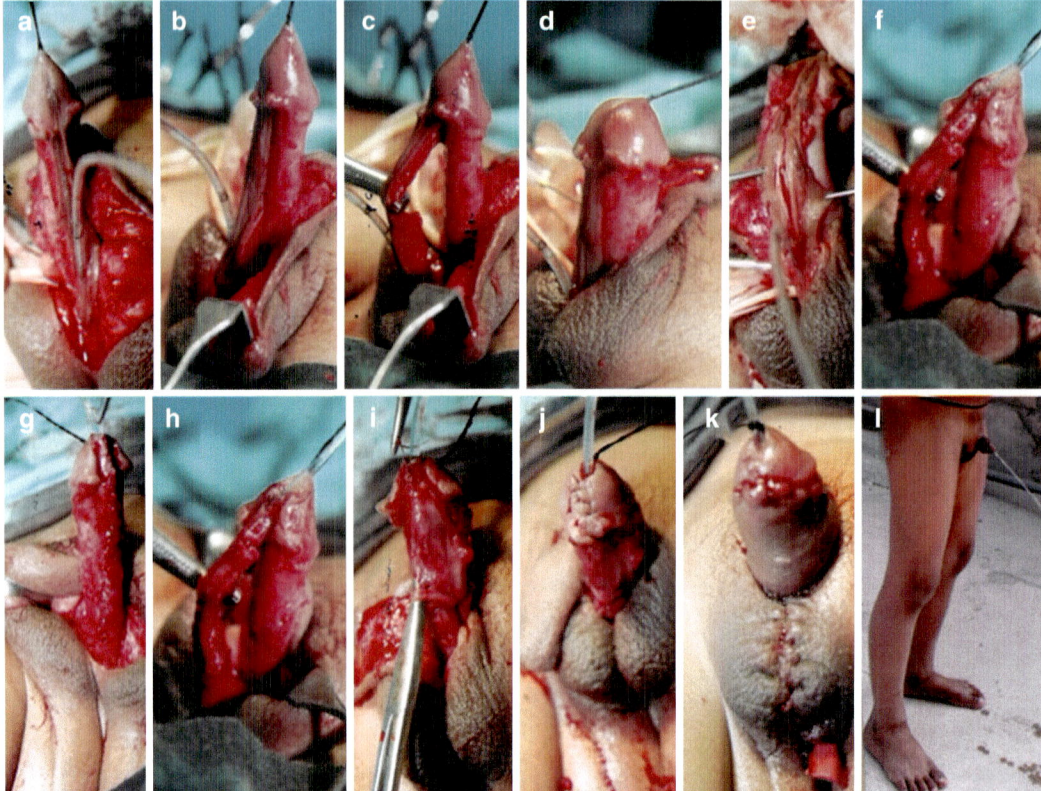

Fig. 10.1 Steps of tubularized incised plate urethroplasty in perineal hypospadias. (**a**) Penile de-gloving. (**b** and **c**) Urethral plate with the corpus spongiosum mobilization. (**d**) Gittes test showing correction of the chordee. (**e**) Incision of the urethral plate. (**f**) Tubularization of the urethral plate. (**g** and **h**) Spongioplasty. (**i**) Coverage of the neourethra with a dorsal dartos flap. (**j**) Glanuloplasty. (**k**) Skin closure. (**l**) Patient projecting the urinary stream from the tip postoperatively. {with permission Bhat et al. [7] copyright @Elsevier}

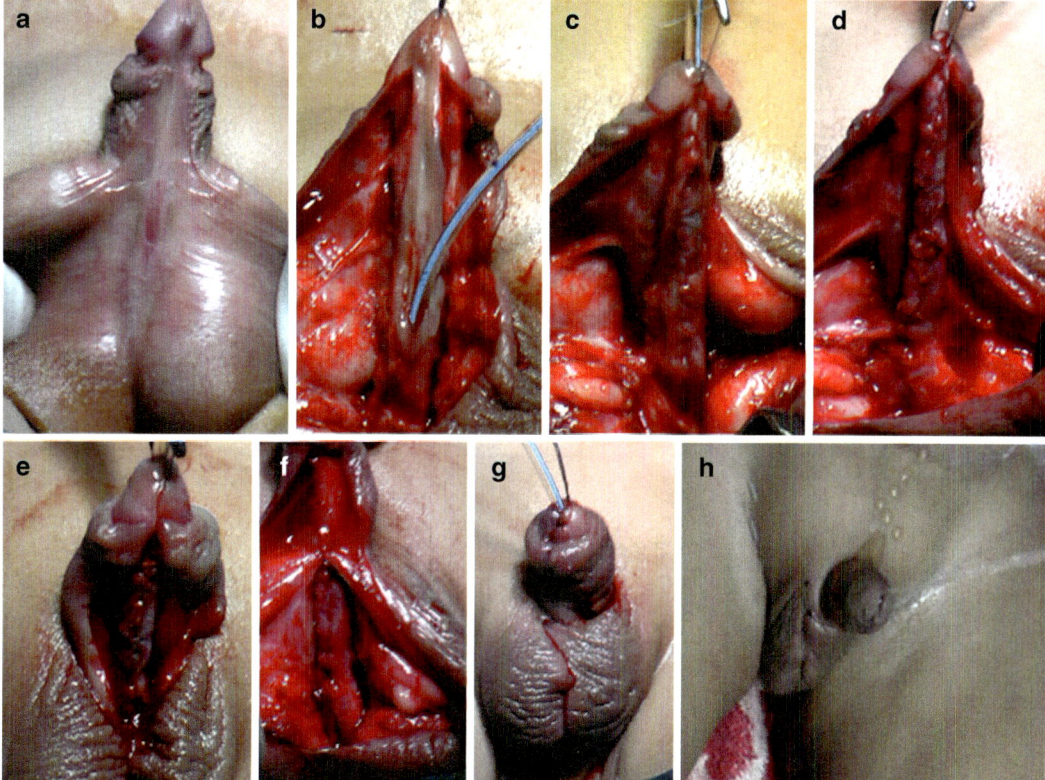

Fig. 10.2 Steps of tubularized incised plate urethroplasty with preputioplasty in perineo-scrotal hypospadias. (**a** and **b**) Penile de-gloving and urethral plate mobilization. (**c**) Tubularization of the urethral plate. (**d**) Spongioplasty. (**e**) Glanuloplasty. (**f**) Coverage of the neourethra with a ventral dartos flap. (**g**) Skin closure and prepucioplasty. (**h**) Patient projecting the urinary stream from the tip postoperatively. {with permission Bhat et al. [7] copyright @ Elsevier}

the margin of the urethral plate in case chordee has been corrected by penile de-gloving or cases with no chordee but under the urethral plate where chordee persists after penile skin de-gloving. Proximal urethra is mobilized on the persistence of chordee, and Gittes test is done to confirm its correction (Fig. 10.1d). If chordee continues, then the single-stitch dorsal plication is made.

Mobilizing the urethral plate into the glans and glanuloplasty is done after raising glanular wings to correct the glanular chordee. The Gittes test confirms the final chordee correction. However, in cases with the spongiosum segment's tethering after mobilization or persist chordee after dorsal plication, the urethral plate is transected at the corona to correct the chordee, and the plan is changed to inner prepucial flap repair or two-stage repair.

10.2.2 Incising the Urethral Plate and Tubularization of it with or Without the Dorsal Inlay

The urethral plate is incised in the midline, taking care not to cut through the urethral plate (Fig. 10.1e) and proximal urethra is calibrated with the largest acceptable catheter to get the size of the urethral stent. The incision in the urethral plate is avoided if the urethra is wide enough to tubularize it over an adequate size urethral stent. Depth of incision depends on the width and development of the urethral plate and spongiosum. The patients whose required width is more; then we supplement it with a dorsal inlay graft (Fig. 10.3) or buccal mucosal graft. Tubularization of the urethral plate is done using 6/0–7/0 PDS

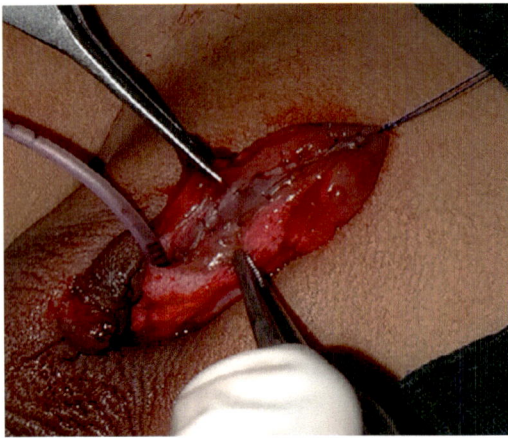

Fig. 10.3 Showing the dorsal inlay skin graft

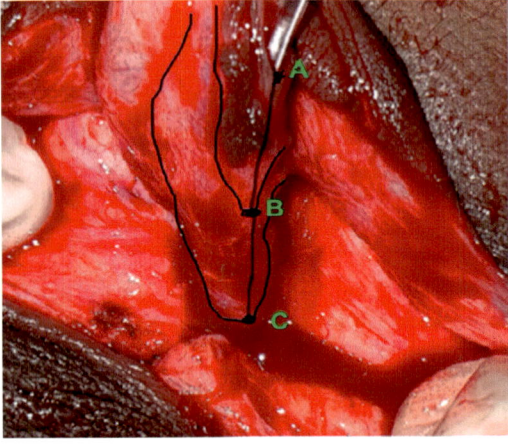

Fig. 10.4 Showing the demarcation and margins of the urethral plate and spongiosum (**a**) Meatus, (**b**). Bifurcation of urethral plate, (**c**). Bifurcation of Spongiosum

to leave any everting margin of the urethral plate and not to buckle neo-urethra.

10.2.3 Spongioplasty and Glansplasty

Suturing of mobilized spongiosum is started proximal to the limit of the tubularization of the urethral plate (Fig. 10.5b) and continued up to neo-meatus through the glans (Figs. 10.1g, h and 10.2d). Reconstructed neourethra by urethral plate tubularization with spongioplasty anatomically resembles a normal urethra with a urothelial layer covered by spongiosum. The neourethra is again covered with a dorsal dartos flap in cases without prepucioplasty (Fig. 10.1i), ventral dartos with prepucioplasty (Fig. 10.2f) or with a tunica vaginalis flap. Thus, neourethra is covered by two healthy interposing tissues, which help prevent fistula and maintain a better blood supply. A 6–10 Fr urethral catheter/infant feeding tube is left in situ depending on the patient's age, smaller than the native urethral calibre. The glanular wings are mobilized deep up to tunica to have wide glanular flaps. Glanuloplasty is done in two layers with 6/0–7/0 PDS suture. The second layer of sutures can be used either subcuticular (Fig. 10.2e) or through the glans (Fig. 10.1l, j). Care is taken to have adequate space between the neourethra and glans wings while ensuring no compromise in blood supply.

continuous/interrupted sutures over a 5–8 Fr stent according to the child's age (Figs. 10.1f and 10.2c). The bifurcation of the spongiosum and the urethral plate is well demarcated and is about 1–2 cms proximal to the meatus (Fig. 10.4) (Urethral plate Bifurcation is marked 'B' and the spongiosum 'C'). The first suture is taken in the glans creating an adequate size meatus. The tubularization is started about one centimetre proximal to the meatus (Fig. 10.5a) and continued up to mid-glans using 6/0/7/0 PDS/Vicryl interrupted/continuous sutures to complete urethroplasty. (Figs. 10.1g and 10.2d). Care is taken not

10.2.4 Scrotoplasty and Skin Closure

Midline scrotal sac is mobilized, and the scrotoplasty is done in two layers (Figs. 10.1k and 10.2f). The scrotoplasty covers the proximal part of the neourethra, which helps in the prevention of fistula. The prepucioplasty is done depending on the available prepucial tissue and patients' or parents' desire. First, prepucioplasty is done in three layers: inner prepucial skin, dartos and outer skin closure. Then skin closure is done (Figs. 10.1k, 10.2f, g), and a pressure dressing is done.

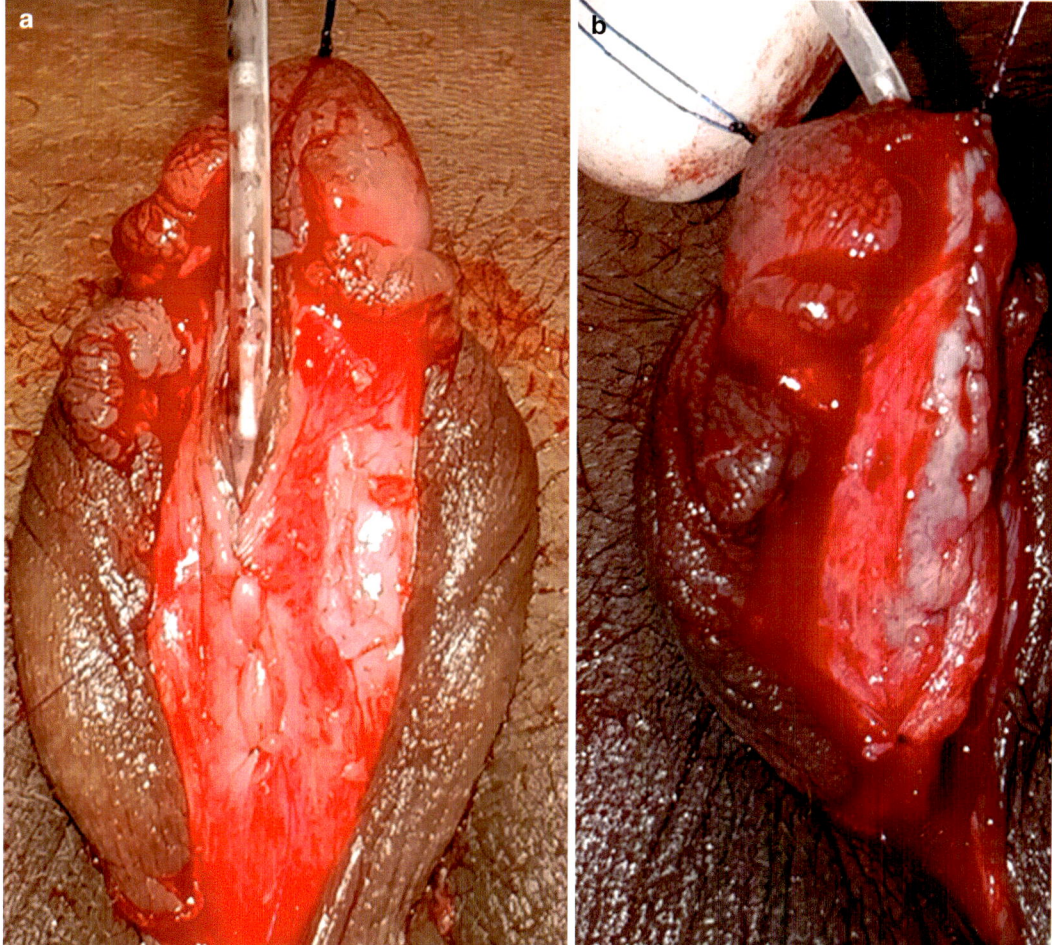

Fig. 10.5 (**a**) The starting of tubularization of urethra plate proximal to the meatus, (**b**). Starting of spongioplasty proximal to the tubularized urethral plate

The urethral catheter is kept for 10–14 days. After that, the patient is called in follow-up at 1, 3, 6 and 12 months postoperatively, and then every year and evaluated for the appearance of the penis and glans meatal stenosis, fistula, stricture and other complications. The visual impression of voiding stream (Fig. 10.1l) and urinary leakage from other sites than the meatus gives the impression of meatal stenosis, stricture and fistula. Besides, the urethra may be calibrated to rule out the urethral stricture and meatal stenosis.

10.3 Why TIPU in Proximal Hypospadias

A rational approach in the management is the application of a urethral plate preservation urethroplasty with spongioplasty. Choosing single-stage or two-stage procedures depend on the training, surgical experience and problems in the particular case of hypospadias. The single-stage technique is more suitable for the patients saving time, money visits to the hospital and less anxiety and mental trauma to the parents. Another important factor that matters in the long-term follow-up is the quality of the urethra with the spongiosum. Aldamanhori and Chapple 2017 in a review article on the failed hypospadias surgery presenting in adulthood, narrated that a narrow or short tube may be created because the neourethra may fail to grow adequately, keeping up with the rest of the genital tissues during puberty [8]. The late complication like stricture may present late because of the rapid genital growth during puberty. Besides, it is assumed that the congenital lack of spongiosum or no spongiosal covering the neourethra during repair in those patients may not provide adequate vascular support to the urethra during the rapid growth of puberty. Similarly, it can be postulated that the neourethra does not tolerate any trauma during erection and sexual activity because of a lack of spongiosum support [8]. The reconstructed urethra with tubularization of urethral plate and spongioplasty in TIPU simulates with the native urethra [9], which is likely to grow with age as genital tissue being responsive to hormones. The urethral plate with spongiosum and proximal urethral mobilization is used to correct the mild to moderate curvature [1]. These steps deal with all the factors responsible for ventral curvature in skin, dartos, Bucks fascia and spongiosum segment [10]. The limitation of the technique is that chordee due to intrinsic corporeal disproportion cannot be corrected. However, further corporeal disassembly can be added to correct the chordee if required. So, patients of corporal disproportion are to be treated with corporotomy, corporoplasty, and penile disassembly. Perovic et al. reported straightening of the penis in 68% of the patients by penile disassembly alone. In 32% of patients, though the curvature's severity decreased significantly it required dorsal plication for corporoplasty. So, the penile shortening was limited [11]. The disassembly technique is extensive and requires the separation corpus spongiosum segment with glans and the neurovascular bundle from copora cavernosa and has the chances of nerve injury. Our technique only involves mobilizing the corpus spongiosum segment without separating the glans and the corpora cavernosa from each other or the neurovascular bundle. We could correct the curvature in 88% of cases which is better compared to penile disassembly [1].

Snodgrass and Lorenzo had 22% fistula and overall 33% complications in mid-shaft to scrotal hypospadias with TIP, but 55% of the cases required dorsal plication for chordee correction [12]. But later on, the addition of spongioplasty reduced the fistula rate 33% to 10% and with tunica vaginalis had nil fistula. Snodgrass 2007 reported an overall 14% complication in 250 mid to proximal hypospadias [13]. Chen et al. reported an overall complication rate of 17.5% with TIPU in 40 cases of proximal hypospadias [14]. Besides, the spongioplasty gives almost a normal shape to the urethra, adds length, helps in chordee correction and the repair is more anatomical [15]. Finally, spongioplasty adds an extra layer of healthy vascular tissue, which helps to prevent fistula.

El Saket (2008) reported their results in 28 cases of proximal hypospadias where they could correct chordee by the mobilization technique in 80% of patients and 30% required the addition of dorsal plication and had overall complication 39% and fistula rate of 14% [16]. Therefore, they opined TIPU as a choice of procedure in mid and proximal hypospadias.

Mobilizing the urethral plate and spongiosum allows corporoplasty in patients of dorsoventral corporal disproportion, preserving the urethral plate. Kajbafzadeh et al. (2007) successfully preserved the plate for TIP urethroplasty in 13–18 cases (perineal six and penoscrotal 12) after correction of severe chordee by corpus spongiosum/urethral plate elevation combined with ventral corporotomy and tunica vaginalis grafting [4].

Snodgrass [2013] had a higher stricture rate 5/29 (17.24%) after the urethral plate and proximal urethral mobilization compared to 0/47 and stated that they have stopped mobilizing the urethral plate [17]. At the same time, stricture reported by Pfistermuller et al. (2015) in a review of 625 cases of proximal hypospadias was 2% (mean). Other complications were the mean fistula rate, 10.3%, meatal stenosis of 4.4% and reoperation rate of 12.2% in a mean follow-up of 16 months [18].

11. Perovic SV, Djordjevic ML, Djakovic NG. A new approach to the treatment of penile curvature. J Urol. 1998;160(3 Part 2):1123–7.
12. Snodgrass W, Lorenzo A. Tubularized incised-plate urethroplasty for proximal hypospadias. BJU Int. 2002;89(1):90–3.
13. Snodgrass W, Yucel S. Tubularized incised plate for mid-shaft and proximal hypospadias repair. J Urol. 2007;177(2):698–702.
14. Chen S, Yang S, Hsieh C, Chen Y. Tubularized incised plate urethroplasty for proximal hypospadias. BJU Int. 2000;86(9):1050–3.
15. Bhat A, Sabharwal K, Bhat M, Saran R, Singla M, Kumar V. Outcome of tubularized incised plate urethroplasty with spongioplasty alone as additional tissue cover: a prospective study. Indian J Urol. 2014;30(4):392.
16. El Saket HA, Fares A, Kaddah SN. Tubularised incised plate urethroplasty for mid penile and more proximal hypospadias repair. Ann Pediatr Surg. 2008;4(3 & 4):94–9.
17. Snodgrass WT, Granberg C, Bush NC. Urethral strictures following urethral plate and proximal urethral elevation during proximal TIP hypospadias repair. J Pediatr Urol. 2013;9(6):990–4.
18. Pfistermullera KLM, MacArdle AJ, Cucknow P. MMeta-analysis of complication rates of the tubularized incised plate (TIP) repair. J Pediatr Urol. 2015;11:54–9.
19. Bhat A, Gandhi A, Saxena G, Choudhary GR. Preputial reconstruction and tubularized incised plate urethroplasty in proximal hypospadias with ventral penile curvature. Indian J Urol. 2010;26(4):507.
20. Sarhan OM, El-Hefnawy AS, Hafez AT, Elsherbiny MT, Dawaba ME, Ghali AM. Factors affecting outcome of tubularized incised plate (TIP) urethroplasty: a single-Centre experience with 500 cases. J Pediatr Urol. 2009;5(5):378–82.

But Snodgrass applies the same principle of mobilization of the urethral plate and proximal urethra to correct curvature in STAG repair. He transects the urethral plate at the corona, mobilizes the urethral plate and urethra in the bulbar region to gain the length and re-attaches the urethra to corpora to correct the curvature. This shows the principle of mobilization is exemplary and should be followed. The blood supply of the urethral plate and urethra is from the bulbar artery, which is maintained as the urethral plate is lifted with the corpus spongiosum, and the proximal and distal ends are kept attached, maintaining the continuity of the corpus spongiosum. It is important not to damage the corpus spongiosum or corpus cavernosum. Care is to be taken not to damage the bulbar artery during the extensive bulbar dissection. We had the strictures in 14.28% of cases of proximal hypospadias repair with TIPU [19]. Our selection of patients with a well-developed wide urethral plate and spongiosum, proper mobilization of the urethral plate and spongiosum, taking care not to damage the blood supply of the urethral plate probably helped us to minimize the incidence of urethral strictures. The very fact that tubularization of the urethral plate without an incision was possible in 35% of cases shows better case selection [1]. Another critical point is not to damage the spongiosum; damage to the blood supply may also cause stricture urethra. A proper plane of dissection is created proximal to meatus at tunica albuginea and taking the deep layer of Buck's fascia with the spongiosum to prevent to damage the spongiosum. We covered the neourethra with spongiosum by spongioplasty and dorsal dartos/tunica vaginalis flaps, which helped us to reduce fistula formation. Similar were observations of Sarhan et al.; They reported a statistically significant lower fistula rate in spongioplasty with dartos in TIPU [20].

10.4 Conclusions

The objective of the hypospadias surgery is to reconstruct the functional urethra. TIPU is feasible in selected cases of proximal hypospadias with chordee, with an acceptable complication rate even in perineal and perineo-scrotal hypospadias, provided the urethral plate is wide, well developed and the corpus spongiosum is moderate to well developed. Chordee can be corrected by preserving the urethral plate with spongiosum and proximal urethral mobilization up to the bulbar region, spongioplasty and glanuloplasty: as it adds about the 2–3.5-centimetre length of to the urethra. The mobilization technique of chordee correction is simple, effective and safe, and enlarges the scope of TIP in proximal hypospadias with good results. Mobilization of spongiosum allows spongioplasty with tension-free sutures, and TIPU with spongioplasty reconstructs near-normal urethra.

References

1. Bhat A. Extended urethral mobilization in incised plate urethroplasty for severe hypospadias: a variation in technique to improve chordee correction. J Urol. 2007;178(3):1031–5.
2. Retik AB. Hypospadias. In: Campbell MF, Retik AB, Walsh PC, editors. Campbell's urology, vol. 4. 8th ed. Philadelphia: WB Saunders Co.; 2008.
3. Upadhyay J, Shekarriz B, Khoury AE. Midshaft hypospadias. Urol Clin. 2002;29(2):299–310.
4. Kajbafzadeh A-M, Arshadi H, Payabvash S, Salmasi AH, Najjaran-Tousi V, Sahebpor ARA. Proximal hypospadias with severe chordee: single-stage repair using corporeal tunica vaginalis free graft. J Urol. 2007;178(3):1036–42.
5. Lam P, Greenfield SP, Williot P. 2-stage repair in infancy for severe hypospadias with chordee: long-term results after puberty. J Urol. 2005;174(4 Part 2):1567–72.
6. Bracka A. A long-term view of hypospadias. Br J Plast Surg. 1989;42(3):251–5. https://doi.org/10.1016/0007-1226(89)90140-9.
7. Bhat A, Singla M, Bhat M, Sabharwala K, Upadhaya R, Kumara V. Incised plate urethroplasty in perineal and perineo-scrotal hypospadias. African. J Urol. 2015;21(2):105–10.
8. Aldamanhori R, Chapple CR. Management of the patient with failed hypospadias surgery presenting in adulthood. F1000Research. 2017;6:1890.
9. Bhat A, Bhat M, Kumar R, Bhat A. Double breasting spongioplasty in tubularized/tubularized incise plate urethroplasty: a new technique. Indian J Urol. 2017;33(1):58.
10. Bhat A, Bhat M, Kumar V, Kumar R, Mittal R, Saksena G. Comparison of variables affecting the surgical outcomes of tubularized incised plate urethroplasty in adult and pediatric hypospadias. J Pediatr Urol. 2016;12(2):108.e101–7.

Spongioplasty in Hypospadias Repair

11

Amilal Bhat

11.1 Introduction

The corpus spongiosum is a spongy tissue that surrounds the urethra. Spongiosum is also termed as the corpus cavernosum urethrae, but this term is rarely used in the day-to-day description. At the proximal-most point, the corpus spongiosum forms a bulb, which is the entrance point of the urethra to the penis. The tissue tapers down all through the length of the penis, finally enlarges again to form the glans. Tubularized Incised Plate Urethroplasty (TIPU) is a widely performed procedure and popular due to its versatility, low complication rate, and good cosmetic results. Since the inception of TIPU, there have been many modifications to improve the functional and cosmetic outcomes. The basic principle in managing any congenital anomaly is to reconstruct an organ with the existing tissue or by addition of the tissue, thereby restoring the anatomy to normal or near normal [1]. Tubularization of the urethral plate with spongioplasty reconstructs a near-normal urethra. So as per surgical principles, spongiosum is a better choice as a healthy interposing tissue in TIPU. Spongiosum prevents urethral compression and closure during the erection of the penis. But unfortunately, it is used less frequently. In the year 2000, S. Beaudoin from France coined the term "spongioplasty" [2], and York's et al. later described the Y-to-I wrap spongioplasty where the spongiosum was separated from the corporal bodies on both sides of the urethral plate [3]. Dodat et al. (2003) introduced a modified spongioplasty approach where spongiosum was separated from the corpora cavernosa from both medial and lateral edge [4]. Since the spongiosum is an integral part of the urethra; so, the spongioplasty should be done to reconstruct a near normal urethra.

A. Bhat (✉)
Bhat's Hypospadias and Reconstructive Urology Hospital and Research Centre,
Jaipur, Rajasthan, India

Department of Urology, Jaipur National University Institute for Medical Sciences and Research Centre,
Jaipur, Rajasthan, India

Department of Urology, Dr. S.N. Medical College,
Jodhpur, Rajasthan, India

Department of Urology, S.P. Medical College,
Bikaner, Rajasthan, India

P.G. Committee Medical Council of India,
New Delhi, India

Academic and Research Council of RUHS,
Jaipur, Rajasthan, India

11.2 Embryology

The development of the male urethra starts with the fusion of the urethral folds in the midline after the sixth week of fetal life. The endodermal derived distal solid urethral plate canalizes to form the glanular part of the urethra. The urethra forms sequentially after the proximal urethral folds fuse, and the mesenchyme within the urethral folds is the precursor of the corpus spongiosum. The mesenchymal tissue which surrounds it becomes denser and forms the troughing of the corpus spongiosum.

The amount of collagen in the corpus cavernosum is lesser than the corpus spongiosum during all fetal periods [5]. The smooth muscle growth in the corpus cavernosum, predominantly in the trabeculae, correlates with a proportional decrease of collagen with increasing gestational age. There is about four times more collagen in the corpus spongiosum than smooth muscle fibers and elastic system fibers during all fetal periods. In the corpus spongiosum, the percentage of smooth muscle fibers and elastic system fibers is equivalent during the fetal period. This corpus spongiosum is the supportive erectile tissue that usually surrounds the urethra and communicates with the erectile tissue of the glans. The deep layer of Buck's fascia covers the corporeal bodies, invests the spongiosum, and is attached to the corporal bodies' midline septum. Dorsally the neurovascular bundles lie deep to the layer of Buck's fascia. Superficial to Buck's layer lies the dartos fascia, the loose subcutaneous layer containing the superficial veins and lymphatics. These structures are formed subsequent to the urethral development by medial fusion of the outer genital folds, starting from the proximal to the distal end of the penis to form the urethra. This development accounts for how a fully formed urethra can have a poorly developed spongiosum with thin overlying skin and ventral tethering, despite the meatus being located at the tip of the glans. The failed urethral fold fusion and ectodermal intrusion develop an abortive spongiosum and abnormal glans in hypospadias. Abortive spongiosum lies deep to the urethral plate and dartos fascia at the lateral margin and over the deep layer of Buck's fascia [6]. The severity of hypoplasia of the corpus spongiosum also depends upon the severity of hypospadias and the proliferation of mesodermal tissue. In 2000, Snodgrass et al. demonstrated by optical microscopy and conventional staining techniques in the biopsies of 17 urethral plates of boys with hypospadias, the well-vascularized connective tissue composed of smooth muscle and collagen [7].

11.3 Identification and Classification of Spongiosum

A well-conducted clinical examination is important to see the spongiosum. Spongiosum is to be looked for both distal and proximal to the meatus. A Y-shaped pillar can be seen in moderately and well-developed spongiosum (Fig. 11.1a), but a poorly developed spongiosum may not be visible through the skin. But after penile degloving, the spongiosum can be identified in all cases, even in poorly developed corpus spongiosum and re-operative cases (Fig. 11.1b). The spongiosum is classified according to development and vascularity on the operating table [7, 8].

1. The corpus spongiosum is missing, resulting in a congenital condition called scaphoid megalourethra (Fig. 11.2a, b).
2. Poorly developed—Thin spongiosal tissue with decreased vascularity; the diameter of the neourethra covered by spongiosum after spongioplasty is less than the proximal healthy urethra (Fig. 11.3a–d).
3. Moderately developed—Average thickness and vascularity of spongiosal tissue; the diameter of the neourethra covered by spongiosum after spongioplasty is almost equal to that of the proximal healthy urethra (Fig. 11.4a–d).
4. Well-developed—Robust and thick spongiosum with good vascularity; the neourethra's diameter after spongioplasty is greater than that of the proximal healthy urethra (Fig. 11.5a–c).

Though the classification done on the operating table is subjective, it gives enough clues about the development of spongiosum. The difference between the moderately and well-developed spongiosum may be marginal, but poorly developed urethra can be identified easily. The classification is useful in predicting the outcome of hypospadias surgery. Ours was the only classification described, but recently Zhang et al. (2020) divided the spongiosum into [9]:

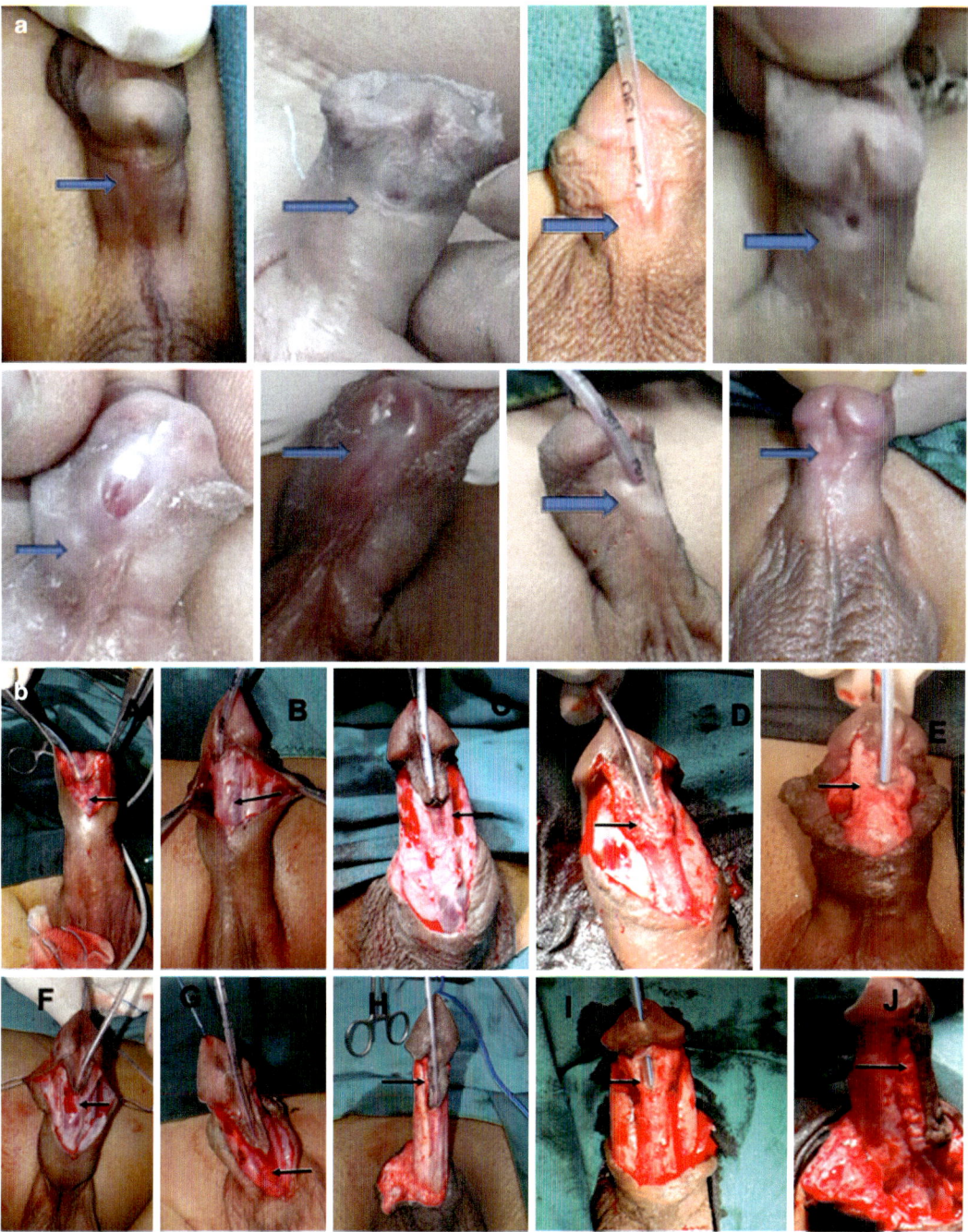

Fig. 11.1 (a) Arrows showing spongiosal pillars. (b) Arrows showing spongiosum after penile degloving. (a–d, f–h) in primary cases. (e, i, j) in re-operative patients

1. Well-developed with light fibrosis.
2. Poorly developed with severe fibrosis.

Zhang et al. classification has a flaw in their description by showing light and severe fibrosis. There is no fibrosis in the spongiosum and urethral plate, which is proved histologically by Snodgrass et al. They demonstrated well-vascularized connective tissues without any evidence of fibrous tissue in excised dartos spongiosum tissues during hypospadias repair [10].

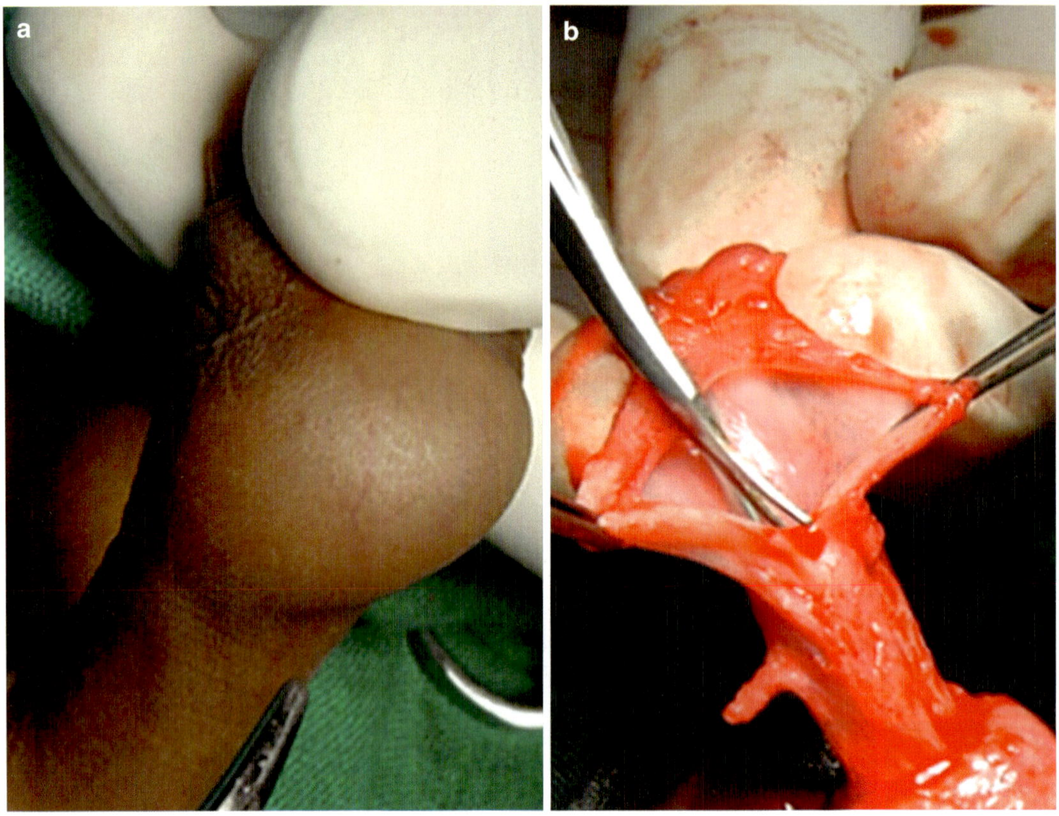

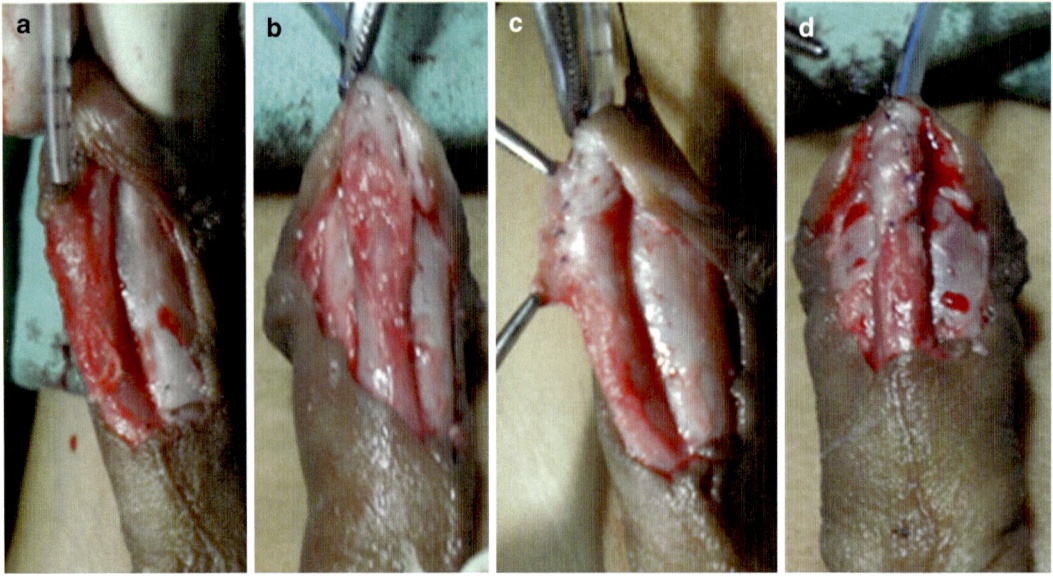

Fig. 11.2 Scaphoid urethra. (**a**) Saline filled urethra. (**b**) Laid open urethra without spongiosum

Fig. 11.3 Poorly developed spongiosum. (**a**) Distal penile hypospadias with mobilized urethral plate and spongiosum. (**b**) Tubularization of urethral plate. (**c**) Spongioplasty in progress. (**d**) Diameter of neo-urethra more than the proximal urethra after Spongioplasty

11 Spongioplasty in Hypospadias Repair

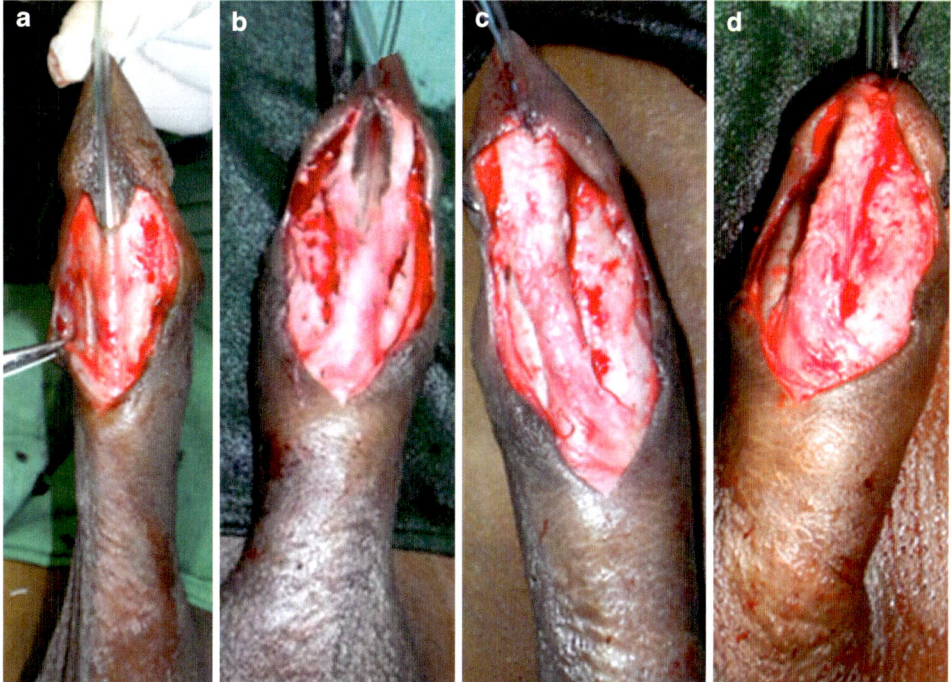

Fig. 11.4 Moderately developed spongiosum. (**a**) Penile degloving with prominent spongiosum pillars in Distal penile hypospadias. (**b**) Mobilized urethral plate with spongiosum. (**c**) Tubularization of urethral plate. (**d**) Diameter of neo-urethra equal to the proximal urethra after Spongioplasty

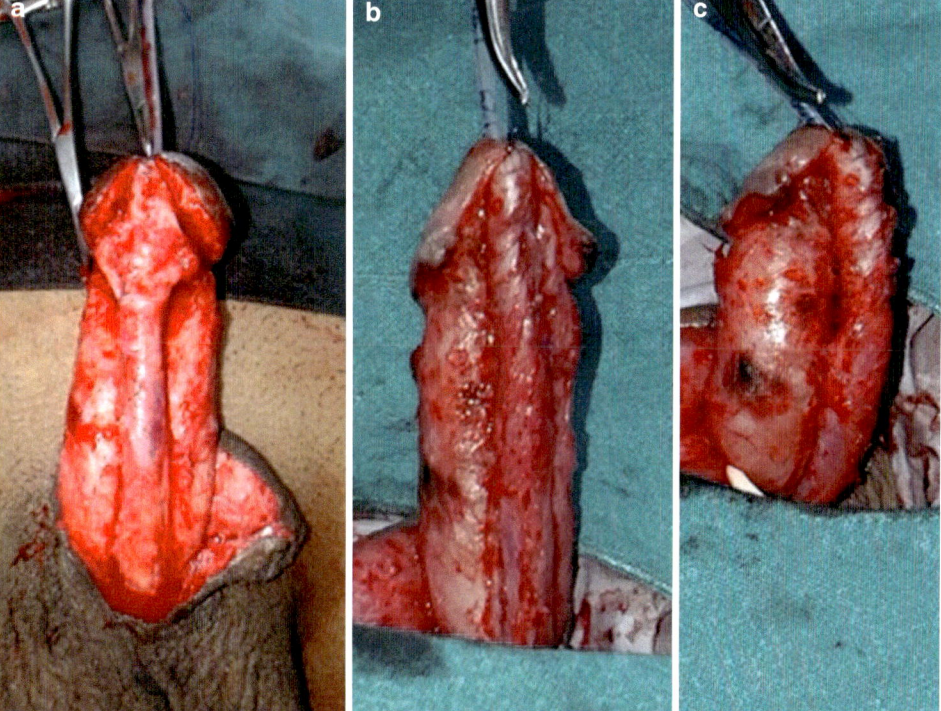

Fig. 11.5 Well-developed spongiosum. (**a**) Spongiosum pillars after tubularization of Urethral plate. (**b** and **c**) Diameter more than the proximal urethra after Spongioplasty

11.4 Co-Relation of the Bifurcation of Spongiosum with the Type of Hypospadias and Chordee

The bifurcation of spongiosum is an important landmark to classify the types of hypospadias. Often the meatus is distal, and the bifurcation of the spongiosum is proximal. The urethra distal to the bifurcation is hypoplastic. Mouriquand et al. reported little or no chordee when the division of spongiosum is distal to meatus in the hypospadiacs [11]. On the other hand, the division of the corpus spongiosum proximal to the meatus is usually associated with chordee, and the distal hypoplastic urethra is adherent to the skin (Fig. 11.6). Orkiszewski M (2012) classified the hypospadias based on the co-relation of the meatus and the bifurcation of corpus spongiosum. The site of external meatus was located above the pubis in 94.1% of the patients, the division of corpus spongiosum was seen above the pubis in 90% only (distal penile 38%, midshaft 25.3%). The distal meatus/urethra was stenotic in 84% and hypoplastic in 86.8%, with true chordee in 10.4%. The urethra distal to the division of the corpus spongiosum was considerably narrower than the proximal urethra in the majority of patients [12]. Therefore, the classification based on the bifurcation of spongiosum as anterior, middle, proximal penile, scrotal, and perineal rather than the meatus' location is better to understand the pathology of hypospadias.

However, there is not much literature on the co-relation of bifurcation of spongiosum with chordee. We found the development of spongiosum directly proportional to the severity of hypospadias ($P = 0.05$). The hypoplastic urethra length is directly proportionate to the severity of the chordee. No chordee: When the meatus is coronal or subcoronal, and bifurcation of the spongiosum is also at the same level, there is no chordee (Fig. 11.7a, b). Mild chordee: When the bifurcation of the spongiosum is mid to distal penile and meatus is at coronal or distal penile level; the hypoplastic urethra from the bifurcation of the spongiosum to the meatus shows mild chordee (Fig. 11.8a, b).

Moderate chordee: When the bifurcation of the spongiosum is mid to proximal penile and meatus is at mid or distal penile level, the hypoplastic urethra from the bifurcation of the spongiosum to the meatus shows moderate chordee (Fig. 11.9a, b).

Severe chordee: Similarly, the more proximal the bifurcation and greater the length of the hypoplastic urethra increases the curvature's severity (Fig. 11.10a, b).

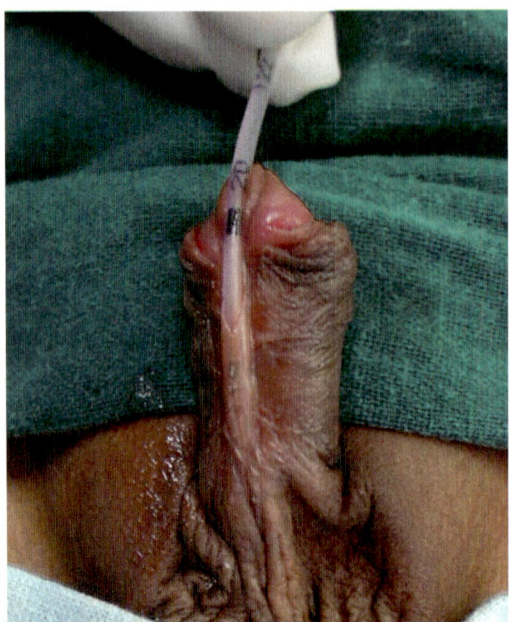

Fig. 11.6 Meatus distal penile with the long hypoplastic urethra

11.5 Surgical Techniques of Spongioplasty

Beaudoin (2000) [2] and Yerkes (2000) [3] described the bifurcated urethral spongiosum, combining these separated two pillars which were used to cover the ventral side of the new urethra, the procedure was termed "spongioplasty." There have been many changes in the technique of spongioplasty to improve the results. Various surgical techniques, their advantages and limitation are as follows:

Fig. 11.7 Distal hypospadias with no chordee. (**a**) Schematic diagram of Subcoronal hypospadias with no chordee. (**b**) Subcoronal hypospadias without hypoplasic urethra

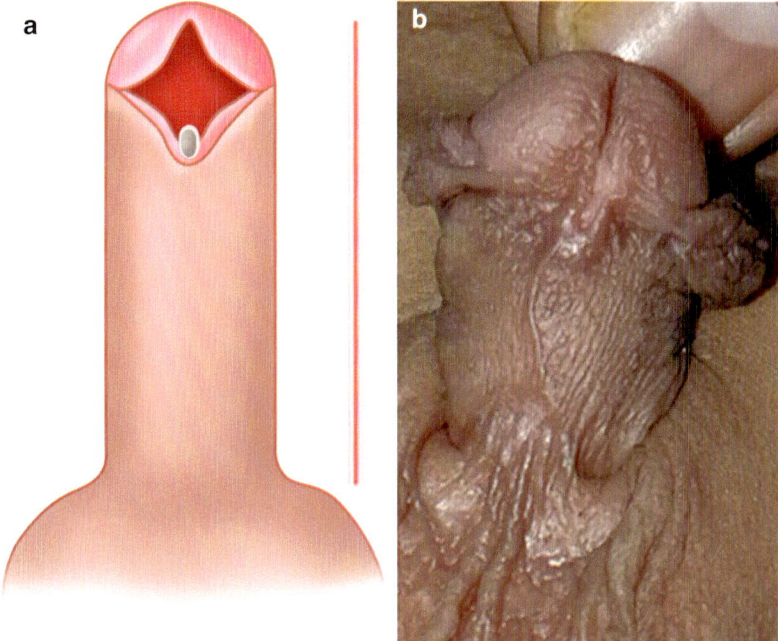

Fig. 11.8 Distal hypospadias with mild chordee, short hypoplastic urethra. (**a**) Schematic diagram of distal hypospadias with mild chordee and small hypoplastic urethra. (**b**) Showing distal hypospadias with mild chordee and small hypoplastic urethra

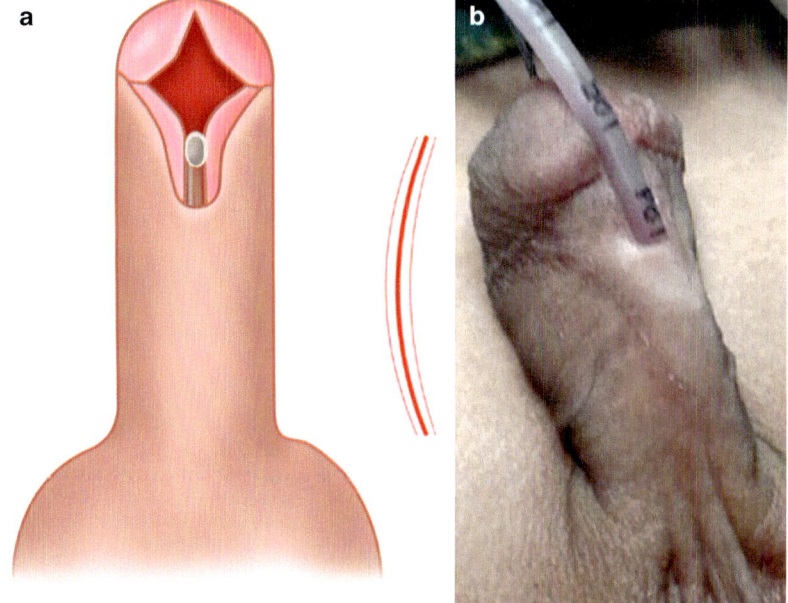

11.5.1 Yerkes Technique
[3] (Fig. 11.11a–c)

Penile degloving is done, and the distal spongiosum is mobilized laterally to the urethral plate. The mobilization of the spongiosum is started lateral to the margin of the corpus spongiosum proximal to the hypospadiac meatus. The spongiosum is then dissected from the underlying corpora cavernosa proximal to the distal and lateral to the medial. The urethral plate with spongiosum is wholly elevated off

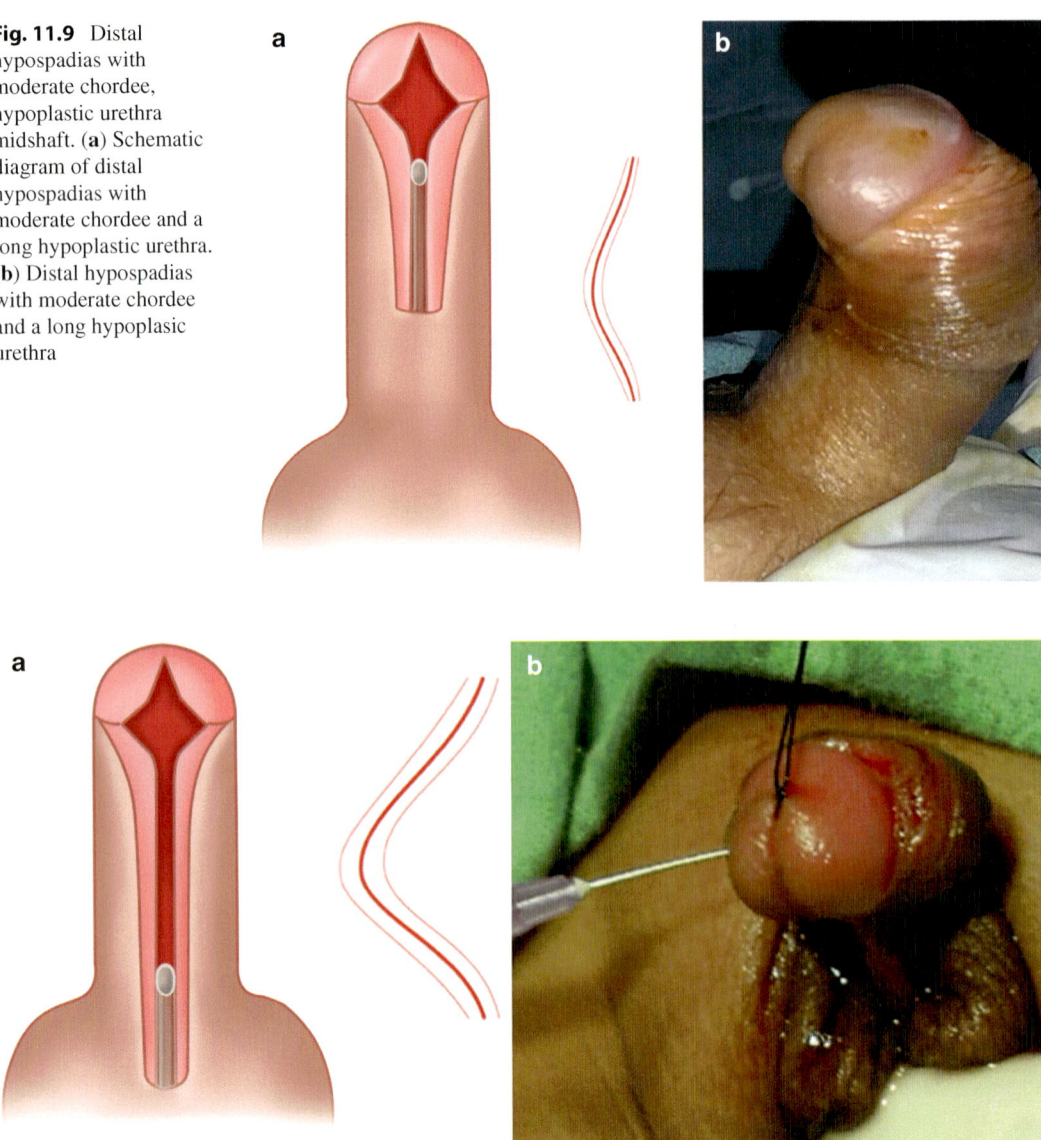

Fig. 11.9 Distal hypospadias with moderate chordee, hypoplastic urethra midshaft. (**a**) Schematic diagram of distal hypospadias with moderate chordee and a long hypoplastic urethra. (**b**) Distal hypospadias with moderate chordee and a long hypoplasic urethra

Fig. 11.10 Proximal hypospadias with severe chordee. (**a**) Schematic diagram of proximal hypospadias with severe chordee and small hypoplastic urethra. (**b**) Proximal hypospadias with severe chordee and small hypoplasic urethra

the urethral plate. Mobilization of the spongiosum is continued distally to the end of the urethral plate. Then the spongiosum is incised transversely at the end for complete spongiosum mobilization and glans release. Thus, the spongiosum is mobilized in the same plane up to the glans preserving the spongiosum distally with the urethral plate and leaving an adequate spongiosal wrap and good glans wings for closure. After the urethroplasty, the mobilized pillars of the distal spongiosum are sutured to cover the neourethra using fine absorbable sutures. The spongiosum is brought together in the midline in most of cases. But it is effective in covering lateral urethroplasty suture lines in flip-flap repair. Urethroplasty by midline suture lines is covered by overlapping the spongiosum in a pants-over-vest fashion. The thickness of the spongiosum may allow approximation in multiple layers.

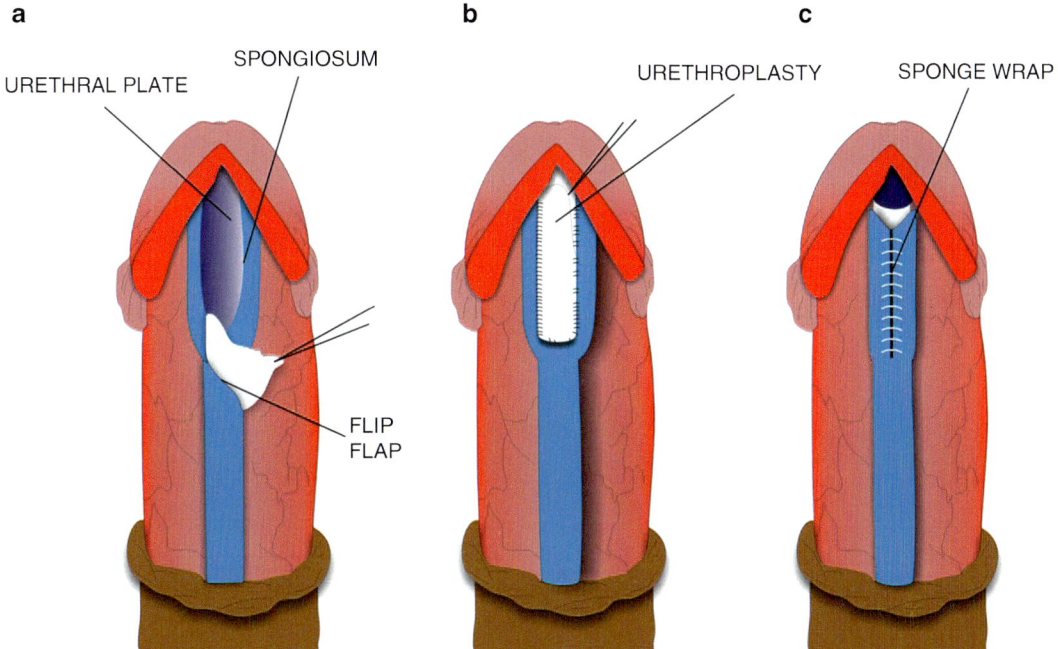

Fig. 11.11 Diagrammatic representation of Yerkes spongioplasty. (−). (**a**) Shwoing flip flap, spongiosum and urethral plate. Spongiosum mobilized, and flap taken in (**b**). Flap sutured, (**c**). Spongioplasty done

Advantage
1. Good mobilization and lifting of the urethral plate with spongiosum lateral to medial allow tension-free suturing.

Limitations
1. Incising spongiosum at corona may increase the chances of fistula at corona.
2. The suture line superimposition of urethroplasty, spongioplasty, and skin closure predisposes to fistula.

11.5.2 Dodat Spongioplasty
(Fig. 11.12a–e) [4]

Technique After putting in the urethral stent, a U-shaped incision encircling the urethral plate is given, and the ventral skin is freed up to the root of the penis. The spongiosum is incised starting from the glans' tip and followed onto the urethral plate's external borders up to the bifurcation of the spongiosal pillars. Next, the incision is given from proximal to distal, extending to the glans' tip and carried deep up to the corpora cavernosum tunica albuginea. That exposes the surface of the corpora cavernosa, inferiorly, up to the glans tip. The urethral plate is then tubularized to complete the urethroplasty with 6–0 or 7–0 absorbable (PDS/Vicryl) sutures. Next, the glans is closed by separate 6–0 sutures achieving hemostasias. Traction on the suture exposes the spongy bifurcation, and then spongioplasty is done by suturing the medial ends of the spongiosum over the neourethra by a 6–0 single suture. Because of the spongy tissue's extensive lateral dissection, this suture is placed with no tension. It should go well above the hypospadiac orifice to conceal the urethra devoid of spongy tissue until it becomes normal. This is followed by suturing the dissected margins of the glans and ensures complete hemostasias. Before releasing the tourniquet, Gittes test is done to confirm chordee correction. Then preputial reconstruction is done if demanded by the parents, or circumcision is performed to complete the surgery. The prepuce after prepucioplasty allows enough penile covering to give an esthetically and physiologically normal appearance [4].

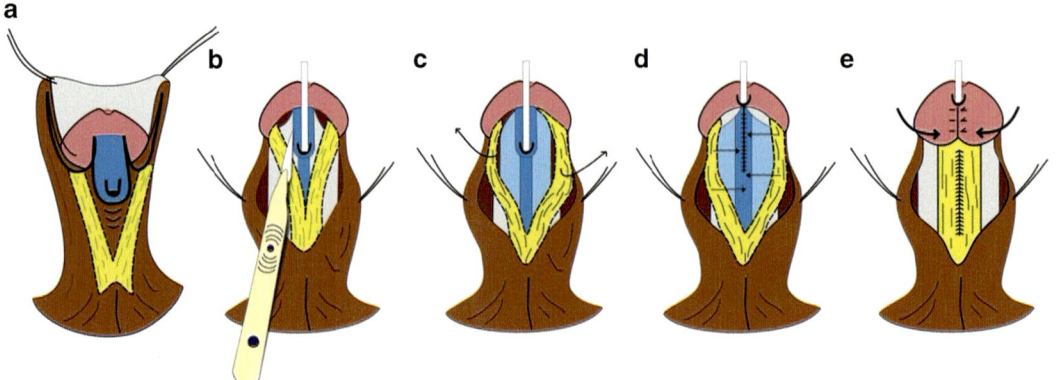

Fig. 11.12 Diagrammatic representation of Dodat spongioplasty. (**a**). Bifurcation of spongiosum, (**b**). Incising the urethral plate and spongiosum, (**c & d**). Mobilization of spongiosal pillar, (**e**). Spongioplasty and glanuloplasty

Advantages
1. Mobilization of both medial and lateral sides allows tension-free approximation of the spongiosum.
2. As the spongiosum posterior to the urethral plate is not mobilized, it preserves both dorsal and ventral surfaces of the spongiosum.
3. Spongioplasty and glanuloplasty increase the length of the penis and also correct mild chordee.

Limitations
1. Mobilization from both medial and lateral ends may compromise the vascular supply.
2. Superimposition of suture lines of urethral plate tubularization, spongioplasty, and skin suture may increase fistula chances.
3. Spongiosum is neither sutured to the neourethra nor to the corpora on the lateral aspect, which leaves the urethra uncovered laterally.
4. A partial cover over the urethra at the bifurcation of the spongiosal pillar may increase fistula chances.

11.5.3 Bhat's Modified Y-I Technique
[7, 8]

Technique: After injecting 1:100000 solution of adrenaline at the incision site, a U-shaped incision is given up to the corona encircling the meatus. Then partial ventral penile degloving is done in patients with mild curvature/torsion. But the incision is extended circumferentially circumcoronal in cases with moderate to severe chordee or torsion, and complete penile degloving is done up to the root of the penis by creating a plane of dissection at the level of Buck's fascia (Fig. 11.13). Then correction of chordee is evaluated by a Gittes test. A dissection plane is created in the healthy urethra proximal to the hypospadiac meatus at tunica albuginea, lifting a deep layer of Buck's fascia with the spongiosum to mobilize the urethral plate with spongiosum (Figs. 11.13 and 11.14a). The dissection is done just lateral to the margin of the corpus spongiosum on the ventral surface of the penile shaft. The spongiosum is dissected from the corpora cavernosa from lateral to medial. The complete mobilization spongiosum with urethral plate is done beneath the urethral plate on both sides, lifting off the midline spongiosum urethral plate from the corpora cavernosa when required, to correct the chordee and torsion [8].

Dissection is performed carefully at Buck's fascia level avoiding damage to the corpus spongiosum or corpus cavernosum. The proximal urethra may be mobilized up to the bulbar region accordingly in case of persistent chordee. The Gittes test confirms the adequacy of curvature correction. The spongiosal pillars spread beneath the glans wings on each side obliquely. Therefore, an oblique incision is given at about 45 degrees along the lateral borders of the spongiosal pillars (Fig. 11.14b, c).

11 Spongioplasty in Hypospadias Repair

Fig. 11.13 Schematic diagram showing cut section of hypospadiac penis with the plane of dissection of penile degloving and mobilization of spongiosum

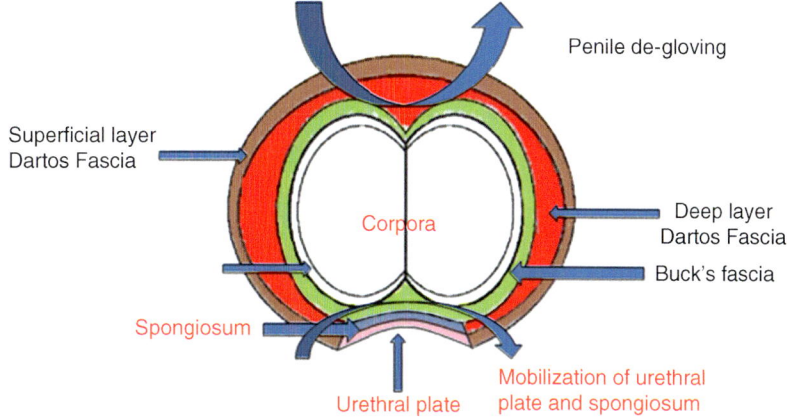

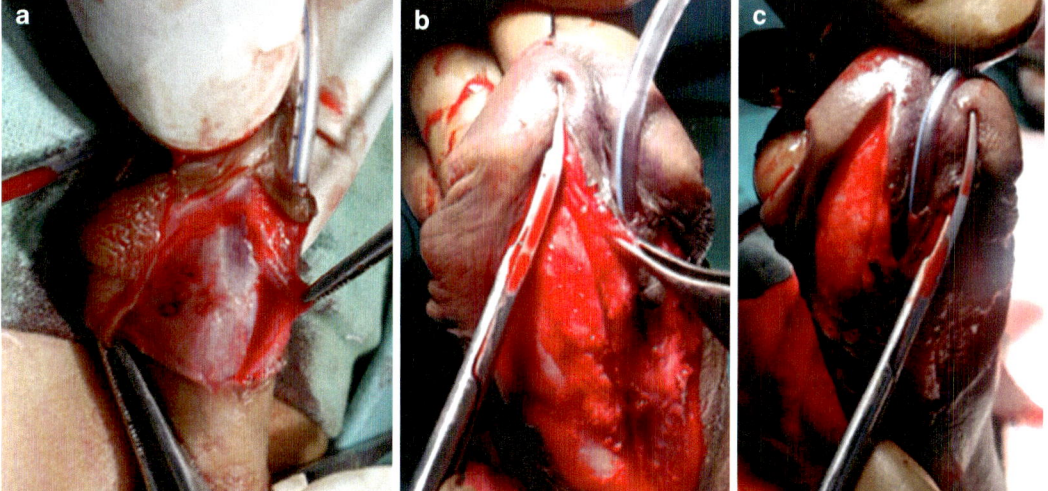

Fig. 11.14 Diagram showing mobilization of urethral plate and spongiosum. (**a**) Lateral to medial mobilization, (**b** & **c**). Mobilization of the spongiosum and urethral plate into glans

Care is taken to keep the dissection at tunica albuginea while mobilizing the glans wings distally. An adequate size, thick glans wings (with an intact spongiosum medially) are raised for glanuloplasty. Gittes test is repeated to see glanular chordee correction. The urethral plate is incised in the case of the narrow urethral plate (Fig. 11.15a). The incision should not be too deep and not to extend through and through the spongiosum. If required, a dorsal inlay graft is placed to achieve adequate width of the urethral plate (Fig. 11.15b). Then the urethral plate is tubularized with a subcuticular 6–0/7–0 polydioxanone (PDS) suture to reconstruct the neourethra (Fig. 11.15c). The mobilized spongiosal pillars are then sutured in the midline with 6–0/7–0 PDS by continuous suturing covering the entire neourethra starting one centimeter proximal to the bifurcation of spongiosum and right up to distal end of the neo-meatus (Fig. 11.15d). According to the patient's age, an adequate size urethral catheter (6–10 Fr) is left in situ. Glandular wings are sutured to complete the glansplasty. Skin is sutured with 6–0/7–0 PDS interrupted sutures and dressing done.

Advantages
1. Suturing the spongiosum is up to neo-meatus, covers the neourethra with healthy spongiosum beyond coronal sulcus, preventing fistula at corona.

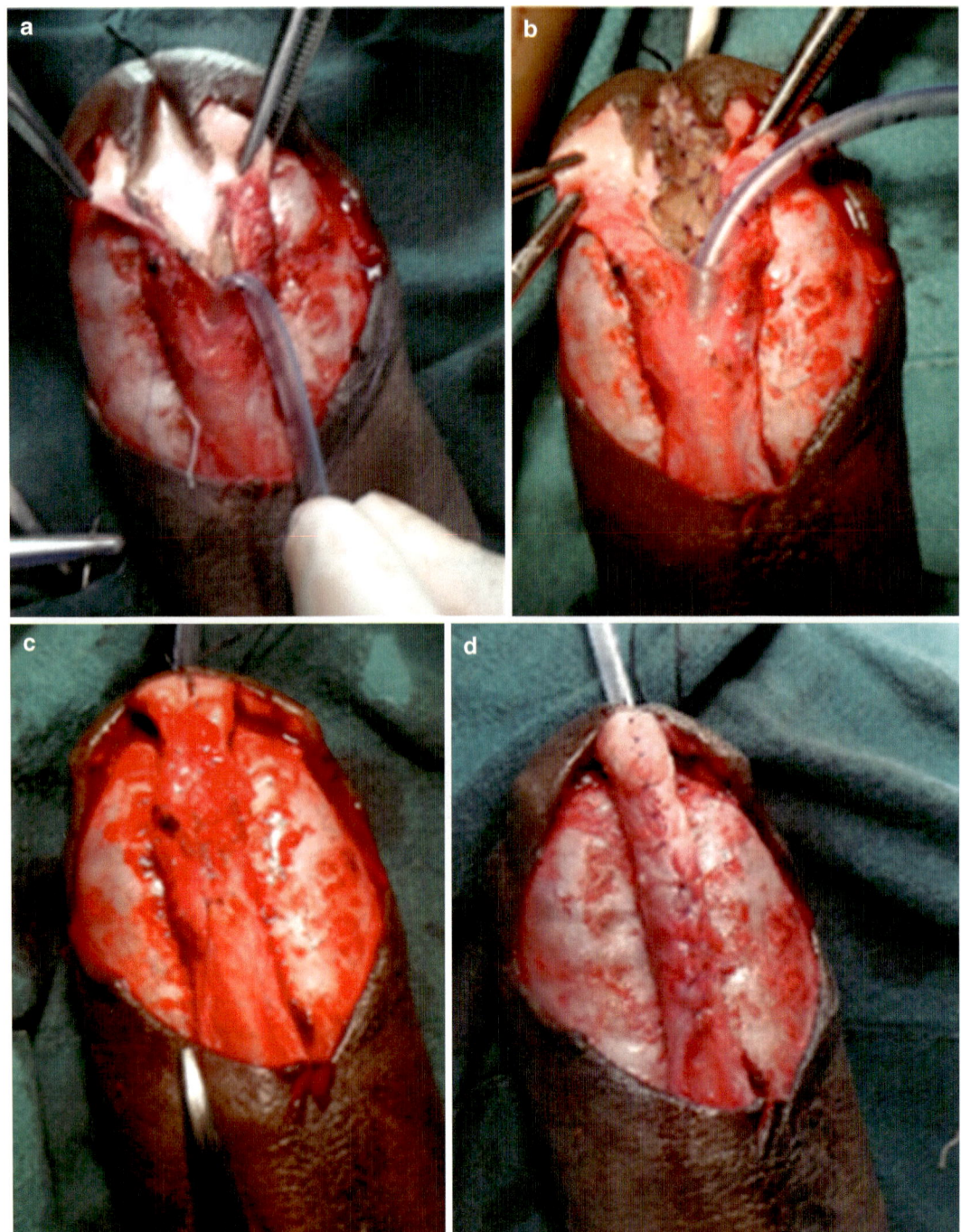

Fig. 11.15 Diagram showing mobilization of urethral plate and dorsal inlay graft. (**a**) Incised urethral plate. (**b**) Quilted inlay skin graft. (**c**) Tubularization of urethral plate. (**d**) Spongioplasty

2. Spongioplasty done after the mobilization and lifting of the spongiosum and urethral plate is tension-free and helps in the correction of chordee/torsion.
3. Dorsal inlay graft can be placed after incising the urethral plate.

Disadvantages of the Technique
1. The superimposition of suture lines of urethroplasty, spongioplasty, and skin sutures.
2. A conical shape of neourethra after spongioplasty.

11.5.4 Double Breasting Spongioplasty (Bhat's Technique) [13]

Technique: Steps of the double breasting spongioplasty are depicted in Fig. 11.16. After penile degloving urethral plate and spongiosum is mobilized (Figs. 11.17a, b & 11.18a). Spongiosum is assessed intra-operatively. If it is moderately or well developed, then double breasting spongioplasty is feasible. Suturing of the spongiosum started proximal to the bifurcation of the spon-

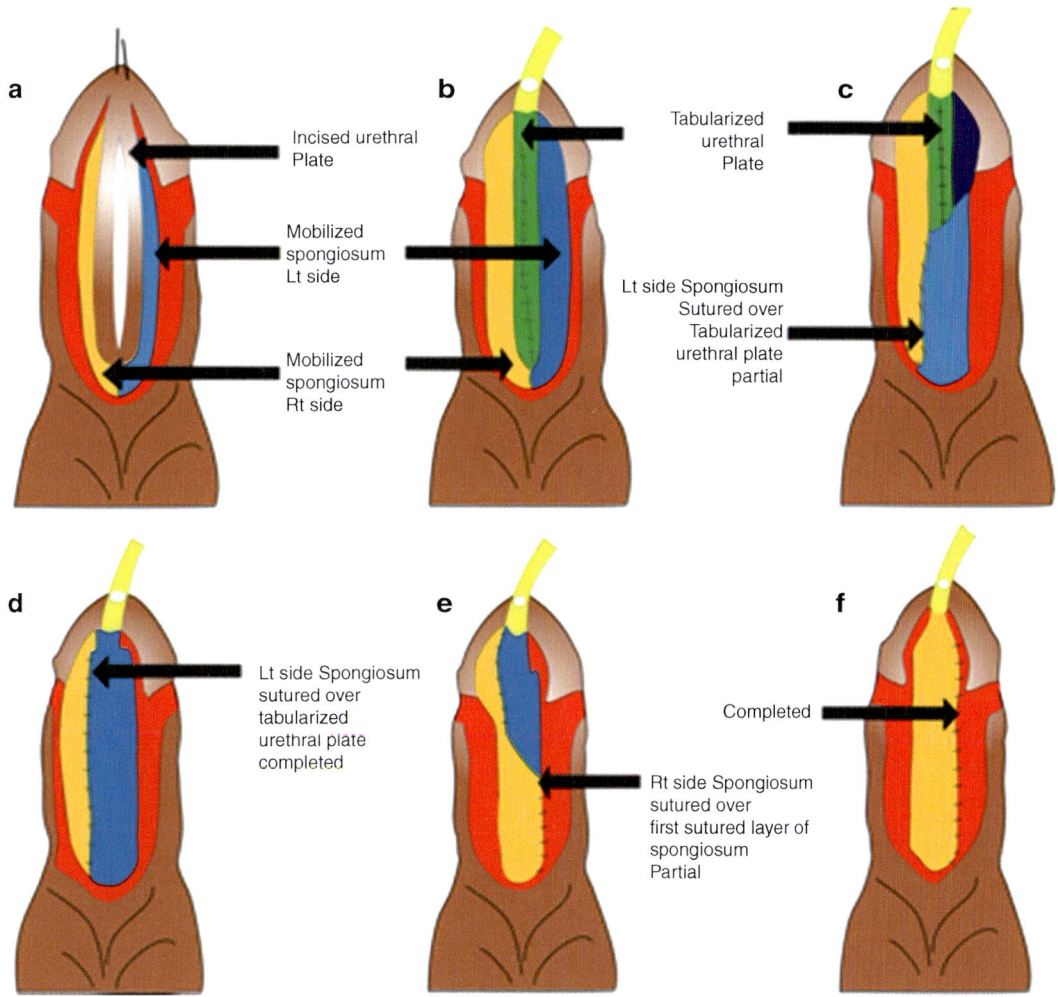

Fig. 11.16 Diagrammatic representation of double breasting. (**a**). Incised urethral plate, (**b**). Tubularized urethral plate, (**c** & **d**). Left side spongiosum sutured laterally to the suture line of tubularized urethral plate. (**e** & **f**). Right side spongiosum sutured to the lateral side as the second layer of double breasting

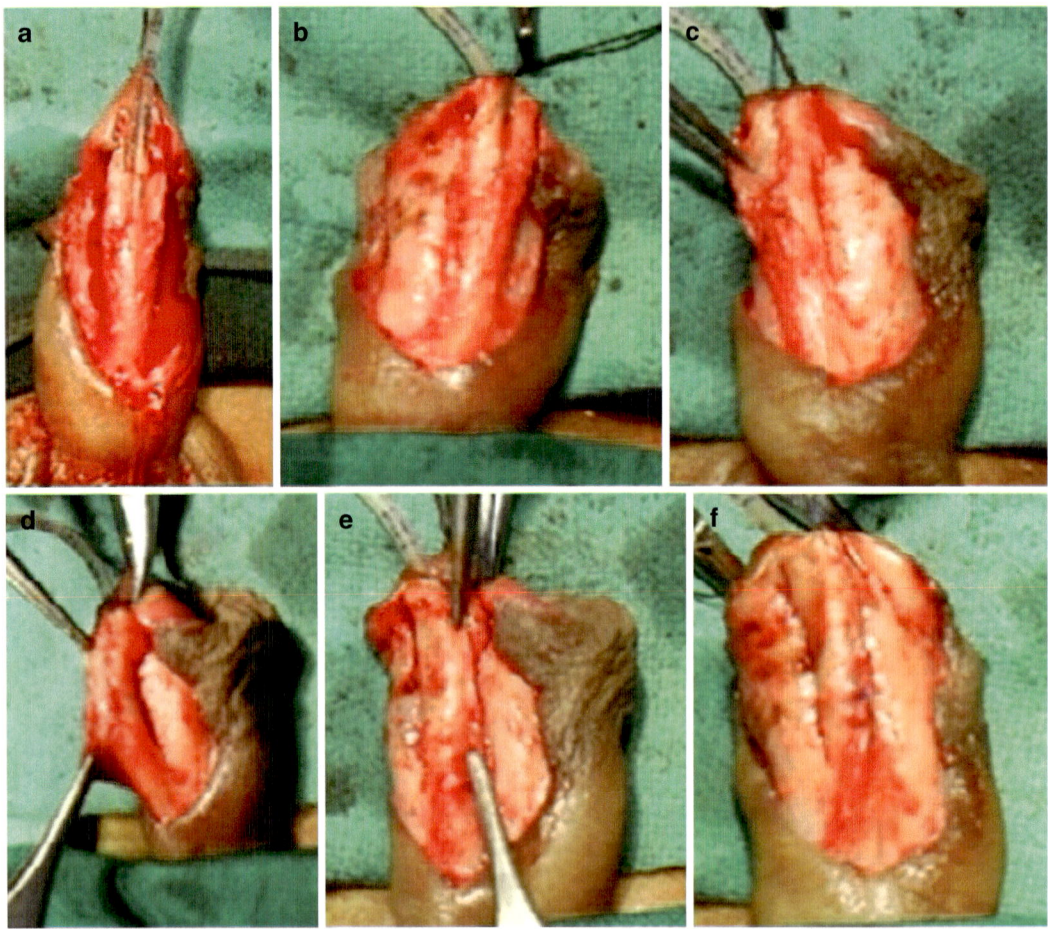

Fig. 11.17 Double breasting spongioplasty. (**a**). Mobilized urethral plate and spongiosum, (**b**). Tubularized urethral plate, (**c** & **d**). Suturing the left Spongiosal pillar lateral to suture line tubularized urethral plate. (**e** & **f**). Suturing the right spongiosal pillar over the sutured left spongiosal pillar covering the suture line

giosum and was done distally into the glans. The first layer of suturing of the spongiosum is done, keeping the suture line towards one side of the neourethral suture line laterally (Figs. 11.17c & d and 11.18b). The second spongiosal layer is sutured to the opposite side over the first layer. The second suture line towards the contralateral side buries the first layer's suture line with no overlapping of suture lines among all three layers (Figs. 11.17e & f and 11.18c, d). Thus, the neourethra is covered by two layers in a double breasting manner. A 6Fr to 10 Fr urethral catheter, depending on patient age, is left in situ. Glansplasty is by suturing the glans wings. Skin closure is done with 6–0/7–0 PDS sutures, and a pressure dressing is done [13].

Advantage

1. Double breasting of the spongiosum covers the neourethra by two layers of healthy spongiosum.
2. The superimposition of suture line of tubularization of the urethral plate, spongioplasty, and skin closure is avoided.
3. Covers the urethra with a double layer of spongiosum at both corona and bifurcation of spongiosum to prevent fistula, these are the commonest site of the fistula.
4. Shape of the neourethra is cylindrical, which is similar to a normal urethra.
5. Preserve a better vascular supply to neourethra and decreases chances of urethral stricture and fistula.

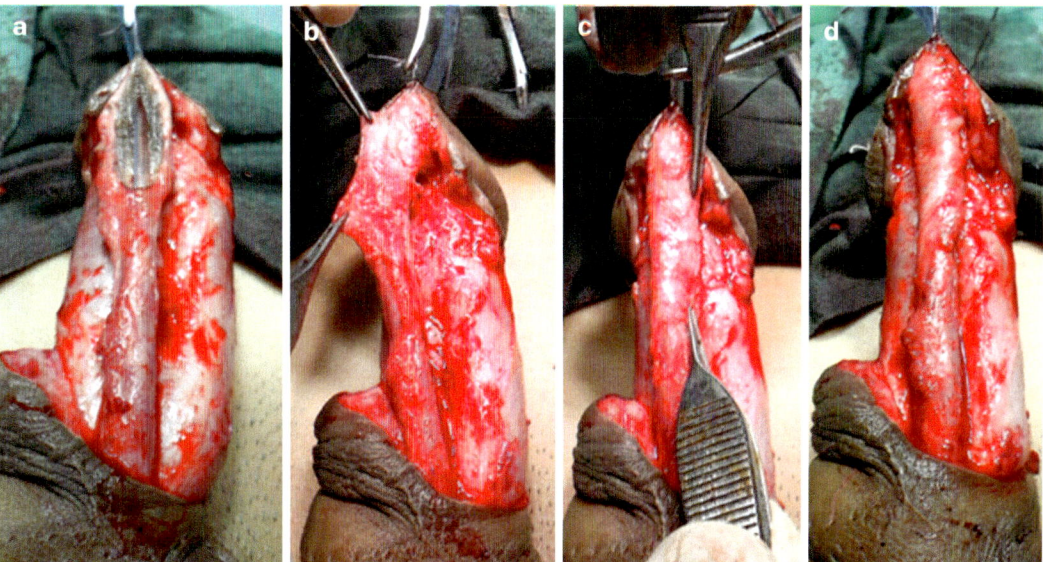

Fig. 11.18 Double breasting spongioplasty in adults. (**a**) Mobilized urethral plate and left side spongiosum sutured as the double breasting layer. (**c** & **d**). Right side spongiosum sutured as the second layer of the double breasting

Limitation

- The spongiosal pillars should be wide enough to make double breasting feasible. Hence, it can be performed only in moderate to well-developed spongiosum.

11.6 Spongioplasty in Transverse Prepucial Island Flap Repairs [14]

Transverse prepucial flap repairs are done in proximal hypospadias with chordee. Stricture and fistula are common complications. Stricture and fistulae in flap repair in severe hypospadias usually occur at the inner prepucial skin tube's anastomosis with the native urethra. Etiology may be poor blood supply of the terminal end of the skin flap and/or poor tissue cover over the anastomotic site. We correct chordee by mobilizing the urethral plate and spongiosum off the corpora from the corona to the urethral meatus instead of resecting it. The dissection is done at the level tunica albuginea, starting distally from the corona to the meatus proximally. The urethral plate with spongiosum is preserved. Correction of chordee with preservation of urethral plate is described in Chap. 6 chordee correction. Urethral mucosa and skin over the urethral plate are resected. The inner prepucial skin tube is anastomosed to the meatus, and the spongiosum is sutured over the anastomosis (Fig. 11.19a & b). Bhat et al. (2017) reported their results of covering the anastomosis with spongiosum. They had a urethrocutaneous fistula in 9.52% of the patients but none was at the anastomotic site [14].

The spongiosum may need to be resected to correct the chordee distal to the meatus in proximal hypospadias cases. In such cases, the spongiosum around the urethral opening and the proximal urethra is mobilized. Skin and mucosa of the urethral plate are resected distal to the meatus, and spongiosum is preserved for spongioplasty. After completing the anastomosis of the skin tube with the urethra, the preserved spongiosum is sutured over it to complete the spongioplasty. If a good spongiosum is not available, then the urethra is mobilized and spatulated dorsally. The urethra mucosa is denuded for 8–10 mm, and then the flap tube is sutured, keeping the skin tube suture line dorsally (Fig. 11.20). The urethral plate's denuded margins are sutured on the corpora's ventral surface to cover the anastomosis by spongiosum [14]. Bhat et al. (2002) reported the results of telescoping the skin tube in the native urethra in 48 patients with a fistula rate of only 4% [15].

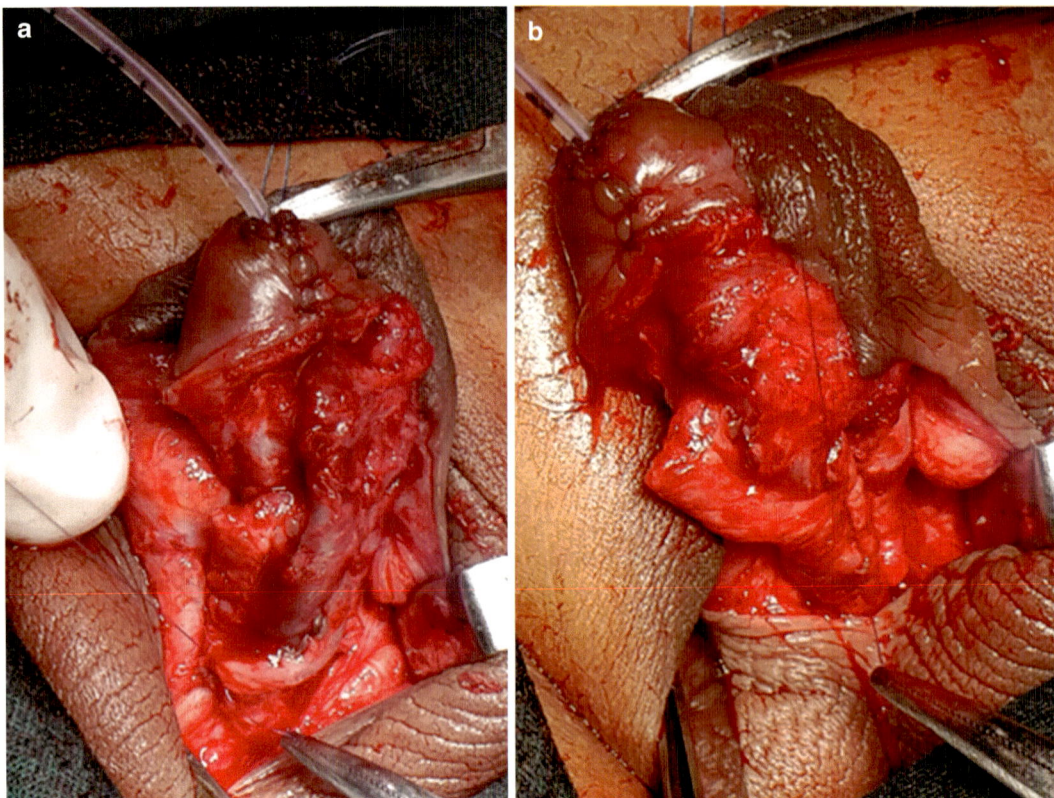

Fig. 11.19 Figure showing covering the anastomosis of the inner skin tube and urethra. (**a**) The anastomosis of the urethra and skin tube, (**b**) Spongioplasty covering the anastomosis

Advantage
1. Covers the anastomosis with healthy spongiosal tissue; so the blood supply of neourethra is maintained and helps in better healing.
2. Anastomosis is waterproof after covering it with spongiosum, reducing the chances of a urethral fistula.
3. Even if few sutures give way, the anastomosis is supported by spongiosum preventing the dehiscence of the anastomosis.

Disadvantage: If the urethral plate is not wide enough, tight suturing over the anastomosis may compress the urethral lumen.

11.7 Spongioplasty in Re-Operative Cases

Availability of spongiosum depends on the previous surgery. Spongiosum is available in all plate preservation procedures. Tubularized incised plate urethroplasty is the most commonly done procedure in distal and mid hypospadias. Common complications requiring a second surgical correction are fistula, chordee, and stricture. Spongiosum is usually well preserved in most TIPU cases, and the residual spongiosum in previous flap procedures may be available in some cases during redo surgery. Spongiosum is identified and mobilized after partial or complete penile degloving. In mild curvature cases, mobilization of spongiosum from corpora is feasible and corrects the chordee (Fig. 11.21). Closure of fistula or tubularization of the available urethral plate is performed with or without dorsal inlay, and then spongioplasty is done to cover the neourethra (Fig. 11.22a–d). A second layer of the healthy tissue of dartos or tunica may be covered to prevent the fistula. Sometimes, spongiosum can be identified in failed flap urethroplasties. That may be used to cover the neourethra with spongiosum (Fig. 11.21a–f).

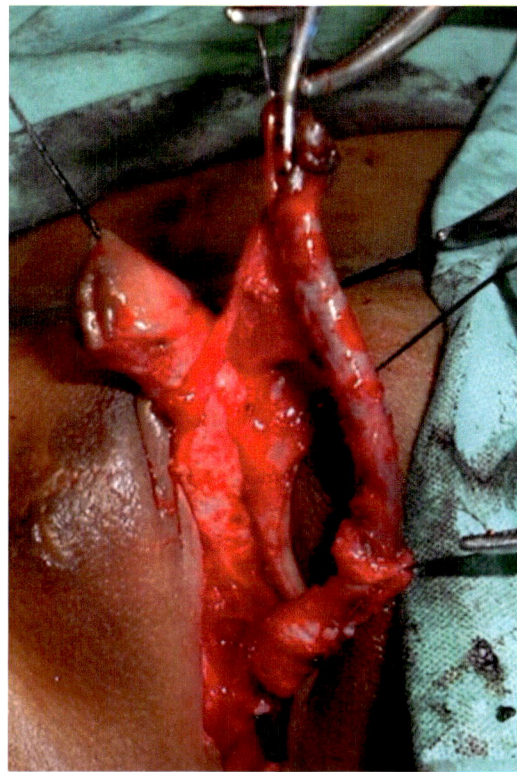

Fig. 11.20 Figure showing the telescoping of skin tube after spongioplasty

11.8 Progressive Modifications in Spongioplasty

Yerkes et al. advised mobilization of the spongiosum with the urethral plate lateral to medial. Then, spongioplasty was performed by suturing the edges to the midline, converting Y of the spongiosum to an I. Initially, this procedure was done in the flip-flap procedure, but now it is done after TIPU [3].

Dodat et al. (2003) introduced a modified spongioplasty technique where both limbs of the spongiosum were separated from the corpora cavernosa from both medial and lateral edges. These mobilized wings were then sutured in the midline over neourethra [4].

The difference in our technique from Yerkes et al. was that we avoided incising the spongiosum transversely at corona but mobilized the spongiosum into glans. Spongioplasty was done up to the neo-meatus, which has the added advantage of covering the neourethra with healthy spongiosum at the corona to prevent fistula. But the disadvantages of all the techniques described above are the superimposition of the suture lines of tubularized urethral plate, spongioplasty, and skin sutures. Additionally, the shape of the neourethra after spongioplasty is conical. Double breasting spongioplasty overcomes all these pitfalls, and Bhat et al. reported their results with this technique in 2017 with a significantly reduced complication rate (1.66%) than reported earlier [13]. The spongioplasty in flap repairs was reported by Bhat et al. in 2002 and 2017 with promising results [13, 15].

11.9 Why Spongioplasty

Tubularized Incised Plate Urethroplasty (TIPU) has widespread popularity by virtue of its versatility, low complication rate, and good cosmetic results. The TIPU repair is well described, but some surgical technique modifications can change the functional and cosmetic results. The commonest complication in all techniques of hypospadias repair is the urethrocutaneous fistula. The interposition of healthy tissue plays an important role to improve the results. Dartos was used as an interposing tissue in the original description to reduce the fistula rate. Various interposing healthy tissue to cover the neourethra have been described are dorsal (lateral, single, or double) dartos flaps, ventral dartos flap, scrotal dartos, de-epithelized local penile skin, preputial flap, paraurethral tissue, spongiosum, and tunica vaginalis flaps. The dorsal dartos flap is most commonly used, but it is not free of complications. The complications are penile torsion, chordee, or skin loss due to extensive dissection between the skin and dorsal dartos. In addition, dorsal dartos flap from one side may add tissue bulk and lead to the penile shaft's asymmetry.

In modern hypospadiology, the cosmetic results have become equally important as that of the functional one. So, the role of the dorsal dartos flap as an interposing tissue has been questioned. However, there is still no universally accepted ideal interposing tissue in TIPU. Tunica vaginalis has its independent supply and is being

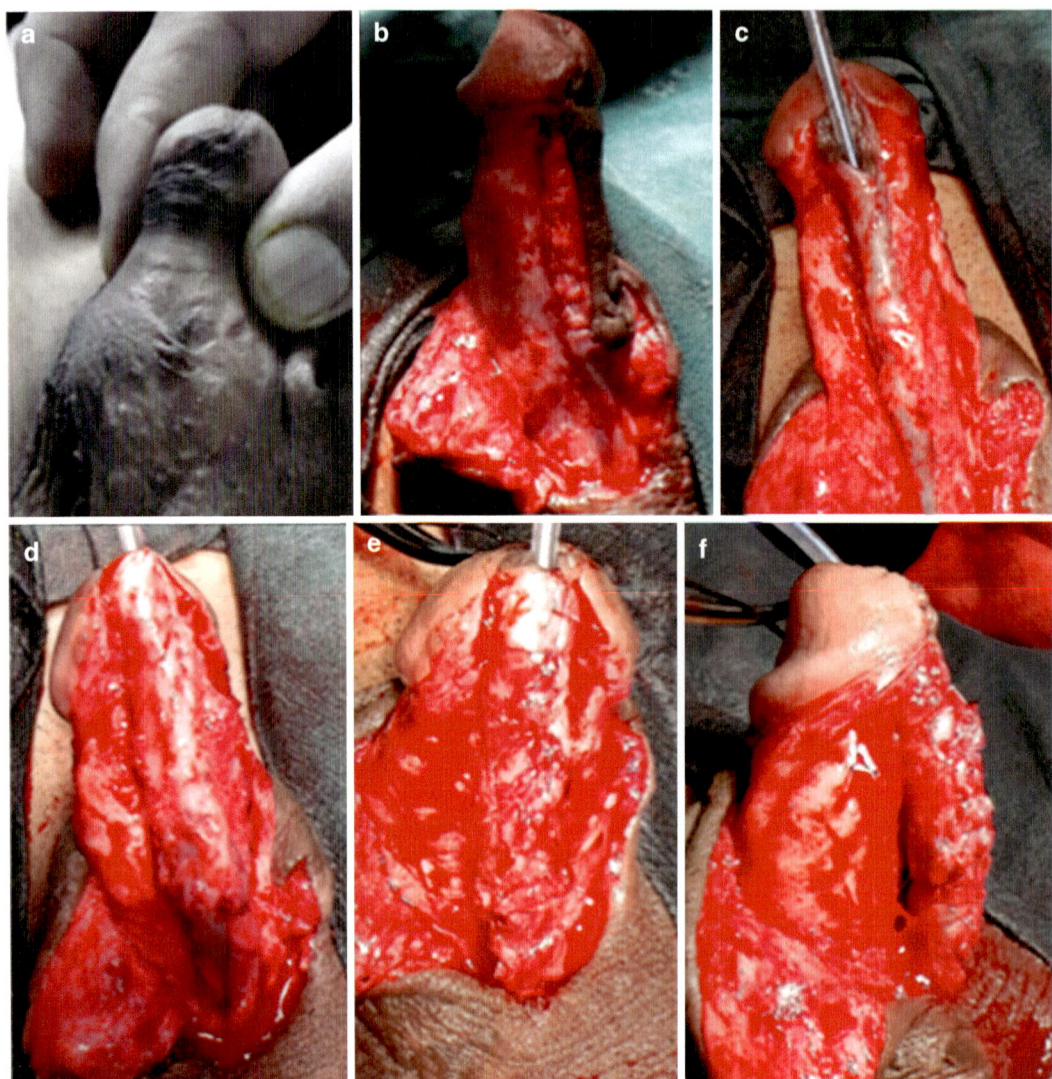

Fig. 11.21 Spongioplasty in re-operative cases. (**a**). Mild chordee with meatus at proximal penile area, (**b**). Mobilization of the midline skin with the urethral plate, (**c**). Skin tube tubularized, (**d** & **e**). Secondary spongioplasty

used as an interposing healthy tissue. This involves the opening of tunica vaginalis, adds time to the procedure, and chances of injury to the spermatic vessels, vas deference, epididymis, or testis. Inadequate mobilization and a short length of the tunica flap is likely to cause torsion. Tunica vaginalis cover is usually considered in cases of proximal, redo, and fistula repair cases. The advantages of spongioplasty are that it reconstructs near-normal functional urethra; the healthy interposing tissue cover is available locally and is very vascular. Therefore, it maintains the vascular supply of the urethral plate. Y to I spongioplasty adds length to the urethra and helps in chordee correction too. Every hypospadias surgeon is afraid of a urethral fistula, and spongioplasty helps reduce the fistula. Y-I spongioplasty is the most commonly used technique among the reported 781 cases of spongioplasty. The urethrocutaneous fistula rate varied from 0 to 14.28%, with an average of 5.12% (Table 11.1). Many authors have reported nil fistula rates following spongioplasty. Yerkes et al. reported no fistula in any of the patients of spongioplasty in

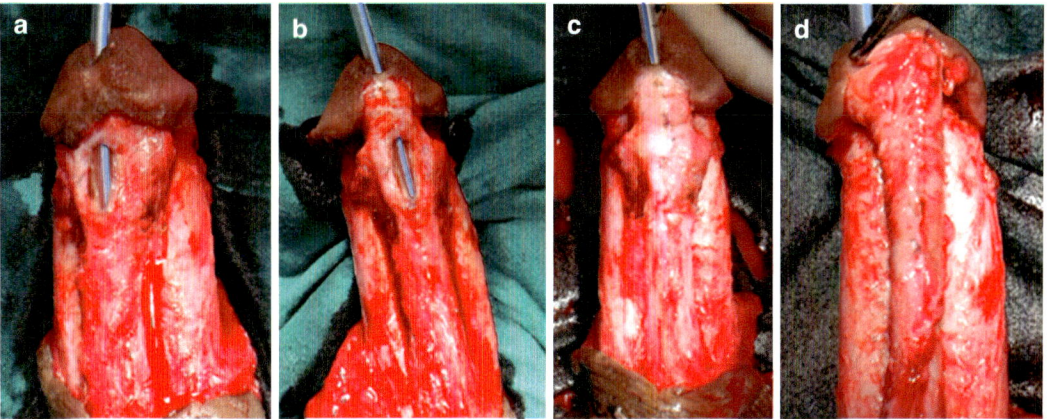

Fig. 11.22 Spongioplasty in redo TIPU. (**a** & **b**). Mobilization of urethral plate and spongiosum, (**c**). Tubularization of urethral plate, (**d**). Spongioplasty

Table 11.1 Showing the reported cases of spongioplasty with complications

SN	Authors	Year	Type of spongioplasty	No of cases	Fistula	Percentage
1	Yerkes [3]	2000	Y-I	25	Nil	0%
2	Dodat et al. [4]	2003	Dodat	51	2	3.92%
3	Bhat A [16]	2007	Modified Y-I	34	3	8.82%
4	Almodhen et al. [17]	2008	Y-I	32	Nil	0%
5	Gamal W M [18]	2009	Y-I	50	2	4.00%
6	Eassa et al. [19]	2011	Y-I	39	5	12.82%
7	Bilici et al. [20]	2011	Y-I	86	Nil	0%
8	Hayashi et al. [21]	2013	Y-I	37	3	8.10%
9	Bhat et al. [8]	2014	Modified Y-I	113	6	5.30%
10	Bhat et al. [23]	2015	Modified Y-I	14	2	14.28%
11	Bhat et al. [22]	2016	Modified Y-I	120	9	7.5%
12	Bhat et al. [13]	2017	Double breasting	60	1	1.66%
13	Zhang B et al. [8]	2020	Y-I	85	2	2.3%
14	Das et al. [24]	2020	Y-I	35	5	14.28%
	Total			781	40	5.12%

flip-flap repair [3]. Later on, Almodhen [17] in 32 cases and Billici [20] et al. in 86 cases reported their results of tubularized urethral plate urethroplasty with Y-I spongioplasty dorsal dartos cover with nil fistula. Dodat et al. in 2003 reported their results of the Duplay procedure and spongioplasty with separation of the corpora cavernosa in 51 patients. There was no fistula in anterior hypospadias (40) but two fistulae (3.92%) occurred in posterior hypospadias. The fistula site was at the base of the urethroplasty because of the insufficient covering by the spongy tissue. They recommended spongioplasty must always cover the area of urethroplasty up to the bifurcation of the spongy tissue [4]. Sarhan [25] et al. performed tubularized urethral plate urethroplasty using dartos flap and dartos with spongioplasty to cover the neourethra reported a statistically significant decrease in fistula rate in patients with spongioplasty. However, Hayashi et al. analyzed their data of 37 patients of TIP with spongioplasty for chordee correction and complication rate and found spongioplasty effective in decreasing chordee in 59% up to 15 degrees but no reduction of complications rate, and concluded that spongioplasty could not replace dartos cover. Unfortunately, spongiosum is used less frequently as a part of hypospadias repair despite such a low fistula rate. We do preserve and utilize the spongiosum in all cases. Y-I Spongioplasty is supported by dorsal or ventral dartos in cases of tubularized urethral plate urethroplasty.

The type of hypospadias, the severity of the chordee, development of the urethral plate and spongiosum are crucial variables in developing the fistula in hypospadias repair. Higher fistula rate has been observed in proximal hypospadias, severe curvature, poor development of spongiosum, and urethral plate. We had higher fistula 9% and 14.28% fistula in severe hypospadias and poorly developed spongiosum. But the exclusion of poorly developed spongiosum and adding double breasting technique fistula rate dropped to 1.66%. Spongiosum is the part of the urethra, and spongioplasty reconstructs a near-normal urethra. So, we recommend spongioplasty should be an integral part of tubularized urethral plate urethroplasty and all plate preservation urethroplasties to make the repair more anatomical. The option of supplementing it with other interposing healthy tissue remains in hand to improve the results.

11.10 Conclusion

Spongioplasty over tubularized urethral plate reconstructs a near-normal urethra. Spongioplasty with thicker and well-developed spongiosum lowers the incidence of fistula and meatal stenosis. Spongioplasty in flap repairs covers the anastomosis, making it waterproof and maintains good blood supply at the anastomotic site, reducing fistula and stricture chances. Double breasting spongioplasty is an excellent technique based on sound surgical principles, covers the neourethra with two layers of spongiosum, avoids the superimposition of suture lines of the urethral plate, spongiosum, and skin, maintains the urethral plate's vascular supply, the shape of the reconstructed urethra is cylindrical and significantly lowers the overall complication rate. Spongioplasty is feasible in redo cases wherever spongiosum is available in failed TIPU and other urethroplasties. Spongioplasty in these cases increases the chances of success rate. We recommend spongioplasty as an essential step in all patients undergoing tubularized incised plate repair for hypospadias.

References

1. Bhat A. General considerations in hypospadias surgery. Indian J Urol. 2008;24(2):188.
2. Beaudoin S, Delaage P-H, Bargy F. Anatomical basis of surgical repair of hypospadias by spongioplasty. Surg Radiol Anat. 2000;22(3–4):139–41.
3. Yerkes EB, Adams MC, Miller DA, Pope JC, Rink RC, Brock JW. Y-to-I wrap: use of the distal spongiosum for hypospadias repair. J Urol. 2000;163(5):1536–9.
4. Dodat H, Landry JL, Szwarc C, Culem S, Murat FJ, Dubois R. Spongioplasty and separation of the corpora cavernosa for hypospadias repair. BJU Int. 2003;91(6):528–31.
5. Gallo CB, Costa WS, Furriel A, Bastos AL, Sampaio FJ. Modifications of erectile tissue components in the penis during the fetal period. PLoS One. 2014;9(8):e106409.
6. Bhat A, Singla M, Bhat M, Sabharwal K, Kumar V, Upadhayay R, Saran RK. Comparison of results of TIPU repair for hypospadias with "Spongioplasty alone" and "Spongioplasty with dorsal dartos flap". Open J Urol. 2014;4(5):41–8.
7. Snodgrass W, Patterson K, Plaire JC, Grady R, Mitchell ME. Histology of the urethral plate: implications for hypospadias repair. J Urol. 2000;164(3 Part 2):988–90.
8. Bhat A, Sabharwal K, Bhat M, Saran R, Singla M, Kumar V. Outcome of tubularized incised plate urethroplasty with spongioplasty alone as additional tissue cover: a prospective study. Indian J Urol. 2014;30(4):392.
9. Zhang B, Bi Y, Ruan S. Reconstructing forked corpus spongiosum to correct glans droop in distal/midshaft hypospadias repair. J Int Med Res. 2020;48(5):0300060520925698.
10. Snodgrass W. A farewell to chordee. J Urol. 2007;178(3):753–4.
11. Mouriquand P, Mure P-Y. Hypospadias. In: Puri P, Höllwarth M, editors. Pediatric surgery. Heidelberg: Springer; 2006. p. 529–42.
12. Orkiszewski M. A standardized classification of hypospadias. J Pediatr Urol. 2012;8(4):410–4.
13. Bhat A, Bhat M, Kumar R, Bhat A. Double breasting spongioplasty in tubularized/tubularized incise plate urethroplasty: a new technique. Indian J Urol. 2017;33(1):58.
14. Bhat A, Bhat M, Sabharwal K, Kumar R. Bhat's modifications of Glassberg–Duckett repair to reduce complications in management severe hypospadias with curvature. Afr J Urol. 2017;23(2):94–9.
15. Bhat A, Saxena G, Prajapat P, Arya M, Patni M. Telescoping of skin tube and urethra to reduce fistula rate in one stage hypospadias repair. Bju International-Supplement. 2002;90(2):67–8.
16. Bhat A. Extended urethral mobilization in incised plate urethroplasty for severe hypospadias: a variation in technique to improve chordee correction. J Urol. 2007;178(3):1031–5.

17. Almodhen F, Alzahrani A, Jednak R, Capolicchio JP, El Sherbiny MT. Nonstented tubularized incised plate urethroplasty with Y-to-I spongioplasty in non–toilet trained children. Can Urol Assoc J. 2008;2(2):110.
18. Gamal W, Zaki M, Rashid A, Mostafa M, Abouzeid A. Tubularized incised plate (TIP) repair augmented by spongioplasty for distal and mid penile hypospadias. Uro Today Int J. 2009;2(3) https://doi.org/10.3834/uij.1944-5784.2009.06.13.
19. Eassa W, Jednak R, Capolicchio JP, Brzezinski A, El-Sherbiny M. Risk factors for re-operation following tubularized incised plate urethroplasty: a comprehensive analysis. Urology. 2011;77(3):716–20.
20. Bilici S, Sekmenli T, Gunes M, Gecit I, Bakan V, Isik D. Comparison of dartos flap and dartos flap plus spongioplasty to prevent the formation of fistulae in the Snodgrass technique. Int Urol Nephrol. 2011;43(4):943–8.
21. Hayashi Y, Mizuno K, Moritoki Y, Nakane A, Kato T, Kurokawa S, Kamisawa H, Nishio H, Kohri K, Kojima Y. Can spongioplasty prevent fistula formation and correct penile curvature in TIP urethroplasty for hypospadias? Urology. 2013;81(6):1330–5.
22. Bhat A, Bhat M, Kumar V, Kumar R, Mittal R, Saksena G. Comparison of variables affecting the surgical outcomes of tubularized incised plate urethroplasty in adult and pediatric hypospadias. J Pediatr Urol. 2016;12(2):108. e101–7.
23. Bhat A, Singla M, Bhat M, Sabharwala K, Upadhaya R, Kumara V. Incised plate urethroplasty in perineal and perineo-scrotal hypospadias. African. J Urol. 2015;21(2):105–10.
24. Das SK, Hasina K, Huq MAU, Adil SA, Alam MM, Alam SS. Spongioplasty with dartos flap coverage in the Snodgrass technique of hypospadias repair. J Bangladesh Coll Phys Surg. 2020;38(2):64–7.
25. Sarhan OM, El-Hefnawy AS, Hafez AT, Elsherbiny MT, Dawaba ME, Ghali AM. Factors affecting outcome of tubularized incised plate (TIP) urethroplasty: a single-Centre experience with 500 cases. J Pediatr Urol. 2009;5:378–82.

Flaps and Grafts in Hypospadias Repair

12

Octavio Herrera and Mohan S. Gundeti

12.1 Introduction

Hypospadias is attributed to the failed fusion of the endodermal urethral folds, resulting in incomplete urethral tubularization. The incomplete tubularization of the urethra results in an ectopic urethral opening that can be found anywhere from the glans to the perineum. About 50% of hypospadias are distal (glans and coronal), 30% are middle (penile shaft), and 20% are proximal (scrotal and perineal). This arrest in development often also causes ventral chordee (penile curvature) and ventral foreskin deficiency, leading to a dorsal "hooded" prepuce. More severe presentations of hypospadias may be accompanied by peno-scrotal transposition, in which the scrotum is abnormally positioned superior and anterior to the penis.

Hypospadias repair should aim to achieve the following three main objectives: voiding in an upright position, an appropriate voiding stream, and normal penile appearance and function.

There are hundreds of operative techniques with slight variations described in the hypospadiology literature with an ultimate goal of achieving normal penile function and cosmesis [1]. These modifications often focus on the method of reconstructing the urethra or correcting penile curvature. Urethral reconstruction for distal hypospadias may not need tissue replacement besides an interposition layer to cover the neo-urethra suture line, such as a dartos flap. Proximal hypospadias more commonly requires additional tissue during reconstruction to compensate for the congenital ventral tissue deficiencies [2]. In this chapter, we will describe the roles, types, and basic principles of flaps and grafts used for urethral substitution, augmentation, primary tissue for penile resurfacing, and interposition in hypospadias repair with current outcomes in literature using comparative studies.

12.2 Patient Examination

Hypospadias should be diagnosed at birth with a thorough physical examination. Establishing a diagnosis during the neonatal period is essential, as performing a neonatal circumcision is contraindicated in these patients. This is because the prepuce is frequently used as a vascularized flap or free graft during the urethral reconstruction. After urologic consultation and shared decision-making with the patient's parents for repair, several factors should be taken into consideration

---

O. Herrera
Class of 2021, Pritzker School of Medicine, University of Chicago, Chicago, IL, USA
e-mail: oherrera@uchicago.edu

M. S. Gundeti (✉)
Pediatric Urology (Surgery), MFM (Ob/Gyn) and Pediatrics, The University of Chicago Medicine & Biological Sciences, Chicago, IL, USA

Pediatric Urology, Comer Children's Hospital, Chicago, IL, USA
e-mail: mgundeti@surgery.bsd.uchicago.edu

prior to repair. A thorough genitourinary examination should be conducted to determine the meatal location, glans volume, penile length, degree of chordee, presence of peno-scrotal transposition, and depth and width of the urethral plate. These operative characteristics, in addition to a surgeon's preference and experience, play a role in the selection of a method of repair and use of pre-operative testosterone therapy for surgical optimization [3].

12.3 Flaps

12.3.1 History and Evolution

A flap is a transfer of tissue with an intrinsic vascular supply from one area of the body to another. Flaps have long been used in surgery for coverage of areas damaged by trauma, burns, radiation, chronic inflammation, and congenital anomalies. In fact, the earliest known description of flap use derives from ancient India [4]. The *Suśrutasaṃhitā*, dated back to almost 900 B.C., contains detailing of ancient Indian physicians using flaps for facial reconstruction. Similar principles of flap use have also been attempted by Aulus Cornelius Celsus (25 B.C.–50 A.D.) in ancient Rome and Oribasius of Alexandria (320–403 A.D.) in ancient Greece. Flap manipulation to replace skin defects has evolved throughout centuries into what is today modern plastic surgery.

One benefit of a flap transfer is that it carries its own blood supply, so it does not rely on the recipient bed for perfusion (Table 12.1). As such, it does not require microsurgical anastomosis with surrounding vessels for neovascularization. This allows for flaps to be used to reconstruct large areas of defect. In addition to the size of the defect, the surgeon must also account for the location, shape, depth, and surrounding skin laxity when planning for reconstruction. Another important consideration includes the local vascular supply that provides viable options for flap coverage, as well as ensuring that the flap is receiving sufficient perfusion. The current method of intraoperatively assessing flap perfusion in hypospadias is through the surgeon's clinical judgment of the tissue color and presence of bleeding. Though, a systematic review of intraoperative flap perfusion in microsurgery reports that fluorescence imaging and laser Doppler are suitable tools for assessment of flap perfusion [5]. These tools may be applicable in hypospadias repair in order to optimize flap survival.

Table 12.1 Broad comparison of characteristics between flaps and grafts in hypospadias repair

	Flaps	Grafts
Vascularity	Intrinsic vascular supply	Relies on recipient bed
Mobility	Limited mobility and rotation around pedicle	No mobile constraints for placement
Recipient site	Can survive on recipient site with questionable supply	Requires robust supply at recipient site for survival
Type of tissue	"Like" penile tissue	"Like," distant, or engineered tissue
Surgical sites	Single surgical site	One or more surgical sites

12.3.2 Flap Classification

Flaps can be classified through various methods such as the vascular supply of tissue, composition of tissue, and movement of tissue. When flaps are described by their vascular supply, they are either termed random or axial [7] (Fig. 12.1). Random flaps are not supplied by a named blood vessel. Rather, they are supplied by the interconnected dermal-subdermal plexuses. These systems of vascular supply are delicate and limited in the size of flap they can sustain. The distal end of a random flap is particularly prone to ischemia. This is due to its increased distance from a reliable blood supply and hyperadrenergic vasoconstrictive response to being incised and elevated [8]. Thus, prompt re-approximation of the flap to a vascularized source of nourishment is essential to optimize survival. Additionally, a 3:1 length-to-width ratio is used as a rule of thumb when harvesting a random flap to promote adequate circulation throughout the entire area. Axial flaps are developed based on angiosomes,

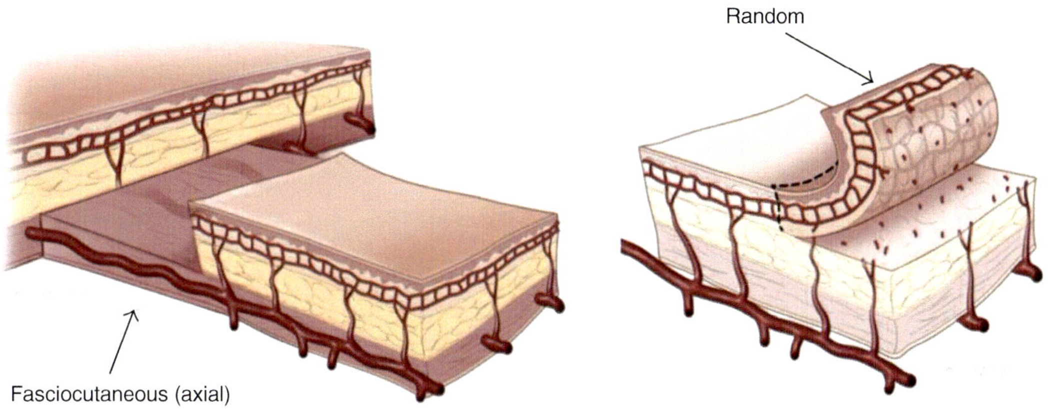

Fig. 12.1 An axial flap has a known blood vessel or vessels traversing its length, which supply the flap tissue directly and through their vascular networks. Random flaps do not contain an axial or named vessel. Instead, they are supplied by interconnected dermal-subdermal plexuses (Reprinted: Wisenbaugh ES, Gelman J. The Use of Flaps and Grafts in the Treatment of Urethral Stricture Disease. *Advances in Urology*. 2015 [6])

or territories of tissue that are vascularized by a specific vessel. The superficial and deep external pudendal arteries and their subdermal arterial plexuses are responsible for supplying the penile skin, prepuce, and subcutaneous tissue, which are all valuable resources in penile reconstruction.

Flaps can also be labeled by their method of transfer. Advancement flaps are transferred along the body parallel to their vascular pedicle. Rotation flaps are rotated around their vascular pedicle. The range of these flaps is limited as to not compromise the vascular supply from excessive rotational compression. Island flaps are used when the tissue bulk surrounding the vascular pedicle prevents adequate rotation. In island flaps, the cuff of tissue surrounding the vascular pedicle is removed to improve the rotational range. Attention must be placed to prevent torsion and kinks in the exposed vascular pedicle. Although these numerous variations encourage surgical innovation in flap use, an important principle is to prevent vascular compromise by minimizing excess flap rotation, pressure, and tension.

a urethra. Numerous methods of flap use have since been developed and implemented in hypospadias repair. Flaps are valuable in hypospadias repair due to ventral penile tissue deficiencies in severe presentations, which puts into question the reliability of the local perfusion and nutrition. When the decision is made to use flaps in hypospadias repair, local penile flaps are preferred as they can be well-mobilized, placed under minimal tension, and have a reliable blood supply. Local penile flaps are also preferred as they provide like tissue, which may provide superior aesthetic and functional results. Various techniques of flap use for urethral reconstruction in hypospadias repair have been described in the literature (Table 12.2). A brief summary of flap outcomes reported in the literature is outlined in Table 12.3. Techniques using penile skin, inner preputial skin, perimeatal tissue, and dartos tissue are implemented for urethral reconstruction. Tunica vaginalis and dartos flaps are used as intermediate healthy layers to cover the neourethra for fistula prevention (Fig. 12.2). Penile skin and scrotal flaps are effective options for skin resurfacing.

12.3.3 Flaps in Hypospadias

Flap use in hypospadias repair was first described by Bouisson in 1861, in which he used a scrotal flap to reconstruct the missing inferior segment of

12.3.4 Onlay Island Flap

Onlay island flap (OIF) entails the use of a dorsal pedicled prepuce or penile skin flap on the ventral

Table 12.2 Brief description of flap technique characteristics, advantages, and disadvantages

Flap	Tissue type	Advantages	Disadvantages
Onlay island flap	Prepuce (inner or outer) or dorsal penile skin	Single-stage Urethral augmentation Use in distal, mid, and proximal repair	Highly variable complication rates reported
Dorsal preputial flap (Byars)	Inner prepuce	Urethral augmentation or substitution Use in severe cases	Two-stage Highly variable complication rates reported
Preputial tubularized island flap	Prepuce	Single-stage Urethral substitution	Severe fistula risk
Perimeatal flap (Mathieu)	Ventral penile skin	Single-stage Urethral augmentation	Poor cosmetic outcome Limited to mid-penile and distal repair

Table 12.3 Summary table of outcomes using different flap techniques reported in the literature

Authors	Meatal location	Technique (n) [# of planned stages]	Total complications	Urethrocutaneous Fistula	Meatal stenosis	Cosmetic complications
ElGanainy [10]	Coronal, subcoronal, distal	OIF (30) [1] Mathieu (30) [1]	0 (0%) 6 (20.0%) p = 0.036	0 (0%) 4 (13.3%)	–	OIF better cosmetically than Mathieu p < 0.001
Braga [13]	Peno-scrotal	OIF (40) [1] TIP (35) [1]	18 (45.0%) 21 (60.0%) p = NS	8 (20.0%) 15 (42.9%) p = 0.03	1 (2.5%) 1 (2.9%) p = NS	–
Long [15]	Proximal	Byars (81) [2]	40 (49.0%)	5 (6.2%)	5 (6.2%)	–
Stanasel [16]	Proximal	Byars (56) [2]	38 (67.9%)	32 (57.1%)	5 (8.9%)	–
McNamara [17]	Proximal	Byars (134) [2]	71 (53.0%)	39 (29.1%)	17 (12.7%)	–
Wiener [20]	Proximal	PTIF (74) [1] OIF (58) [1]	27 (36.5%) 18 (31.0%) p = 0.64	10 (13.5%) 10 (17.2%) p = 0.73	3 (4.1%) 2 (3.4%)	1 (1.4%) 3 (5.2%)
Ghali [21]	Distal, mid-penile, proximal	Mathieu (216) [1] PTIF (148) [1] OIF (42) [1]	33 (15.3%) 48 (32.4%) 3 (7.1%)	19 (8.8%) 22 (14.9%) 1 (2.4%)	1 (0.5%) 17 (11.5%) 0 (0%)	22 (14.9%) 3 (7.1%)
Wilkinson [28]	Distal	Mathieu (1496) [1] TIP (1872) [1]	–	79 (5.3%) 72 (3.8%) p = 0.03	7/1050 (0.7%) 57/1861 (3.1%) p < 0.001	–

aspect of the penis. This technique was popularized by Elder et al. in 1987 as a method for repairing mid-penile and distal hypospadias, as well as hypospadias that is too proximal to be repaired with the Mathieu technique [8]. This is performed by making a U-shaped incision along the urethral plate that extends proximal to the hypospadic meatus followed by a subcoronal circumferen-

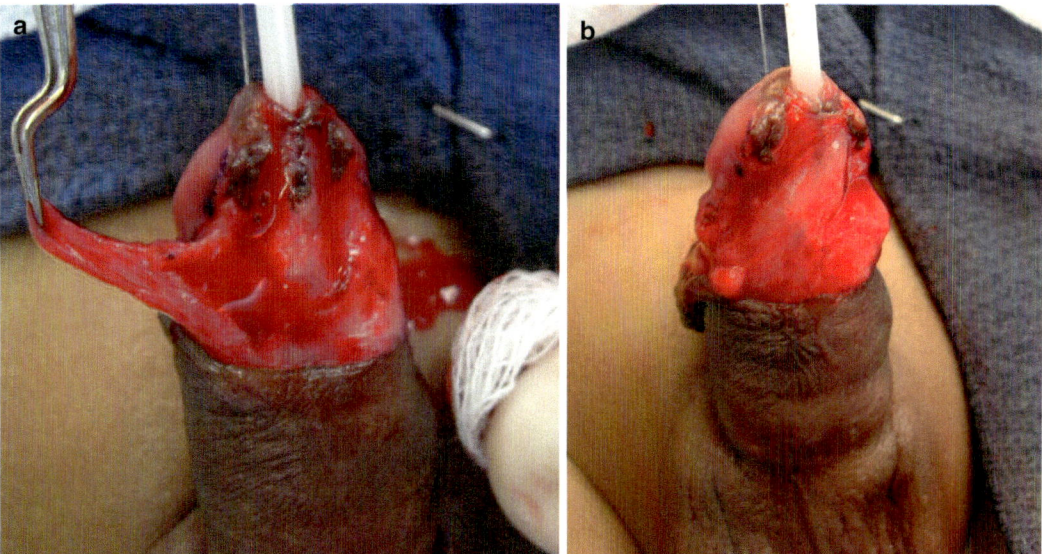

Fig. 12.2 Dartos flaps. (**a**) Lateral dartos flap harvested to cover the suture line at the neourethra in a distal hypospadias repair. (**b**) The suture line is covered. Glans flaps will then be re-approximated over the flap

tial incision. A pedicled skin flap is created on the dorsal penis using stay sutures to expose the junction between the inner and outer layers of the prepuce and then incising at this junction just beneath the inner preputial skin (Fig. 12.3) [9]. A longitudinal incision is made through the proximal dartos fascia to free the flap while preserving its vascular pedicle. The flap pedicle is dissected down to the penopubic junction to prevent tension during flap mobilization. The flap is then transposed over its pedicle onto the ventral aspect by placing the glans through the longitudinal incision via a buttonhole maneuver. The onlay island flap is then sutured to the bilateral edges of the urethral plate, covered with a second layer of vascularized inner preputial tissue, and then ventral skin and glans are re-approximated [10, 11]. OIF is an appropriate and reliable technique for urethral augmentation in hypospadias given its favorable post-operative outcomes and normal cosmetic appearance [12, 13].

12.3.5 Dorsal Preputial Flap

In many cases of severe hypospadias, the robustness of the ventral dartos tissue and urethra is insufficient for a successful single-stage hypospadias repair. A two-stage procedure may be more effective, as it allows an opportunity to use a graft or flap to provide sufficient vascularity and tissue prior to urethroplasty. The first stage entails orthoplasty, or straightening of the penis, followed by harvesting and placing a graft or flap. The second stage is comprised of urethroplasty, glansplasty, and a layered closure. Here we will discuss the use of dorsal preputial flaps during the first stage of repair.

The use of dorsal preputial flaps for hypospadias repair was popularized by Byars in 1951 [14]. During the first stage, a midline incision is made which extends to the hypospadic meatus (Fig. 12.4) [9]. A circumferential incision is then made proximal to the coronal sulcus. The penis is then degloved to its base to correct the chordee. Further orthoplasty techniques such as dorsal plication, ventral fairy cuts, or urethral mobilization may be necessary if chordee persists. Once the penile curvature correction is satisfactory, the glans is divided in the midline and dissected laterally in order to separate the ventral aspect off of the corpora cavernosa. The Byars technique is performed by extending the dorsal foreskin, which is then divided in the midline to allow for

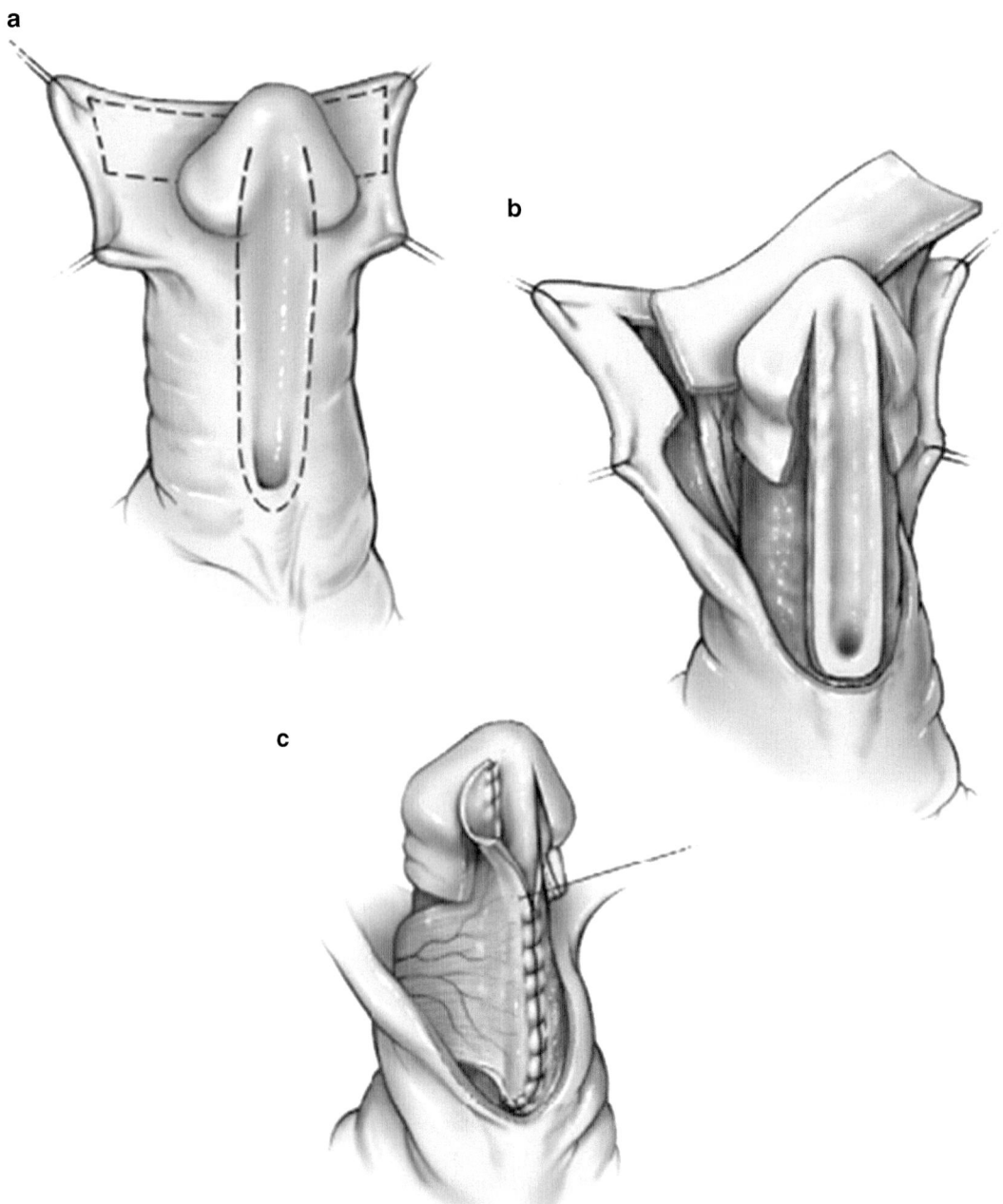

Fig. 12.3 Onlay island flap. (**a**) Incisional lines are outlined on the inner prepuce and the urethral plate. (**b**) The inner preputial flap is dissected along its vascular pedicle for mobilization. (**c**) The mobilized flap is transposed ventrally, either through a buttonhole maneuver or laterally. The flap is then sewn to the urethral plate for urethral augmentation (Reprinted with permissions from: Campbell-Walsh Urology tenth ed. Wein AJ, Kavoussi LR, Novick AC, Partin AW, Peters CA. Hypospadias. Fig. 130–12 p. 3515. Copyright Elsevier Health Sciences 2011)

ventral mobilization. The dorsal preputial flaps are rotated ventrally and sutured into the glanular cleft and distal urethral bed. The purpose is to establish a supple dartos bed for a safe and effective second-stage urethroplasty. The ventral skin is then closed at the midline. The second-stage urethroplasty should be performed after at least 6 months to allow for proper healing. Urethroplasty

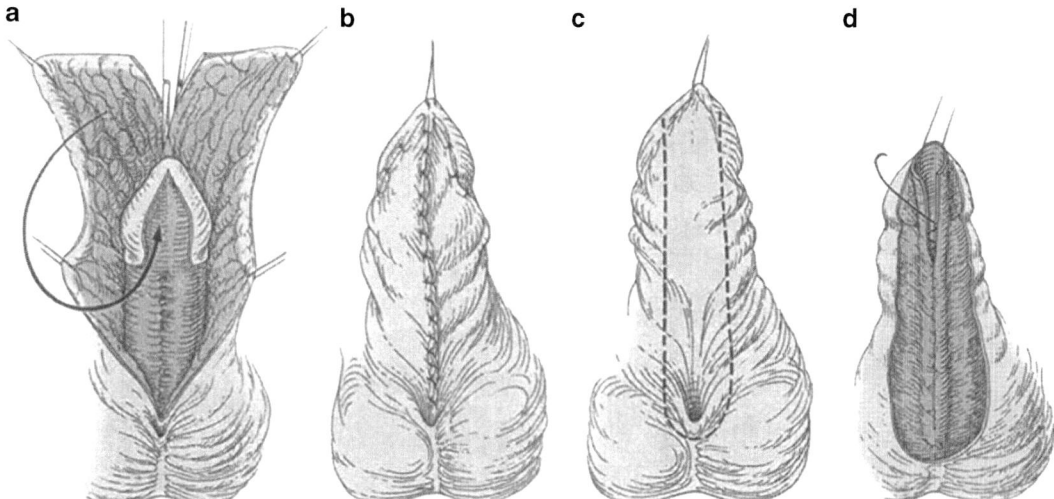

Fig. 12.4 Byars flaps. (**a**) Midline incision is made extending to the hypospadic meatus, followed by a circumferential incision proximal to the coronal sulcus. The penis is then degloved to its base to correct the chordee. Upon satisfactory chordee correction, the glans is divided in the midline. The dorsal foreskin is then extended and divided in the midline to allow for ventral mobilization. (**b**) The dorsal preputial Byars flaps are rotated ventrally and sutured into the glanular cleft and distal urethral bed. The ventral skin is closed at the midline. (**c**) Six months are allowed for proper healing after the first stage. In the second stage, U-shaped incision is made, which extends proximal to the meatus. (**d**) The strip is tubularized to create a neourethra (Reprinted with permissions from: Campbell-Walsh Urology tenth ed. Wein AJ, Kavoussi LR, Novick AC, Partin AW, Peters CA. Hypospadias. Fig. 130–17 p. 3520. Copyright Elsevier Health Sciences 2011)

may be performed using the surgeon's preferred technique. Thiersch-Duplay or TIP is currently the most widely-preferred method.

Urethrocutaneous fistula is often the most frequently reported complication. Other commonly reported complications include glans dehiscence, urethral stricture, urethral diverticulum, and meatal stenosis. When interpreting high complication rates for proximal hypospadias, it is important to remember that multi-stage procedures are used to repair the most complex and severe presentations and should not be compared to distal hypospadias outcomes [15–17]. Dorsal preputial flaps are viable options for embedding ventral penile vascularized tissue prior to urethroplasty.

> *Author's perspective*—When used for proximal hypospadias, Byars skin flaps create a midline scar. This may complicate the second-stage tubularization and may impair the outcomes.

12.3.6 Preputial Tubularized Island Flap

Significant tissue deficiency in the urethral plate may require transection and replacement with a more robust substitute to create a neourethra. The preputial tubularized island flap (PTIF) was first described by Duckett in 1980 for a one-stage repair of severe hypospadias [18]. This technique involves a subcoronal circumferential incision, degloving the penis to its base, and orthoplasty. A dorsal transverse island flap is dissected from the inner prepuce that is equal or slightly longer in length to the distance between the hypospadic meatus and the glanular tip (Fig. 12.5) [9]. The flap is mobilized around its axial pedicle to allow for tension-free ventral transposition. The native urethra distal to healthy spongiosa is transected and removed. The flap is then tubularized over an appropriately-sized stent and anastomosed proximally to the spatulated native urethra. The neourethra is fixed at the new meatal opening through an artificially created glans channel. Another layer of dartos is used to cover the neourethra prior to re-approximating the ventral skin and glans [19]. The preputial tubularized island flap method has been noted to have higher complication rates than other techniques [20, 21] and should be reserved for severe and refractory presentations of hypospadias.

> *Author's perspective*—Tubularized flaps have high attrition rates, which may lead to common complications such as urethrocutaneous fistulas.

12.3.7 Perimeatal Flap

Perimeatal flaps involve the use of healthy ventral penile shaft skin as a flap for hypospadic urethral augmentation. The most popularized technique for perimeatal flaps was described by Mathieu in 1932 [22]. The Mathieu procedure entails using a U-shaped incision beginning at the glans and extending proximal to the hypospadic meatus to raise a flap on the ventral aspect of the penis. The length of the flap proximal to the meatus should be equal in length as the distance from the meatus to the glanular tip. Notably, the length of the flap should not be more than double the width, which limits the use of this technique to mid-penile or distal hypospadias. The flap is folded or flipped over distally to cover the hypospadic meatus (Fig. 12.6) [23]. The urethroplasty is completed by bilateral anastomosis of the onlay perimeatal flap to the urethral plate. The ventral skin and glans are re-approximated and closed over the flap. The Mathieu technique creates a round, horizontal meatus, which is cosmet-

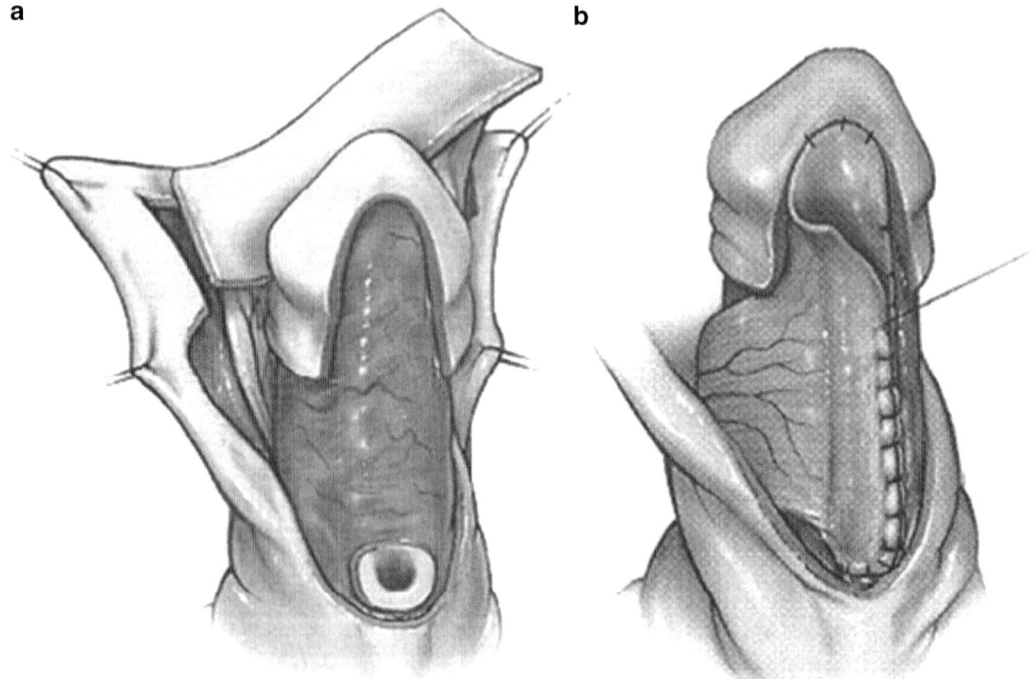

Fig. 12.5 Preputial tubularized island flap. (**a**) After adequate chordee correction, a dorsal transverse island flap is dissected from the inner prepuce. The flap should be equal or slightly longer to the distance between the hypospadic meatus and the glanular tip. The flap should be sufficiently mobilized to allow for tension-free ventral transposition. The native urethra distal to healthy spongiosa is removed. (**b**) The flap is tubularized over an appropriately sized stent and anastomosed proximally to the spatulated native urethra. The neourethra is fixed at the new meatal opening through an artificially created glans channel. A dartos flap should cover the neourethra prior to skin closure (Reprinted with permissions from: Campbell-Walsh Urology tenth ed. Wein AJ, Kavoussi LR, Novick AC, Partin AW, Peters CA. Hypospadias. Fig. 130–15 p. 3519. Copyright Elsevier Health Sciences 2011)

ically unfavorable compared to the normal vertical, slit-like meatus [24, 25]. Multiple technical modifications have been developed in order to create a vertical, slit-like meatus, such as hinging the urethral plate and a V-shaped incision on the flap apex [26, 27]. Fistulas are believed to be more common [28] after the Mathieu procedure due to the flap requiring two suture lines to approximate to the urethral plate. Though cosmetically unfavorable, Mathieu procedure can be an effective method of distal and mid-penile hypospadias repair using a perimeatal flap.

> *Author's perspective*—Recession of the meatus and high fistula rates discourages the use of perimeatal flaps.

12.3.8 Intermediate Layer Flap

Urethrocutaneous fistula is one of the most commonly reported complications in the hypospadias literature [29]. The use of an additional waterproofing layer of vascularized tissue to cover the neourethra suture line has been shown to lower the fistula rate [30]. Dartos (DF) and tunica vaginalis (TVF) flaps are the most widely used sources of interposition layers due to their vascular reliability and accessibility. DF can be harvested from the dorsal or ventral penile skin, prepuce, or scrotum. TVF is harvested by opening the anterior and distal aspect of the scrotum with a transverse incision. When isolating the flap, two longitudinal incisions are made along the transverse incision while taking great care to preserve the spermatic cord and vascular supply from the cremasteric artery. The TVF is brought to the suture line through a subcutaneous tunnel [31]. The decision between these two tissue materials is left to surgeon preference. However, a recent meta-analysis compared 353 patients who received primary hypospadias repair using the TIP technique and either DF or TVF as intermediate layers [32]. Patients with TVF intermediate layers had better total post-operative complication, urethrocutaneous fistula, and wound-related complication rates than those with DF. Another systematic review supports using a TVF as the first-choice for urethral coverage [33]. Worse outcomes with a DF may be a result of damage to the blood supply of the neourethra and penile skin during flap dissection, which does not occur with a TVF. Ultimately, a vascularized intermediate layer flap should be used to

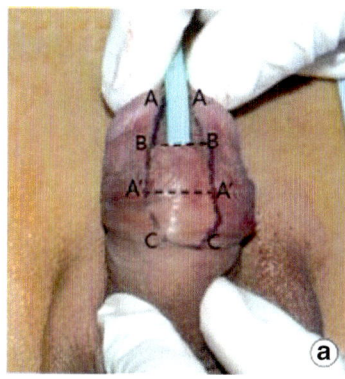
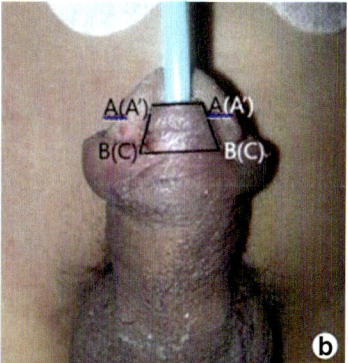
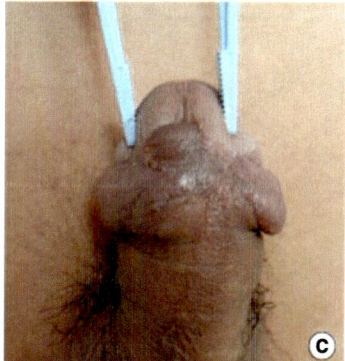

Fig. 12.6 Perimeatal flap. (**a**) The Mathieu procedure is started with a U-shaped incision from the glans that extends proximal to the hypospadic meatus to create a flap on the ventral aspect of the penis. The length of the flap proximal to the meatus should be equal in length to the distance from the meatus to the glanular tip. Chordee should be corrected as necessary after penile degloving. The flap is folded over distally to cover the urethral plate, followed by bilateral anastomosis of the onlay perimeatal flap to the urethral plate. The ventral skin and glans are re-approximated and closed over the flap. (**b**) Two weeks post-operation. (**c**) Three months post-operation (Reprinted with permissions from: Bae SH, Lee JN, Kim HT, Chung SK. Urethroplasty by Use of Turnover Flaps (Modified Mathieu Procedure) for Distal Hypospadias Repair in Adolescents: Comparison With the Tubularized Incised Plate Procedure. *Korean J Urol.* 2014;55(11):750–755)

limit post-operative complications, with recent studies supporting the use of TVF.

> *Author's perspective*—Interposition is the most important step in hypospadias surgery to prevent urethrocutaneous fistula. Most of the time, a dartos flap is available and adequate for interposition. There is rarely a need for a TVF.

12.3.9 Resurfacing of Skin

Ventral tissue deficiencies are characteristic of hypospadias and are typically more severe in proximal presentations. In most of these cases, Byars flaps or local penile skin flaps are sufficient for skin resurfacing [34]. A dorsal relaxing incision or Z-plasty may be necessary to allow for adequate tissue rearrangement. However, patients who have undergone multiple failed repairs often have more drastic tissue deficiencies. Not only is the recipient bed damaged due to the compromised vascularity and scarring of the skin and urethra [35], but the local tissue may also be affected and not usable for skin coverage. Scrotal flaps are fasciomyocutaneous flaps that can be rotated towards the penis for skin coverage. Scrotal flaps have an extensive arterial supply, making them a reliable option for skin resurfacing [36]. This is done by raising a flap from one hemiscrotum without crossing the midline and rotating it to cover the ventral penile skin defect [34]. A 2:1 length-to-width ratio is ideal for vascular preservation. Though cosmetic defects like dog-ears or hairy skin may occur, the favorable overall results demonstrate scrotal flaps are a dependable option where others are not available.

12.4 Grafts

12.4.1 History and Evolution

Free grafts are sheets of tissue that are detached from their vascular supply and placed in a new area of the body. Relative to skin flaps, graft use throughout history is not as extensive [37]. Early attempts for systematic trials of grafting on animals were noted by Thomas Birch throughout the seventeenth century, although these resulted in failure. In 1804, Giuseppe Baronio (1758—1814) published successful results from his skin grafting experiments on rams and other large animals. He noted using adhesive tape to fix the graft edges and gradual restoration of blood flow during healing. In 1874, Karl Thiersch (1822—1895) famously published his grafting findings. He described an adhesive material (fibrin) between the graft and recipient bed, revascularization of grafts, and improved success with thin grafts. He also described learning of an ancient Indian technique for graft preparation, in which the donor tissue was softly pounded to stimulate an inflammatory reaction prior to removal. This technique, termed "flagellation," was thought to improve graft survival. Thiersch's work throughout his life had a significant impact on the field of plastic surgery, as well as hypospadiology through his contribution to the Thiersch-Duplay technique.

Grafts are a valuable tool for reconstruction where local tissue availability is limited and flaps are not a viable option. Grafts are used in reconstruction due to their function as protective barriers for mechanical damage and fluid loss. Further, they provide the recipient site with improved tissue robustness after healing occurs.

12.4.2 Graft Characteristics

Skin and mucosa are the most frequently derived sources of tissue for engraftment. Skin grafts are classified as either full thickness or split thickness. Full-thickness skin grafts (FTSG) include all the layers of the epidermis and dermis. These are harvested by raising the dermis from the subcutaneous tissue using a scalpel and usually include hair follicles in that region. Split thickness skin grafts (STSG) include the epidermis and only a portion of the dermal layers. These are harvested using either a knife or a dermatome with an adjustable depth gauge. The key difference in physiologic characteristics between these two types of graft is the amount of dermis present [38]. Within the dermis are sweat glands, sebaceous glands, hair follicles, and increased amounts of elastin. These characteristics, along with increased overall thickness, lead to greater metabolic requirements and a higher risk for primary contraction in FTSG. Primary contraction is the immediate recoil after a graft is harvested and is correlated to the amount of elastin in the dermis layers. However, STSG are more likely to undergo secondary and overall contraction. Secondary contraction is caused by increased myofibroblast activity leading to graft contracture. FTSG have lower rates of secondary contraction due to the increased dermal layers, which shorten the life cycle of myofibroblasts and decrease their effect on graft survival [39]. Further, FTSG are advantageous in that they provide superior texture and aesthetic results at both donor and recipient sites compared to STSG [40]. However, STSG can be used to cover larger areas of defect and can be re-harvested from donor sites due to skin regeneration. Mucosal grafts differ from skin grafts in that they lack keratin, hair follicles, sweat glands, and sebaceous glands, which are sources of chronic inflammation when present in the urethra [41]. They may be obtained from the inner cheek, tongue, palate, bladder, and small intestine. The unique secretory epithelium of mucosal grafts makes them ideal options for urethral reconstruction. Of note, much of the knowledge and principles related to grafting in hypospadias is assumed from the skin grafting literature in plastic surgery. Future studies may focus on the specific physiologic processes of tissue materials and their recipient bed in hypospadias repair.

12.4.3 Graft Take

Since grafts are not attached to their own vascular supply, they rely on an adequate wound bed to survive. It is believed the graft must lie within 1–2 mm of the recipient vascular supply in order to successfully undergo the processes necessary for graft survival: plasmatic imbibition, vascular inosculation, and neovascularization [42] (Fig. 12.7) [43]. Plasmatic imbibition is the exchange of gas and nutrients from the wound bed to the graft during the first 48 h of tissue transfer. This occurs as the plasma diffuses from the recipient capillary bed into the graft vessels, thereby sustaining the graft and preventing immediate graft ischemia. Inosculation is described as the growth of a fine vascular network from the wound bed that interfaces with the dermis of the graft after 48–96 h of tissue transfer. These new capillary buds serve as the foundation for more dependable vascularization. Then, neovascularization occurs in which new blood vessels invade the graft and undergo a dual process of anastomoses with existing vascular channels and creation of new vasculature. Neovascularization establishes a permanent vascular supply to provide the nourishment necessary for healing. The need for adequate blood supply from the wound bed to the graft requires great care to achieve the equilibrium between hemostasis and perfusion. Due to this delicate process, grafts are typically only used in staged procedures in order to allow the graft to heal or "take" before continuing with reconstruction.

12.4.4 Grafts in Hypospadias

Grafts have been proven to be useful in hypospadias repair as there may be significant deficiencies in ventral tissue or scarring secondary to previous repair. The first description of graft use in hypospadias repair was in 1897 when Nové-Josserand tubularized a free skin graft for urethroplasty. There are various sources and techniques for grafting described in the current hypospadias literature, including autografts, allografts, and xenografts (Table 12.4). Autografts are derived from the same individual. Allografts are derived from the same species but a different individual. Xenografts are derived from completely different species. Preputial skin and buccal mucosa are the most commonly used graft material in urethroplasty. Bladder mucosa and posterior auricular skin have also been described for urethroplasty, however, it is used significantly less frequently due to their associated complica-

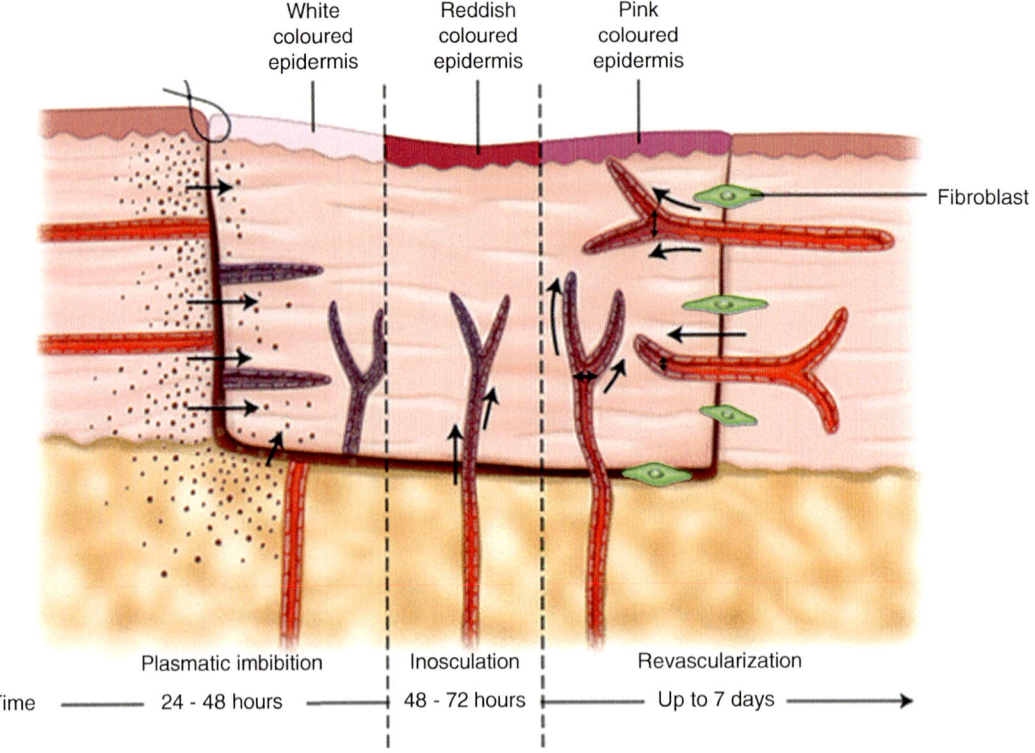

Fig. 12.7 Illustration demonstrating the 3 stages of graft healing. First, plasmatic imbibition occurs in which gas and nutrients diffuse between the recipient bed and the graft. Next, capillary buds begin to develop within the graft during inosculation. Finally, new blood vessels invade the graft and establish a permanent vascular network to revascularize the new graft tissue (Reprinted with permissions: Fortier JL, Castiglione CL, Guo L. Skin Grafting. In: Orgill DP, ed. *Interventional Treatment of Wounds: A Modern Approach for Better Outcomes.* Springer International Publishing; 2018:123–142)

tions. A brief summary of graft outcomes reported in the literature is outlined in Table 12.5. Lastly, several ventral lengthening techniques for chordee correction have been described with a variety of tissue material used including both flaps and grafts.

12.4.5 Preputial Skin Graft

Preputial skin is a commonly used source of flaps and autografts. Many surgeons prefer the use of preputial skin flaps over grafts due to the proximity of the flap to the urethra, which allows the flap to be rotated around its pedicle to preserve vascularity and optimize flap survival. However, an advantage of using preputial skin as a graft is that dissection becomes simpler since there is not a pedicle to be mobilized and preserved [44]. Further, there is relatively less bulkiness when using a graft compared to a flap, which may facilitate ventral skin closure. Though the preputial skin is typically hairless, it does have the potential to grow hair in the future [41]. The presence of hair follicles, as well as sebaceous and sweat glands, may cause neourethral complications due to chronic inflammation [41]. Preputial grafts are harvested from the inner prepuce and de-fatted prior to placement. Graft length should correspond to the length of urethral defect, beginning at the proximal aspect of the hypospadic urethral meatus to the glanular tip when the penis is fully stretched. Graft width depends on whether it will be used as an inlay or onlay. If it is to be used as

Table 12.4 Brief description of graft types and their respective advantages and disadvantages

Graft type	Advantages	Disadvantages
Preputial skin graft	Accessible Single surgical site Low complication rates	Sebaceous and sweat glands Possible luminal hair growth
Inner preputial skin graft	Hairless, accessible Single surgical site	Often not adequate for urethral replacement
Buccal mucosa graft	Hairless, accessible Histologically similar to urethra Highly vascularized Low complication rates	Two surgical sites Oral pain after graft harvest Contracture and facial deformities previously reported
Bladder mucosa graft	Histologically resembles urethra Accustomed to urine exposure	Invasive procedure Metaplasia upon air exposure Higher meatal complication rates
Post-auricular Wolfe graft	Accessible	Two surgical sites Fine hair in lumen Chronic inflammation in FTSG

an inlay for urethral augmentation in an atretic dorsal urethral plate, the width should be about 10 mm, or enough to lay within the incised urethral plate [45, 46]. This technique is effective in widening the urethral plate [47]. If the graft is used as an onlay in urethral augmentation, the width of the graft plus the dorsal urethral plate should be about 2 mm greater than the circumference of the proximal urethra [44]. The slightly greater width accounts for the suture line.

Preputial skin can also be used in multi-stage repairs when ventral tissue deficiencies or ventral chordee is not optimal for a single-stage repair. The Bracka technique is a widely accepted method for two-stage repair using the inner prepuce as a graft [48]. In this method, the urethral plate and glans are divided using a midline incision extending to the proximal meatus. The graft is quilted onto the ventral defect as a dorsal inlay graft (Fig. 12.8). The second stage is comprised of urethroplasty using the Thiersch-Duplay or TIP techniques. It is recommended to wait at least 6 months between stages to allow the new urethral plate to heal and become well-vascularized prior to tubularization.

Initial concerns regarding grafting in hypospadias questioned the ability for grafts to "take" and be functional, especially in severe cases where the recipient vascular bed may be insufficient. Meatal stenosis and neourethral strictures are complications that are thought to be related to ischemic donor tissue secondary to poor graft take, though these rates are reportedly low when using preputial grafts [49, 50]. This low rate of ischemia-related urethroplasty complications demonstrate the ability for preputial grafts to take, even in severe cases of hypospadias. In addition to implementation for primary repair, the Bracka technique using a preputial graft is highly regarded and more commonly performed for re-operation when the urethral plate is scarred and unlikely to re-epithelialize. A preputial skin graft is accessible, versatile, and adaptable, making it a favorable tool in hypospadias repair.

> *Author's perspective*—The two-stage urethroplasty using the free inner preputial skin graft has given consistent results across the board. When the graft is placed during the first stage, it is important to remove all scar tissue from the graft bed to optimize graft take. The graft quilting and dressing are critical for uptake.

12.4.6 Buccal Mucosa Graft

Buccal mucosa autografts are sheets of oral mucosa that are harvested from the inner cheek. Buccal mucosa grafts have the distinct advantage of having a rich submucosal vascular or pan laminar plexus that facilitates plasmatic imbibition and inosculation, thereby enhancing graft uptake and survival. Further, this mucosa is de-keratinized and its epithelial surface is accustomed to a moist environment, making it a suitable substitute in the urethra. A buccal mucosa graft is harvested by

Table 12.5 Summary table of outcomes using different graft material and techniques reported in the literature

Authors	Meatal location	Technique (n) [# of planned stages]	Total complications	Urethrocutaneous Fistula	Meatal stenosis	Cosmetic outcomes
Kolon [45]	All locations	Inlay, prepuce (32) [1]	2 (6.3%)	–	–	–
Cambareri [44]	Distal, mid-penile, proximal	Onlay, prepuce (62) [1]	22 (35.5%)	21 (33.9%)	3 (4.8%)	–
Ferro [49]	Proximal, scrotal, perineal	Bracka, prepuce (34) [2]	8 (23.5%)	2 (5.9%)	0 (0%)	0 (0%)
Markiewicz [52]	Not specified	Onlay, buccal (362) [1&2] Tube, buccal (55) [1&2]	71 (19.6%) 29 (49.1%) $p < 0.001$	–	–	–
Manasherova [41]	Peno-scrotal, scrotal, perineal	Bracka, prepuce (108) [2] Bracka, buccal (112) [2]	33 (30.6%) 23 (20.5%) $p = 0.092$	22 (20.4%) 15 (13.4%) $p = 0.21$	0 (0%) 0 (0%)	Buccal better cosmetically than prepuce
Lanciotti [53]	Peno-scrotal, scrotal, perineal	Bladder (50) [2]	23 (46.0%)	9 (18.0%)	4 (8.0%) *7 (14.0%)	8 (16.0%)
Nitkunan [56]	All locations	Bracka, PAWG (29^) [2]	2 (6.9%)	1 (3.4%)	0 (0%)	–
Pfistermüller [57]	All locations	Bracka, PAWG (66^)	6 (9.1%)	–	–	–

*Meatal prolapse complications; ^Secondary repairs

placing two stay sutures at the upper and lower cheek to optimize exposure (Fig. 12.9). An anesthetic is injected into the graft submucosal space. The required length of graft is measured and dissected sharply with great care to avoid injuring Stensen's duct. Bipolar electrocautery may be used for hemostasis. The harvest site may be left open or sutured closed, as both have similar outcomes for pain and complications [51]. The graft is then thinned, shaped, and immersed in an antibiotic solution prior to its use as a graft. In terms of use as a graft in single-stage procedures, buccal mucosa may be used as an onlay or inlay graft for urethral augmentation or as a tube graft for urethral substitution. A systematic review found greater success when used as an onlay graft compared to tube graft (80.4% vs 52.7%) [52].

Buccal mucosa grafts may also be used in two-stage repair via the Bracka technique. The Bracka technique, as described previously, originally intended for the use of a preputial graft to repair severe proximal hypospadias. However, buccal mucosa grafts have become increasingly favorable as an extragenital option due to the previously described characteristics [41]. Though the type of tissue differs compared to the rest of the techniques, the types of complications associated with buccal mucosa remain the same. These complications include urethrocutaneous fistula, meatal stenosis, and graft contracture. There is concern for surgical infection due to the oral microbiome that is introduced to the urethra. When appropriate, patients are started on prophylactic chlorhexi-

12 Flaps and Grafts in Hypospadias Repair

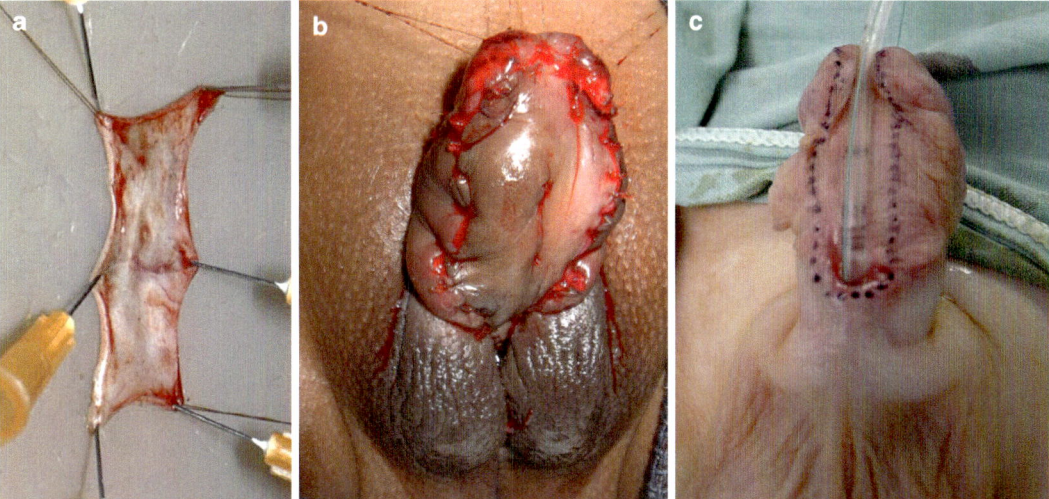

Fig. 12.8 Inner preputial graft. (**a**): Free graft derived from inner preputial skin. The graft has been thinned and prepared to cover the ventral penile defect in the first stage of a Bracka two-stage repair. (**b**) The graft has been quilted into place on the ventral penile shaft. The graft for this peno-scrotal hypospadias penis will be covered with a protected tie-over dressing and given 6 months to heal prior to the second stage. (**c**) Six-month follow-up of a different patient with proximal hypospadias after undergoing the first stage of a Bracka repair using inner preputial skin. The patient had excellent graft take and will undergo neourethral tubularization during the second stage

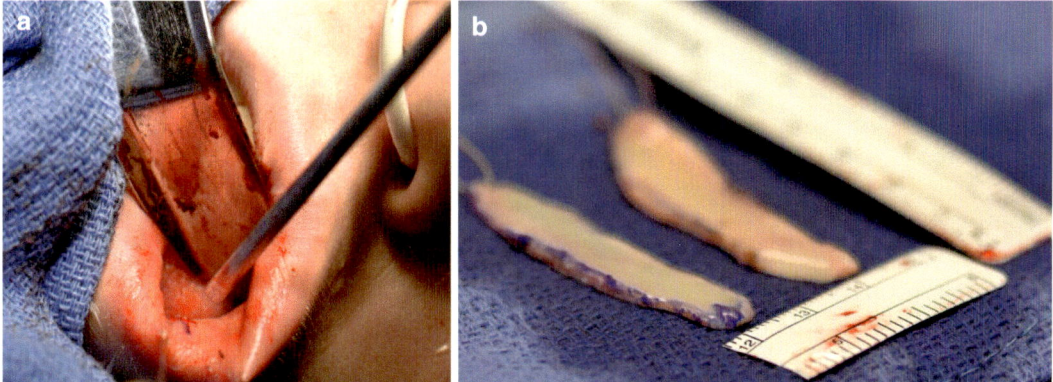

Fig. 12.9 Buccal mucosa graft. (**a**) The mouth is first disinfected with a mucosa-specific solution. Two traction sutures are in place at the border between the buccal mucosa and lip skin. A retractor is used to better expose the buccal mucosa. Metzenbaum scissors are used to lift the graft by dissecting in the plane between the mucosa and buccal fat, with great care to avoid injuring Stensen's duct. The donor site may be closed or left open. (**b**) The buccal mucosa will be de-fatted using curved scissors, shaped, and disinfected prior to being used as a graft

dine mouthwash 3 days prior to surgery, as well as broad-spectrum intravenous antibiotics the day before surgery to minimize this risk. Many surgeons favor buccal mucosa grafts due to the lower complication rates and histologic structure similarities between buccal mucosa and the native urethra [41]. Further, these grafts do not contain foreign structures such as sweat or sebaceous glands that lead to chronic inflammation and possible scar contraction of the graft [41]. Buccal mucosa is a favorable option for grafting in urethroplasty given its structural resemblance to native urethra, accessibility, and promising outcomes.

> *Author's perspective*—Buccal mucosa is the best tissue for urethroplasty if the inner prepuce or foreskin is unavailable. Precautions during harvesting should be taken, and avoid the lip if possible. Long-term contractures and facial deformities have been reported. Otherwise, this graft has excellent outcomes in all regards.

12.4.7 Bladder Mucosa Graft

In theory, bladder mucosa is well-suited for free autograft material in urethroplasty due to its functional resemblance to native urethra. Similar to buccal mucosa, bladder mucosa is de-keratinized and accustomed to moist environments. The bladder urothelium is continuously exposed to urine, making the graft a suitable substitute to the urethra. A bladder mucosa graft is obtained through a small Pfannenstiel incision. The bladder is filled via a bladder catheter and distended to facilitate identification of the anterior aspect. Once the anterior surface is identified, a deep incision is made through the detrusor muscle until enough mucosa is exposed to obtain a proper-sized graft [53]. The size of the graft depends upon the length of the defect as well as the repair technique of choice. Various methods have been described for bladder mucosa graft use such as an onlay patch for urethral augmentation or tubularization for urethral substitution.

Although the composition of bladder mucosa is comparable to that of native urethra, its use as a graft is limited for several reasons. Obtaining a bladder mucosa graft is much more invasive than harvesting a graft or flap from penile skin, preputial skin, and buccal mucosa. For that reason, bladder mucosa is rarely used for primary repair. Instead, it is typically only used in urethroplasty when nearby penile and preputial tissue has limited availability, such as in severe hypospadias or revision repairs. In these cases, it is more common practice to obtain a graft from the buccal mucosa due to the advantageous accessibility and histologic similarities. Another downfall for bladder mucosa as a urethral graft are the physiologic changes that occur when it comes in contact with air. Air exposure causes these grafts to undergo columnar metaplasia and develop mucinous glands leading to hyperplasia and edema [54]. As a result, bladder mucosa grafts are more likely to result in meatal complications, such as meatal prolapse or stenosis, due to the meatus enduring increased air exposure relative to the rest of the graft. Modifications have been made to avoid meatal and distal urethral complications secondary to air exposure [53]. Combined bladder mucosa and skin grafts, in which the distal urethra is a tubularized skin graft or flap, have been proven to be effective [55]. Overall, bladder mucosa grafts should not be considered the primary option in urethroplasty.

> *Authors perspective*—Bladder mucosa grafts are historical and not used in current practice due to the morbidities that are unique to bladder mucosa grafts and the availability of other widely accepted techniques.

12.4.8 Post-Auricular Wolfe Grafts

Post-auricular Wolfe grafts (PAWG) are another extragenital option for graft material in 2-stage repairs. PAWG is a readily-available, full-thickness skin graft. It is considered an option in hypospadias repair due to the absence of thick hair in the area, though fine hair of unknown clinical significance may be present [56]. The data for PAWG is limited, as many urologists prefer using preputial skin or buccal mucosa when managing urethral defects. The literature regarding grafting with PAWGs describes keloid formation at both the donor and recipient sites [56, 57]. These issues arise secondary to chronic inflammation when using full-thickness skin grafts in the urethra, as well as the creation of a separate surgical site during graft harvesting. As such, preputial skin and buccal mucosa are currently the preferred tissue material for urethral reconstruction.

> *Author's perspective*—PAWGs are very thick and difficult for tubularization. They may cause scarring at the donor site.

12.5 Ventral Lengthening

Severe chordee correction that is refractory to penis degloving can be repaired through multiple approaches, including ventral lengthening. Ventral lengthening is a highly considered technique in correcting severe chordee due to its ability to address the significant disproportion in length between the ventral and dorsal corporal bodies. The flap or graft used to cover the ventral defect in the tunica albuginea is what allows for ventral lengthening, as opposed to a dorsal plication which results in penile shortening. Ventral lengthening is associated with significantly lower rates of ventral curvature recurrence compared to dorsal plication (9.4% vs 27.9%) [58]. Various materials for ventral lengthening are described in the literature such as tunica vaginalis and dermis. Commercially available acellular matrix materials have also been studied, including small intestinal submucosa (SIS) and dermis.

Ventral lengthening is started by mobilizing the urethral plate off of the underlying corpora cavernosa [58]. A transverse incision is made through the tunica albuginea on the ventral aspect. It is essential to sufficiently extend this incision laterally to allow for complete release of chordee. The tunica albuginea is then lifted off the underlying tissue carefully through both proximal and distal dissection. A flap or graft of the surgeon's choice is then used to cover the ellipsoid defect. When harvesting a graft, the surgeon should ensure that it is 20–30% larger than the defect in order to avoid graft contracture and consequently recurrent curvature [59]. A tunica vaginalis flap or graft is often preferred when performing a ventral lengthening technique due to its easy accessibility. Dermal autografts are harvested from the inguinal crease, which allows for enough dermis to be removed as well as achieve cosmetic closure of the donor site [60]. The epidermis is removed from dermal grafts prior to detaching the graft from the underlying tissue. The flap or graft is anastomosed to the ellipsoid defect in the tunica albuginea, which then covers the corporal defect.

The viability of the donor tissue should be prioritized in corporoplasty, as poor attrition may result in tissue contracture and ventral curvature recurrence. Sufficient tissue vascularity is essential for optimizing tissue survival and preventing chordee recurrence, which highlights the issue of using flaps or grafts for ventral lengthening. One study compared tunica vaginalis flaps and grafts for ventral tunica albuginea defect coverage in rabbits [61]. There was no contracture in the flaps at 3 months, meanwhile 42% of the grafts had contracted by this point. Microscopic examination of three flaps all showed an intact blood supply and no evidence of tissue necrosis. In contrast, examination of three grafts all showed necrosis and granulation tissue at 2 weeks, which were replaced by collagenized fibrous tissue at 6 weeks. The reliable vascularity and lack of necrosis support the use of tunica vaginalis flaps in ventral lengthening. Further, reports have shown a 95% success rate when using tunica vaginalis flaps to correct penile curvature in hypospadias [59]. Dermal grafts may be considered when tunica vaginalis is unavailable, such as in patients with bilateral cryptorchidism or inguinal hernias [59]. However, experiences with dermal grafts have varied among hypospadias surgeons. Some hypospadiologists report excellent cosmetic and functional outcomes in 100% of patients with dermal grafts [60], while others report less than 60% success with a single dermal graft repair [62].

Xenografts and allografts are commercially available, pre-packaged graft materials that spare the need for additional donor site dissection and closure. Small intestinal submucosa xenografts are porcine-derived and composed of extracellular matrix bioscaffolds with type 1 collagen, which facilitates constructive remodeling of tissues [63, 64]. SIS grafts come pre-packaged as acellular, freeze-dried, and sterile. This graft type relies on inoculation and imbibition for vascular ingrowth and replacement of the graft by host tissue. There is limited literature published for outcomes after SIS graft use for chordee correction in hypospadias repair. The data thus far is unclear, as some authors report successful chordee correction with SIS corporal grafting [65], meanwhile others have found long-term complications of corporal scarring and dense fibrosis with SIS grafts [66]. Complications result due to graft rejection resulting in an inflammatory reaction and eventually fibrosis. An acellular dermal matrix allograft is also available for corporal grafting (Fig. 12.10) [67]. This human cadaveric-derived graft material has regenerative properties that have proven to function in other types of reconstructive surgeries [67]. Regeneration occurs through growth factors and vascular channels within the collagen scaffold that facilitate tissue infiltration, fibroblast proliferation, and neovascularization [68]. The data on ventral lengthening using acellular dermal matrices is limited, but one case series of 7 patients reports no recurrent ventral curvature after over a 1-year follow-up [67]. They report using grafts 20% larger than the defect to allow for contraction. Though there are various options for corporal grafting in ventral lengthening, there is not a clearly superior choice, leaving the decision for the surgeon's preference.

> *Authors perspective*—The long-term outcomes are not yet known, especially venous leak and erectile function when these materials are used to cover the defect in corporotomies. Xenografts pose the challenge of infection.

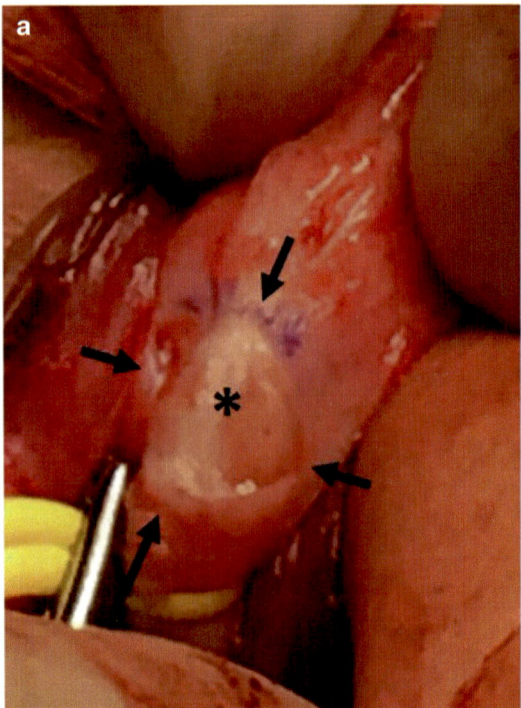
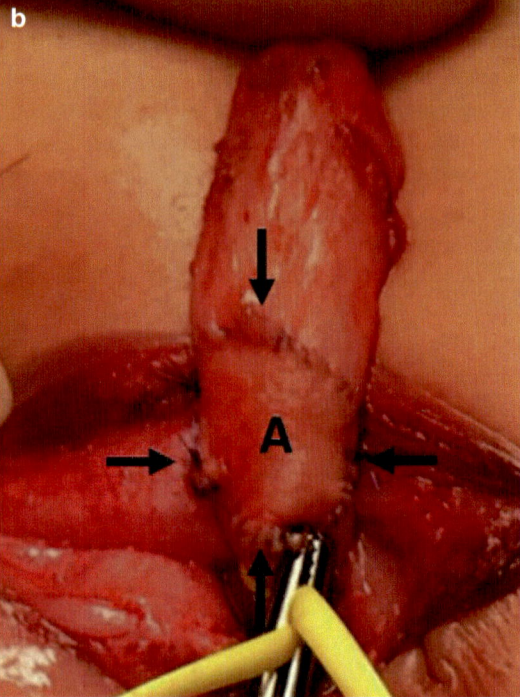

Fig. 12.10 Acellular dermal matrix graft. (**a**) The penis is completely degloved and an incision is made in the tunica albuginea, leaving a 180-degree ellipsoid defect outlined by the arrows. (**b**) An acellular dermal matrix graft is placed in the defect and sutured along its edges (Reprinted with permissions: Palmer LS, Palmer JS. The use of Alloderm® for correction of severe chordee in children: An initial experience. *Journal of Pediatric Urology*. Published online June 14, 2020)

12.6 Future Direction

Tissue engineering (TE) is a rapidly advancing field that aims to restore tissue and organ function. Scientists in TE draw principles from fields such as cell biology, material science, and biomedical engineering to develop natural and synthetic matrices to facilitate the regeneration of human tissue. In alignment with plastic surgery principles, the tissue material should possess similar biologic, physical, and mechanical properties to the native tissue. Though, there are a lack of tissue substitutes that perfectly resemble the native urethra and corpus spongiosum [69]. Other important qualities for optimizing scaffold success include adequate porosity, regenerative capacity, biodegradability, flexibility, and firmness [70]. One group reported using an amniotic membrane layer in proximal and revision hypospadias repairs, though results are not reported [71]. The amniotic membrane layer serves as collagen-based architecture and provides active growth factors, stem cells, and other biomolecules to stimulate healing and regeneration of tissue. Another group performed urethral defect repairs in 5 boys using tubularized 50:50 polyglycolic acid:poly (lactide-co-glycolide acid) mesh scaffolds seeded with autologous bladder smooth muscle and urothelial cells [72]. Though it was not hypospadias repair, there were no functional complications with the neourethras after a median 71-month follow-up. These favorable results are promising for tissue engineering for hypospadias repair.

Tissue engineering in hypospadias may evolve with the advancement of nanotechnology and 3-D bioprinting [69]. Nanotechnology allows engineers to regulate the microenvironment on a cellular level. The nanofibers composed of natural and synthetic polymers can sense cellular migration and control drug delivery, which work to directly influence local inflammation, angiogenesis, and healing [69]. Advances in 3-D bioprinting may enable for the creation of neourethras from scaffolds with precisely seeded cells [69]. The continued development of this innovative technology is promising for the future of hypospadias repair.

12.7 Conclusion

The use of flaps and grafts in modern hypospadias repair continues to be a valuable tool for pediatric urologists. Despite slight variation in the success rates and the availability of data for the techniques described, these methods are all seen as viable options in hypospadias repair. Ultimately, the pediatric urologist must weigh their options given the individual characteristics of the patient and their own technical experiences when deciding their method of reconstruction.

References

1. Stein R. Hypospadias. Eur Urol Suppl. 2012;11(2):33–45.
2. Wallis MC, Braga L, Khoury A. The role of flaps and grafts in modern hypospadiology. Indian J Urol. 2008;24(2):200–5.
3. Snodgrass WT, Villanueva C, Granberg C, Bush NC. Objective use of testosterone reveals androgen insensitivity in patients with proximal hypospadias. J Pediatr Urol. 2014;10(1):118–22.
4. Santoni-Rugiu P, Sykes PJ. Skin Flaps. In: Santoni-Rugiu P, Sykes PJ, editors. A history of plastic surgery. Berlin: Springer; 2007. p. 79–119.
5. Smit JM, Negenborn VL, Jansen SM, et al. Intraoperative evaluation of perfusion in free flap surgery: a systematic review and meta-analysis. Microsurgery. 2018;38(7):804–18.
6. Wisenbaugh ES, Gelman J. The use of flaps and grafts in the treatment of urethral stricture disease. Adv Urol. 2015;2015:8.
7. Ridenour BD, Larrabee WF. Skin flap design: physiology and biodynamics. In: Meyers A, editor. Biological basis of facial plastic surgery. New York: Thieme Medical; 1993.
8. Elder JS, Duckett JW, Snyder HM. Onlay island flap in the repair of mid and distal penile hypospadias without chordee. J Urol. 1987;138(2):376–9.
9. Snodgrass WT. Hypospadias. In: Wein AJ, Kavoussi LR, Novick AC, Partin AW, Peters CA, editors. Campbell-Walsh urology. 10th ed. Philadelphia, PA: Elsevier Health Sciences; 2011.
10. ElGanainy EO. A modified onlay island flap vs. Mathieu urethroplasty for distal hypospadias repair: a prospective randomised study. Arab J Urol. 2015;13(3):169–75.
11. Perović S, Vukadinović V. Onlay Island flap urethroplasty for severe hypospadias: a variant of the technique. J Urol. 1994;151(3):711–4.
12. Mohajerzadeh L, Mirshemirani A, Rouzrokh M, et al. Evaluation of Onlay Island flap technique in

shallow urethral plate Hypospadiasis. Iran J Pediatr. 2016;26(1):e660.
13. Braga Luis HP, Pippi Salle Joao L, Lorenzo AJ, et al. Comparative analysis of Tubularized incised plate versus Onlay Island flap urethroplasty for penoscrotal hypospadias. J Urol. 2007;178(4):1451–7.
14. Byars LT. Functional restoration of hypospadias deformities; with a report of 60 completed cases. Surg Gynecol Obstet. 1951;92(2):149–54.
15. Long CJ, Chu DI, Tenney RW, et al. Intermediate-term follow-up of proximal hypospadias repair reveals high complication rate. J Urol. 2017;197(3 Pt 2):852–8.
16. Stanasel I, Le H-K, Bilgutay A, et al. Complications following staged hypospadias repair using transposed preputial skin flaps. J Urol. 2015;194(2):512–6.
17. McNamara ER, Schaeffer AJ, Logvinenko T, et al. Management of proximal hypospadias with 2-stage repair: 20 year experience. J Urol. 2015;194(4):1080–5.
18. Duckett JW. Transverse preputial island flap technique for repair of severe hypospadias. Urol Clin North Am. 1980;7(2):423–30.
19. Sowande AO, Olajide AO, Salako AA, Olajide FO, Adejuyigbe O, Talabi AO. Experience with transverse preputial island flap for repair of hypospadias in Ile-Ife, Nigeria. Afr J Paediatr Surg. 2009;6(1):40.
20. Wiener JS, Sutherland RW, Roth DR, Gonzales ET. Comparison of onlay and tubularized island flaps of inner preputial skin for the repair of proximal hypospadias. J Urol. 1997;158(3 Pt 2):1172–4.
21. Ghali. Hypospadias repair by skin flaps: a comparison of onlay preputial island flaps with either Mathieu's meatal-based or Duckett's tubularized preputial flaps. BJU Int. 1999;83(9):1032–8.
22. Mathieu P. Traitement en un temps de l'hypospadias balanique et juxtabalanique. J Chir. 1932;39:481–4.
23. Bae SH, Lee JN, Kim HT, Chung SK. Urethroplasty by use of turnover flaps (modified Mathieu procedure) for distal hypospadias repair in adolescents: comparison with the Tubularized incised plate procedure. Korean J Urol. 2014;55(11):750–5.
24. Oswald J, Körner I, Riccabona M. Comparison of the perimeatal-based flap (Mathieu) and the tubularized incised-plate urethroplasty (Snodgrass) in primary distal hypospadias. BJU Int. 2000;85(6):725–7.
25. Ververidis M, Dickson AP, Gough DCS. An objective assessment of the results of hypospadias surgery. BJU Int. 2005;96(1):135–9.
26. Rich MA, Keating MA, Snyder HM, Duckett JW. Hinging the urethral plate in hypospadias meatoplasty. J Urol. 1989;142(6):1551–3.
27. Boddy S-A, Samuel M. A natural glanular meatus after 'Mathieu and a V incision sutured': MAVIS. BJU Int. 2000;86(3):394–7.
28. Wilkinson DJ, Farrelly P, Kenny SE. Outcomes in distal hypospadias: a systematic review of the Mathieu and tubularized incised plate repairs. J Pediatr Urol. 2012;8(3):307–12.
29. Hardwicke JT, Bechar JA, Hodson J, Osmani O, Park AJ. Fistula after single-stage primary hypospadias repair - a systematic review of the literature. J Plast Reconstr Aesthet Surg. 2015;68(12):1647–55.
30. Basavaraju M, Balaji DK. Choosing an ideal vascular cover for Snodgrass repair. Urol Ann. 2017;9(4):348–52.
31. Pescheloche P, Parmentier B, Hor T, et al. Tunica vaginalis flap for urethrocutaneous fistula repair after proximal and mid-shaft hypospadias surgery: a 12-year experience. J Pediatr Urol. 2018;14(5):421.e1–6.
32. Yang H, Xuan X, Hu D, et al. Comparison of effect between dartos fascia and tunica vaginalis fascia in TIP urethroplasty: a meta-analysis of comparative studies. BMC Urol. 2020;20(1):161.
33. Fahmy O, Khairul-Asri MG, Schwentner C, et al. Algorithm for optimal urethral coverage in hypospadias and fistula repair: a systematic review. Eur Urol. 2016;70(2):293–8.
34. Fam MM, Hanna MK. Resurfacing the penis of complex hypospadias repair ("hypospadias cripples"). J Urol. 2017;197(3, Part 2):859–64.
35. Amukele SA, Stock JA, Hanna MK. Management and outcome of complex hypospadias repairs. J Urol. 2005;174(4 Pt 2):1540–2. discussion 1542–1543
36. Mendez-Fernandez MA, Hollan C, Frank DH, Fisher JC. The scrotal Myocutaneous flap. Plast Reconstr Surg. 1986;78(5):676–8.
37. Santoni-Rugiu P, Sykes PJ. Skin Grafts. In: Santoni-Rugiu P, Sykes PJ, editors. A history of plastic surgery. Berlin: Springer; 2007. p. 121–39.
38. Thakar HJ, Dugi DD. Practical plastic surgery: techniques for the reconstructive urologist. In: Brandes SB, Morey AF, editors. Advanced male urethral and genital reconstructive surgery. Current clinical urology. New York: Springer; 2014. p. 69–82.
39. Rudolph R. Inhibition of myofibroblasts by skin grafts. Plast Reconstr Surg. 1979;63(4):473–80.
40. Iwuagwu FC, Wilson D, Bailie F. The use of skin grafts in postburn contracture release: a 10-year review. Plast Reconstr Surg. 1999;103(4):1198–204.
41. Manasherova D, Kozyrev G, Nikolaev V, et al. Bracka's method of proximal hypospadias repair: preputial skin or buccal mucosa? Urology. 2020;138:138–43.
42. Converse JM, Smahel J, Smahel J, Ballantyne DL, Harper AD. Inosculation of vessels of skin graft and host bed: a fortuitous encounter. Br J Plast Surg. 1975;28(4):274–82.
43. Fortier JL, Castiglione CL, Guo L. Skin Grafting. In: Orgill DP, editor. Interventional treatment of wounds: a modern approach for better outcomes. Cham: Springer International Publishing; 2018. p. 123–42.
44. Cambareri GM, Yap M, Kaplan GW. Hypospadias repair with onlay preputial graft: a 25-year experience with long-term follow-up. BJU Int. 2016;118(3):451–7.
45. Kolon TF, Gonzales ET. The dorsal inlay graft for hypospadias repair. J Urol. 2000;163(6):1941–3.
46. Asanuma H, Satoh H, Shishido S. Dorsal inlay graft urethroplasty for primary hypospadiac repair. Int J Urol. 2007;14(1):43–7.

47. Gundeti M, Queteishat A, Desai D, Cuckow P. Use of an inner preputial free graft to extend the indications of Snodgrass hypospadias repair (Snodgraft). J Pediatr Urol. 2005;1(6):395–6.
48. Bracka A. The role of two-stage repair in modern hypospadiology. Indian J Urol. 2008;24(2):210–8.
49. Ferro F, Zaccara A, Spagnoli A, Lucchetti MC, Capitanucci ML, Villa M. Skin graft for 2-stage treatment of severe hypospadias: back to the future? J Urol. 2002;168(4 Part 2):1730–3.
50. Castagnetti M, El-Ghoneimi A. Surgical management of primary severe hypospadias in children: systematic 20-year review. J Urol. 2010;184(4):1469–75.
51. Rourke K, McKinny S, St. Martin B. Effect of wound closure on buccal mucosal graft harvest site morbidity: results of a randomized prospective trial. Urology. 2012;79(2):443–7.
52. Markiewicz MR, Lukose MA, Margarone JE, Barbagli G, Miller KS, Chuang SK. The oral mucosa graft: a systematic review. J Urol. 2007;178(2):387–94.
53. Lanciotti M, Betti M, Elia A, et al. Proximal hypospadias repair with bladder mucosal graft: our 10 years experience. J Pediatr Urol. 2017;13(3):294.e1–6.
54. Ransley PG, Duffy PG, Oesch IL, Van Oyen P, Hoover D. The use of bladder mucosa and combined bladder mucosa/preputial skin grafts for urethral reconstruction. J Urol. 1987;138(4, Part 2):1096–8.
55. Fu Q, Deng C-L. Ten-year experience with composite bladder mucosa-skin grafts in hypospadias repair. Urology. 2006;67(6):1274–7.
56. Nitkunan T, Johal N, O'Malley K, Cuckow P. Secondary hypospadias repair in two stages. J Pediatr Urol. 2006;2(6):559–63.
57. Pfistermüller KLM, Manoharan S, Desai D, Cuckow PM. Two-stage hypospadias repair with a free graft for severe primary and revision hypospadias: a single surgeon's experience with long-term follow-up. J Pediatr Urol. 2017;13(1):35.e1–7.
58. Braga LHP, Lorenzo AJ, Bägli DJ, et al. Ventral penile lengthening versus dorsal plication for severe ventral curvature in children with proximal hypospadias. J Urol. 2008;180(4):1743–8. Published online October 2008
59. Braga LHP, Pippi Salle JL, Dave S, Bagli DJ, Lorenzo AJ, Khoury AE. Outcome analysis of severe chordee correction using tunica vaginalis as a flap in boys with proximal hypospadias. J Urol. 2007;178(4S):1693–7.
60. Pope JC, Kropp BP, McLaughlin KP, et al. Penile orthoplasty using dermal grafts in the outpatient setting. Urology. 1996;48(1):124–7.
61. Hafez AT, Smith CR, Mclorie GA, et al. Tunica vaginalis for correcting penile chordee in a rabbit model: is there a difference in flap versus graft? J Urol. 2001;166(4):1429–32.
62. Lindgren BW, Reda EF, Levitt SB, Brock WA, Franco I. Single and multiple dermal grafts for the management of severe penile curvature. J Urol. 1998;160(3 Part 2):1128–30.
63. Badylak SF. The extracellular matrix as a biologic scaffold material. Biomaterials. 2007;28(25):3587–93.
64. Elmore JM, Kirsch AJ, Scherz HC, Smith EA. Small intestinal submucosa for corporeal body grafting in severe hypospadias requiring division of the urethral plate. J Urol. 2007;178(4, Supplement):1698–701.
65. Weiser AC, Franco I, Herz DB, Silver RI, Reda EF. Single layered small intestinal submucosa in the repair of severe chordee and complicated hypospadias. J Urol. 2003;170(4, Part 2):1593–5.
66. Soergel TM, Cain MP, Kaefer M, et al. Complications of small intestinal submucosa for corporal body grafting for proximal hypospadias. J Urol. 2003;170(4, Part 2):1577–9.
67. Palmer LS, Palmer JS. The use of Alloderm® for correction of severe chordee in children: an initial experience. J Pediatr Urol. 2020;16(4):446.e1–5. Published online June 14, 2020
68. Chauviere MV, Schutter RJ, Steigelman MB, Clark BZ, Grayson JK, Sahar DE. Comparison of Allo Derm and AlloMax tissue incorporation in rats. Ann Plast Surg. 2014;73(3):282–5.
69. Chan YY, Bury MI, Yura EM, Hofer MD, Cheng EY, Sharma AK. The current state of tissue engineering in the management of hypospadias. Nat Rev Urol. 2020;17(3):162–75.
70. Zhang Y, Yoo JJ, Atala A. Chapter 46 - Tissue engineering: bladder and urethra. In: Lanza R, Langer R, Vacanti JP, Atala A, editors. Principles of tissue engineering (fifth edition). New York: Academic Press; 2020. p. 845–62.
71. Oottamasathien S, Hotaling JM, Craig JR, Myers JB, Brant WO. Amniotic therapeutic biomaterials in urology: current and future applications. Transl Androl Urol. 2017;6(5):943–50.
72. Raya-Rivera A, Esquiliano DR, Yoo JJ, Lopez-Bayghen E, Soker S, Atala A. Tissue engineered autologous urethras for patients who need reconstruction: an observational study. Lancet. 2011;377(9772):1175–82.

The Surgical Approach to Two-Stage Hypospadias Repair

13

Christopher J. Long, Aseem R. Shukla,
and Mark R. Zaontz

13.1 Background, Epidemiology, and Introduction

Hypospadias is amongst the most common congenital male anomalies, with an incidence ranging from 1:150 to 250 of male births [1, 2]. The vast majority of boys present with a mild, distal variant, and surgical reconstruction, when indicated, is highly successful [3, 4]. Proximal hypospadias is reported to occur in 10–25% of patients with hypospadias, and its increased severity presents several unique management challenges to the surgeon [5, 6]. In addition to worsened curvature and shorter penile length, anatomic studies have found less elastic tissue and relative androgen resistance in boys with proximal hypospadias, suggesting more dysplastic tissue which further complicates surgical reconstruction [7–9]. Although traditionally thought to have a complication rate ranging up to 25%, recent publications indicate a significantly higher complication rate for proximal hypospadias repair, with secondary surgery rates as high as 70%, and many of these complications presenting after puberty, and into adulthood [10–13]. This high complication rate demands that we focus our efforts on identifying risk factors to improve our outcomes for these patients. For these reasons, we consider proximal hypospadias a different disease process when compared to distal hypospadias, one that warrants unique considerations for assessment, management, and follow-up.

13.2 Indications and Considerations for Surgical Repair

Proximal hypospadias can present in a variety of ways. One is the classic appearance with obvious severe curvature and a proximal meatus (Fig. 13.1). The surgeon must also be aware of other variants. A boy can present with a distal meatus, but a more severe proximal variant is identified in the operating room (Fig. 13.2). These pictures suggest hypoplastic ventral penile shaft skin and severe ventral penile curvature after degloving. This boy would benefit from a two-stage repair.

Because of these variants, the surgeon should never enter the operating room with a rigid plan for a hypospadias repair, instead of keeping their plan fluid as the anatomy unfolds in the operating room. Indications for utilizing a two-stage repair at our institution include severe penile curvature (defined as 30 degrees or greater after penile

---

C. J. Long · A. R. Shukla (✉) · M. R. Zaontz
Division of Urology, Department of Surgery, The Children's Hospital of Philadelphia, Perelman School of Medicine, University of Pennsylvania, Philadelphia, PA, USA
e-mail: Longc3@chop.edu; shuklaa@chop.edu; zaontz@chop.edu

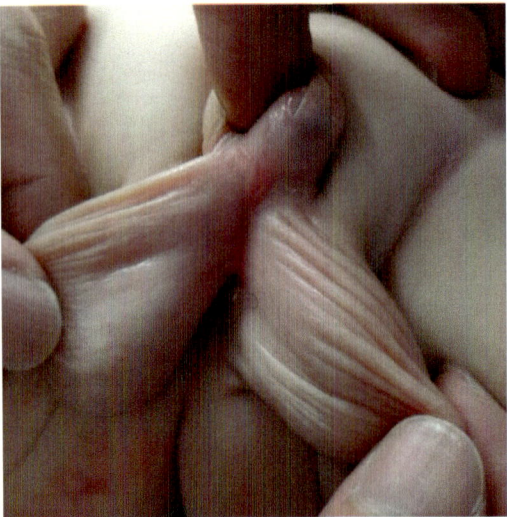

Fig. 13.1 A boy with proximal hypospadias. The meatus is located at the penoscrotal junction, there is severe curvature and severe penoscrotal transposition

degloving) and/or a lack of penile tissue that would prohibit a tension-free repair. A step-wise approach should be used to assess penile curvature, beginning with penile degloving and excision of chordee tissue. Artificial erection is then performed. This can be challenging in this patient population, especially if penile concealment is present. One must be aware of proximal penile curvature that may be obscured with a tourniquet. If a ventral corporal lengthening procedure is required, we feel that a staged repair should be performed, regardless of the initial location of the urethral meatus. We believe that the priority is to correct the penile curvature at the first stage, while at the same time establishing a healthy bed of tissue on the ventral penile shaft for the second stage repair and urethroplasty. As the management of a simple distal variant contrasts greatly with the approach and complication rate for a two-stage repair, the surgeon must educate the parents properly at the time of the office consultation, particularly given the longer recovery process and the possibility of requiring a secondary procedure.

The traditional approach of grading the complexity of hypospadias based solely on the location of the meatus is an inadequate exercise. Staging the phenotype is a vital exercise in understanding the full spectrum or the degree of severity of hypospadias and allows us to convert the art form of hypospadias into a common language for comparison sake. Staging systems such Glans-Urethral Meatus-Shaft (GMS) score objectively assess the penile anatomy with measurement of the glans width, assessment of the quality of the urethral plate, the degree of chordee, and the location of the urethral meatus, and correlate a higher score with an increased complication risk [14]. We believe that the universal acceptance of the GMS or a similar standardized evaluation system such as the Hypospadias International Society scoring system will advance our understanding of hypospadias in hopes of improving our outcomes. Regardless of the method used, one must incorporate the location of the meatus, the quality of the ventral penile shaft tissue, the degree of penile curvature, and any associated anomalies in their assessment.

13.3 Preoperative Assessment

As mentioned above, the office assessment begins the process of evaluating the degree of penile curvature, the quality of the ventral penile shaft skin, the width and quality of the glans, and the urethral plate to determine the potential need for a staged procedure. Patients must also be screened for the presence of undescended testes as this may indicate the presence of a disorder of sexual development, particularly in patients with proximal hypospadias. This will guide the preoperative discussion with the family, including the possible need for a karyotype or additional testing to identify a complicating underlying disorder. Given the high risk for postoperative complications after a proximal hypospadias repair, it is imperative that the family is counseled on the potential for a secondary procedure as in our experience this discussion in the preoperative period guides family expectations.

A glans width <15 mm has been associated with an increased risk of urethroplasty complication development [15]. Supplemental testosterone administration prior to the procedure can increase

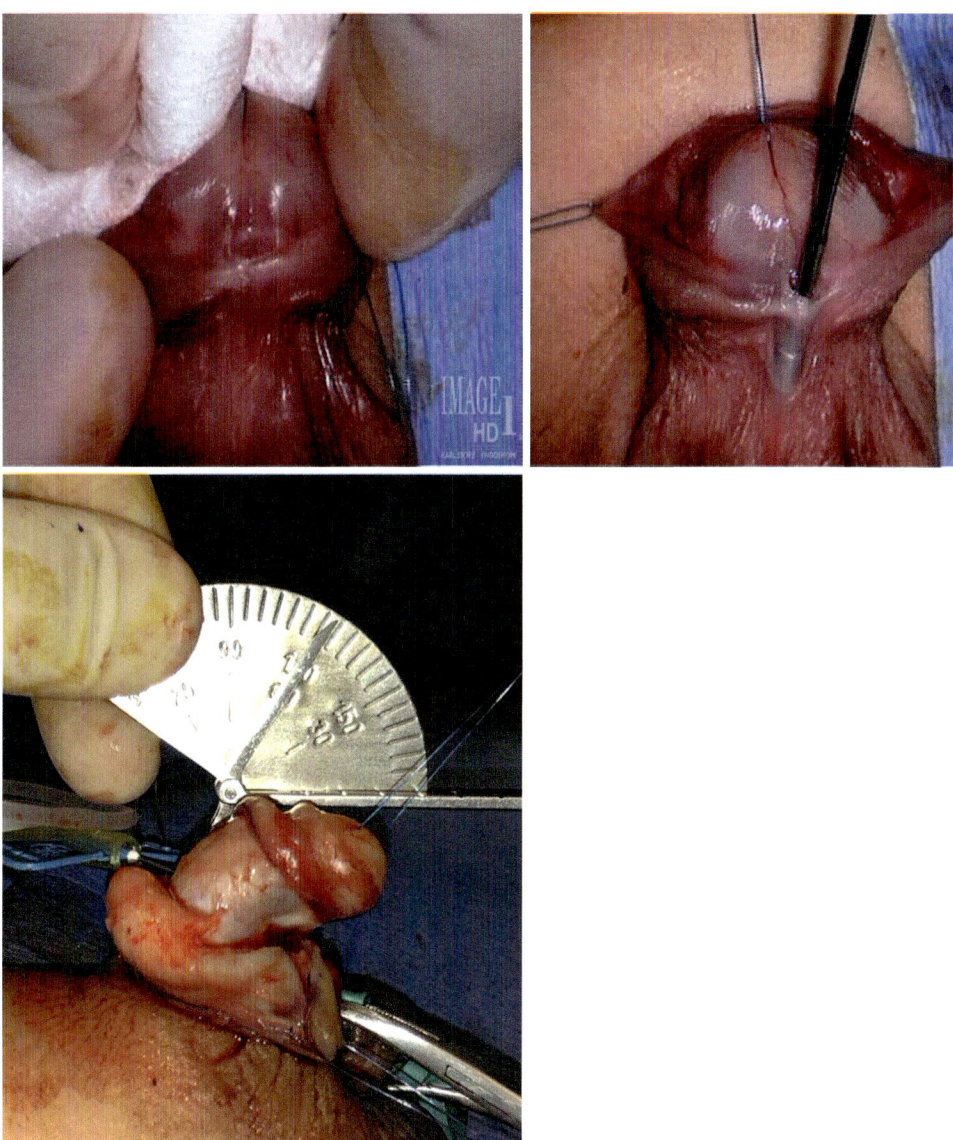

Fig. 13.2 A boy that presented with a distal urethral meatus but after further assessment in the operating room was identified as true proximal hypospadias with poor ventral penile tissue

glans width in pre-pubertal boys [16, 17]. Its use is controversial as some feel that there is little benefit or even a risk of worse surgical outcomes when administered [18]. Others have raised concerns about a blunted response to testosterone in those with a severe form of proximal hypospadias due to androgen insensitivity [9]. Our personal experience does not mirror the aforementioned negative concerns regarding testosterone supplementation, and we feel that testosterone enhances our technique with no increase in complications compared to the literature.

Our use of testosterone in this patient population has changed over time and is patient dependent. Our typical practice is to administer preoperative testosterone 5 and 2 weeks prior to the planned surgery date to boys with a glans with <15 mm. In patients with a small penis with limited penile shaft skin, we administer preoperative testosterone prior to the first stage repair. If glans width remains an issue at the second stage, this can be repeated.

Finally, the preoperative consultation is an important time to center patient and parental expectations. The ultimate goal in any penile reconstruction is to have a functional penis that will act as a sufficient conduit for normal voiding and to achieve full sexual potential in adulthood. Achievement of the so-called perfect penis in distal hypospadias, with a slit-like meatus within the distal glans is much more attainable than it is in proximal hypospadias [3]. Given the degree of dysplasia of the penile tissue in proximal hypospadias, it may not be possible to achieve the same cosmetic results attainable in distal hypospadias. Placing the urethral meatus within the coronal margin, although not the normal anatomic location, may result in a normal functional penis and forestall complications such as meatal stenosis that may complicate attempts to place the meatus within the glans in cases where the glans is underdeveloped. We pursue the approach of placing a urethral meatus in a coronal or proximal glans location in the patients of a narrow urethral plate and glans that otherwise would prohibit glans closure. Consideration must be given to balancing what we may think is a "perfect penis" as surgeons and what ultimately will result in the optimal outcome for patients. Alternatively, we may plan for a dorsal inlay graft at the time of the second stage of the repair to widen the glans in order to advance the meatus into a more distal location [19]. These possible outcomes are conveyed to families in order to set expectations.

13.4 Elements of Surgical Repair

The sequence of surgical decision-making begins with an assessment in the operating room prior to making an incision. The location of the true urethral opening and the quality of the associated ventral shaft tissues is assessed to determine if a more severe variant is present. Although often obvious on the exam, proximal hypospadias can masquerade as distal hypospadias with severe penile curvature and hypoplastic ventral shaft skin. The surgeon must recognize this in the operating room to ensure that the appropriate repair is performed.

The circumcising incision is made, and the penis is degloved to the penoscrotal junction. Care should be taken to develop a mucosal collar, rotating redundant dorsal hooded foreskin to the ventrum as this will aid in ventral shaft skin coverage and yield an improved cosmetic result [20]. One can also leave a shorter mucosal collar in order to preserve inner preputial skin for ventral shaft coverage. It is important to resect all dysplastic tissue on the penile shaft during the degloving process. Once degloved, an objective assessment must be performed as the degree of penile curvature is a major deciding factor between proceeding with a single versus two-stage repair (Fig. 13.3). After degloving and resection of chordee tissue, an artificial erection is performed, and the degree of penile curvature is determined. We use a goniometer to objectively measure the degree of curvature, although we encourage any objective measure of curvature to obtain the most objective assessment [21]. Most surgeons would perform a dorsal plication for curvature <30° [22]. If curvature persists after plication or is ≥30°, the next step would involve either mobilization or division of the urethra. Persistent curvature ≥30° at this point would warrant a corporal lengthening the procedure by incising the ventral corporal tunica albuginea and placing a graft to cover the defect [23]. Options include autologous tissue (dermal graft [24], tunica vaginal flap [25] or graft) or non-autologous tissue (Alloderm, small intestinal submucosa (SIS) [26, 27]). Alternatively one could perform ventral fairy cuts or several ventral incisions through the tunica albuginea to release the ventral curvature without an additional graft or flap insertion to close the gap [28]. Completion of the first stage of the repair is outlined in the next section and is dependent upon the approach taken.

Alternatively, a corporal lengthening procedure utilizing a tunica vaginalis flap, followed by urethroplasty and glansplasty can be performed to complete a single-stage repair utilizing inner

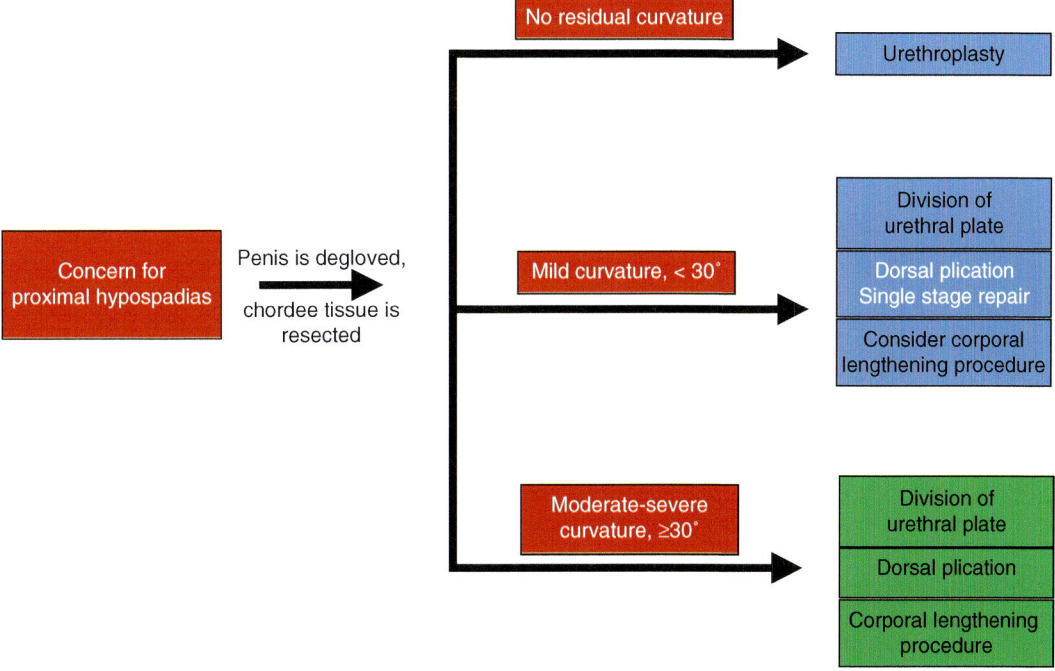

Fig. 13.3 Algorithm for assessment and repair of penile curvature

preputial tissue as a flap, or tubularizing a mobilized urethral plate [25]. We have concerns about the healing potential of a simultaneous graft overlying a flap and feel that this will place both tissues at risk for scarring and poor wound healing [29]. Our preferred approach in the setting of persistent curvature ≥30° is the two-stage repair in order to maximize the healing potential of both the corporoplasty and the subsequent urethroplasty.

Regardless of the approach to corporal lengthening, it is important to ensure that it is corrected fully at the time of the first stage, which can be verified with repeat artificial erection after correction. If necessary, a plication can be performed at the time of the second procedure to correct minor recurrent curvature. The timing between surgical reconstructions should range from a minimum of 6 months to allow sufficient graft take. We often allow 8–12 months between procedures, with interval exams to ensure satisfactory graft uptake, to monitor for recurrent curvature, and to determine if the ventral skin is supple enough for second-stage urethroplasty closure.

13.4.1 Surgical Techniques for Two-Stage Hypospadias Repair

Modern technical approaches to the two-stage repair of proximal hypospadias can be divided into three categories, each separated by technical variations on the approach to urethroplasty. The first procedure addresses penile curvature with the differences outlined below.

The Bracka two-stage repair utilizes a free graft, harvested from either the inner prepuce or the buccal mucosa, which is placed into the ventral penile shaft for eventual closure at the second stage (Fig. 13.4) [30, 31]. The Staged Tubularized Autograft Repair (STAG) is a variation of this technique and has been popularized more recently [28]. The urethral plate is divided, and a midline incision is made within the glans to act as a receiving bed for the graft. The graft can then be quilted into place on the ventral penile shaft to prevent hematoma formation and to facilitate graft take. The second stage is performed at least 6 months later, during which a U-shaped incision, similar to the Thiersch–Duplay approach, is made and the

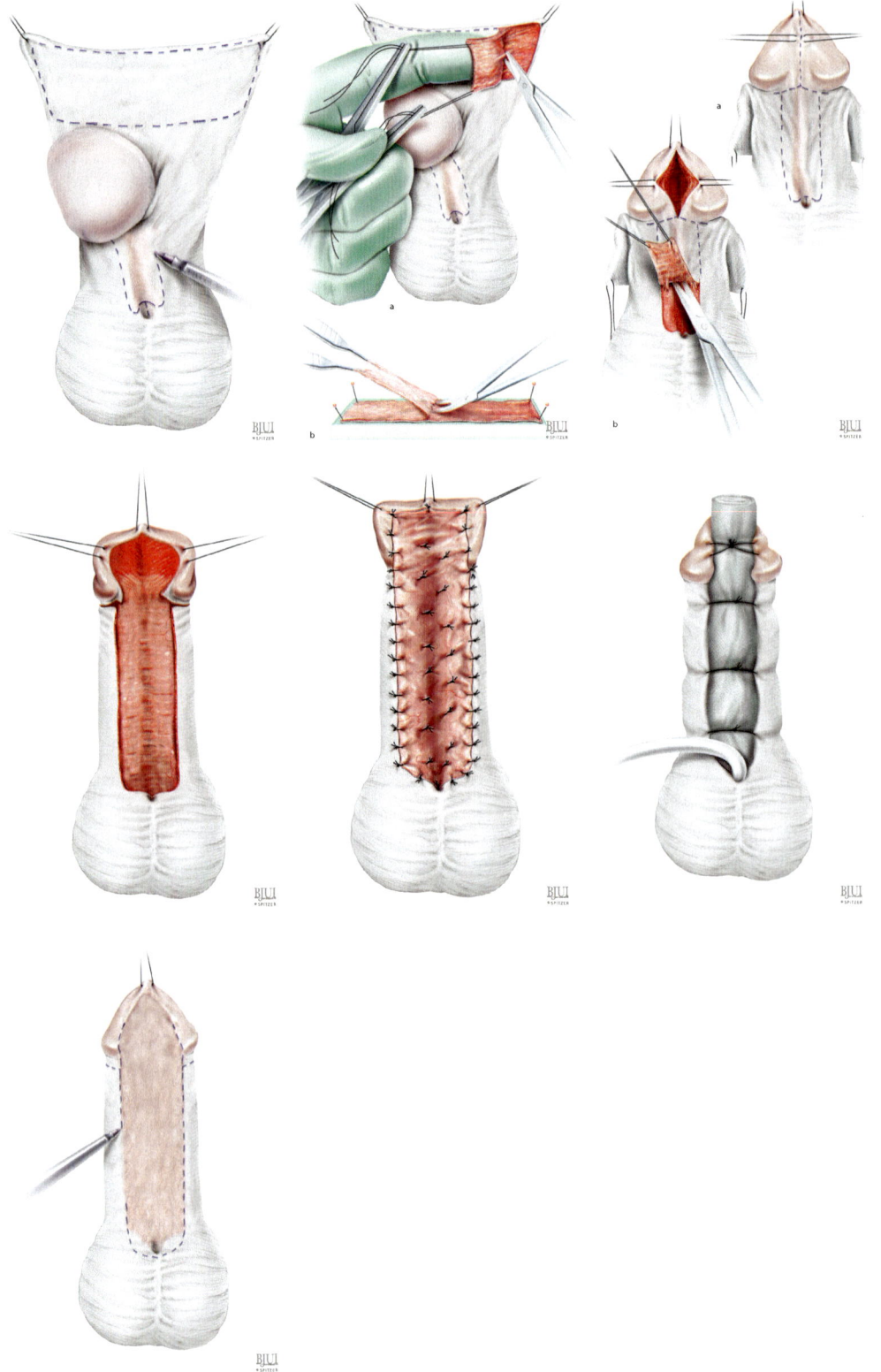

Fig. 13.4 Bracka two-stage repair

urethra is tubularized, and the glans is closed [31]. Multilayer closure is performed to maintain vascular flow to aid the healing process. This technique is ideal for patients in whom a previous circumcision was performed, or a lack of foreskin is present to perform an alternate repair. With the STAG repair, an inner preputial free graft is harvested in lieu of a buccal mucosa graft. In the setting of severe penile curvature requiring a corporal graft procedure, we do not recommend this approach as overlap will impede graft uptake [29]. Graft contracture, particularly over open corporotomies, has been reported to increase graft loss and would require additional procedures.

The Byars flap procedure utilizes redundant dorsal preputial skin, which is incised in the midline dorsally and rotated ventrally at the first procedure, as the scaffold to form the urethra (Fig. 13.5) [32, 33]. Similar to the Bracka repair, at the second stage, the neourethra is closed by making a long-U-shaped incision with glansplasty using a standard Thiersch–Duplay technique. Some key technical components include a water-tight closure and establishing a lumen of equal caliber throughout the length of the urethroplasty. A two-layer urethroplasty, followed by multiple layers of adjacent dartos tissue as an overlay is required to ensure that the neourethra

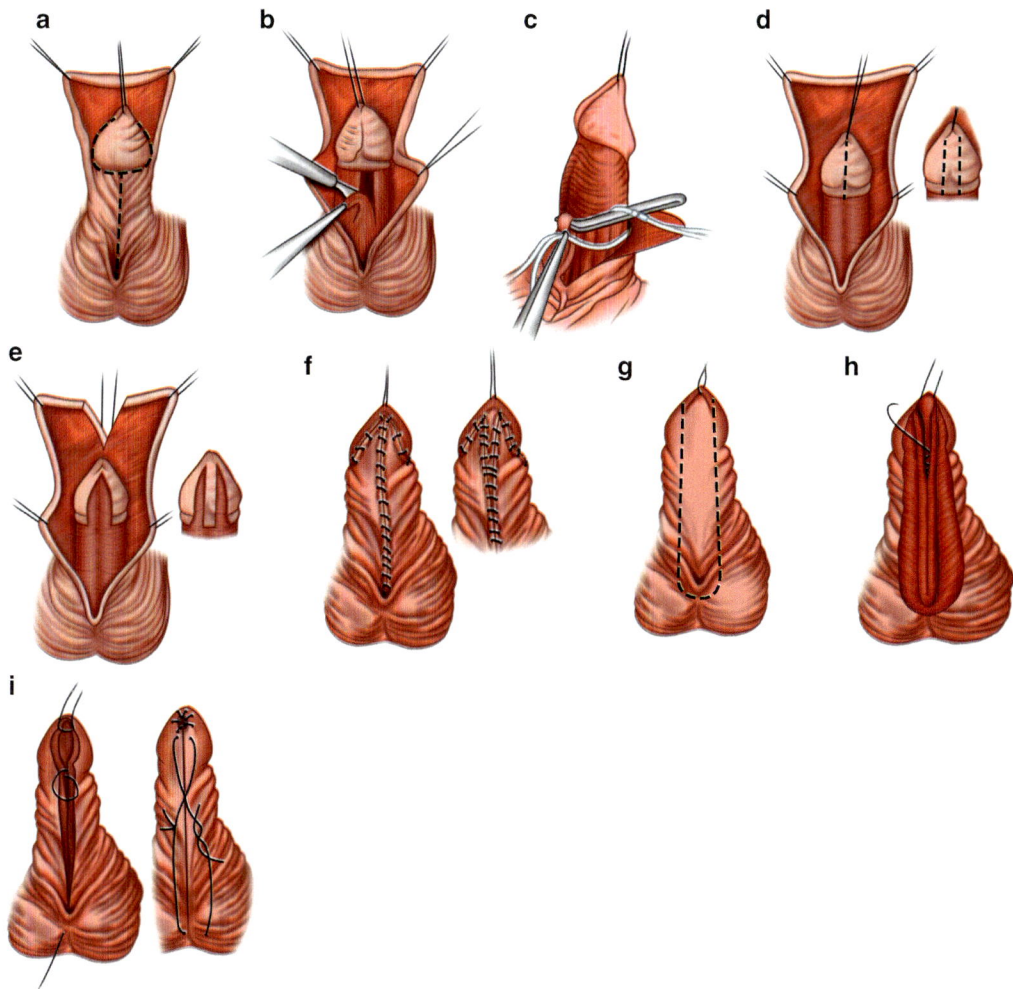

Fig. 13.5 2-stage Byars flap repair. The penis is marked and circumscribing incision is made (**a**). The penis is degloved and the urethral plate is divided (**b**). Artificial erection is performed to confirm that curvature is corrected (**c**). The glans can be incised to allow for flap placement as part of the first stage repair (**d**, **e**). The flap is secured in the mid-line of the penile shaft (**f**). AT teh time of the 2nd stage repair, a ventral U shaped incision is marked and incised (**g**). The urethroplasty is performed (**h**), followed by skin closure (**i**)

maintains adequate blood supply. In particular, establishing a supple dartos bed overlying the corporoplasty at the first stage will provide sufficient vascular flow to allow safe urethroplasty at the second stage.

The third approach involves correction of the penile curvature, closure of the distal urethra and glans, and rotating an interposing flap or graft to replace the urethra at the first stage repair (Fig. 13.6). For the distal urethra, one approach

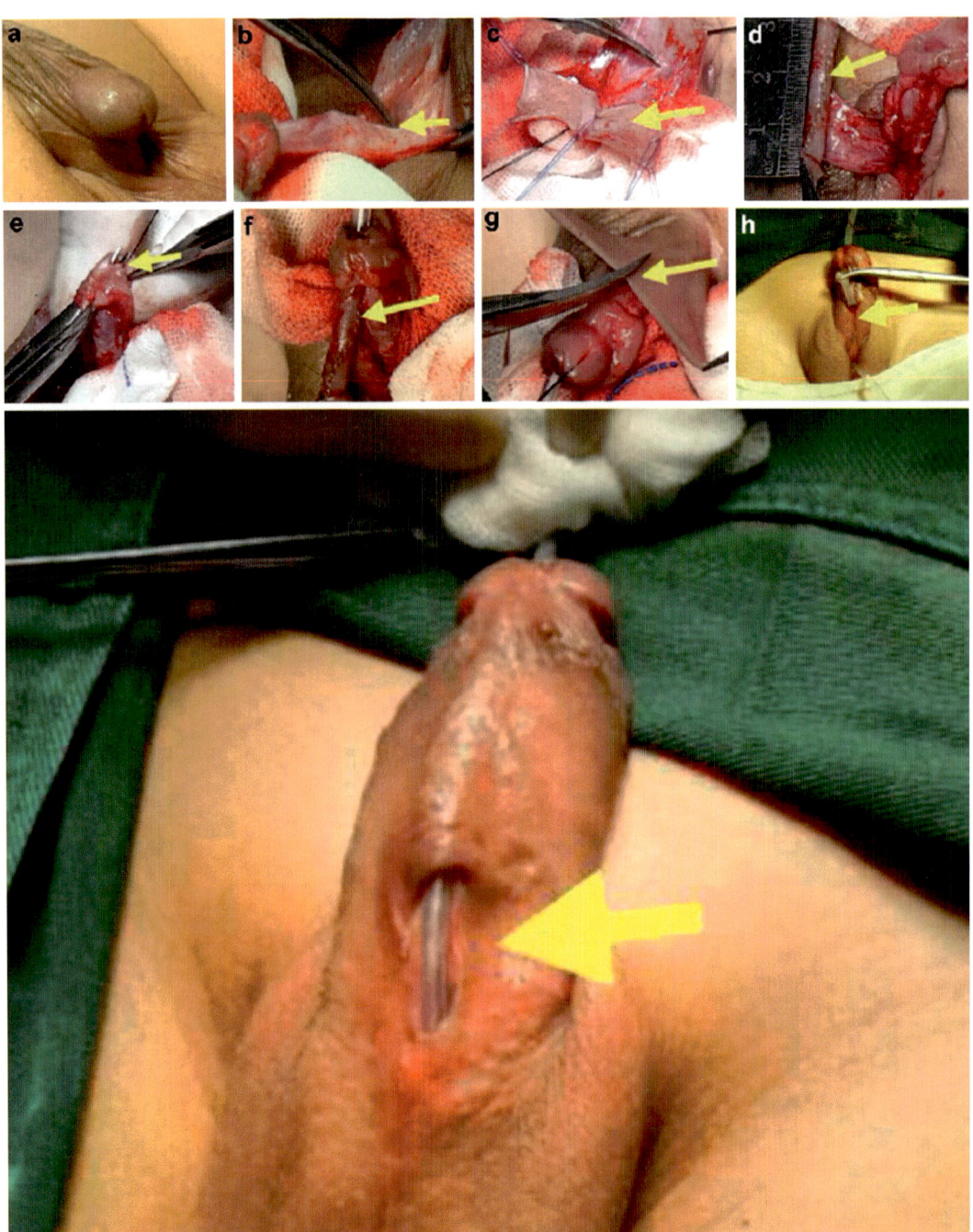

Fig. 13.6 Patient with a severe, proximal hypospadias (**a**). Penis is degloved (**b**). An inner preputial island flap is developed (**c**) and tubularized (**d**). The glans is incised and the tubularized flap is tunneled into the glans (**e, f**). The dorsal penile shaft skin is incised in the midline, creating Byars flaps (**g**). The Byars flaps were rotated ventrally to close the penile shaft skin, leaving a gap between the native urethral meatus (proximal) and the distal, tubularized urethra (**h**)

includes a tubularized incised plate type of closure urethra and glans [34]. Alternatively, in the Ulaanbaatar repair, a transverse island interposition tube can be developed from the preputial skin, which is tunneled into the distal portion of the glans [35]. For both of these variants, the urethra is matured into a proximal position, and Byars flaps are rotated ventrally to allow for completion urethroplasty of the interposing portion of the urethra at the second stage of the closure.

13.4.2 Postoperative Care and Follow-Up

The immediate postoperative period consists of urethral diversion with a stent and compressive dressing. In our practice, a compression dressing is left for 72 h, after which time the stent is removed with the compression dressing, and petroleum jelly is applied to facilitate grafts and/or flaps healing. If a Buccal mucosa graft is performed, we suture a compression dressing 5–7 days directly over the graft to minimize the risk of hematoma formation and subsequent graft loss. A suprapubic tube can be placed, if desired, to maximize urinary diversion, particularly in the setting of a buccal mucosa graft. We utilize this approach more commonly in toilet trained children.

Urinary diversion at the time of urethroplasty is typically done for 7–14 days. Prolonged stent duration has been shown to decrease complication rates although one must determine if this is applicable for all patients and must be balanced against the risk for infection, patient discomfort, and the potential for stent encrustation [36]. Antibiotic prophylaxis is typically given while the stent is in place, although this is controversial [37].

Flap or graft care is a key aspect of the postoperative period. Topical petroleum jelly application with a digit and manual pressure to the ventral penile shaft can help prevent contracture and uneven healing. We initiate this process within 2 weeks of the procedure and continue for 6–8 weeks after the first stage repair. Topical steroid application can be performed if there is skin contraction or other healing concerns.

A minimum of 6 months should separate the first and second stage surgeries to allow sufficient graft and flap uptake and neovascularization and the surgeon should not hesitate to wait an additional time to ensure proper healing has occurred. A critical evaluation is a thorough postoperative assessment to examine for appropriate skin fit, monitoring for persistent curvature, and to determine the viability of the ventral penile shaft skin for potential urethroplasty. The viability of the graft and/or flaps should determine if additional procedures are necessary and the appropriate timing for the next procedure.

13.4.3 Outcomes with Brief Pertinent Literature

Successful outcomes in distal hypospadias are high, ranging from 87 to 95% [3, 4, 38]. Unfortunately, proximal hypospadias reveals a much higher complication rate—and complications may become manifest several years after the initial repair [10–13, 39]. The degree of associated tissue hypoplasia and severity of the phenotype increases with more proximal hypospadias likely explains the higher predilection for complications with proximal hypospadias, since the smaller width of the glans and longer length of the urethroplasty are contributors to this increased complication rate.

Comparison of technical approaches to curvature correction is difficult. Curvature assessment is often subjectively assessed by the surgeon and is categorized into mild, moderate, or severe variants which limits our ability to compare techniques across institutions. Only recently has the focus shifted toward a more objective approach to defining the degree of curvature, which if incompletely corrected, has the potential to create long-term concerns or complex surgical reconstructions [40]. One study directly compared dorsal plication versus penile lengthening procedures to correct curvature in patients with proximal hypospadias [27]. The rate of recurrent curvature at 17 months of follow-up was higher for dorsal plication versus penile lengthening (27.9% vs 9.4%, $p = 0.03$), with insufficient shaft skin the etiology for the latter group suggesting adequate correction of corporal disproportion with a lengthening procedure.

Regardless of technique, the rate of recurrent penile curvature for the two-stage repair of proximal hypospadias in the current literature is thought to be relatively low, ranging from 0 to 5% of patients [10–13, 28]. Two-stage repair with corporoplasty was associated with increased penile length and improved cosmetic results [41]. Penile length is an important aspect in the repair, particularly with proximal hypospadias, as a survey of adult patients after infant repair reveals concerns primarily for shortened penile length [42].

The Bracka repair, or technical variations thereof, has an overall reported complication rate of <25% [28, 41, 43]. The most common complication encountered was glans dehiscence and/or urethrocutaneous fistula. The rate of recurrent penile curvature is low. Additional layers of closure, increasing the local blood supply, have been shown to decrease the complication rate [44]. A comparison of four approaches to proximal hypospadias repair, including tubularized incised play, island preputial onlay, and a two-stage Bracka repair, found that the repair approach did not correlate with complication development [41]. Concerns for a skin graft incorporation over a corporal graft can be circumvented with dorsal plication techniques combined with proximal urethral mobilization to correct the majority of curvature [45]. Otherwise, if severe curvature persists, a corporal graft should be performed, and this would increase the risk for skin graft loss.

Several reports have recently indicated a high complication rate associated with the Byars flap two-stage repair [10–13]. Complication rates ranged from 30 to 70%, with urethrocutaneous fistula representing the most common complication noted, followed by glans dehiscence. Urethral diverticulum is also a potential complication, thought to occur as a result of a combination of a lack of spongiosum and lack of fixation of the flap onto the ventral penile shaft at the time of the urethroplasty. Compared to the graft utilized for the ventral penis in the Bracka repair, the theory would suggest that the improved vascularity of the preputial flaps should improve wound healing. However, the high complication rates suggest a yet unknown cause for complications. One technical modification, the advancement of the urethra to the coronal margin, may prove to decrease the complication rate after the second stage repair.

Although mostly represented by case series, the two-stage approach incorporating distal urethra closure and correction of curvature at the first stage has reportedly favorable outcomes [34, 35]. The authors have not seen a comparative increase in concerns for distal urethral stricture or stenosis, a concern given the increased likelihood of a small glans at the time of the initial procedure and the lack of urine flow through this area after the initial procedure.

To the best of our knowledge, no direct comparison of the three approaches above has been performed that would determine the ideal approach to proximal hypospadias with severe ventral penile curvature. Regardless of the approach taken, long-term outcomes in the literature are lacking and only raise the possibility that more complications will be captured as these patients are followed over time [46, 47]. We strongly agree with this principle and have modified our follow-up protocols accordingly to extend follow-up for these boys well into the pubertal period.

13.4.4 Future Advances and Directions

Much work remains to be completed in the advancement of surgical reconstruction of severe hypospadias [48]. These efforts need to focus on improving the relatively high complication rate, extending our routine follow-up into adulthood, and using long-term analysis to guide patient and parental expectations of the repair.

A survey of the literature reveals a limited number of studies with patients undergoing hypospadias repair with follow-up that into puberty. This severely limits our ability to determine the real outcomes and complications of our repairs. Extending our follow-up will allow us to answer several persistent questions concerning hypospadias repair. The first is to determine the ideal approach to correction of penile curvature, specifically which approach maintains effectiveness through the accelerated penile growth during the pubescent period and into adulthood. If a boy has a straight penis as a child but has painful, curved erections as an adult, then we would argue that we have failed that patient. If it is determined that dorsal plication in a patient with 20° of ventral curvature is associated with a higher rate of recurrence as an adult, then this approach must be abandoned. In a similar fashion if corporal grafting results in a higher rate of erectile dysfunction due to increased venous leak as an adult, then we must consider this when a repair is performed.

In addition to surgeon assessment of outcomes into adulthood, the patient-reported outcomes must also become increasingly important. Unification of patient-reported outcomes with surgical outcomes will advance our understanding of our surgical penile reconstruction. Questions to be answered include the correlation of cosmetic features with functional outcomes. Are patients happy with a urethral meatus located at the coronal margin in the setting of proximal hypospadias? If the patient is able to stand to void with a strong urinary stream and has straight erections sufficient for intercourse, will it matter if the meatus is slightly lower than normal? This question is an important one in the sense that the creation of the so-called perfect penis, with a slit-like meatus within the distal glans, in the setting of proximal hypospadias may be detrimental to the patient. Extension of the meatus into the distal glans may be responsible for, at least in some part, the high complication rates we are seeing in proximal hypospadias. We theorize that the relative rigidity of the spongiosum of the glans acts as a bottleneck for urine passage, increasing proximal voiding pressure, and driving complications such as a urethrocutaneous fistula and diverticulum, amongst others. Finally, as proximal hypospadias is associated with severe tissue dysplasia, we need to determine what normal sexual and voiding function is for these patients as they enter adulthood [49]. Doing so will allow us to fully determine the course of the repair of this complex disease process in infancy in order to translate into achieving its maximal potential as an adult.

13.5 Conclusion

Proximal hypospadias is a complex variant with a high risk for complications. Proper anatomic assessment and determination of complexity is a crucial aspect of the repair. The two-stage repair has emerged as a more reliable approach to ensure adequate correction for chordee at the first stage of the repair, optimizing graft or flap healing in preparation for urethroplasty at the second procedure. Many unanswered questions about hypospadias, and it is clear that long-term follow-ups of these patients into adulthood is not only suggested but should be mandatory.

References

1. Springer A, van den Heijkant M, Baumann S. Worldwide prevalence of hypospadias. J Pediatr Urol. 2015;
2. Elliott CS, Halpern MS, Paik J, Maldonado Y, Shortliffe LD. Epidemiologic trends in penile anomalies and hypospadias in the state of California, 1985-2006. J Pediatr Urol. 2011;7(3):294–8.
3. Pfistermuller KL, McArdle AJ, Cuckow PM. A meta-analysis of complication rates of the tubularized incised plate (TIP) repair. J Pediatr Urol. 2015;11(2):54–9.
4. Rushton HG, Belman AB. The split prepuce in situ onlay hypospadias repair. J Urol. 1998;160(3 Pt 2):1134–6; discussion 7.
5. Bergman JE, Loane M, Vrijheid M, Pierini A, Nijman RJ, Addor MC, et al. Epidemiology of hypospadias in Europe: a registry-based study. World J Urol. 2015;33(12):2159–67.
6. Manzoni G, Bracka A, Palminteri E, Marrocco G. Hypospadias surgery: when what and by whom? BJU Int. 2004;94(8):1188–95.
7. Camoglio FS, Bruno C, Zambaldo S, Zampieri N. Hypospadias anatomy: elastosonographic evaluation of the normal and hypospadic penis. J Pediatr Urol. 2016;
8. Bush NC, DaJusta D, Snodgrass WT. Glans penis width in patients with hypospadias compared to healthy controls. J Pediatr Urol. 2013;9(6 Pt B):1188–91.

9. Snodgrass WT, Villanueva C, Granberg C, Bush NC. Objective use of testosterone reveals androgen insensitivity in patients with proximal hypospadias. J Pediatr Urol. 2014;10(1):118–22.
10. Long CJ, Chu DI, Tenney RW, Morris AR, Weiss DA, Shukla AR, et al. Intermediate-term followup of proximal hypospadias repair reveals high complication rate. J Urol. 2017;197(3 Pt 2):852–8.
11. Stanasel I, Le HK, Bilgutay A, Roth DR, Gonzales ET Jr, Janzen N, et al. Complications following staged hypospadias repair using transposed preputial skin flaps. J Urol. 2015;194(2):512–6.
12. Pippi Salle JL, Sayed S, Salle A, Bagli D, Farhat W, Koyle M, et al. Proximal hypospadias: a persistent challenge. Single institution outcome analysis of three surgical techniques over a 10-year period. J Pediatr Urol. 2015;
13. McNamara ER, Schaeffer AJ, Logvinenko T, Seager C, Rosoklija I, Nelson CP, et al. Management of proximal hypospadias with 2-stage repair: 20-year experience. J Urol. 2015;194(4):1080–5.
14. Merriman LS, Arlen AM, Broecker BH, Smith EA, Kirsch AJ, Elmore JM. The GMS hypospadias score: assessment of inter-observer reliability and correlation with post-operative complications. J Pediatr Urol. 2013;9(6 Pt A):707–12.
15. Bush NC, Villanueva C, Snodgrass W. Glans size is an independent risk factor for urethroplasty complications after hypospadias repair. J Pediatr Urol. 2015;11(6):355 e1–5.
16. Gearhart JP, Jeffs RD. The use of parenteral testosterone therapy in genital reconstructive surgery. J Urol. 1987;138(4 Pt 2):1077–8.
17. Luo CC, Lin JN, Chiu CH, Lo FS. Use of parenteral testosterone prior to hypospadias surgery. Pediatr Surg Int. 2003;19(1–2):82–4.
18. Menon P, Rao KLN, Handu A, Balan L, Kakkar N. Outcome of urethroplasty after parenteral testosterone in children with distal hypospadias. J Pediatr Urol. 2017;13(3):292 e1–7.
19. Kolon TF, Gonzales ET Jr. The dorsal inlay graft for hypospadias repair. J Urol. 2000;163(6):1941–3.
20. Firlit CF. The mucosal collar in hypospadias surgery. J Urol. 1987;137(1):80–2.
21. Villanueva CA. Ventral penile curvature estimation using an app. J Pediatr Urol. 2020;16(4):437 e1–3.
22. Springer A, Krois W, Horcher E. Trends in hypospadias surgery: results of a worldwide survey. Eur Urol. 2011;60(6):1184–9.
23. Steven L, Cherian A, Yankovic F, Mathur A, Kulkarni M, Cuckow P. Current practice in paediatric hypospadias surgery; a specialist survey. J Pediatr Urol. 2013;9(6 Pt B):1126–30.
24. Devine CJ Jr, Horton CE. Use of dermal graft to correct chordee. J Urol. 1975;113(1):56–8.
25. Braga LH, Pippi Salle JL, Dave S, Bagli DJ, Lorenzo AJ, Khoury AE. Outcome analysis of severe chordee correction using tunica vaginalis as a flap in boys with proximal hypospadias. J Urol. 2007;178(4 Pt 2):1693–7; discussion 7.
26. Castellan M, Gosalbez R, Devendra J, Bar-Yosef Y, Labbie A. Ventral corporal body grafting for correcting severe penile curvature associated with single or two-stage hypospadias repair. J Pediatr Urol. 2011;7(3):289–93.
27. Braga LH, Lorenzo AJ, Bagli DJ, Dave S, Eeg K, Farhat WA, et al. Ventral penile lengthening versus dorsal plication for severe ventral curvature in children with proximal hypospadias. J Urol. 2008;180(4 Suppl):1743–7; discussion 7-8.
28. Snodgrass W, Bush N. Staged tubularized autograft repair for primary proximal hypospadias with 30-degree or greater ventral curvature. J Urol. 2017;
29. Mattos RM, Araujo SR, Quitzan JG, Leslie B, Bacelar H, Parizi JL, et al. Can a graft be placed over a flap in complex hypospadias surgery? An experimental study in rabbits. Int Braz J Urol. 2016;42(6):1228–36.
30. Altarac S, Papes D, Bracka A. Two-stage hypospadias repair with inner preputial layer Wolfe graft (Aivar Bracka repair). BJU Int. 2012;110(3):460–73.
31. Bracka A. Hypospadias repair: the two-stage alternative. Br J Urol. 1995;76(Suppl 3):31–41.
32. Retik AB, Bauer SB, Mandell J, Peters CA, Colodny A, Atala A. Management of severe hypospadias with a 2-stage repair. J Urol. 1994;152(2 Pt 2):749–51.
33. Byars LT. Functional restoration of hypospadias deformities; with a report of 60 completed cases. Surg Gynecol Obstet. 1951;92(2):149–54.
34. Cheng EY, Kropp BP, Pope JC, Brock JW III. Proximal division of the urethral plate in staged hypospadias repair. J Urol. 2003;170(4 Pt 2):1580–3; discussion 4.
35. Dewan PA, Erdenetsetseg G, Chiang D. Ulaanbaatar procedure for tubularization of the glans in severe hypospadias. J Urol. 2004;171(3):1263–5.
36. Daher P, Khoury A, Riachy E, Atallah B. Three-week or one-week bladder catheterization for hypospadias repair? A retrospective-prospective observational study of 189 patients. J Pediatr Surg. 2015;50(6):1063–6.
37. Kim JK, Chua ME, Ming JM, Braga LH, Smith GHH, Driver C, et al. Practice variation on the use of antibiotics: an international survey among pediatric urologists. J Pediatr Urol. 2018;14(6):520–4.
38. Perlmutter AE, Morabito R, Tarry WF. Impact of patient age on distal hypospadias repair: a surgical perspective. Urology. 2006;68(3):648–51.
39. Lucas J, Hightower T, Weiss DA, Van Batavia J, Coelho S, Srinivasan AK, et al. Time to complication detection after primary pediatric hypospadias repair: a large, single-centre, retrospective cohort analysis. J Urol. 2020;204(2):338–44.
40. Menon V, Breyer B, Copp HL, Baskin L, Disandro M, Schlomer BJ. Do adult men with untreated ventral penile curvature have adverse outcomes? J Pediatr Urol. 2016;12(1):31 e1–7.

41. Castagnetti M, Zhapa E, Rigamonti W. Primary severe hypospadias: comparison of reoperation rates and parental perception of urinary symptoms and cosmetic outcomes among four repairs. J Urol. 2013;189(4):1508–13.
42. Moriya K, Nakamura M, Nishimura Y, Kitta T, Kanno Y, Chiba H, et al. Factors affecting post-pubertal penile size in patients with hypospadias. World J Urol. 2016;
43. Ferro F, Zaccara A, Spagnoli A, Lucchetti MC, Capitanucci ML, Villa M. Skin graft for 2-stage treatment of severe hypospadias: back to the future? J Urol. 2002;168(4 Pt 2):1730–3; discussion 3.
44. Telfer JR, Quaba AA, Kwai Ben I, Peddi NC. An investigation into the role of waterproofing in a two-stage hypospadias repair. Br J Plast Surg. 1998;51(7):542–6.
45. Warwick RT, Parkhouse H, Chapple CR. Bulbar elongation anastomotic meatoplasty (BEAM) for subterminal and hypospadiac urethroplasty. J Urol. 1997;158(3 Pt 2):1160–7.
46. Grosos C, Bensaid R, Gorduza DB, Mouriquand P. Is it safe to solely use ventral penile tissues in hypospadias repair? Long-term outcomes of 578 Duplay urethroplasties performed in a single institution over a period of 14 years. J Pediatr Urol. 2014;10(6):1232–7.
47. Spinoit AF, Poelaert F, Groen LA, Van Laecke E, Hoebeke P. Hypospadias repair at a tertiary care centre: long-term follow-up is mandatory to determine the real complication rate. J Urol. 2013;189(6):2276–81.
48. Long CJ, Canning DA. Proximal hypospadias: we aren't always keeping our promises. F1000Res. 2016;5
49. Tack LJW, Springer A, Riedl S, Tonnhofer U, Weninger J, Heiss M, et al. Psychosexual outcome, sexual function, and long-term satisfaction of adolescent and young adult men after childhood hypospadias repair. J Sex Med. 2020;17(9):1665–75.

14

Modifications in Inner Prepucial Flap Repair of Hypospadias

Amilal Bhat

14.1 Introduction

TIP urethroplasty is the standardized approach for most distal and middle hypospadias. But the management of severe hypospadias remains the "Holy Grail" of hypospadiology [1]. Surgical technique in single-stage and two-stage repairs is described for the management of severe hypospadias with variable results. However, two-stage repairs are not free of complications. A recent review shows comparable results of one and two-stage repair. The urethral plate should be preserved and used in the modern approach for any hypospadias repair if possible [2]. Recently tubularized incised plate urethroplasty is being chosen more frequently for proximal hypospadias repair [3]. Other techniques for these patients are onlay flap urethroplasty, transverse island flap urethroplasty, and multiple stage repair. The urethral plate is usually transected and resected to correct chordee in proximal hypospadias. And transverse flap or skin graft urethroplasty is done for a single-stage repair.

If the prepucial flap falls short, it forcing the surgeon to go for a two-stage repair in some of the cases. Glassberg (1987) used an augmented Duckett repair for these cases. First, a part of the neo urethra is constructed with midline skin and is anastomosed to the inner prepucial skin tube [4]. The complications are very high, varying from 25% to 42%, as reported in the literature [5, 6]. The flap procedures and two-stage approach are preferred in proximal hypospadias with severe curvature and poor urethral plate, re-operative hypospadias and balanitis xerotica obliterans [7–9]. The chordee is corrected by resecting the urethral plate in the first stage and is substituted with either a genital (prepuce) or extra-genital graft (Buccal mucosa or post-auricular skin). The second stage, urethroplasty, reconstructs the neourethra with a substituted urethral plate after 6 months. Long-term cosmetic results of the two-stage inner prepucial skin graft urethroplasty and buccal mucosal grafts are reported to be good. Still, voiding and ejaculatory problems have been reported in up to 40% of the cases [8].

Disadvantages of the two-stage repairs are multiple surgeries causing the loss of patient's or parents' time and money. There are chances of some late complications such as post-void dribble,

A. Bhat (✉)
Bhat's Hypospadias and Reconstructive Urology Hospital and Research Centre,
Jaipur, Rajasthan, India

Department of Urology, Jaipur National University Institute for Medical Sciences and Research Centre, Jaipur, Rajasthan, India

Department of Urology, Dr. S.N. Medical College,
Jodhpur, Rajasthan, India

Department of Urology, S.P. Medical College,
Bikaner, Rajasthan, India

P.G. Committee Medical Council of India,
New Delhi, India

Academic and Research Council of RUHS,
Jaipur, Rajasthan, India

splaying of the stream, anejaculate and milking of the ejaculate. The advantages of a single-stage repair are the availability of unscarred healthy skin, less financial burden, cost-effectiveness, a decreased anesthesia risk and separation anxiety, and a better psychological impact [10, 11]. The complication rates in single-stage procedures using inner prepucial flap have been reported from 17% to 42%, with an average of 32% [5, 12, 13]. The repair offers greater convenience, comfort, and ease to the patients' parents and the surgeon.

Flap repair in hypospadias has a very long history. Bouisson (1861) was the first to describe flap use in hypospadias repair [14]. Inner Prepucial flap repairs were the mainstay of treatment in the nineteenth century. There have been many modifications in the flap repairs from time to time.

Island flap technique (Asopa 1971) [15], transverse prepucial island flap procedures (Duckett 1980) [16], and double island flap technique (Asopa 1984) [17] were frequently performed for proximal hypospadias in the 1980s and 1990s. These time-tested procedures have lost their sheen, even to the extent that the Tubularized Duckett tube was considered history in a recent round table discussion by Hypospadiologists [7]. But, the procedures are in practice even today. Unfortunately, a high incidence of late complications brought the flap procedures to disrepute. Though flaps have better blood supply, but the flap results were poorer than grafts, and two-stage procedures have replaced the flap procedures with Buccal Mucosal and Skin grafts. We prefer a single-stage procedure in severe hypospadias because of comparable results of one stage or two stages of urethroplasty. Some modifications in the flap procedures to reduce the complications have been suggested utilizing the concept of urethral plate preservation in hypospadias repair and providing a functional urethra up to the penoscrotal junction [1]. So we modified the flap repairs to improve the results.

14.2 Modified Flap repair (Surgical Technique) [1]

The steps of modified flap repair are:

1. Chordee correction
2. Raising inner prepucial flap and tubularization of skin flap
3. Tubularization of mobilized and preserved urethral plate
4. Bringing the skin tube ventrally
5. Inner prepucial skin tube is anastomosed to the tubularized urethral plate and covering it with spongiosum
6. Anastomosis of inner prepucial skin tube to glans tip
7. The inner prepucial skin tube is covered with dartos and fixed to corpora
8. Scrotoplasty and skin closure

14.2.1 Chordee Correction

An adrenaline solution of 1:100,000 is injected at the proposed incision site, and a circum-coronal circumferential incision is given. Penile skin degloving is done by dissecting at Buck's fascia. The urethral plate transaction is done at the corona, and the urethral plate with spongiosum is mobilized proximally up to the meatus dissecting at the tunica albuginea. The mobilized urethral plate and spongiosum are preserved for the proximal segment of the neo-urethra (Fig. 14.1a–d). Gittes test is done to confirm chordee correction. Midline and lateral dissection of Buck's fascia correct the ventral curvature if persist, and the same is ensured by penile erection test. Dorsal plication is done if persisted chordee is less than 30 degrees & superficial corporotomies/corporoplasty for more than 30 degree. Gittes test is repeated to ensure the complete correction rather than relying on the visual impression of chordee correction alone.

Step-by-step correction of chordee is done in the patients in whom a urethral plate preservation procedure is planned. Chordee correction is being attempted by the urethral plate with the spongiosum and urethra mobilization; the urethral plate is still attached to glans and chordee can still not be corrected because of short spongiosum segment due to tethering of the urethral plate (Fig. 14.2a–d). The urethral plate is transected at the corona to correct the curvature (Fig. 14.2e), and the plan is changed to flap urethroplasty. Gitte's Test is done to confirm the

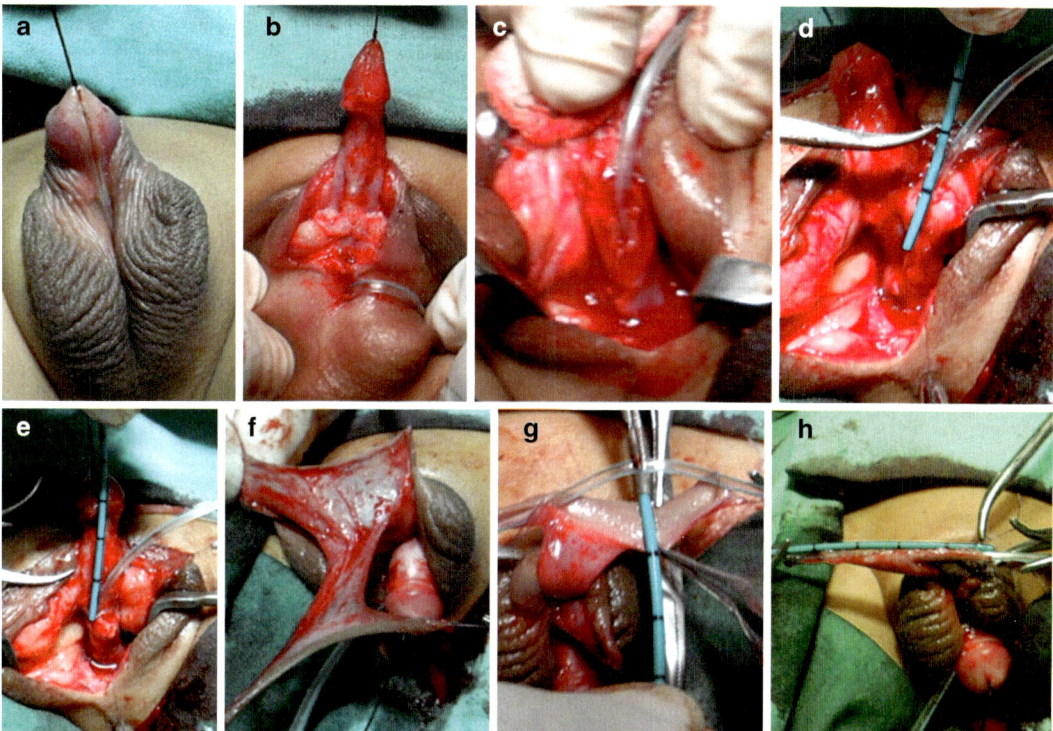

Fig. 14.1 Showing the correction of chordee, length of required neo-urethra, raising & measuring. (**a**) Scrotal hypospadias with bifid scrotum. (**b**) Penile skin degloving and urethral plate with spongiosum mobilization. (**c**) and (**d**) Measuring the length of mobilized and preserved urethral plate. (**e**) Measuring the required length of the flap. (**f**) Mobilization of the inner prepucioplasty flap. (**g**) Measuring the flap width. (**h**) Measuring the flap length

chordee correction (Fig. 14.2f), and residual curvature (if any) is again corrected by midline dissection of corporeal bodies, lateral dissection of Buck's fascia with or without superficial corporotomies/dorsal plication. Chordee correction is always confirmed at its completion by the Gittes test. Minimal electrocautery should be used to avoid postoperative fibrosis.

14.2.2 Mobilization of Inner Prepucial Flap and Tubularization

A dissection plane is created between the two layers of dartos fascia in the de-gloved penis & the pedicle is dissected up to the penis root to prevent the penile torsion (Fig. 14.1f). The required length is measured from the tip of the glans to the receded meatus after chordee correction. The flap is measured slightly longer than this length after stretching the skin (Figs. 14.1e, g, h and 14.2g, h), the width of the flap is measured according to the size of the urethra as per the age of the child, and measurement is done after stretching the flap to a distance of 1–2 cm to have the same width over the whole length (Figs. 14.2i, j and 14.3a–c). Measuring the width of the unstretched skin flap may result in a larger size of the flap (Fig. 14.4a–d), leading to diverticula formation. Figure 14.4 shows a 5–8 mm difference in width when measured on stretching. Skin is trimmed to have an adequate width of the flap to prevent urethral diverticula. The mobilized inner prepucial flap is tubularized with 6-0 or 7-0 PDS sutures over a 6-8 Fr urethral stent. The sutures are taken in a sub-cuticular inverting fashion, either interrupted or continuous. Sutures at both ends are always taken interrupted to allow trimming of the skin tube if required. Trimming the skin tube is done if the

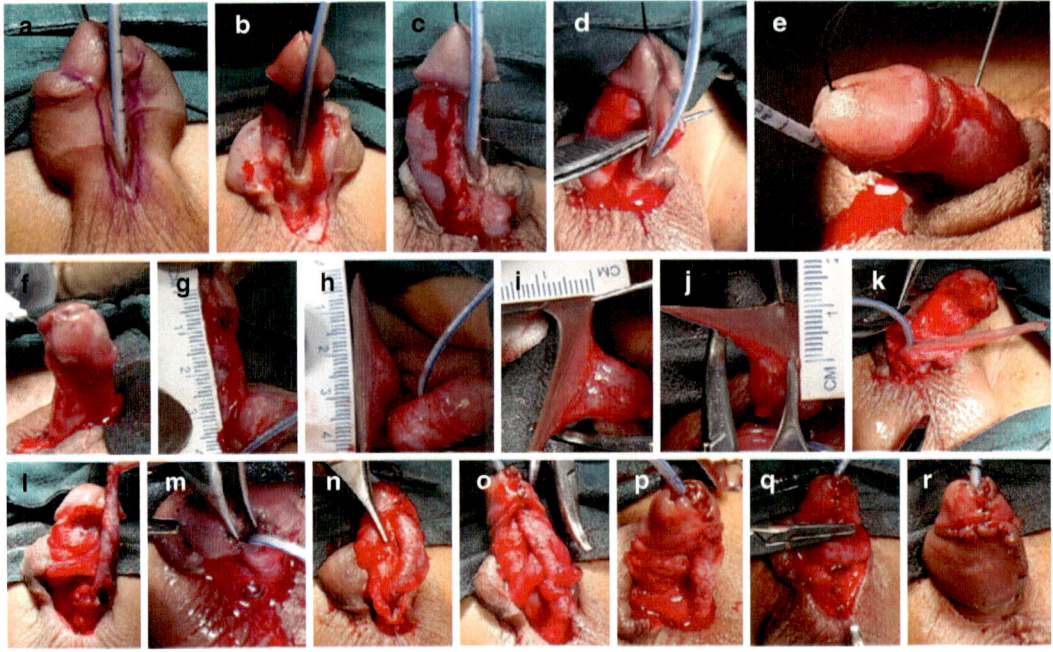

Fig. 14.2 Showing the steps of modified flap repair. (**a**) Penoscrotal hypospadias with moderate chordee. (**b**) Penile Skin degloving. (**c**) and (**d**) Urethral plate and spongiosum mobilization. (**e**) Gittes test showing persistence of chordee. (**f**) Gittes test showing chordee correction after urethral plate transection at corona. (**g**) Measuring the required length of the neourethra. (**h**) Measuring the flap for required neo-urethra length. (**i**) Measuring width at different places. (**k**) Anastomosis of the flap to the urethra. (**l**) Tubularization of the inner prepucial flap. (**m**) Distal anastomosis to the glans margins. (**n**) Glanuloplasty. (**o**) Spongioplasty over the anastomosis. (**p**) and (**q**) Dartos cover over the skin tube. (**r**) Final picture after skin closure

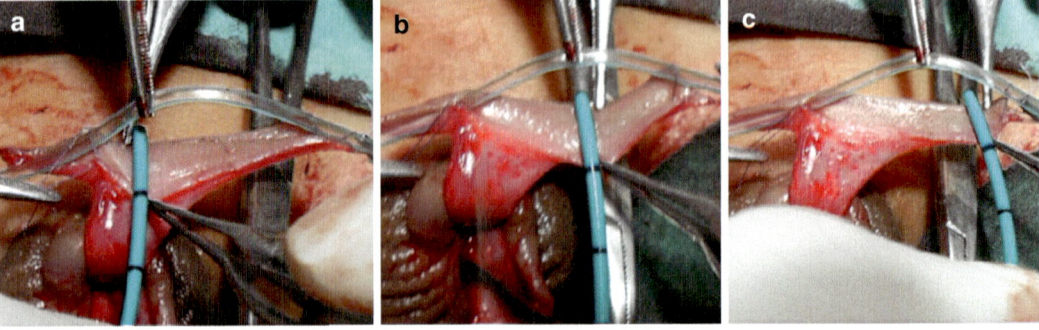

Fig. 14.3 Showing the measurement of the flap width at 2 cm distance. (**a**) Measuring flap width on left end of flap, (**b**) Measuring flap width on mid-part of flap, (**c**) Measuring flap width on right end of flap

terminal portions' vascular supply is questionable or the flap is excessive. Bucking of the neo-urethral tube is avoided if continuous sutures are used. The other skin flap tubularization technique is to complete the skin flap's anastomosis to the urethral plate and then tubularize it on the dorsal side (Fig. 14.2k, l).

14.2.3 Tubularization of Preserved Urethral Plate and Spongioplasty

The preserved urethral plate's length may vary 1–2 cm (Fig. 14.1d). The mobilized urethral plate is tubularized with continuous 6-0 or 7-0 PDS or

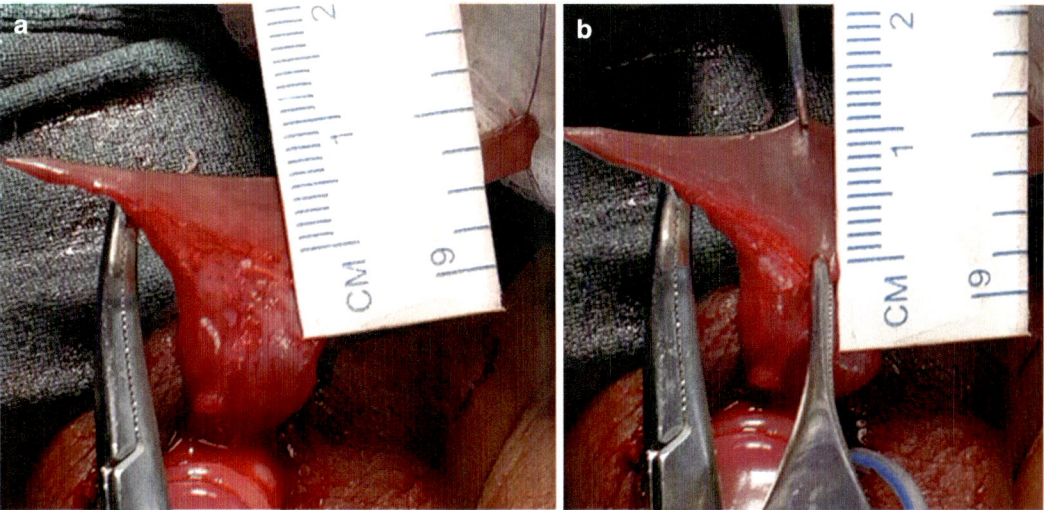

Fig. 14.4 Showing the difference in width un-stretched and stretched flap. (**a**) Un-stretched width center 7 mm. (**b**) 11 mm after stretching

5-0, 6-0 Vicryl/PDS suture to construct the proximal urethral segment with spongiosum as long as possible. Preferably the proximal neo-urethra segment with spongiosum should be reconstructed up to the penoscrotal junction. If needed, the proximal urethra can be mobilized up to the bulbar region to increase the proximal urethral length (Fig. 14.1c). Addition of this tubularized urethra with spongiosum reduces the required length of skin tube and reduces the complications. The addition of this tubularized urethral plate segment enhances the chances of a successful single-stage repair in cases where inner prepucial skin falls short. The longer the segment of tubularized urethral plate with spongioplasty, the fewer chances of late complications.

14.2.4 Bringing the Inner Prepucial Flap Ventrally

Traditionally, the skin flap is brought ventrally from one side of the shaft, which is likely to cause traction on the pedicle and torsion of the penis. We make a hole in the dartos flap sparing the vessels, and the skin tube is brought ventrally, keeping one-half of dartos on each side. Extra care is taken not to damage the pedicle vessels. This will prevent traction on the vascular pedicle, maintain the skin flap's vascular supply, and the shaft's symmetry (Fig. 14.5a, b).

14.2.5 The Anastomosis of the Tubularized Inner Prepucial Skin Flap & the Tubularized Urethral Plate Covering it with Spongiosum

The urethral plate's mucosa preserved is denuded to about 8–10 mm from the margin of the urethral plate. In cases with a very narrow and poorly developed urethral plate, the urethral mucosa is resected, preserving the spongiosum to cover the anastomosis and the skin tube. The anastomosis of the neo-urethras is done in an elliptical shape with 6-0 PDS or Vicryl interrupted inverting sutures, with the spongiosum spared to cover the anastomosis keeping the stent in situ (Fig. 14.1c). The anastomosis is covered with spongiosum to prevent fistula at the site of anastomosis (Fig. 14.1d). In case of tension on the suture line, the spongiosum is sutured to the dartos flap to cover the anastomosis with healthy tissue of the spongiosum and dartos. It is important to protect the anastomosis with healthy vascular tissue to ensure proper healing (Fig. 14.6a–c).

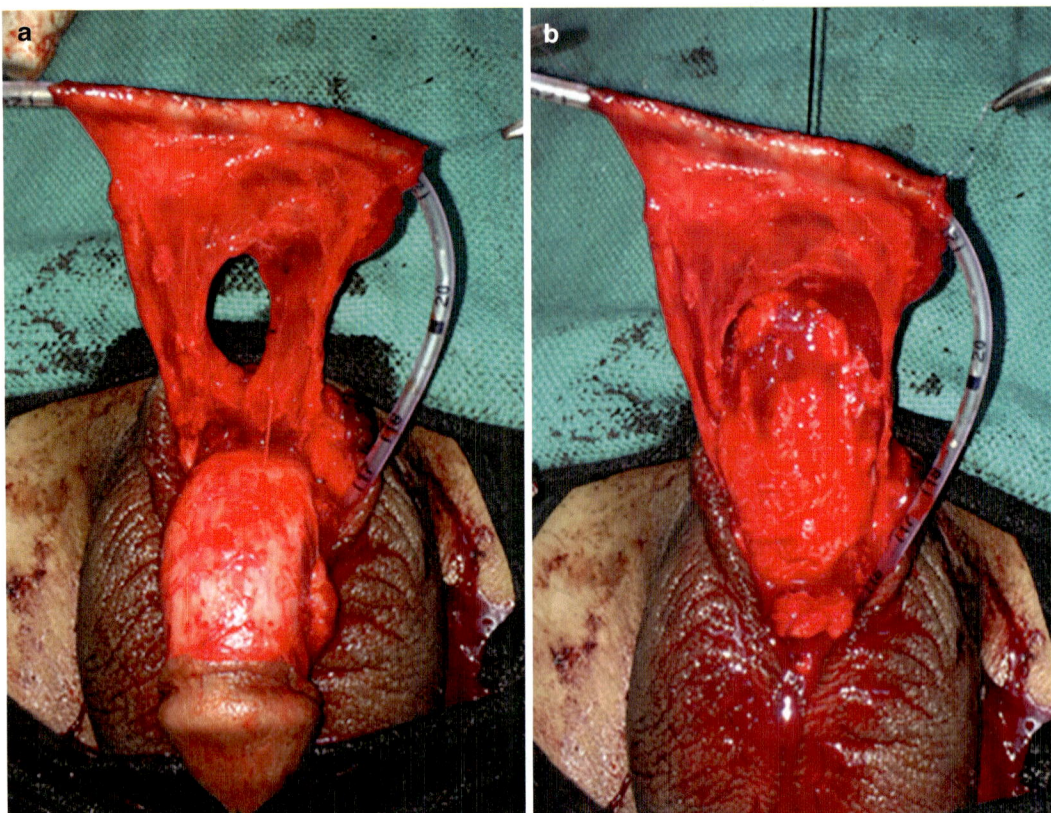

Fig. 14.5 (**a**) Showing Button holing in the pedicle of the flap. (**b**) Flap brought ventrally taking penis above though the hole

14.2.6 Distal Anastomosis

Glanular wings are dissected deep up to the tunica albuginea and laterally to raise wide glanular wings. These glanular flaps have intact mucosa inside. The anastomosis of the transverse island flap skin tube is done 5–8 mm proximal to the glans' tip with 6-0 PDS/Vicryl, (Fig. 14.7a) thus preventing the skin's protrusion on the glans. The glanular wings are sutured to reconstruct a wide natural-looking meatus to reduce the chances of meatal and sub-meatal stenosis (Fig. 14.1e and Fig. 14.7a–c). There should be adequate space between the skin tube and sutured glanular wing to avoid vascular compromise and postoperative edema.

14.2.7 Covering of Skin Tube with Dartos and its Fixation to Corpora

The suture line of the skin tubularization is kept dorsally opposing the corporal bodies, and few interrupted sutures are taken to fix it to the corpora. The skin tube is covered by suturing the dartos pedicle from both sides, sparing the vessels, and the skin tube is fixed to the corpora on both sides to decrease the laxity of the tube. Proximally, the dartos is sutured to the spongiosum. Thus, the whole length of the tubularized skin tube is covered either with the dartos or the spongiosum (Fig. 14.8a, b).

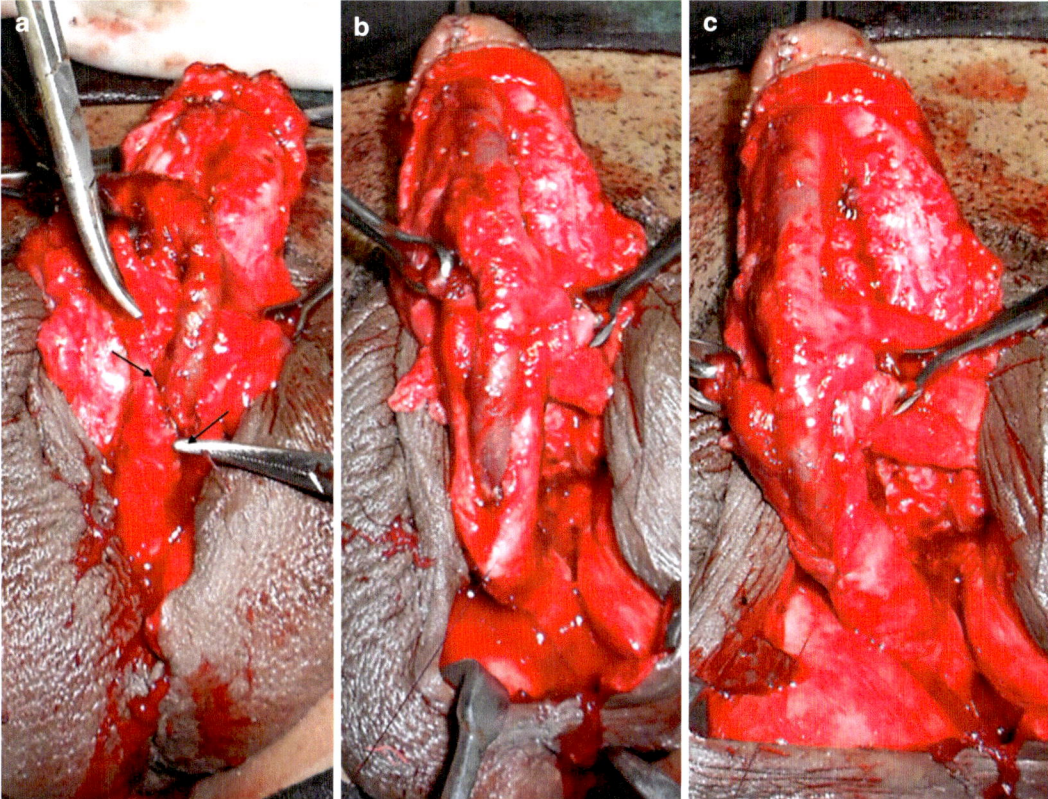

Fig. 14.6 Showing anastomosis of neourethra with urethra and covering it spongiosum. (**a**) Elliptical anastomosis of neo-urethra and urethra. (**b**) and (**c**) Covering the anastomosis with spongiosum (with permission Bhat et al. [1] @ copyright Elsevier)

14.2.8 Scrotoplasty and Skin Closure

Depending upon the severity of penoscrotal transposition, scrotoplasty is done. In mild penoscrotal transposition, scrotal skin is mobilized & the midline skin is excised. The scrotal sac is also mobilized then sutured in the midline over the neo-urethra in two layers, and then skin closure is done (Fig. 14.8c). In severe penoscrotal transposition, scrotal flaps and then scrotal sacs are mobilized on both sides and sutured in the midline in three layers after excising the midline skin. Thus, the proximal neo-urethral anastomosis is covered by the reconstructed scrotum, which prevents the fistula at the proximal anastomosis. Skin closure is done after putting in a drain tube and the stent; the drain tube is taken out in 2–3 days, and the urethral stent is removed after 10–14 days.

14.2.9 Postoperative Protocol

The patients are asked to follow up 1, 3, 6, and 12 months after the surgery and then yearly. They are evaluated for the urinary stream, uroflowmetry, and cosmetic function (Fig. 14.9) and complications are noted and rectified accordingly.

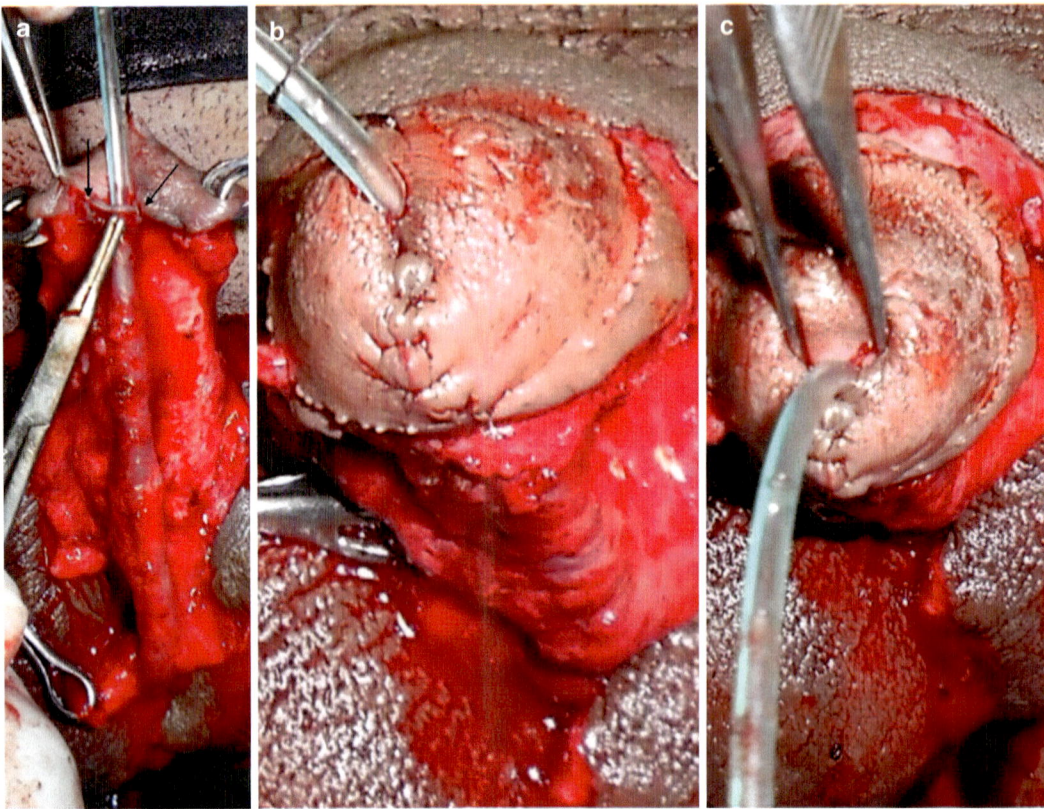

Fig. 14.7 Showing distal anastomosis of skin tube and glanular wings. (**a**) Anastomosis of skin tube with glanular wings. (**b**) and (**c**) Completed anastomosis and glanuloplasty with the large meatus (with permission Bhat et al. [1] @ copyright Elsevier)

The meatus is calibrated at 6 and 12 months. If uroflow is poor and meatus is found narrow, then these cases are identified as meatal stenosis. Meatoplasty is considered if meatal dilatation is required beyond 6 months. Urethrogram is done in suspected cases of the urethral stricture and diverticula and managed accordingly.

14.3 Prevention of Complications in Flap Repairs

Common complications that led the flap repair to disrepute are high fistula rate, diverticula, torsion, asymmetry of the shaft, and greater disfigurement than two-stage repairs. Results of two-stage repair are claimed to be better than the tubularized skin repair in one stage. Let us see the technical differences in the two-stage and the one-stage flap repair. The graft is stretched and fixed to the corpora in two-stage repair that facilitate keeping the exact width and length of the urethral plate in the second stage of the repair. Fixity of the graft helps in ensuring a good blood supply. While in flap tube repairs, wider flap tube than required, skin tube is not fixed, allowing the turbulence in the urine flow, leading to diverticula and fistula. Another technical point is to bring the skin tube pedicle from one side of the penile shaft responsible for torsion and asymmetry of the penile shaft. The dartos covers neourethra in two-stage repair, but in flap repair, it lies just below the skin lacking the dartos support that may be responsible for fistula and diverticula. There is no anastomosis in two stages but in one stage two anastomoses, skin tube with urethra and glans skin distally. A circular anastomosis may cause stricture and meatal stenosis and,

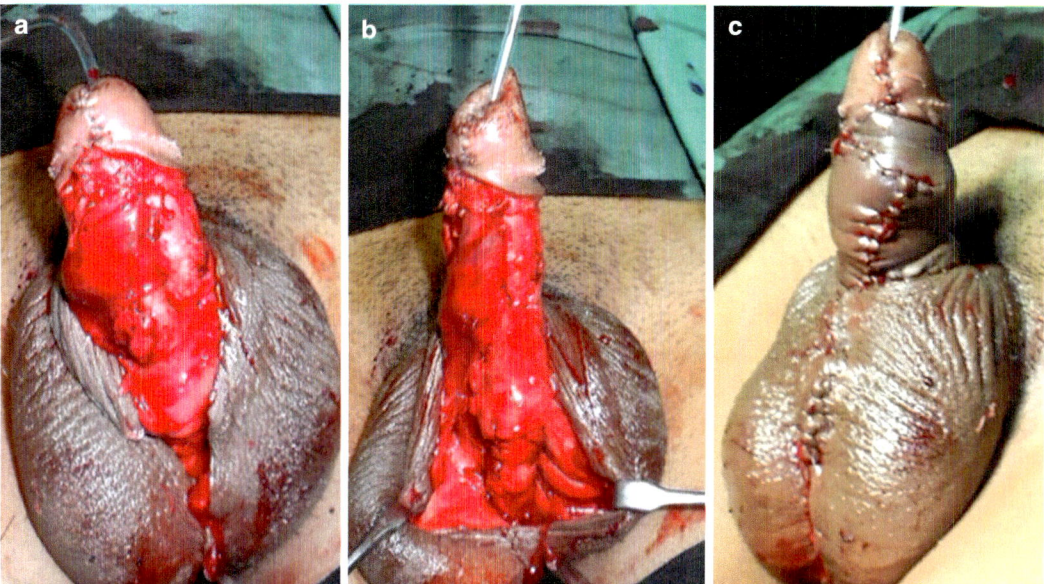

Fig. 14.8 Showing healthy tissue cover over the skin tube and Scrotoplasty. (**a**) and (**b**) Proximally spongiosum and distally with dartos over the neo-urethra. (**c**) Scrotoplasty and skin closure (with permission Bhat et al. [1] @ copyright Elsevier)

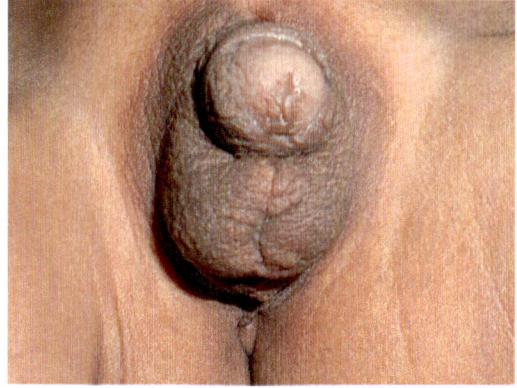

Fig. 14.9 Postoperative straight penis with the normal-looking meatus

poor healthy tissue cover over proximal anastomosis may lead to fistula. Modified flap repair eliminates all these pitfalls of flap repairs. The modifications are:

1. Rather than excising the urethral plate and spongiosum, we mobilize, preserve, and utilize it.
2. Measuring the length and width of flap after stretching the skin.
3. The vascular pedicle is brought ventrally by making a Buttonhole in the middle sparing the vessels.
4. Proximal segment of the urethra is reconstructed by the preserved urethral plate tubularization and spongioplasty, reducing the required length of the skin tube.
5. Skin tube is fixed to the ventral surface of the corpora.
6. Skin tube is covered in its whole length by the dartos pedicle.
7. Ugly skin outside the external urethral meatus can be prevented by anastomosis 5–8 mm proximal to the meatus to create a wide meatus.

14.3.1 Fistula

The fistula's commonest site in a single stage with inner prepucial flap urethroplasty is at anastomosis of the tubularized skin tube and urethra

[18, 19]. However, it may form anywhere along the whole length of the urethra. Predisposing risk factors for fistula formation are failure to invert all epithelial edges during anastomosis of the urethra and skin tube and the lack of healthy tissue support over the anastomosis [11]. The skin flap tube under the skin without the support of dartos is one of the causes of a higher fistula rate. With the modifications, the anastomosis is covered by the spongiosum, and the skin tube is covered with dartos which provides an additional protective layer and support to the reconstructed neo-urethra. Thus, the entire length of the neo-urethra is covered by a healthy interposing tissue layer, which helps preserve the neo-urethral blood supply and reduces fistula chances. Proximal anastomosis and urethra are covered by the overlying scrotal tissue, which again lowers fistula chances.

14.3.2 Penile Torsion

Penile torsion is one of the common complications of flap repairs. The vascular pedicle is brought down by one side of the shaft. The causes of torque are traction on the vascular pedicle and improper adjustment of skin flaps during skin closure. Inadequate mobilization of the vascular pedicle is the cause of the traction. The flap is mobilized up to the root of the penis to release the traction on the pedicle and brought ventrally by making a hole in the dartos pedicle, dividing the dartos into two halves to prevent torsion. Patel et al. (2005) brought the flap by creating a 'buttonhole' through the vascular pedicle at the penopubic junction minimizing the risk of penile torque [20]. Another vital step to avoid penile torsion is adjusting skin flaps during skin closure [21]. The dorsal dartos pedicle is slit in the midline to split into two equal parts. This maintains the aesthetic symmetry of the shaft and prevents torsion.

14.3.3 Diverticula

The possible factors for diverticula in flap repairs are

1. A larger width and/or length of the unstretched dartos-based flap
2. The laxity of the dartos-based flap
3. The lack of fixation of the flap to the corpora
4. The lack of support to the skin tube
5. Meatal stenosis due to a circular anastomosis at the meatus

The second stage of the two-stage urethroplasty is done with the well-stretched graft fixed to the corpora cavernosa allowing the adequate length to be measured. While in the transverse island flap, urethroplasty, the flap is dartos based, and the dartos contracts during surgery; so, unstretched measuring will give a larger width. The modification, measuring the width after stretching the flap at a distance of 1–1.5 cm in the whole length of the flap, ensures an adequate flap width. There is a significant difference in width (about 0.8–1 cm) when measuring the flap without stretching it (Fig. 14.3c, d). Another modification, the skin tube is covered with the dartos pedicle to ensure adequate support and is also fixed to the corpora. Fixing the skin tube to the corpora and covering it with a dartos vascular flap provides stability to the skin tube, a major pitfall in the Duckett/Asopa repair. Similar to our technique Patel et al. (2005) did the modification in transverse flap urethroplasty to fix the flap. The flap's medial margin is anchored longitudinally to corpora cavernosa just right or left to the midline. These subcuticular sutures do not pass through the epithelium of the flap—(Fig. 14.10). Then the flap is tubularized, trimming the excessive skin [20].

A normal-looking wide meatus is reconstructed by anastomosing the skin 5–8 mm proximal to the glans margin. Anastomosis of the skin

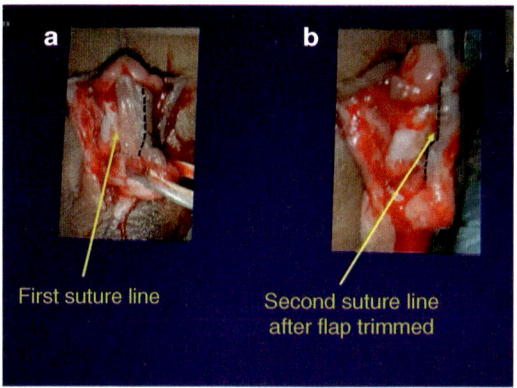

Fig. 14.10 Showing the flap fixation to the corpora. (**a**) Fixing the flap to create a urethral plate. (**b**) Urethral plate tubularization to construct the neourethra (by courtesy Prof D. Canning CHOP USA)

to mucosa provides better healing, resulting in good cosmetic results and the prevention of meatal stenosis, which also helps prevent diverticula.

14.3.4 Residual Curvature

Residual chordee is a known complication of flap procedures. To prevent residual curvature, complete curvature correction is confirmed before proceeding for urethroplasty. The neourethra's adequate required length is achieved after measuring both by tubularized inner prepucial flap and having a proper neo-urethra length. A good vascular flap provides adequate blood supply to the skin tube, avoiding the tube contracture and curvature. Minimal electrocautery is used on the ventral surface of corpora to prevent fibrosis. Many a time, infection leads to fibrosis which may be the cause of residual curvature. The excessive plications will shorten the penis, while excessive ventral dissection will leave a raw area vulnerable to later scarring. The recurrent curvature on many occasions develops years later. A clear message is that do not over excise or dissect extensively to prevent scarring and curvature.

14.3.5 Meatal Stenosis

Wide glanular flaps are raised by dissecting deep up to the tip of the corpora. The circular anastomosis of the skin tube too far distally on the glans may lead to skin protruding outside the meatus and increase meatal stenosis risk. The prepucioplasty tube is sutured 5–8 mm proximal to the glans' tip, creating a wide slit-like meatus with no skin protrusion outside, provides better cosmetic results, and decreases the risk of meatal stenosis. Meatal stenosis is a significant risk factor in fistula and diverticula formation [16], prevention reduces fistula and diverticula chances.

14.3.6 Post Void Dribble and Ejaculate

Long and unsupported neourethra by spongiosum cannot propel semen and the last drops of urine. This sequalae is seen in one-stage flap as well as in two-stage repairs. Bracka reported high long-term complications, 40% urine dribble, 33% dribble of ejaculate, and 45% retained ejaculate [8]. These can be minimized with modifications, as the proximal neo-urethra is covered with spongiosum up to the penoscrotal junction by tubularization of the preserved urethral plate. The proximal extended urethral mobilization can be done to bring the urethra up to the penoscrotal junction to increase the length of the urethra (about 2–3.5 cm) [22]. The dartos pedicle also supports the distal urethra. Thus, it creates a comparatively functional proximal segment instead of a lax skin tube that does not propel semen and leads to ejaculate problems.

14.4 Discussion

Transverse prepucioplasty island flap and double island flap are vascular pedicles based on sound surgical principles. Yet, they did not yield the long-term expected results, likely because of the wrong case selection or some technical inadequacy. Some modifications were published to improve the results. Prof. Canning group reported an important modification of fixing the skin tube to corporal bodies, and they brought the flap ventrally by making a hole in dartos pedicle. They fixed the flap lateral to the midline and the spatulated urethra and fixed flap to the ventral surface of corpora and then tubularized, thus fixing the tube, and overcoming the flap's flaw of mobility & torsion of the penis [20]. We used the principle of fixing the skin tube differently, taking a few sutures through the dartos pedicle sparing the vessels. Glassberg modified the Duckett technique by augmenting a midline tubularized skin tube to a tubularized inner prepucial tube. They corrected the chordee by resecting the spongiosum. The complication rates of Glassberg's procedure have been reported to vary from 26% to 42% [4–6]. The hair can grow at adulthood in the hair-bearing area included with the margins of non-hair-bearing midline skin. The proximal skin tube without supporting tissue will increase the risk of diverticula as well as fistula formation. Our modification preserving and utilizing the urethral plate and spongiosum to create a spongiosum supported urethra up to the penoscrotal junction will have fewer complications like fistula and diverticula. We also do an elliptical anastomosis of skin tube proximal 1 cm urethral plate margin and cover it with spongiosum. The overall complication rate of the inner prepucial tube used for single-stage repair of proximal hypospadias was reported to vary from 17% to 42%, with an average of around 32% [5, 12, 13]. We had an acceptable complication rate (19%) with the modified inner prepucioplasty flap repair. These modifications are likely the bring back lost shine to the flap urethroplasties.

14.5 Conclusions

Flaps have a better blood supply than grafts; still, flap repairs have poorer results than graft repairs. However the technique still has an important place in the management of hypospadias repair. The results can be improved by critical analysis of the flaws and rectifying them by modifications. Mobilized and preserved urethral plate is tubularized to bring the urethra up to the penoscrotal junction. This functional urethra helps in the prevention of postvoid dribble and retained ejaculate. Mobilizing the vascular pedicle up to the root of the penis and bringing it ventrally by splitting it midline prevents the torsion and constructs an aesthetically symmetric penile shaft. Covering the elliptical anastomosis with spongiosum helps in reducing fistula and stricture. Measuring the stretched skin flap adequate width and length; covering the neo-urethra with dartos pedicle, and fixing it to corpora help prevent diverticula. The distal anastomosis of the skin tube is done 5–8 mm proximal to the glans margin to create a wide slit-like normal-appearing meatus and prevent meatal stenosis. The modified flap urethroplasty for treating severe hypospadias is feasible with an acceptable complication rate and can avail the advantages of one stage repair; cost-effectiveness, less mental trauma to patients and parents, and saving the patient's time.

References

1. Bhat A, Bhat M, Sabharwal K, Kumar R. Bhat's modifications of Glassberg–Duckett repair to reduce complications in management severe hypospadias with curvature. Afr J Urol. 2017;23(2):94–9.
2. Upadhyay J, Shekarriz B, Khoury AE. Midshaft hypospadias. Urol Clin. 2002;29(2):299–310.
3. Manzoni G, Bracka A, Palminteri E, Marrocco G. Hypospadias surgery: when and by whom? BJU Int. 2004;94(8):1188–95.
4. Glassberg KI. Augmented Duckett repair for severe hypospadias. J Urol. 1987;138(2):380–1.

5. MacGillivray D, Shankar K, Rickwood A. Management of severe hypospadias using Glassberg's modification of the Duckett repair. BJU Int. 2002;89(1):101–2.
6. Tiryaki T. Combination of tubularized island flap and ventral skin flap techniques in the single-stage correction of severe proximal hypospadias. Urol Int. 2010;84(3):269–74.
7. Snodgrass W, Macedo A, Hoebeke P, Mouriquand PDE. Hypospadias dilemmas: a round table. J Pediatr Urol. 2011;7(2):145–57. https://doi.org/10.1016/j.jpurol.2010.11.009.
8. Bracka A. A long-term view of hypospadias. Br J Plast Surg. 1989;42(3):251–5. https://doi.org/10.1016/0007-1226(89)90140-9.
9. Bracka A. The role of two-stage repair in modern hypospadiology. Indian J Urol IJU: J Urol Soc India. 2008;24(2):210.
10. Kajbafzadeh A-M, Arshadi H, Payabvash S, Salmasi AH, Najjaran-Tousi V, Sahebpor ARA. Proximal hypospadias with severe chordee: single-stage repair using corporeal tunica vaginalis free graft. J Urol. 2007;178(3):1036–42.
11. Moursy EE. Outcome of proximal hypospadias repair using three different techniques. J Pediatr Urol. 2010;6(1):45–53.
12. Ghali A. Hypospadias repair by skin flaps: a comparison of onlay preputial island flaps with either Mathieu's metal-based or Duckett's tubularized preputial flaps. BJU Int. 1999;83:1032–8.
13. Shukla AR, Patel RP, Canning DA. THE 2-STAGE HYPOSPADIAS REPAIR. IS IT A MISNOMER? J Urol. 2004;172(4, Suppl):1714–6. https://doi.org/10.1097/01.ju.0000138926.26530.f9.
14. Fossum M, Svensson J, Kratz G, Nordenskjöld A. Autologous in vitro cultured urothelium in hypospadias repair☆. J Pediatr Urol. 2007;3(1):10–8.
15. Asopa H. One-stage correction of penile hypospadias using a foreskin tube, a preliminary report. Int Surg. 1971;55:435–40.
16. Duckett J. Transverse preputial island flap technique for repair of severe hypospadias. 1980.
17. Asopa R, Asopa H. One-stage repair of hypospadias using double island preputial skin tube. Indian J Urol. 1984;1(1)
18. Kwon T, Song GH, Song K, Song C, Kim KS. Management of urethral fistulas and strictures after hypospadias repair. Korean J Urol. 2009;50(1):46–50.
19. Retik AB, Atala A. Complications of hypospadias repair. Urol Clin North Am. 2002;29(2):329–39. https://doi.org/10.1016/s0094-0143(02)00026-5.
20. Patel RP, Shukla AR, Christopher A, Canning DA. Modified tubularized transverse preputial island flap repair for severe proximal hypospadias. Br J Urol. 2005;95:901–4.
21. Bhat A, Mandal AK. Acute postoperative complications of hypospadias repair. Indian J Urol IJU: J Urol Soc India. 2008;24(2):241.
22. Bhat A. Extended urethral mobilization in incised plate urethroplasty for severe hypospadias: a variation in technique to improve chordee correction. J Urol. 2007;178(3):1031–5.

Management of Chordee Without Hypospadias

Amilal Bhat

15.1 Introduction

The literal interpretation word "chordee" is curvature, and the chordee without hypospadias (CWH) is applied "when the urethral meatus is at the glans penis tip, a ventral penile curvature coexists, and the prepuce is well-formed" [1]. Congenitally, the abnormalities are of the skin, fascial coverings of the penis, corpus spongiosum, or combined. Synonyms for the chordee without hypospadias are the congenital short urethra, congenital penile curvature, Hypospadism without hypospadias, and corporeal disproportion [1, 2]. The most commonly used among these terms is congenital penile curvature. But Devine and Horton preferred the term chordee without hypospadias as the most suitable and accurate for the anomaly description [3]. The earliest depiction of penile curvature dates back to Galen (130–199 AD) [4]. Siever first reported the entity in 1962 and described the cause of penile curvature because of "the skin tethering implicating subcutaneous tissue" [5], since then, various classifications have been advocated for it. This is a comparatively rare condition, and its incidence varies from 4% to 10% of cases of hypospadias. "Chordee without hypospadias" has recently been grouped in two, and the term used for it helps to clarify these groups. The first group is "hypospadias variants" (type I, II, or III), and in the second group, the urethra is normal but has a chordee, and the term is used "congenital ventral penile curvature." They present late in adolescence and adulthood with penile curvature during erection."

A. Bhat (✉)
Bhat's Hypospadias and Reconstructive Urology Hospital and Research Centre,
Jaipur, Rajasthan, India

Department of Urology, Jaipur National University Institute for Medical Sciences and Research Centre,
Jaipur, Rajasthan, India

Department of Urology, Dr. S.N. Medical College,
Jodhpur, Rajasthan, India

Department of Urology, S.P. Medical College,
Bikaner, Rajasthan, India

P.G. Committee Medical Council of India,
New Delhi, India

Academic and Research Council of RUHS,
Jaipur, Rajasthan, India

15.2 Embryology

Embryologically, the condition is missed hypospadias, where the curvature persists without displacement of the urethral meatus. The exact etiology of congenital curvature is not well described to date. However, various anatomical changes related to chordee with and without hypospadias are well accepted. Penile development starts at 9 weeks of gestational age. The genital tubercle undergoes enlargement to form the penis. The glans become distinguishable by the appearance of coronary sulcus with the growth of the phallus. The prepuce is created by reduplication of the ectoderm covering the distal part of the phallus. The formation of the urethra starts as an epithelial groove in the middle of the ventral surface of the developing penis. As the genital tubercle enlarges, two sets of tissue folds develop on its ventral surface, on either side of a developing trough, the urethral groove having two folds. The fusion of the more medial endodermal urethral folds in the ventral midline forms the male urethra. The lateral ectodermal urethral folds merge over the developing urethra and form the penile shaft skin & the prepuce. The fusion of the urethral tube and formation of the urethra eventually reaches the tip of the glans penis during normal development. Proliferating mesenchyme surrounds the urethral tube, separates it from the skin, and differentiates to form the corpus spongiosum, Buck fascia, and Dartos fascia. These two layers fuse from posterior to anterior, and they leave behind a skin line forming the median raphe. In chordee without hypospadias, there is a fusion of both endodermal and ectodermal urethral folds. There is some problem with the proliferation of mesenchymal tissue between the endodermal and ectodermal folds leading to major hypoplasia of tissues forming the ventral surface. The molecular mechanisms that regulates this mesenchymal differentiation likely depending on epithelial-mesenchymal interaction. The development of the mesenchymal tissue in the penis may be deficient or abnormal and result in dysgenetic and in-elastic fascial layers. As fusion is posterior to anterior, any anomaly with fusion may lead to disproportional development of dorsal and ventral surfaces, which may be responsible for chordee without hypospadias.

A recent theory in the development shows that ventral chordee is a normal stage of embryogenesis, & the arrest in penile development represents the chordee without hypospadias. Human demonstrated in their fetal studies a ventral curvature is a normal state of penile development at the 16th week of gestation and resolves during the 20–25th week [6]. Currently, three main theories of penile curvature are (1) Abnormal development of urethral plate; (2) Abnormal fibrotic mesenchymal tissue at the urethral meatus; (3) Differential growth of dorsal and ventral corporal tissue. The genital tubercle becomes cylindrical and is now called the phallus. The spongiosum division is the key criteria to define the severity of this congenital penile anomaly. The urethral defect in this anomaly is missing. The causes of ventral chordee, i.e., tethering the hypoplastic glans to the underlying hypoplastic urethra, tethering the hypoplastic urethra onto the underlying corpora cavernosa & a split corpus spongiosum. The cause of the curvature may reside in the skin, facial covering, short spongiosum segment or short corpora or because of a combination of the factors.

15.2.1 Incidence

The incidence of hypospadias in the general population is approximately 1 in 300 [7], and one-fourth of them will have chordee. The true incidence of chordee without hypospadias varies from 4% to 10% [8]. We found an incidence of 7.69% and among these type I 32%, type II 44% and 24 % had type III cases [1] while Tang et al. reported type I 35.4%, type II 27.8%, type III 12.7%, and type IV 24.1% in a study of 79 children [9]. Donnahoo et al. reported etiology in 87 patients of isolated chordee and found the skin tethering (32%), fibrotic fascia (33%), dorsoventral corporal disproportion (28%), and a congenitally short urethra (7%) [10].

15.2.2 Associated Anomaly

Common anomalies associated with hypospadias are undescended testis, inguinal hernia, webbed penis, penoscrotal transposition, hydrocele and penile torsion. Rarely the upper tract anomalies and urethral diverticula are found.

15.3 Classification

Chordee without hypospadias is classified according to etiological factors and the degree of curvature.

15.3.1 Congenital

Devine and Horton, and Kramer [3, 11] (Fig. 15.1) classified into:

1. Type I: Corpus spongiosum, Buck's and Dartos fascia distal to the division of spongiosum are Deficient
2. Type II: The Bucks and Dartos fascia are deficient, and the urethra is surrounded by normal corpus spongiosum.
3. Type III: Deficient Dartos fascia, and the corpus spongiosum and Buck's fascia are normal
4. Type IV: Discrepancy in development of the dorsal and ventral aspects of corpora cavernosa
5. Type V: Congenital short urethra

The mentioned classification was widely adopted until 1998, But Donnahoo et al. [10] grouped the 87 patients with penile curvature without hypospadias according to the structural defect and surgical steps. The step-wise treatment algorithm defines the cause of isolated chordee in chordee without hypospadias and thus minimizes the need for urethral replacement.

15.3.2 Modified Donnahoo Classification

Group 1 (Type II & III) When chordee is corrected by simple penile skin degloving, the patient is considered to have "skin chordee." The cause is abnormal dartos fascia tethering of the skin and Buck's fascia. This corresponds to type II and Type III of the Devine Horton classification.

Group 2 (Type I) When penile curvature persists, any dysgenetic chordee tissue is excised, and the whole urethra is mobilized if necessary. Patients in whom chordee is corrected at this step are considered to have fibrotic Bucks and dartos fasciae as the etiology of chordee. This is the same as that of Type I, according to the Devine and Horton classification.

Group 3 (Type IV) Patients with residual chordee after the steps mentioned above and no evidence of urethral tethering are treated with a procedure to correct corporeal disproportion with either dorsal placation or ventral corporotomy with grafting.

Group 4 (Type V) Patients having a truly tethered urethra after complete urethral mobilization; they need urethral division and a tubularized preputial interposition graft, which is called a congenital short urethra.

Group 5 (Type V) Urethra is normally developed but short and is called the congenital short urethra. Surgical correction requires division of the urethra to correct the chordee and reconstruct the urethra.

Group 6 (Type I, IV, V) When multiple factors like hypoplastic urethra and coverings of penile shaft with or without dorso-ventral corporal disproportion coexist and requires division/resection of the hypoplastic urethra. Resection of chordee tissue with ventral corporoplasty or dorsal plication.

15.3.3 Acquired

The original word chordee originated from ventral bending of the penis because of urethral stricture following gonococcal urethritis. The causes of secondary chordee are fibrosis after trauma, stricture, and degenerative causes like Peyronie's disease.

Degree Chordee is classified as:

1. Mild up to 30 degrees
2. Moderate 30–60 degrees
3. Severe more than 60 degrees

15.4 Assessment of Curvature

External genitalia of the child is examined during the erection of the penis, and adults should be asked to have a photograph during erections.

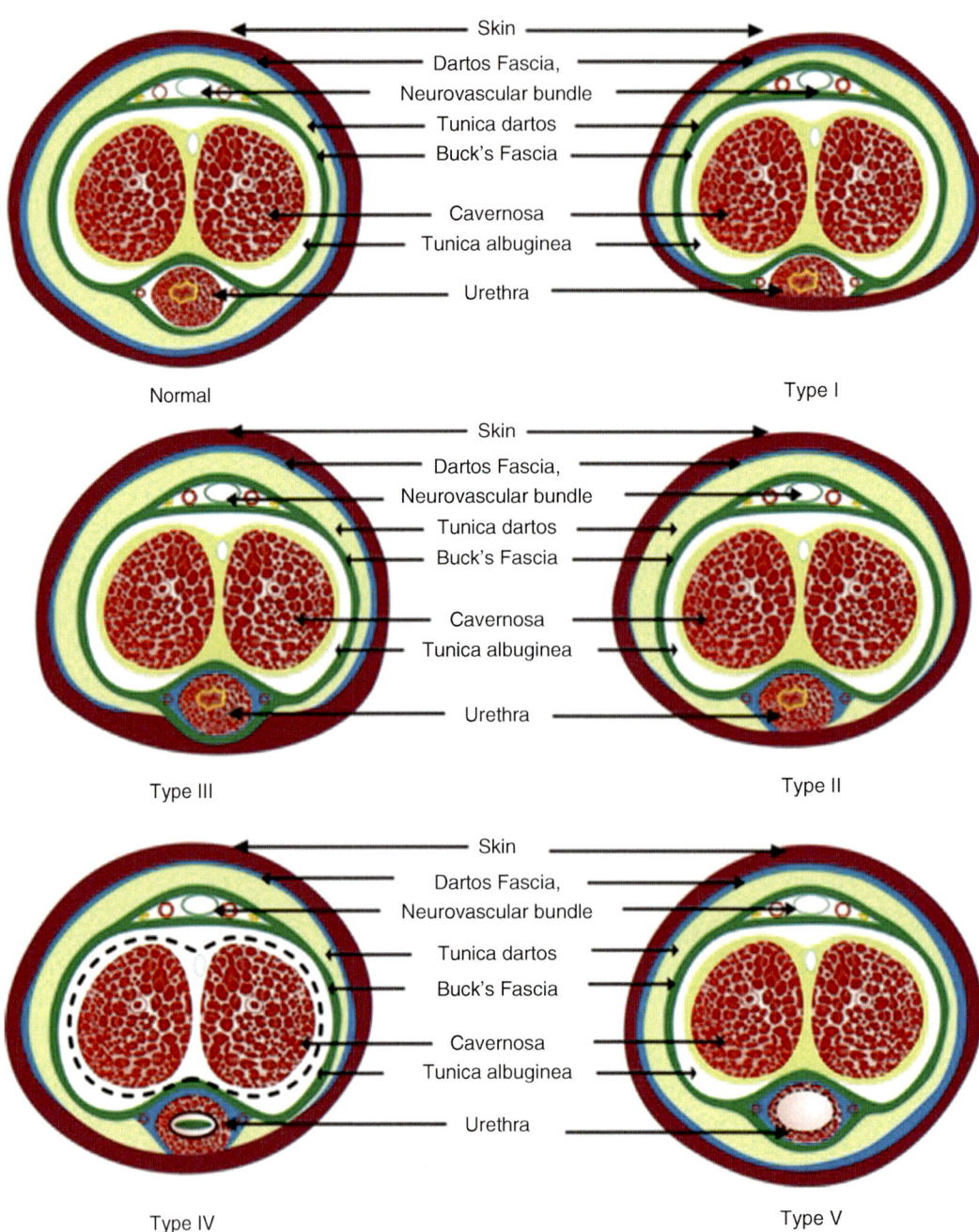

Fig. 15.1 Classification of chordee without hypospadias

The degree of curvature is assessed and recorded. During surgery, the erection test is performed either by artificial erection or pharmacological erection. Maclaghlin and Gittes first described the artificial erection test in 1974 and is now universally accepted for artificial erection during surgery [12]. The test is performed by injection saline into corpora by piercing the needle into one of the corporal bodies or through glans (Fig. 15.2).

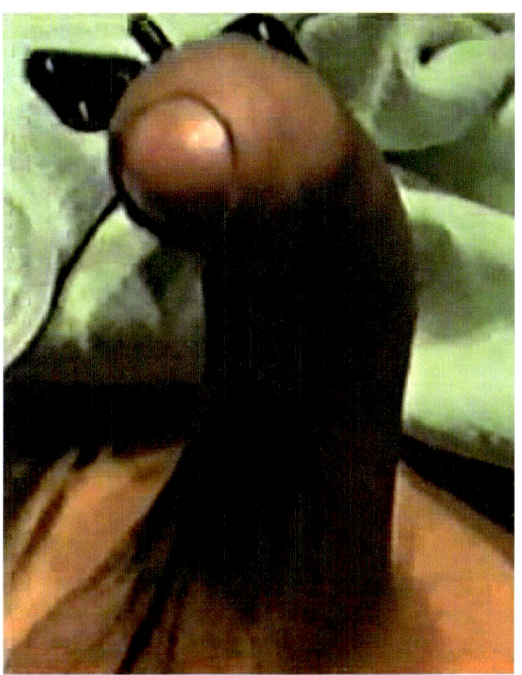

Fig. 15.2 Showing the Gittes test with moderate chordee

Injection through glans avoids hematoma in the penile shaft. The test is done at the beginning of surgery and the final correction of curvature. Pharmacological erection is done by injecting the arterial vasodilator prostaglandin E1 intracavernously during hypospadias surgery. The erection is more physiological, allows an accurate and continued assessment of chordee before, during, and after chordee correction.

15.5 Clinical Presentation

Healthy young men of chordee without hypospadias usually present between the ages of 18 and 30 years. Many of these patients have had noticed chordee before puberty but have presumed it to be normal. However, in adolescence, when they become sexually aware and active, discover that the curvature impedes their efforts, they observe an abnormal curvature. Patients with true congenital curvature usually have a long phallus, and curvature correction is recommended in the case of functional impairment. The parents bring children with severe curvature to the hospital. Examination of these patients is very important, and erection may be created in children by gently stimulating the penis. The parents may be asked for pictures during erection at the next visit. Careful examination of prepuce dorsally and bifurcation/deviation of median raphe may give a hint about the severity of chordee without hypospadias (Fig. 15.3a–f). Retraction of the prepuce provides a clue about the shortening of the skin and covering of the penile shaft.

15.6 Controversy

There is no Conesus and agreement on both the etiology or surgical management of this congenital. Young opined this anomaly due to congenital short urethra and advised to be managed by transection of the hypoplastic urethra and replacement urethroplasty [13]. In contrast to it, Devine and Horton in 1973 thought it to be due to abnormal development of fascial layers of the penis. The majority of these could be treated with resection of fibrous tissue for chordee correction; the transaction of the urethra is rarely required [3]. Nesbit expressed a dilemma in these cases " whether to lengthen the short ventral surface or shorten the longer dorsal one," and he opted for the shortening one and described the excisional plicating procedures [14]. Hurwitz et al. [15] thought that the paper-thin urethra of type I with an abnormal meatus requires excision of the entire dysplastic urethra, and replacement urethroplasty. If the meatus is normal, clinical judgments dictate the type of urethra that may be preserved or reconstructed [9]. In the lack of uniformity on management guidelines of chordee management, controversy continues whether to shorten the dorsal surface or lengthen the ventral surface and transect/resect or preserve the hypoplastic urethra. The management dispute is almost resolved in the management of chordee without hypospadias by the step-by-step management approach.

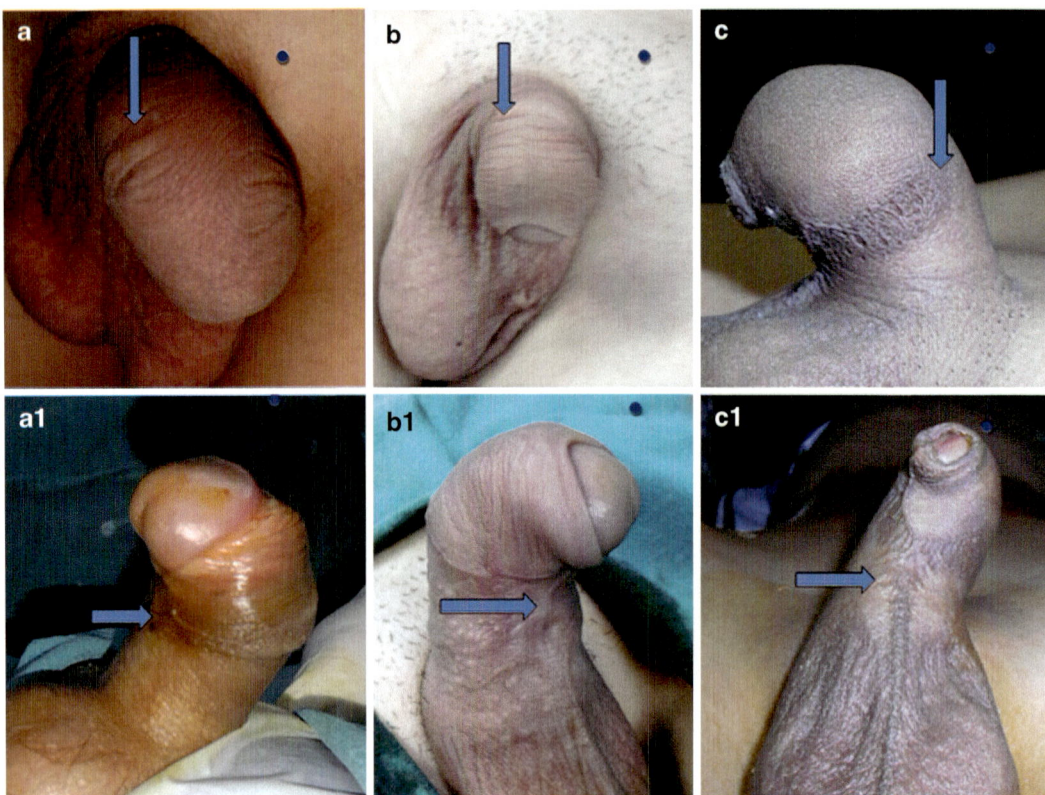

Fig. 15.3 Showing the site of embryological event. (**a, b, c**) Dorsal surface showing Bull's eye, (**a1, b1, c1**) Ventral surface showing bifurcation of the median raphe

15.7 Management

15.7.1 Goals

Surgical management of the anomaly aims to provide a straight penis without migration of urethral meatus proximally. The cause of the underlying defect is ascertained accurately. Accordingly, an appropriate and specific surgical procedure is planned to achieve the goal. Since the main aim in chordee without hypospadias repair is to correct the curvature, the causes of curvature are to be identified in the individual case. Various causes of penile curvature are skin tethering, short-covering of the penile shaft, hypoplastic spread out corpus spongiosum, bowstring effect of the hypoplastic urethra, and corporal disproportion. The step-by-step approach by Bhat et al. resolves the question: whether to go for dorsal shortening or ventral lengthening and preserve the hypoplastic urethra or resecting it [1].

15.7.2 Indications and Age of Surgery

More than 20 degrees curvature is considered significant by most pediatric urologists and is an indication of surgery. A dorsal approach of dorsal plication is preferred in cases of less than 30-degree curvature, while the ventral approach of penile lengthening manages cases of chordee more than 30-degrees. The penile development process begins in fetal life and continues until the end of puberty. Cendron and Melin proposed the surgery is to be done after puberty [16]. They believed that the curvature would improve spontaneously with age, and early surgery might disturb the growth of the penis by altering the tunica of corpora cavernosa. But others advocate that if diagnosed in childhood, correction should be at the time of the first diagnosis. In Type III chordee without hypospadias with mild to moderate chordee, it is logical to wait but type II and type I should be operated in the same age group as hypospadias or whenever the child presents to the hospital [1].

15.7.3 Methods of Chordee Correction

The methods for chordee correction are:

1. Penile degloving
2. Dorsal Shortening Procedure
   (a) Nesbit' technique
   (b) Tunica Albuginea Plication (TAP)
   (c) Dorsal Midline tunica Plication
   (d) Multiple Parallel Suture tunica Plication (MPP)
   (e) Essed Schroeder Technique
3. Ventral Lengthening Procedures
   (a) Corporeal Rotation
   (b) Division of Hypoplastic Urethra
   (c) Extended Urethral mobilization
   (d) Perovic partial Penile Disassembly
   (e) Ventral Grafts
      Tunica Vaginalis Free Graft
      Dermal Graft
      Small intestine mucosal graft

But most commonly used methods are penile degloving, dorsal tunica plication, transection and resection of the hypoplastic urethra and replacement urethroplasty. The application of the mentioned procedures is not according to the etiological factors. However, the step-by-step approach deals with the etiological factors, so it is a preferred approach in managing this entity. The Steps of the approach are:

1. Penile de-gloving
2. Hypoplastic urethra with spongiosum mobilization up to the corona
3. Hypoplastic urethra with spongiosum mobilization into the glans
4. Proximal urethral mobilization
5. Midline dissection of corporal bodies
6. Lateral mobilization of Buck's fascia
7. Superficial ventral corporotomy(ies)
8. Corporal rotation/Dorsal plication
9. Transection and or Resection of Hypoplastic urethra
10. Penile disassembly/Corporoplasty.

15.8 Surgical Technique: Hypoplastic Urethra and Spongiosum and Proximal Urethral Mobilization [1]

1 in 100,000 solution of adrenaline is injected into the proposed site of the incision and stay suture. An infant feeding tube is passed, and a stay suture is taken in the glans. Assessment of chordee is done with the Gittes test (Fig. 15.4a, b). A circumferential circumcoronal incision is given, and penile skin degloving (at the level of Buck's fascia) is done up to the root of the penis. Then the Gitte's test is repeated to see the degree of correction achieved (Fig. 15.4c, d). Then, a plane of dissection is created just proximal to the hypoplastic urethra. The spongiosum is mobilized up to the corona (Fig. 15.4e), and the Gittes test confirms chordee correction (Fig. 15.4f). If chordee persists, the urethra is mobilized into the glans, and the penile erection test reassesses the chordee to confirm chordee correction (Fig. 15.4g, h). The urethra is further mobilized proximally up to the bulbar urethra in case of the persistence of chordee, and correction is assessed by Gittes test. A single stitch dorsal plication is

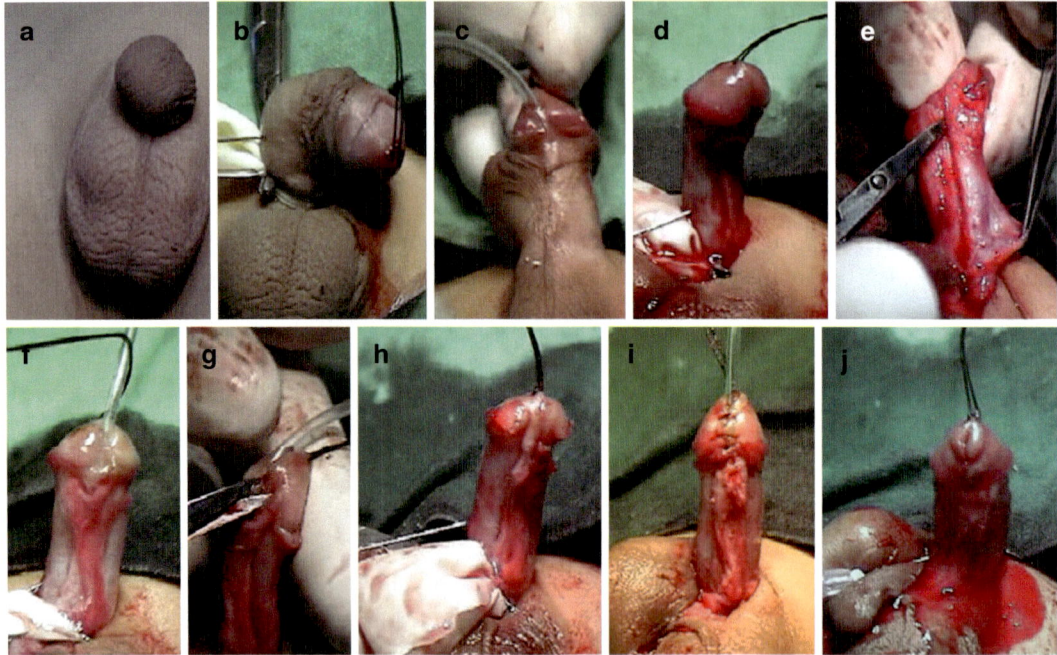

Fig. 15.4 Steps of chordee correction for type I without hypospadias with torsion. (**a**) Type III chordee without hypospadias with torsion. (**b**) Severe chordee on Gittes test without hypospadias. (**c**) Skin adherent to the hypoplastic urethra. (**d**) Moderate chordee on Gittes test after penile degloving. (**e**) Mobilization of urethra and corpus spongiosum. (**f**) Minimal glanular chordee after mobilization of the urethra with corpus spongiosum on Gittes test. (**g**) Mobilization of the urethra into glans. (**h**) Complete correction of chordee after mobilization of the urethra into glans. (**i**) Glanuloplasty and spongioplasty. (**j**) Complete correction of chordee on Gittes test after glanuloplasty and spongioplasty (with permission Bhat et al. [1] @ copyright Elsevier)

done if the chordee is less than 30 degrees and the ventral transverse superficial corporotomies/corporoplasty, when it is more than 30 degrees. With the complete correction of chordee, the meatus recedes down, so glanular wings are raised, the urethral plate is tubularized, and spongioplasty is done by suturing the mobilized corpus spongiosum over the hypoplastic urethra, starting from the normal urethra to the tip of glans. The Y-shaped corpus spongiosum is sutured in midline I shape, reconstructing a near-normal urethra. Glanuloplasty is done by approximating the glanular flaps with interrupted sutures. That brings the meatus to the tip, and the final Gittes test confirms chordee correction (Fig. 15.4i, j). Then skin closure is done by utilizing the prepucial skin to cover the deficit of the short ventral skin. The prepucioplasty is performed whenever feasible, and the pressure dressing is done. The per-urethral stent is put in and kept for 3–5 days.

The extent of the proximal urethral mobilization depends on the degree of curvature and the type of chordee without hypospadias. Mild to moderate chordee in type III chordee without hypospadias, can be corrected by penile degloving at the level of tunica albuginea up to the penoscrotal junction and mobilization of hypoplastic urethra only (Figs. 15.5a–h and 15.6a–f). Similarly, type II chordee without hypospadias with moderate curvature mobilization of urethral up to penoscrotal junction proximally and up to mid-glans distally may correct the curvature

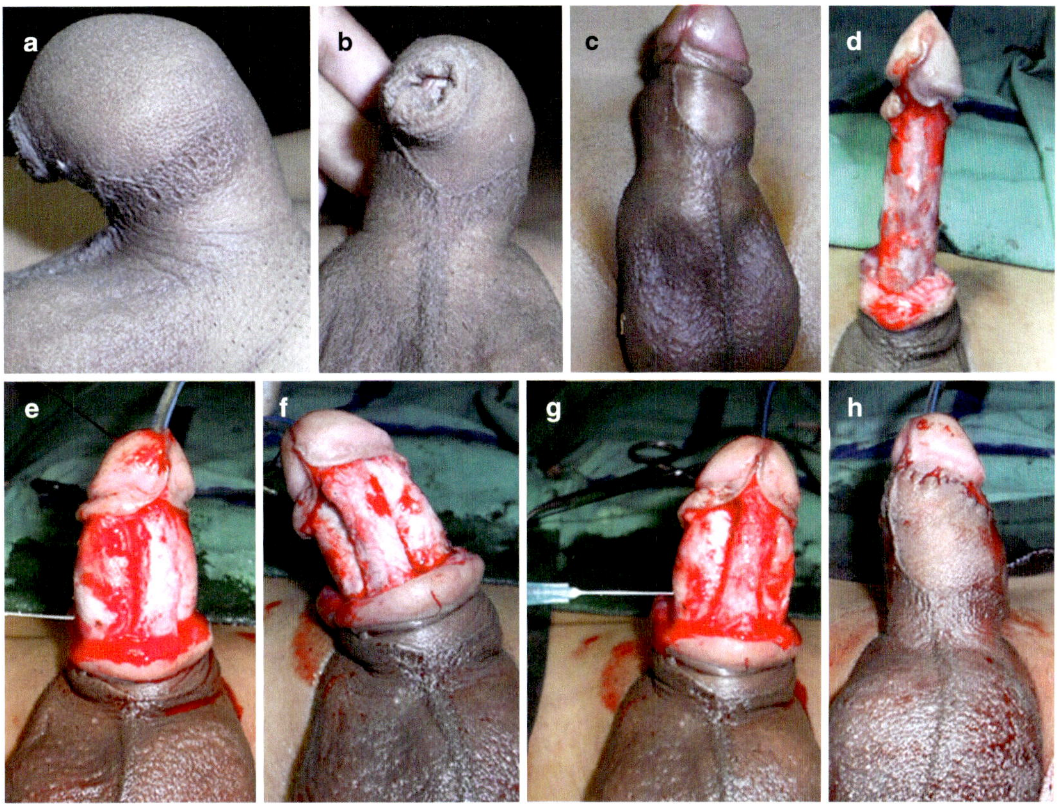

Fig. 15.5 Correction of moderate chordee in type III chordee without hypospadias. (**a**)–(**c**) Showing chordee without hypospadias (type III) with moderate curvature. (**d**) Gittes test showing mild curvature after penile skin degloving. (**e**, **f**) Showing hypoplastic urethra with spongiosum mobilization. (**g**) Gitte's test showing correction of curvature. (**h**) Skin closure

(Fig. 15.7a–i). But if curvature persists, then dorsal plication is needed. (Fig. 15.8a–p). Type IV and V chordee without hypospadias with congenital short urethra and/or dorso-ventral corporal disproportion may require the transection (Fig. 15.9) or resection of the hypoplastic urethra and replacement urethroplasty with or without corporoplasty. In most cases, after mobilization of the proximal urethra, the residual curvature is less than 30 degrees which can be managed by single stitch dorsal plication. Torsion associated with the chordee without hypospadias can also be managed with the technique of hypoplastic urethra and spongiosum mobilization (Fig. 15.1). Based on the etiological factors, an algorithm is proposed for the management of chordee without hypospadias (Fig. 15.10).

15.9 Methods of Penile Curvature Correction in Chordee Without Hypospadias

15.9.1 Penile De-gloving

Skin tethering may be the only factor in chordee without hypospadias is called skin chordee and is type III of Devine and Horton classification. Penile degloving is a simple and easy technique that can be done even by the beginner and is

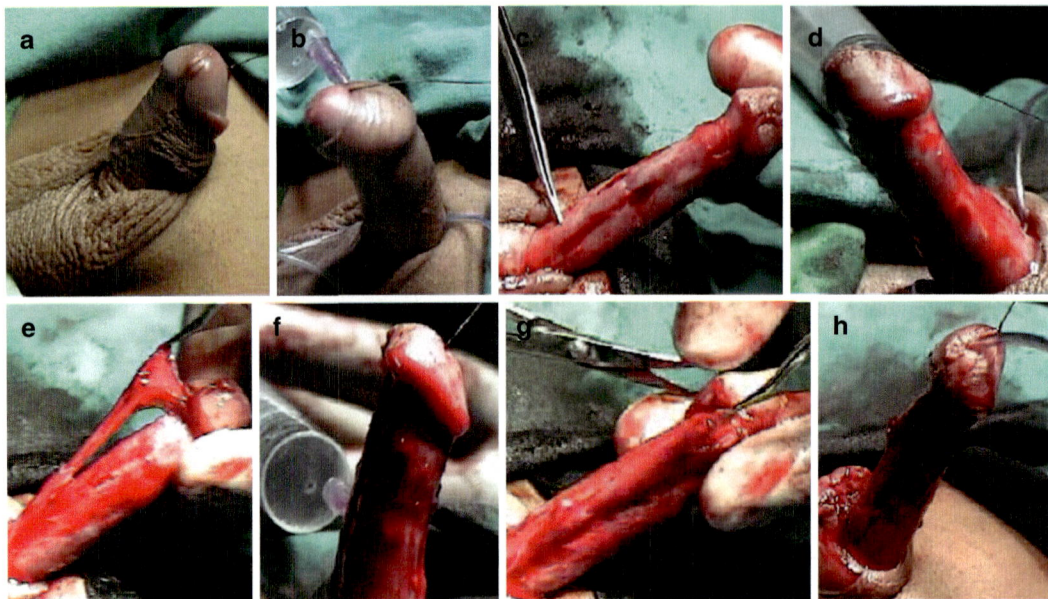

Fig. 15.6 Correction of chordee in type III chordee without hypospadias. (**a**) Showing chordee without hypospadias Type III with moderate curvature. (**b**) Gittes test showing Moderate curvature. (**c**) Penile skin degloving. (**d**) Mild glanular chordee on Gittes test. (**e**) Urethra and corpus spongiosum mobilization from corporal bodies. (**f**) Gittes test showing complete chordee correction. (**g**) Raising of glanular flaps. (**h**) Glansplasty done with complete correction of chordee (with permission Bhat et al. [1] @copyright Elsevier)

effective in such cases. If ventral skin is short, then the ventral transfer of skin after penile degloving corrects the curvature. In patients with severe curvature requiring the transection of the hypoplastic urethra, ventral transposition of skin helps correct curvature and is utilized for urethroplasty in the second stage. The limitation of the technique is its effectivity only in mild curvature. This falls under type III of Devine Horton classification and group 2 Donnahoo.

15.9.2 Release of Dartos

Dartos is released during penile degloving in most cases if the dissection plane is kept between the dartos and Bucks fascia dorsally and ventrally between the dartos fascia, whatever coverings of the urethra. In some cases, the skin may be stuck to Buck's fascia with no intervening dartos, while skin is directly adherent to the skin in type I. The skin is very thin, and there are chances of injury and buttonholing during the dissection. Often these thin areas of skin require excision. Saline injection at the site of adherent skin may help dissect the adherent urethra (Fig. 15.11a–f). Dissection and resection of the thickened, tethering, inelastic dartos bands are carried out until the penis is free. A more extensive ventral dissection is needed in some cases, especially along the urethra and corpora cavernosa. If the curvature is corrected by releasing the dartos, then these cases may be of type II and grouped in group 2.

15.9.3 Mobilization of Urethra & Spongiosum

Devine (1991) [17], Mollard (1994) [18], and more recently Bhat (2008) [1] advocate performing mobilization and preserving the hypoplastic urethra. Proximal urethral mobilization up to the bulbar region adds about 2–3.5 cm length to the spongiosal segment, which helps in chordee correction. Y-I spongioplasty after the divergent corpus spongiosum mobilization is done covering

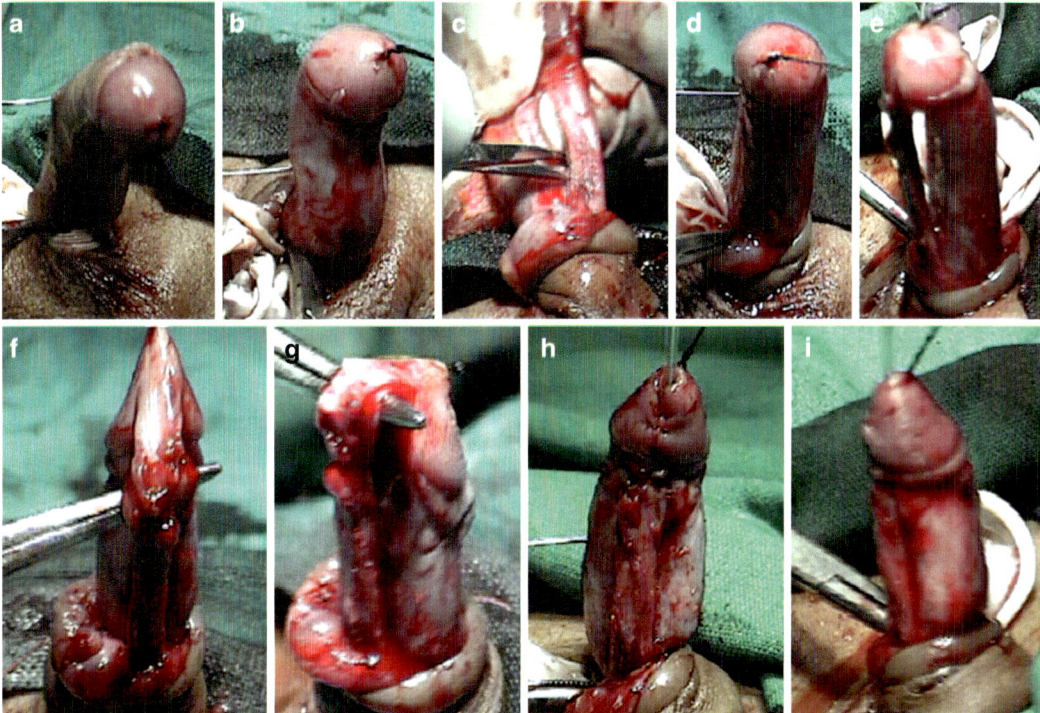

Fig. 15.7 Correction of chordee in type II hypospadias. Steps of chordee correction for Type II without hypospadias. (**a**) Moderate chordee on Gittes test. (**b**) Moderate chordee on Gittes after penile degloving. (**c**) Mobilization of urethra and corpus spongiosum. (**d**) Mild glanular chordee on Gittes test after mobilization of the urethra. (**e**) Mild glanular chordee on Gittes test after mobilization of the urethra, lateral view. (**f**) Mobilization of the urethra into glans. (**g**) Corpus spongiosum segment longer than corpus cavernosum. (**h**) Complete correction of chordee on Gittes test after spongioplasty. (**i**) Complete correction of chordee on Gittes test after spongioplasty, lateral view (with permission Bhat et al. [1] @copyright Elsevier)

the hypoplastic urethra reconstruct a nearer to "normal" urethra. The main aim of spongioplasty is to obtain an anatomical reconstruction as well as prevention of fistulas formation and also helps in the correction of curvature. The extent of urethral mobilization is done to the penoscrotal junction or up to the bulbar region according to the length needed for chordee correction keeping the ratio of 4:1. However, Atala et al. recommended a 5:1 ratio to prevent blood supply compromise to the urethra in hypospadias [19]. But it is possible to mobilize a little more proximally since mobilization is with corpus spongiosum and the distal end of the urethra remains attached to the glans keeping both blood supplies intact in chordee without hypospadias. The penis can be straightened without transecting the hypoplastic urethra by applying the steps mentioned above.

Urethral mobilization can easily be carried out by dissecting directly on top of the tunica albuginea. The mobilization is started in the healthy urethra proximal to the hypoplastic urethra after creating a plane between Buck's facia and tunica albuginea. Mobilization of the urethra is difficult in type I as it is adherent to both corpora and the skin. There is a risk of urethral fistula in these cases because of injury to the hypoplastic urethra during dissection. Creating a plane of dissection around the normal urethra proximally and then dissecting distally helps in mobilizing the urethra along with corpus spongiosum, with less risk of bleeding and injury to the urethra. Injecting saline or adrenaline solution helps in the dissection of the skin from the hypoplastic urethra. Then extended distally into glans and proximally as required. Gross et al. [20] reported their

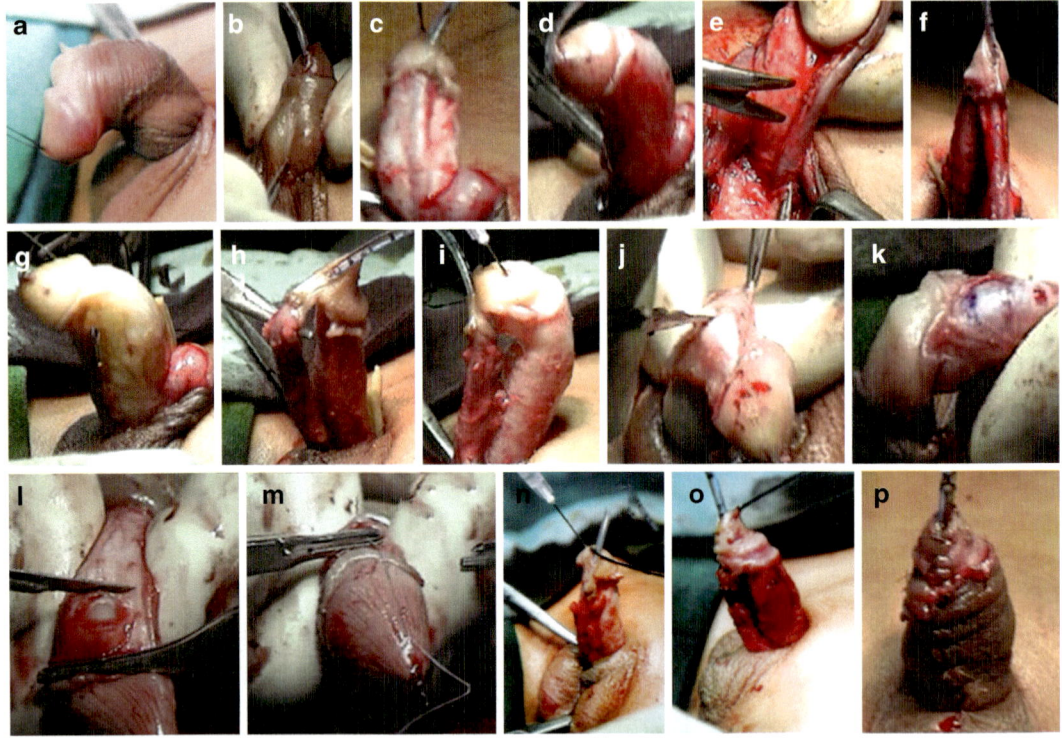

Fig. 15.8 Steps of chordee correction for Type II without hypospadias. (**a**) Moderate chordee on Gitte's test without hypospadias. (**b**) Midline incision on the ventral surface. (**c**) Penile degloving and poorly developed corpus spongiosum. (**d**) Moderate chordee Gittes test after penile degloving. (**e, f**) Mobilization of the hypoplastic and proximal urethra. (**g**) Moderate chordee Gittes test after mobilization of the urethra. (**h**) Mobilization of the urethra into glans. (**i**) Minimal chordee after mobilization of the urethra into glans. (**j**) Mobilization of the neurovascular bundle. (**k**) Site and size of incision for tunica albuginea plication. (**l**) Incision in tunica albuginea. (**m**) Suture for plication in tunica albuginea. (**n**) Complete correction of chordee after tunica plication on Gittes test. (**o**) Complete correction of chordee after spongioplasty and glanuloplasty. (**p**) Complete correction of chordee and skin closure (with permission Bhat et al. [1] @copyright Elsevier)

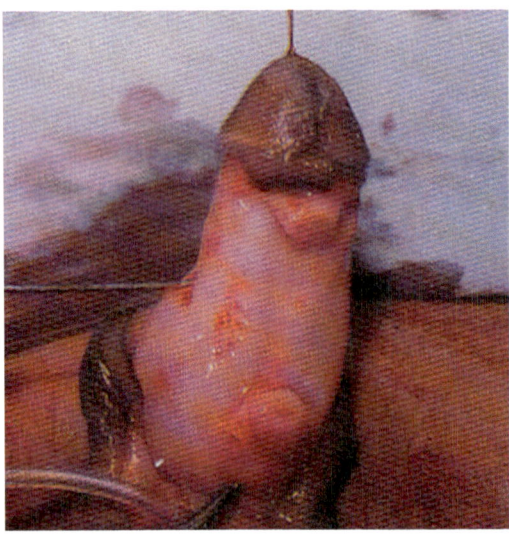

Fig. 15.9 Showing transection of the hypoplastic urethra for correction of chordee

experience with comprehensive mobilization of the urethra to correct the chordee and single-stage repair of chordee without hypospadias. Dipaola et al. managed chordee patients without hypospadias with dorsal plication in type III, extensive mobilization of the urethra in type II, and vascularized neo-urethra in type I cases in a study of 26 cases [21]. We could correct the chordee in 76% of cases by mobilizing the urethra, and only 8% of patients needed dorsal plication [1]. There is less risk of shortening the penis if dorsal tunica plication is done after mobilization of the urethra, as partial correction of chordee is achieved by mobilization of the urethra. Only 16% required division of hypoplastic urethra and 4% of these were due to damage that occurred to the hypoplastic urethra during mobilization. We routinely do spongioplasty and glanuloplasty in

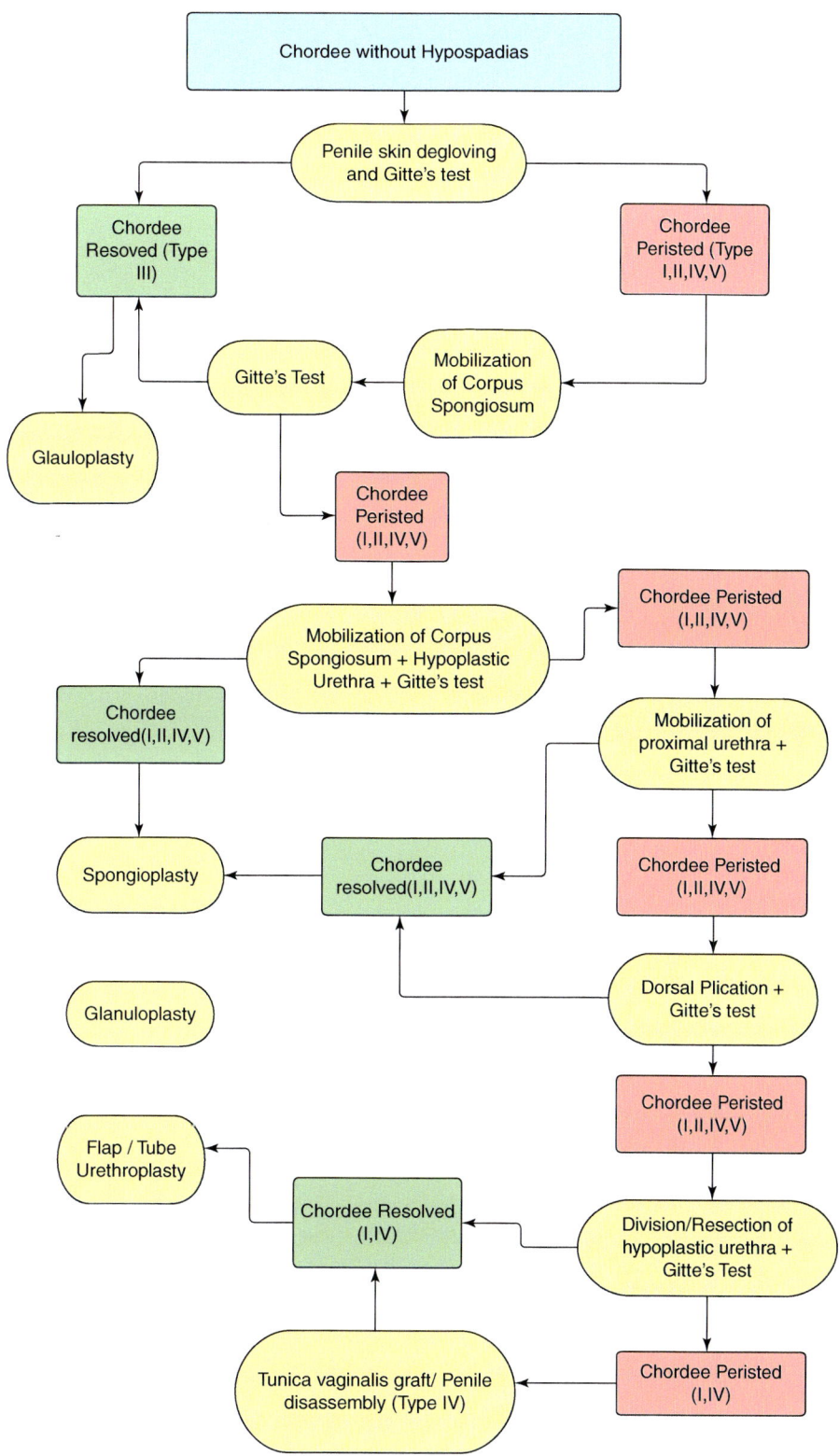

Fig. 15.10 Showing the algorithm for management of chordee without hypospadias

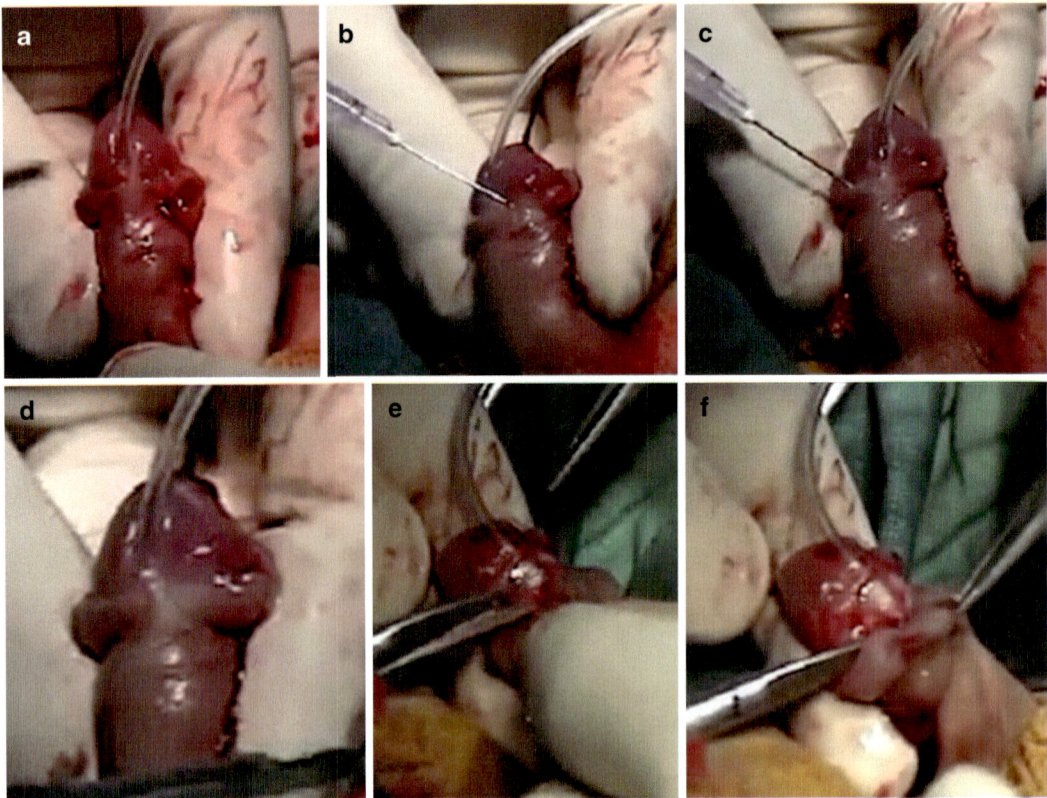

Fig. 15.11 Showing mobilization of adherent skin to the hypoplastic urethra. (**a**) Type I chordee without hypospadias. (**b**)–(**d**). Injection of saline to dissect the skin from the hypoplastic urethra. (**e, f**) Dissection and separation of skin from the hypoplastic urethra

all cases. Spongioplasty adds to the length of the urethra and so helps in the correction of the chordee. Mobilization of the hypoplastic urethra and spongioplasty reconstructs a near-normal urethra, repairing as per anatomical principles of surgery, corrects the chordee, and helps prevent urethral fistulae [1]. Glanuloplasty has a dual advantage of correcting the glanular part of the chordee and giving a conical shape to the glans. Utilizing the advantages mentioned above, we propose an algorithm (Fig. 15.10) to manage chordee without hypospadias, which defines etiology and guidelines for managing this congenital anomaly according to the etiology. Mobilization of the urethra along with the corpus spongiosum for correction of chordee is the best option, eliminating the complications mentioned above and having the advantage of utilizing the hypoplastic urethra with spongioplasty.

15.9.4 Plication and Corporeal Rotation Procedures

The principle of plication and the technique is the simplest one for correcting the curvature, but unfortunately, the recurrence rate is high. The plication is done opposite to the point of maximum curvature marked after the Gittes test. The cut edges in incisional or excisional plication heal better and hold approximation tension better than the shortening without it; yields better results. Chertin et al. reported a success rate of 85–100% with the dorsal plication corporoplasty for correcting chordee. They claimed it to be a simple, effective method without injury to neurovascular bundles or a detrimental effect on erection [22]. The limitation of the techniques is only effective in mild to moderate curvature. The long-term results reported by the others are contrary to it, with a high recurrence rate [23]. The disadvantages of the plication procedures are shortening of the penis, blood loss, chances of injury to corpora, and neurovascular bundle causing psychosexual problems. Corporal volume and elasticity of tunica may be compromised due to excessive folding or excision of tunica. More so, these are against the anatomical principles of surgery as rather than lengthening the pathological ventral surface, the normal dorsal surface is shortened. We use dorsal plication only when we find chordee less than 30 degrees after mobilization of the urethra by a single midline stitch or one or two sutures without much folding of the tunica.

15.9.5 Resection of the Hypoplastic Urethra and Replacement Urethroplasty

The resection of the hypoplastic urethra and urethroplasty is one of the options for managing chordee without hypospadias. Young advocated the resection of the hypoplastic urethra and replacement urethroplasty. But the disadvantages are it being an extensive procedure having higher complications. Urethral fistula, stricture, diverticula, penile torsion, stenotic and retrusive meatus are seen in flap procedures and chances of graft contracture if the free graft is used for urethroplasty.

15.9.6 Penile Disassembly and Corporoplasty

In case of the persistence of chordee even after the hypoplastic urethral transection or resection, the option of superficial corporotomy with or without corporoplasty may be considered. First, Corporotomy is done by fairy cuts, the superficial transverse incisions through the deep layer of the tunica. Snodgrass and Prieto reported good results with these fairy cuts without any recurrences. Then, they advocated performing three transverse ventral corporotomies at the point of maximal curvature, cutting through the tunica albuginea, but not into the erectile tissue, without any additional ventral grafting [24]. The next step is the Corporoplasty with dermal, tunica vaginalis graft, and SIS graft as ventral lengthening. The complications like erectile dysfunction due to venous leak, aneurysmal dilatation, penile instability, predisposition to penile fracture are reported in corporoplasty [25]. Penile disassembly is the last resort, which with/without corporoplasty corrects the curvature in almost all types of curvature. But this is an extensive procedure and requires vast experience. In our experience, we did not need penile dis-assembly for chordee correction in chordee without hypospadias.

15.10 Conclusions

The chordee without hypospadias is a group of conditions where the urethral meatus is at the glanular tip and has a variable degree of ventral penile curvature. Type III chordee without hypospadias with mild to moderate chordee may be operated at adolescence, but type II and type I should be operated in the same age group as hypospadias or whenever the child presents to the hospital. Mild chordee (30 degrees) is managed by dorsal approach while moderate to severe one with ventral lengthening. Surgical management with a single correct approach is difficult as the surgery is influenced by preference and opinion. The surgeon must be trained in hypospadias surgery and must understand the expected complications during and after surgery while mobilizing the hypoplastic urethra. At the same time, the step-by-step approach from simple to more complex solve the problem in most cases. The complexity of the problem will become apparent only after exposure of the urethra for mobilization. The surgery may turn out to be quick and straightforward or a long and complicated repair. Mild to moderate curvature in chordee without hypospadias may be corrected simply by penile degloving or with the addition of the hypoplastic urethral mobilization. Moderate to severe chordee requires extensive procedures like extended urethral mobilization, dorsal plication, or corporoplasty. Dorsal plication should be chosen in cases less than 30 degrees after urethral mobilization. Corporoplasty/corporotomy is preffered in more than 30 degrees cases to prevent penile shortening. The hypoplastic urethra and proximal extended urethral mobilization add length (2–3.5 cm) to the spongiosum segment, that helps in chordee correction. Spongioplasty with the mobilization of divergent corpus spongiosum and glanuloplasty reconstructs an anatomically near-normal urethra, adds length to correct the chordee, and eliminates the fear of preserving the hypoplastic urethra. An algorithm is proposed to preserve the urethra in a step-by-step approach.

References

1. Bhat A, Saxena G, Abrol N. A new algorithm for management of chordee without hypospadias based on the mobilization of the urethra. J Pedtr Urol. 2008;4(1):43–50.
2. Daskalopoulos EI, Baskin L, Duckett JW, Snyder III HM. Congenital penile curvature (chordee without hypospadias). J Urol. 1993;42(6):708–12.
3. Devine CJ, Horton CE. Chordee without hypospadias. J Urol. 1973;110(2):264–71.
4. Montag S, Palmer LS. Abnormalities of penile curvature: chordee and penile torsion. Scientific World J. 2011;11:1470–8.
5. Azmy AF. Chordee (penile Curvature). Hypospadias surgery. Springer; 2004. p. 115–8.
6. Kaplan GW, Lamm DL. Embryogenesis of chordee. J Urol. 1975;114(5):769–72.
7. Chen YC, Woolley Jr PV. Genetic studies on hypospadias in males. J Med Genet. 1971;8(2):153–9.
8. Culp OS. Struggles and triumphs with hypospadias and associated anomalies: a review of 400 cases. J Urol. 1966;96(3):339–51.
9. Tang YM, Chen SJ, Huang LG, Wang MH. Chordee without hypospadias: report of 79 Chinese prepubertal patients. J Androl. 2007;28:630–3.
10. Donnahoo KK, Cain MP, Pope JC, Casale AJ, Keating MA, Adams MC, et al. Etiology, management and surgical complications of congenital chordee without hypospadias. J Urol. 1998;160(3 Part 2):1120–2.
11. Kramer SA, Aybin G, Kelalis PP. Chordee without hypospadias in children. J Urol. 1982;128(3):559–61.
12. Gittes R, McLaughlin A. Injection technique to induce penile erection. Urology. 1974;4(4):473–4.
13. Young HH. Genital abnormalities: hermaphroditism and related adrenal diseases. The Williams and Wilkins; 1937.
14. Nesbit RM. Congenital curvature of the phallus: report of three cases with description of corrective operation. J Urol. 1965;93(2):230–2.
15. Hurwitz RS, Ozersky D, Kaplan H. Chordee without hypospadias: complications and management of the hypoplastic urethra. J.urol. 1987;138(2):372–5.
16. Cendron J, Melin YJ. Congenital curvature of the penis without hypospadias. UCNA. 1981;8(3):389–95.
17. Devine Jr CJ, Blackley SK, Horton CE, Gilbert DA. The surgical treatment of chordee without hypospadias in men. J Urol. 1991;146(2):325–9.
18. Mollard P, Castagnola C. Hypospadias: the release of chordee without dividing the urethral plate and onlay island flap (92 cases). J Urol. 1994;152(4):1238–40.
19. Atala AJ. Urethral mobilization and advancement for midshaft to distal hypospadias. J Urol. 2002;168(4 Part 2):1738–41.
20. Gross M, Fein R, Waterhouse K. Single stage correction of chordee without hypospadias and coronal hypospadias. J Urol. 1969;102(1):70–4.
21. Dipaola G, Spalletta M, Balducci T, Giacomello L, Camoglio FS, Bianchi S, et al. Surgical treatment of chordee without hypospadias. Eur Urol. 2000;38(6):758–61.
22. Chertin B, Koulikov D, Fridman's A, Farkas AJBi. Dorsal tunica albuginea plication to correct congenital and acquired penile curvature: a long-term follow-up. BJU Int. 2004;93(3):379–81.
23. Hendren WH, Caesar RE. Chordee without hypospadias: experience with 33 cases. J Urol. 1992;147(1):107–9.
24. Snodgrass W, Prieto J. Straightening ventral curvature while preserving the urethral plate in proximal hypospadias repair. J Urol. 2009;182(4S):1720–5.
25. Dason S, Wong N, Braga LH. The contemporary role of 1 vs 2-stage repair for proximal hypospadias. Transl Androl Urol. 2014;3:347–58.

Management of Female Hypospadias

16

Amilal Bhat, Akshita Bhat, and Madhu Bhat

Abbreviation

UTI   Urinary Tract Infection

16.1 Introduction

Hypospadias in females is a rare but well-defined congenital anomaly due to arrest of the development of the sinus urogenitalis. The term "hypospadias feminis" means a congenital false urethral opening/fissure of the posterior (lower) wall of the urethra in the anterior vaginal wall proximal to the hymenal ring [1]. Male hypospadias is more common, and the male to female ratio reported is 150:1. Female hypospadias, however, seems to have attracted much less attention and many cases go undiagnosed, and most of these are case reports only. Nevertheless, when the patients were evaluated for incontinence, the incidence was much higher than reported. In the study by Hoebeke et al. (1999), 288 girls were referred for correlation between the functional voiding disorders and the meatal anomaly. Eighty-eight of them presented with meatal anomalies (24 hypospadias and 64 covered hypospadias) [2]. In another study of 12,739 patients evaluated in Neuro-urology department, 131 patients met the inclusion criteria, and 18 (13.74%) were diagnosed as cases of hypospadias [3]. This shows that the anomaly is underreported. Though the diagnosis and management of the female hypospadias are simple, the condition is easily overlooked as physicians are unaware of female hypospadias. Usually, it becomes significant only as a result of difficulty during catheterization because of the inability to localize the meatus. All variants of female hypospadias should be surgically corrected by transposition of the external opening of the urethra from the vagina on the perineum under the clitoris to cure the chronic urethritis, cystitis and vulvovaginitis and chronic/recurrent UTI with hypospadias.

A. Bhat
Bhat's Hypospadias and Reconstructive Urology Hospital and Research Centre,
Jaipur, Rajasthan, India

Department of Urology, Jaipur National University Institute for Medical Sciences and Research Centre,
Jaipur, Rajasthan, India

Department of Urology, Dr. S.N. Medical College,
Jodhpur, Rajasthan, India

Department of Urology, S.P. Medical College,
Bikaner, Rajasthan, India

P.G. Committee Medical Council of India,
New Delhi, India

Academic and Research Council of RUHS,
Jaipur, Rajasthan, India

A. Bhat
Department of Surgery, Swai Man Singh Medical College, Jaipur, India

M. Bhat (✉)
Department of obstetrics and Gynecology,
S.M.S. Medical College, Jaipur, India

16.2 Embryology

True hypospadias with failure of fusion of the urethral folds cannot occur in females since that portion of the urethra does not develop. However, the urethral meatus opens high up in the anterior vaginal wall and assumes a hypospadiac position. The etiology of this condition remains obscure. Embryologically, it is believed to be due to abnormal development of the urogenital sinus in distal hypospadias, or a lack of differentiation of Wolff's tissue, when it is proximal. The lower part of the urethra and the vagina has a common origin from the lower part of the urogenital sinus, and failure of the normal development of this structure may explain hypospadias formation. In an experimental study (Miyagawa et al.) in the mice, hypospadias was induced by injecting diethylstilbestrol [4]. Doses response analysis indicated that 0.03 g diethylstilbestrol for 5 days is the lowest known critical dose for hypospadias induction. The authors have shown that diethylstilbestrol-induced female hypospadias onset may primarily be the result of changes in developing dorsal urethral epithelial cell apoptotic and proliferative activity. The location of diethylstilbestrol-induced hypospadias formation is dependent on age at the time of exposure. Sometimes a part of hymen covers the hypospadiac opening and is called webbed hypospadias. The urinary stream in these cases may be directed anteriorly.

Other congenital anomalies of the urogenital septum like bicornuate uterus, vaginal septum, and vaginal atresia may be associated with hypospadias. Urethral abnormalities like urethral atresia, urethral stenosis, urethral duplication, and dorsal urethral epispadias may also be associated with female hypospadias.

16.3 Classification

16.3.1 Congenital

Most of the time, the urethral opening is in anterior vaginal wall proximal to introitus; the patient is vaginal voider and presents with incontinence (Fig. 16.1a, b). But the hypospadiac opening is often partially covered by hymen, and the urinary stream is directed anteriorly. The web cover may be partial (Fig. 16.2a) or complete (Fig. 16.2b).

16.3.2 Acquired Hypospadias

The cause of female hypospadias in the older age group may not be congenital. The urethral meatus in such cases may become drawn up due to fibrosis after atrophic vaginitis or surgery on the urethra (Fig. 16.3a, b). Sometimes the patient may be subjected to female genital mutilation during early childhood, which is a tradition practiced in West African Yoruba tribe, and this may cause the urethral opening in hypospadiac location [5]. The long-term catheterization and poor catheter management in neurogenic bladder or old bedridden patient may lead to ventral urethra erosion and pooling the meatus high up in the vagina.

16.3.3 Blum Classification [6]

He divided these cases into three groups:

1. A longitudinal communication between the posterior wall of the urethra and the anterior wall of the vagina.
2. A persistent urogenital sinus, where the vagina enters into the urethra, but the hymen lies deep in the urogenital sinus.
3. The urethra opening into the vagina proximal to a normal hymen.

16.3.4 Solov'ev Classification [7]

1. Vestibular (partial)
2. Vestibulovaginal (subtotal)
3. Vaginal (total)

16.3.5 Clinical Classification

The clinical classification consists of complete (type I) and incomplete (type II); urethral subtypes are II-a, short wide, and II-b, standard urethral diameter.

16 Management of Female Hypospadias

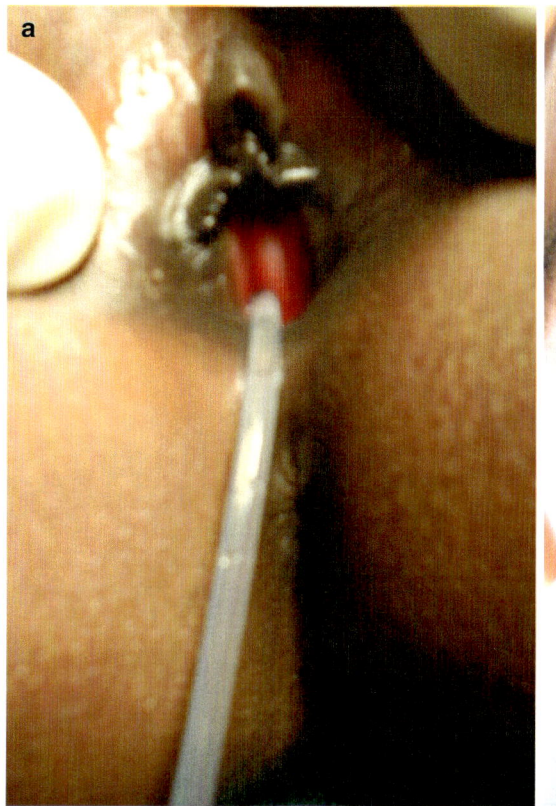 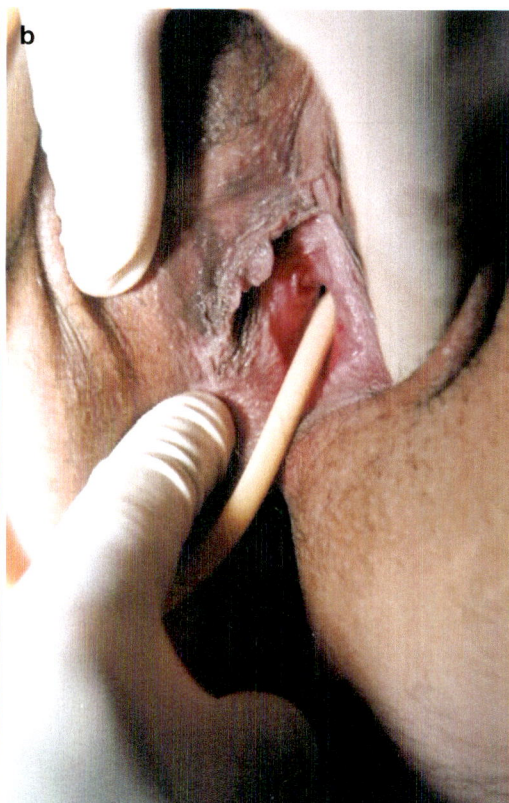

Fig. 16.1 Congenital female hypospadias in childhood and adult. (**a**) Congenital hypospadias with a catheter in hypospadiac opening high in the vagina in a child. (**b**) Congenital hypospadias with a catheter in hypospadiac opening high in the vagina in an adult

16.3.6 Derevianko Classification of Anatomic Variants of Female Hypospadias [8]

1. Low vaginal ectopia: Ectopia of the external urethral opening still outside the introitus
2. High vaginal ectopia of the external opening of the urethra lying inside the introitus
3. Urovaginal (vesicovaginal) fusion of the neck of the urinary bladder with vagina accompanied with enuresis, whole urethra is opened
4. Ectopia of the external urethral opening in the urogenital sinus, i.e. urogenital sinus in females
5. Any of the above variants of female hypospadias in combination with false or true hermaphroditism.

16.4 Presentation

Most of the time, female hypospadias goes unnoticed. It needs a high index of suspicion to diagnose the female hypospadias. Female hypospadias should be suspected in the following conditions:

1. Urinary incontinence
2. Recurrent UTI
3. Chronic UTI
4. Urethral syndrome
5. Dysfunctional voiding
6. Dyspareunia
7. Urethritis, cystitis, and vulvovaginitis
8. Cervico-vaginitis, endometritis, and secondary infertility

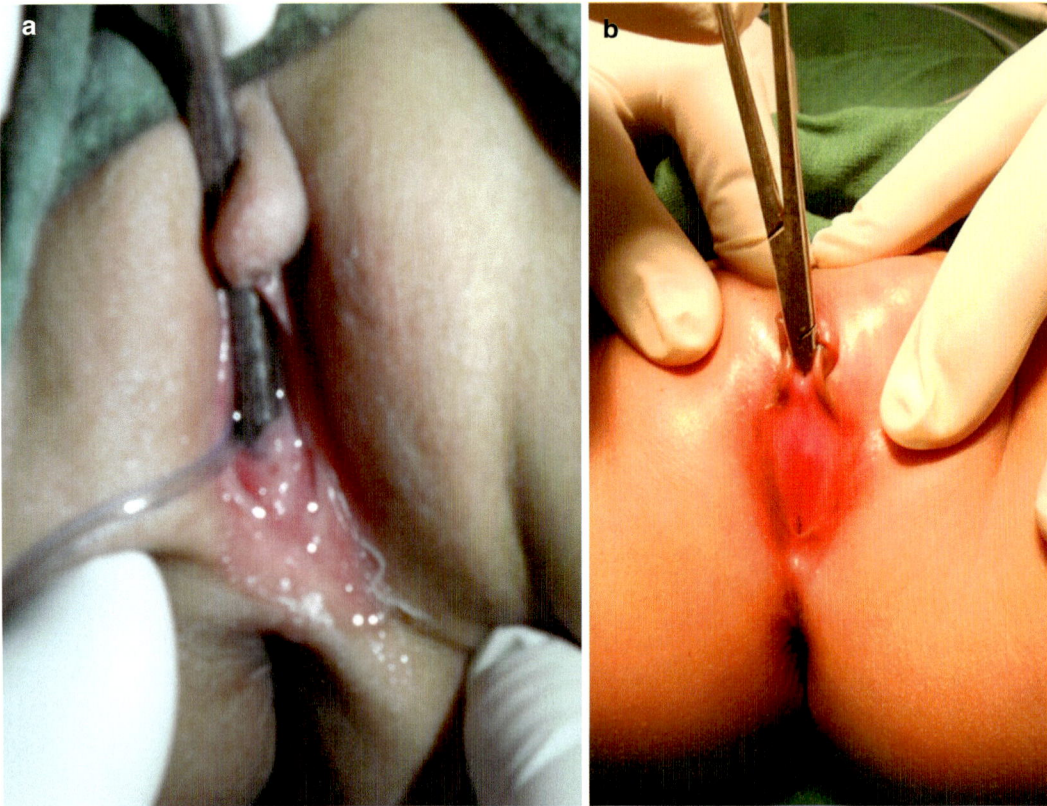

Fig. 16.2 Congenital webbed female hypospadias. (**a**) Partial/incomplete webbing with a catheter in hypospadiac opening. (**b**) Complete webbing with imperforate hymen Hemostat showing the common opening just below the clitoris

A urethra of standard caliber without meatal stenosis may be asymptomatic, coming to light only when an attempt is made to catheterize the patient. Incontinence of urine is an important sign of female hypospadias. Incontinence can be true, determined by a short urethra on which the pelvic muscular complex could not act at best and can be pseudo-incontinence or post micturition incontinence, imperfect control caused by vaginal voiding. They can have urethral syndrome (frequency, dysuria, urgency), recurrent UTI, and dyspareunia presenting when a sexually active life has started. If the urethra is narrow, the presentation is more likely to have signs of urinary outflow obstruction, distended urinary tract, urinary tract infection, obstructive nephropathy, and hypertension. Webbed hypospadias may present with the direction of the stream towards the face. The web may cover the meatus completely with imperforate hymen or may cover the meatus partially. So important observation of the parents may be that baby soils the chest and face by the urinary stream, or the baby does not pass urine in stream.

16.5 Diagnosis

Diagnosis is usually by clinical examination to locate the meatus, and hardly any investigation is required. Inability to locate the meatus for catheterization should raise the suspicion of the hypospadias. Failed catheterization in a female is a cardinal sign in the diagnosis of hypospadias. Examination of the external genitalia of the baby may show leakage of urine from the vagina with an absence of urethral opening (Fig. 16.4a, b).

Per speculum examination is required to locate the meatus in the anterior vaginal wall in adults (Fig. 16.3b). Intravenous Urogram or CT Urogram is advisable to rule out the upper tract

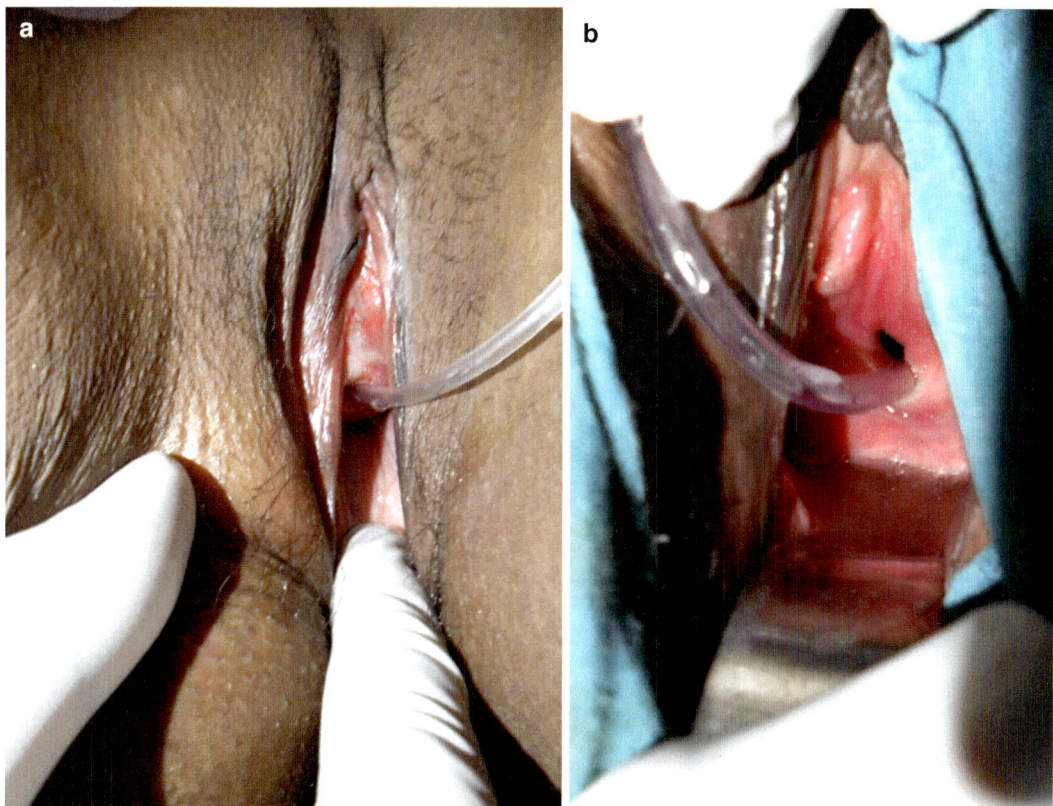

Fig. 16.3 Acquired female hypospadias. (**a**) Urethral opening high in the vagina with atrophic changes. (**b**) Urethral very opening high in the vagina just at the bladder neck

abnormalities. Micturating cystourethrogram may give of vaginal spillage of dye but seems to be an academic exercise. Cystoscopy or catheterization clichés the diagnosis, showing short urethra lying urethral opening high in the vagina (Fig. 16.1).

16.6 Female Hypospadias and Dysfunctional Voiding

Female hypospadias is rare, and many a time patient present as a urethral syndrome. A majority of the women with the urethral syndrome have had dysfunctional voiding since childhood. This suggests a causal association between dysfunctional voiding and minimal meatal deformities. A variety of hypotheses have been proposed to explain this association [2]. The bulbocavernosus reflex that is usually absent during voiding. However, it is generally elicited by genital stimulation. In patients with anterior deflection of the urinary stream, the stream passes the clitoris and can stimulate the bulbocavernosus reflex, which in turn can initiate sphincter activity during voiding. Strong vaginal voiding in cases of female hypospadias could provoke the same reflex. In neurogenic bladder with detrusor sphincter dyssynergia, where the neurological lesion deletes normal inhibition of the bulbocavernosus reflex during voiding; it is similar to the mechanism as seen in female hypospadias. In girls with dysfunctional voiding, this inhibition might not be obtained because of the minimal anatomic deformity. The only defiance against voiding over the rim of the toilet may be a bent posture, that precludes good relaxation of the pelvic floor muscles during voiding, thus creating a functional obstruction during voiding in girls with anterior deflection of the urinary stream. And in girls with hypospadias, extreme vaginal voiding can cause further urine loss after voiding. To prevent this,

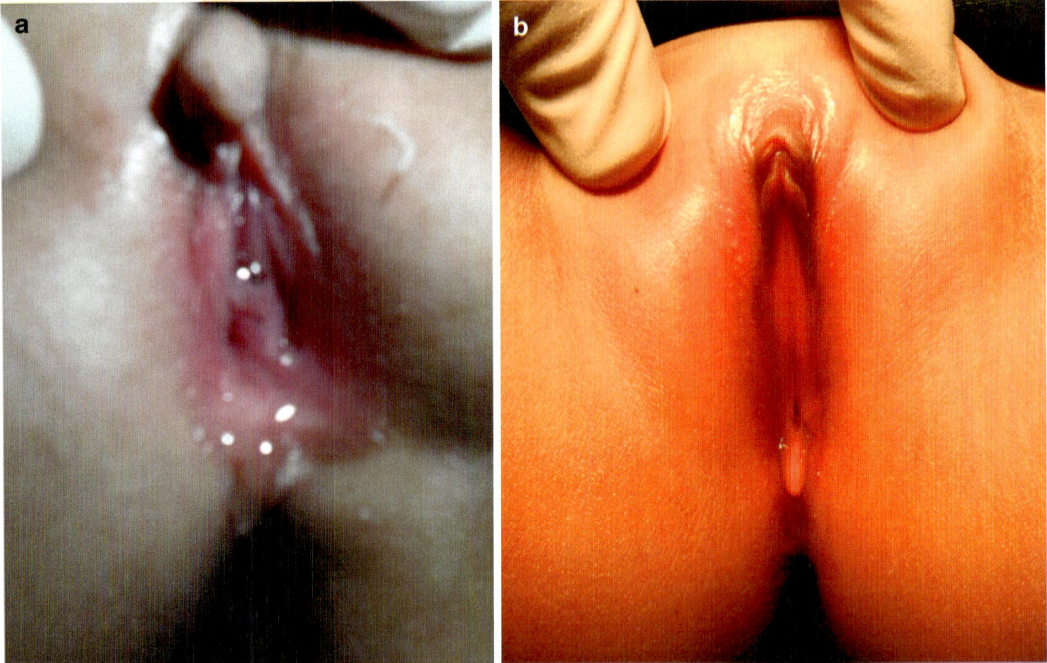

Fig. 16.4 (**a** and **b**) Congenital female hypospadias with urinary leakage and absent urethral meatus in childhood

the girls may contract their sphincter intensely several times a day, which might be responsible for sphincter hypertrophy, finally resulting in dysfunctional voiding. Vaginal filling during voiding can even stimulate the bulbocavernosus reflex.

16.7 Urinary Incontinence in Female Hypospadias

Patients of female hypospadias may have stress incontinence, pseudo-incontinence and even genuine incontinence. Patients are the vaginal voider, so such patients never void in-stream which may be elicited on detailed interrogation while taking history. Urine pooled in vagina later soils the undergarments giving the impression in incontinence, but that is pseudo-incontinence (Fig. 16.4a, b). Many patients of female hypospadias present as stress incontinence after vaginal delivery and sometimes with total incontinence. The total incontinence in severe hypospadias is due to the location of meatus at bladder neck making it incompetent. Genuine incontinence and stress are more common in urethra-vesical and high vaginal hypospadias.

16.8 Vaginal Stones

Vaginal stone with hypospadias is a rare condition; only one case has been reported. Urethral opening high in anterior vaginal wall proximal to hymen will lead to voiding in the vaginal cavity, so much so that patients never voids in a stream. With an intact hymen, there is stagnation of urine in the vagina which may lead encrustation in the vaginal cavity. If a patient is not managed in time, then there may be stone formation and stone may take the shape of the vaginal cavity (Fig. 16.5). Neglected patients with a vagina full of rocks may have coital difficulty and dyspareunia. The vaginal examination may reveal a stone palpable in the vagina and if it enlarges in size and may protrude out of the introitus. We came across one such case who was married and presented with dyspareunia [1].

16.9 Infertility

Female hypospadias may be an unusual cause of infertility. Voiding urine in the vaginal cavity and stagnation of urine in the vagina adversely affect

16 Management of Female Hypospadias

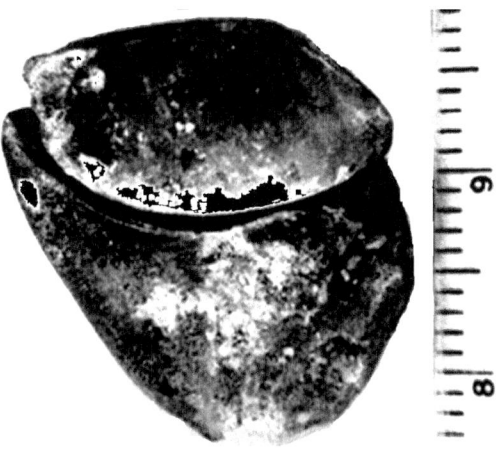

Fig. 16.5 Vaginal cavity shaped stones removed from the vagina (copy from Bhat et al. [1] with permission)

the normal vaginal flora and cause infection in the vaginal cavity. Presence of infected urine in the vagina spreads it to cervix and uterus. The repeated cervicovaginal infections may even lead to chronic or intermittent endometritis and infertility. Secondly, urine washes the vaginal secretion, which will lead to vaginal dryness leading to dyspareunia and contributes to the risk of infertility. Vaginal flap urethroplasty prevents urination into the vaginal cavity and vaginal infection. Control of cervico-vagino-uterine infection and vaginal lubrication with normal secretions reduces the dyspareunia, which helps cure secondary infertility.

16.10 Management

Surgery is the treatment of choice in symptomatic female hypospadias. Both in primary and secondary hypospadias, urethral reconstruction should be done to prevent the sequelae and complication of the hypospadias. Hymenotomy in infants and children may cure the recurrent urinary tract infection.

16.10.1 Vaginal Flap Urethroplasty

A vaginal flap urethroplasty is performed, keeping the patient in a frog-leg position/lithotomy position under general anesthesia. An inverted U-shaped incision is given around the urethral meatus and then extended into the anterior vaginal wall after putting in the catheter (Fig. 16.6a, b, c). Anterior vaginal wall mucosal flaps are raised on both sides of the incision (Fig. 16.6d, e). A urethral tube is constructed by tubularization of vaginal flaps to bring the external meatus to the base of the clitoris over an adequate size catheter. The incision is extended deep into the muscle layer of the anterior vaginal wall, and this surrounding tissue along the muscle is stitched over the newly constructed urethral tube as a second layer. Vaginal mucosal flaps are dissected on both sides of the incision and sutured with interposition of a pedicled adipose tissue flap (Fig. 16.6f). The neo-meatus is reconstructed between the introitus and the clitoris (Fig. 16.6g).

Figure 16.7 The diagrammatic presentation of vaginal flap urethroplasty. In most of the simple cases of the vaginal flap, urethroplasty is sufficient to control the symptoms. Still, surgical management of cases of female hypospadias with stricture may be technically more difficult, as the stricture would further shorten the already short hypospadiac urethra. A combination of urethrolysis, urethral transposition, and urethroplasty, or some other cumbersome amalgam of procedures may be needed for satisfactory resolution of the symptoms.

16.10.2 Hymenotomy/Web Incision

In cases with a meatal mucosal web, the web is incised longitudinally and closed transversely with three interrupted polyglactin 6/0 sutures, which corrects the direction of the urinary stream (Fig. 16.8a). Partial hymenotomy/incision in the hymen is given to open up the meatus (Fig. 16.8b) which corrects the urinary stream pointing forward, and vaginal collection of urine is corrected (Fig. 16.8c). If later on problem persists, then vaginal flap urethroplasty may be required.

16.11 Our Experience and a Brief Review

We published four cases of female hypospadias; one of them having vaginal stones in 2010 [1].

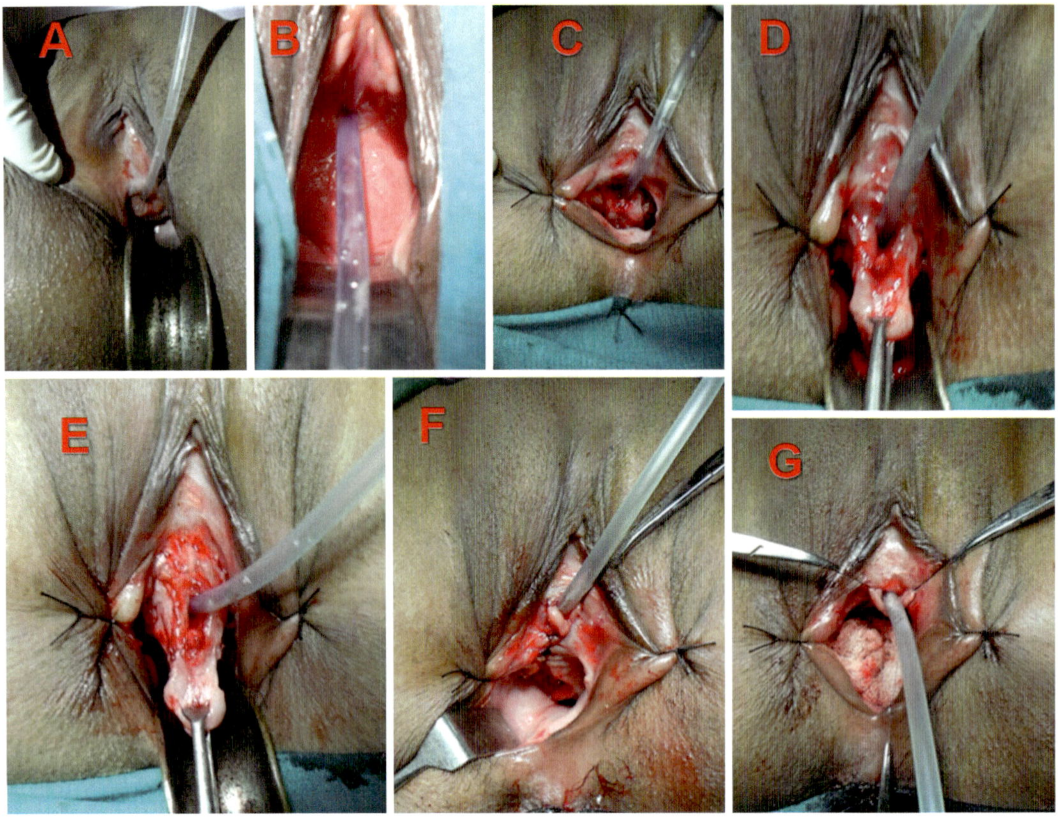

Fig. 16.6 Vaginal flap urethroplasty in acquired hypospadias. (**a**) and (**b**) Atrophic vagina with urethral opening high in the vagina almost at the bladder neck. (**c**) Inverted U-shaped incision in the anterior vaginal wall. (**d**) Vaginal wall flap raised. (**e**) Similar flap marked dorsal to the meatus. (**f**) Both sutured together to bring the meatus at the usual location and vaginal wall sutured over it. (**g**) Vaginal wall closure and wide normal located meatus

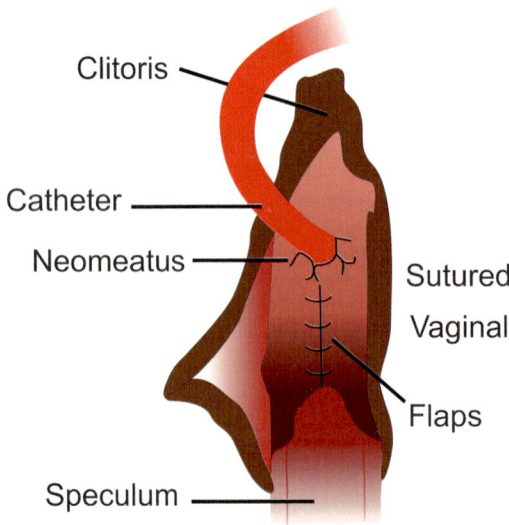

Fig. 16.7 Diagrammatic representation of vaginal flap urethroplasty

Later on, we retrospectively reviewed of cases sheets of females presenting with recurrent UTI, chronic UTI, incontinence, and vaginal discharge from 2012 to 2019. During this period, we had a total of nine (five congenital and four acquired) cases of female hypospadias. Clinical history details were obtained, and thorough clinical examinations, urinary catheterization, and cystoscopy were done. Genitalia examination, observing leakage of urine from vagina, catheterization, and/or cystoscopy clinched the diagnosis. Management was done on a case to case-based, and results were recorded. Age of the patients ranged from 6 months to 25 years in congenital and 55 years to 68 years in acquired cases with a mean age of 29.6 years—all of the patients presented with recurrent UTI and recurrent UTI. One of the patients had stream directed towards the abdomen, and two had leak-

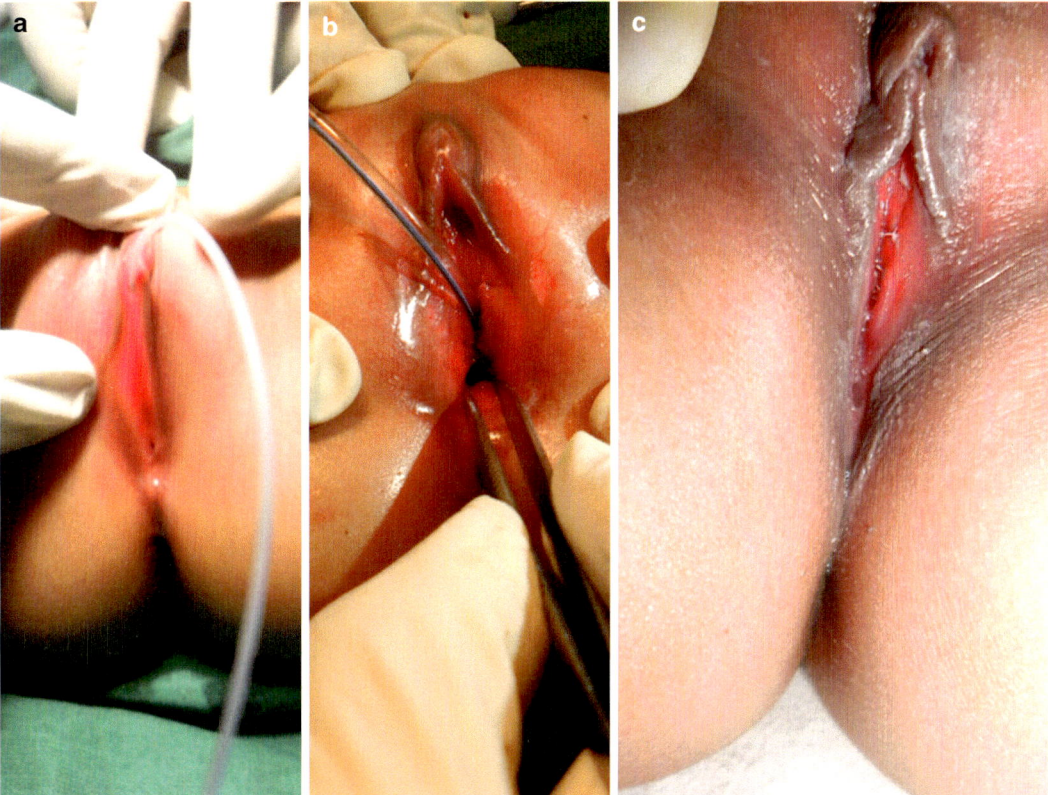

Fig. 16.8 Hymenotomy in hypospadias with imperforate hymen in a patient with a urinary stream directed to face. (**a**) Intact hymen with an opening just below the clitoris. (**b**) Hymen incised to open up the urethral meatus and catheter in the meatus. (**c**) Postoperative, after 3 weeks, meatus still high in the anterior vaginal wall

age of urine from the vagina. Two of the patients had urinary incontinence since birth and recurrent attacks of UTI. The fourth patient complained of dyspareunia. The diagnosis of female hypospadias was made by catheterization, culdoscopy, voiding cystourethrogram, and pan-endoscopy. The patient was put in a frog-leg position, and a peri-urethral vaginal flap urethroplasty was done in three layers. Excellent results were seen in three cases. Two of the patients were managed by partial hymenotomy, the release of the fused membrane was done in two, and supra-pubic cystostomy had to be performed in two cases with urethral erosion. Postoperative period was uneventful, and sterile urine culture was obtained up to 24–36 months of follow-up. Patients of partial hymenotomy are still under follow-up for any problem requiring urethroplasty.

Review of the literature shows that most of the cases are case reports, go undiagnosed and are diagnosed secondary to morbid complication. The studies conducted for evaluation of the patients of incontinence, recurrent UTI, and the incidence of hypospadias in girls with abnormal urodynamic ; the incidence has been as high as 15% of hypospadias which shows that anomaly is not as rare as has been reported. Diagnosis in most of the cases is made either in adulthood with some complication of hypospadias is again an important fact. Urinary incontinence is the commonest symptom, followed by recurrent/chronic UTI. Commonest complication observed was a renal failure due to late diagnosis and treatment. Vaginal pooling of urine may lead to a rare complication of vaginal stones. Once the diagnosis has been confirmed, the outcome of surgery and management had been successful. Salient feature and results of the reported cases in the literature are shown in Table 16.1.

Table 16.1 Reported cases management and results

S.N.	Authors	Year	No of cases	Age (Years)	Presentation	Complication / Sequalae	Procedure / management	Result
1.	Bhat A et al [1]	2010	4	1. 18-65 Years	incontinence of urine, recurrent UTIs since childhood and dysparcunia Inability to Catheterize. Retention of urine	Vaginal stone	Vaginal flap urethroplasty Urethral dilatation and catheterization	Good
2	OEBEKE P [2]	1999	24 Hypospadias 64 covered hypospadias		Urinary incontinence, Neurogenic bladder	-	-	-
3	Ronzoni G et bal [9]	2001	32	Mean age 22 range 16-38	diurnal nocturnal frequency, dysuria, urgency, suprapubic pain and sometimes urge incontinence. Failed medical treatment	-	Urethral translocation	Good
4	Van Bogaert L J [10]	1992	6	Adult females	Urethral Syndrome Failed medical treatment	-	Tranlocation of meatus	Good
5	Ayed M et al. [11]	1995	3	Adult	Urinary incontinence Vaginal Atresia	-	Vaginal Flap urethroplasty	Re- operation -1
6	Antolak et al [12]	1969	2	2 Years 3 Months	Urethral Calibration Vaginal flap urethroplasty Urethral calibration	Pooling of urine in vagina	Vaginal flap urethroplasty	Nil
7	Bouty A et al [13]	2016	2	< 5 Years	Associated with urethral duplication		1.Dorsal urethra resection & Hypospadiac urethral dilatation. 2.Partial urogenital sinus mobilization	Good
8	D'Cunha AR, et al [14].	2016	1	1. 4 Years	Straining during micturition, Ambiguous genitalia	Renal failure	Vesicostomy	Renal function improved
9	Ravichandran R et al [15]	1995	2	3 and 9 Years	Incontinence of urine	Neurogenic bladder	Mitrofanoff operation and CIC	Good
10	Tsujimoto Y et al. [16]	1984	1	24 Years	Urinary frequency and incontinence	Left NFK	Bladder neck and urethral narrowing & suspension bladder neck	Good
11	Sarin YK Kumar P [17]	2019	1	6 Years	Urinary incontinence		external urethral lengthening	Satisfactory
12	Patil N A et al [18]	1995	1	7 Years	Urinary incontinence	Small capacity bladder	Vaginal Flap urethroplasty	Good
13	Lima M. et al [19]	2018	1	5 Years	Recurrent UTI and VU reflux	Vu reflux	-Vaginal flap urethroplasty and ureteric reimplantation	Good
14	Niyagi T et al [20]	2020	1	21 Years	secondary infertility, dysparcunia, and urge symptom	Secondary infertility	Vaginal flap urethroplasty	Good
15	Midburger H et al [21]		1	1 Years	With supra-pubic diversion due to wrong diagnosis of occult neurogenic outlet obstruction and diagnosed during investigation and un-diversion was done.		Undiversion ,And catherization	Good
16	Gaurav Prakash et al [22]	2016	1	11 Years	Chronic retention of urine with CRF Failed per urethral catheterization	Chronic Renal Failure	Suprapubic Catheterization ,Antegrade cystoscopy and catheterization	Good
17	Bello OJ et al [23]	2012	1	68 Years	Obstructive uropathy Stricture urethra CRF	Chronic Renal Failure	Urethral dilatation and CIC	Good

16.12 Conclusions

A high index of suspicion is required to diagnose hypospadias, especially in patients presenting with an abnormal urinary stream, vaginal discharge, urinary incontinence, urethral syndrome, recurrent UTI, and chronic UTI. Senile atrophic vaginitis and urethral erosion and loss may be the cause of secondary hypospadias in patients on long-term catheterization. Absence of urethral opening with vaginal voiding or urinary dribble is a cardinal sign of hypospadias in a female child. Diagnosis is made during catheterization and/or lower tract endoscopy. Vaginal voiding leads to urinary stagnation in the vagina, causing urinary pseudo-incontinence and vaginal infection. A good outcome is expected by early diagnosis and management. Vaginal flap urethroplasty and approximation of peri-urethral smooth muscle help in continence by creating a pseudo-sphincter.

References

1. Bhat A, Saxena R, Bhat MP, Dawan M, Saxena G. Female hypospadias with vaginal stones: a rare congenital anomaly. J Pediatr Urol. 2010;6(1):70–4.
2. Hoebeke P, Van Laecke E, Raes A, Van Gool J, Vande WJ. Anomalies of the external urethral meatus in girls with non-neurogenic bladder sphincter dysfunction. BJU Int. 1999;83(3):294–8.
3. Salga M, Guinet-Lacoste A, Demans-Blum C, Thomas-Pohl M, Weglinski L, Amarenco G. Urethral meatus deformities and urethra hypospadias in women: prevalence, problems and definitions. Study of 12,739 patients. Prog Urol. 2014;24(17):1093–8. https://doi.org/10.1016/j.purol.2014.10.005.
4. Miyagawa S, Buchanan DL, Sato T, Ohta Y, Nishina Y, Iguchi T. Characterization of diethylstilbestrol-induced hypospadias in female mice. Anatomic Rec. 2002;266(1):43–50.
5. Odukogbe A-TA, Afolabi BB, Bello OO, Adeyanju AS. Female genital mutilation/cutting in Africa. Transl Androl Urol. 2017;6(2):138.
6. V. B. Die hypospadie der weiblichen Harnohre. Monatsber Urol. 1904;9:522–44.
7. Se AE. The diagnosis and treatment of hypospadias in girls. Urol Nefrol (Mosk). 1993;6
8. Derevianko IMDT, Ryzhkov VV. Hypospadias in females. Urologiia. 2007;3:26–8.
9. Ronzoni G, Giovanni DE, Weir L, Pasqui JM, Menchinelli F. Transposing the urethral meatus in the treatment of recurrent and postcoital cystitis in women with hypospadias. BJU Int. 2001;87:894–6.
10. Van Bogaert LJ. Surgical repair of hypospadias in women with symptoms of urethral syndrome. J Urol. 1992;147:1263–4.
11. Ayed M, Ben Abid F, Lousssief H, Ben Hassine L, Jemni M. Female hypospadias apropos of 3 cases. J Urol (Paris). 1995;101:244–7.
12. Antolak SJ, Smith JP, Doolittle KH. Female hypospadias. J Urol. 1969;102:640.
13. Bouty A, Lefevre Y, Haper L, Dobremej E. Urethral duplication in girls: three cases associating epispadias urethra and a main hypospadiac urethra. JPed Urol. 2016;12:209.
14. D'Cunha AR, Kurian JJ, Jacob TJK. Idiopathic female pseudohermaphroditism with urethral duplication and female hypospadias. BMJ Case Rep Published online. https://doi.org/10.1136/bcr-2015-214172.
15. Ravichandran R, Sripathi V, Ramanathan S, et al. Female hypospadias with neurogenic bladder. Pediatr Surg Int. 1995;10:572–3. https://doi.org/10.1007/BF00566505.
16. Tsujimoto Y, Nakamura M, Tada Y, Sakurai T. A case of hypospadias in a woman whose incontinence was repaired surgically. Hinyokika Kiyo. 1984;30(1):29–33.
17. Sarin YK, Kumar P. Female hypospadias-need for clarity in definition and management. J Indian Assoc Pediatr Surg. 2019;24:141–3.
18. Patil NA, Patil SB, Kundargi VS, Biradar AN. Female urethral anomalies in the pediatric age group: uncovered. J Surg Tech Case Rep. 2015;7:14–6.
19. Lima M, Di Salvo N, Gargano T, Ruggeri G. Female hypospadias and urinary incontinence: surgical solution of a little-known entity. Int Arch Urol Complic. 2018;4:049. https://doi.org/10.23937/2469-5742/1510049.
20. Niyagi T, Mehmat AS, Murat Y, Guldeniz T. An unusual cause of female secondary infertility: hypospadias. Turk J Obstet Gynecol. 2020;17:233–5.
21. Marberger M, Altwein JE, Straub E, et al. The Lich—Gregoir antireflux plasty: experiences with 371 children. J Urol. 1978;120:216–9.
22. Prakash G, Singh M, Goel A, et al. Female hypospadias presenting with urinary retention and renal failure in an adolescent: uncommon and late presentation with significant hidden morbidity. Case Rep. 2016;bcr2016215064.
23. Bello JO, Ododo BI, Bello HS. Female hypospadias and urethral stricture disease in a circumcised postmenopausal African woman: diagnosis and management. Uro Today Int J. 2013;

Management of Megmeatus Intact Prepuce/Concealed Hypospadias

Amilal Bhat

Abbreviations

GAP	Glanular approximation procedure
MAGPI	Meatal advancement and glanuloplasty
MIP	Megameatus intact prepuce
TUPU	Tubularized urethral plate urethroplasty
TIP	Tubularized incised plate urethroplasty

17.1 Introduction

Juskiewenski et al., in 1983, first time reported the description of the anomaly, a variant of hypospadias [1], and the terminology of Mega-meatus

A. Bhat (✉)
Bhat's Hypospadias and Reconstructive Urology Hospital and Research Centre,
Jaipur, Rajasthan, India

Department of Urology, Jaipur National University Institute for Medical Sciences and Research Centre, Jaipur, Rajasthan, India

Department of Urology, Dr. S.N. Medical College, Jodhpur, Rajasthan, India

Department of Urology, S.P. Medical College, Bikaner, Rajasthan, India

P.G. Committee Medical Council of India,
New Delhi, India

Academic and Research Council of RUHS,
Jaipur, Rajasthan, India

Intact Prepuce was first coined by Duckett and Keating [2]. This anomaly is also termed Concealed Hypospadias/Hidden Hypospadias. A deep glans groove characterizes MIP, a large meatus, and the glans is entirely covered by an intact prepuce. This unusual anterior hypospadias variant contributes approximately 3–6% of total hypospadias cases [2–5]. Concealed hypospadias is usually missed and presents late because it is covered by the prepuce. Many patients, who are un-noticed, may come to the clinician for any other medical problem because they usually do not have symptoms. Recognition at the time of circumcision in newborns and patients seeking advice for phimosis is likely to diagnose the entity. The diagnosis is often made during routine health checkups before the defence or any other services. The critical features identified in the diagnosis are (1) meatus located close to or just below the coronal margin; (2) A wide, splayed-out glans; (3) A deep glans cleft; (4) An abnormal urinary stream if witnessed. Duckett and Keating [2] recognized the distinct surgical challenges of the MIP variant first time in 1989. The controversy continues whether to operate on these patients or not [6]. But in modern-day hypospadiology, with more concern on the cosmesis, surgery is preferred. The techniques described are the "Pyramid procedure, Glans Approximation technique, Meatal Advancement and Glanuloplasty (MAGPI), Mathieu the peri-meatal-based flap technique, TIP and TIPU". The distinct anatomic features of the concealed hypospadias have led to the emergence of several techniques. Good cosmetic and functional results are preferred compared to those achievable with perimeatal-based flaps and MAGPI [7]. The glans approximation procedure (GAP) came into practice to overcome the challenges of a wide, deep glanular groove and a non-compliant fish mouth with the methods mentioned above [8]. Reconstruction of neourethra without dissection of glanular flaps in the GAP technique creates a neourethra with different diameters depending on the depth of the glanular cleft. The diameter of the neourethra may not match the original one, and the difference in caliber may cause pressure differentials that may predispose to fistula formation [3]. An intermediate tissue interposing layer is not used in the original GAP procedure; so, the two suture lines of glans overlie, increasing the fistula chances. The tubularized incised plate urethroplasty (TIPU) technique is the most commonly done procedure for distal hypospadias repair because of its better cosmetic and functional results. Now the same is being used for its MIP variant repair. As the urethral plate in MIP is very wide, so it does not require the incision in the urethral plate. Bhat et al. (2019) reported the excellent results of Tubularized Urethral Plate Urethroplasty (TUPU) in 13 cases of MIP in a retrospective study [9].

17.2 Embryology

The embryologic basis of the MIP variant of hypospadias is not clearly defined. The urethra develops by the fusion of the urethral plate from proximal to distal. The distal urethra is also a part of the urethral plate but grows from the tip of the glans to meet the proximal penile urethra at the coronal sulcus. A cuff of tissue lies at the margin of the sulcus from the prepuce. The arrest in the development and failure of fusion of the urethral plate results in hypospadias with a hooded prepuce. Duckett and Keating [2] postulated that a misdirected clefting of the glans proceeds down the already fused urethra creating the megameatus after normal folding of the proximal penile urethra and normal prepucial formation. The development of prepuce is independent of the glanular urethra, in their opinion. Nonomura et al. [10] proposed a deformation theory, i.e., ischemic or compressive change after completion of a normal urethra may result in a megameatus and a normally occurring prepuce. Megameatus Intact Prepuce is due to external compression of the penis in utero after completion of penis formation. The urethral plate is always wide and elastic, usually without chordee. Others feel it is embryologically related to the Megalo-urethra. But both of these theories fail to explain the embryology of Megmeatus Intact Prepuce. Bhat et al. [9] proposed the theory of both canalization and tubularization to develop the glanular urethra. Both canalizations of glans and closure of glanular plate are needed for the normal development of the glanular urethra, as opposed to the canalization alone. Thus, when dorsal canalization and the overlying prepucial tubularization are complete, but ventral urethral plate closure remains incomplete, that results in Megameatus Intact Prepuce (Figs. 17.1a, b and 17.2). But when canalization and tubularization do not meet to complete the normal urethra, then it may lead to partial duplication of the urethra with or without hypospadias (Fig. 17.1c).

17.3 Classification [9]

The Megameatus Intact Prepuce is divided based on site of meatus into:
1. Glanular: The meatus is usually wide, and the frenulum is well-formed. A deep groove can be seen clearly. The stream is well-formed, and the appearance of the penis is almost normal (Figs. 17.1b and 17.3a)
2. Coronal: The meatus is located at the corona, two grooves are well seen, and the frenulum is attached proximally to the meatus. The urinary stream is well-formed (Fig. 17.3b)
3. Sub-coronal: Meatus just proximal to corona, frenulum not well-formed, and urinary stream is splayed (Fig. 17.3c)

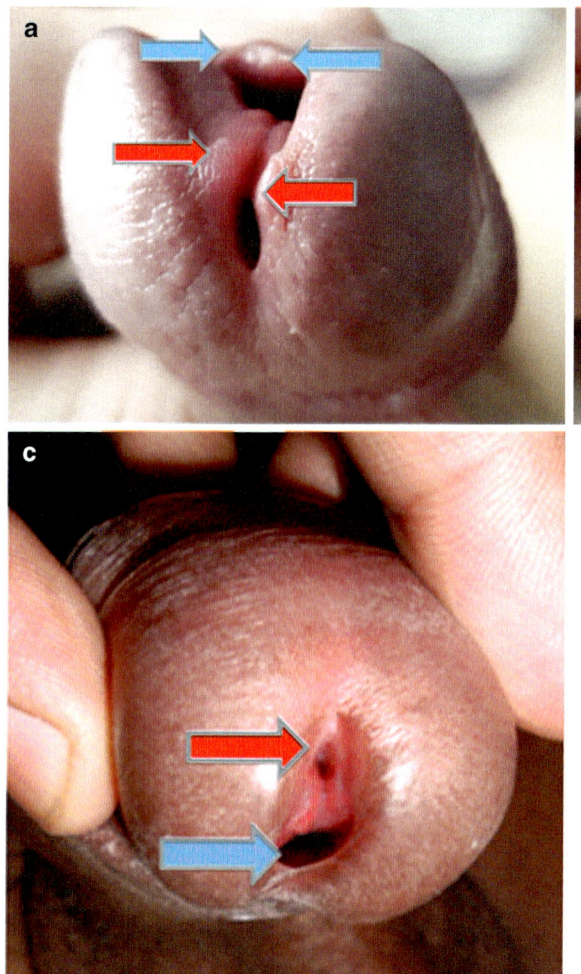

Fig. 17.1 Landmarks of incomplete development of the distal urethra. (**a, b**) Dorsal canalization is complete red arrows showing margins canalized urethra and ventral urethral plate closure remains incomplete tubularization as shown by the blue arrow. (**c**) Dorsal red arrow showing dorsal incomplete canalization leading to duplication of the urethra and a blue ventral arrow showing incomplete tubularization of Glanular hypospadias

4. Distal penile: This is the most severe form of MIP, meatus is located in the distal penile shaft, and the urinary stream is splayed (Fig. 17.3d)

17.4 Diagnosis

Hypospadias diagnosis is made at birth because of an incomplete prepuce, but this anomaly is frequently missed, as it is hidden due to the preputial covering. Many patients who are un-noticed may present for any other problem because they usually do not have symptoms. Recognition is common at the time of religious circumcision in newborns but may be diagnosed at adulthood, clinician's visit for another disease or during catheterization. Though it was reported that the anomaly is not associated with chordee, we found the anomaly is associated with dorsal curvature (Fig. 17.4a), sometimes may have ventral curvature (Fig. 17.4b), partial urethral duplication (Fig. 17.1c), and penile torsion (Fig. 17.5a, b).

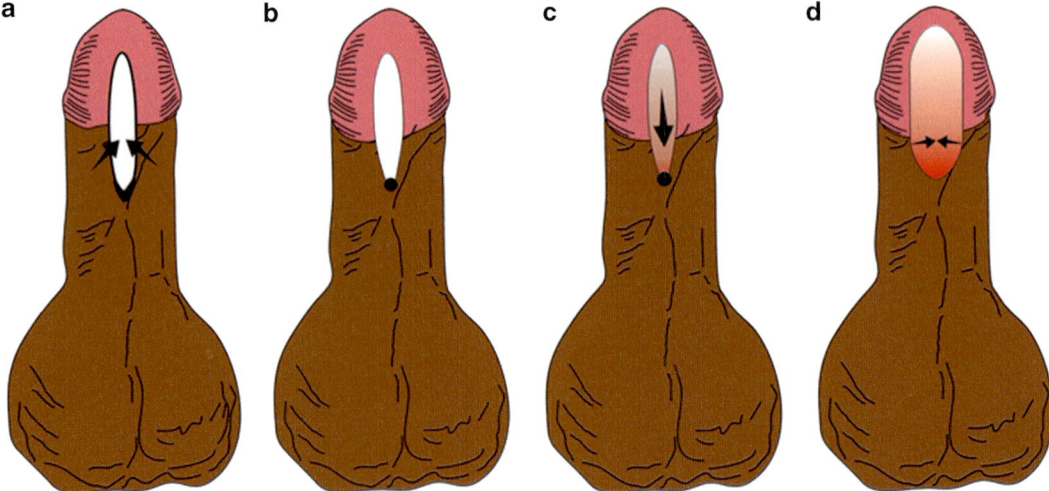

Fig. 17.2 Diagrammatic representation of the development of Megameatus Intact Prepuce. (**a**) Proximal to distal Closure of urethral fold. (**b**) The arrest of urethral fold closure and prepucial closure ventrally forms hypospadias (splayed glans and hooded prepuce). (**c**) Canalization of the glanular plate started and proceeded proximally. (**d**) Complete fusion of the urethral and prepuce fold. Canalization of glanular plate completed up to corona. However, there is no closure of glanular folds (incomplete tubularization)—Results in megameatus intact prepuce

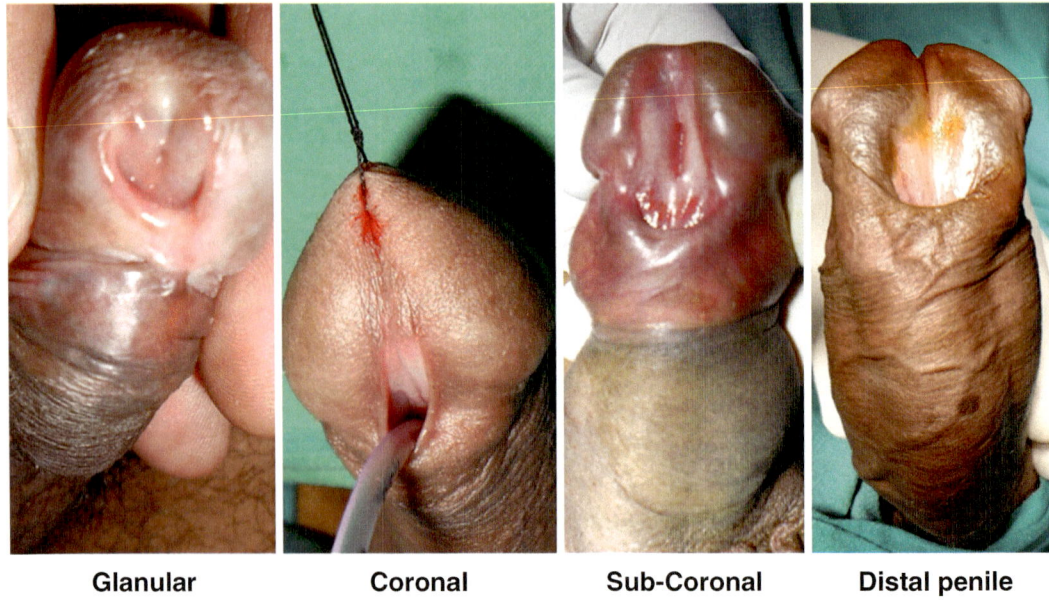

Glanular **Coronal** **Sub-Coronal** **Distal penile**

Fig. 17.3 Showing the classification of Megameatus Intact Prepuce

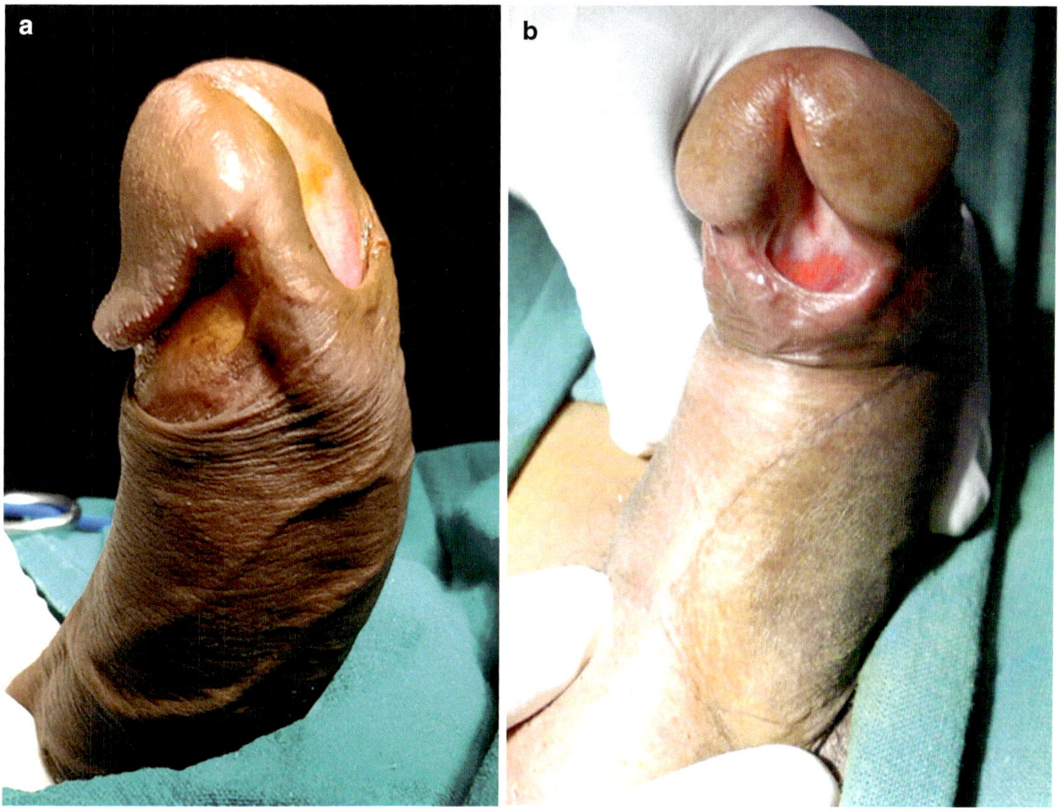

17 Management of Megmeatus Intact Prepuce/Concealed Hypospadias

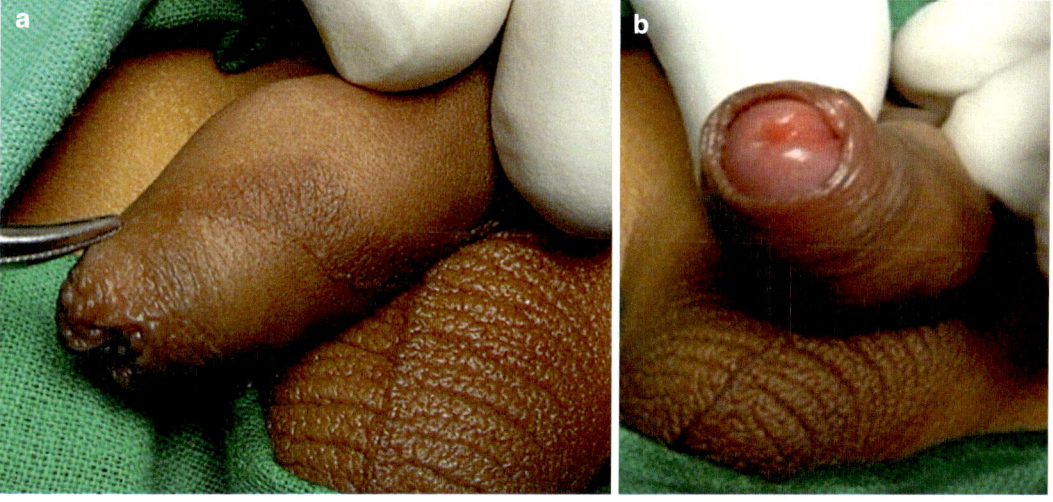

Fig. 17.4 Showing the associated Chordee with Megameatus Intact Prepuce. (**a**) Associated with dorsal curvature. (**b**) Associated with Ventral Curvature

Fig. 17.5 Showing the associated penile torsion with Megameatus Intact Prepuce. (**a**) Median raphe going dorsally indicative of 180 degrees. (**b**) Showing partially retracted prepuce showing meatus dorsally

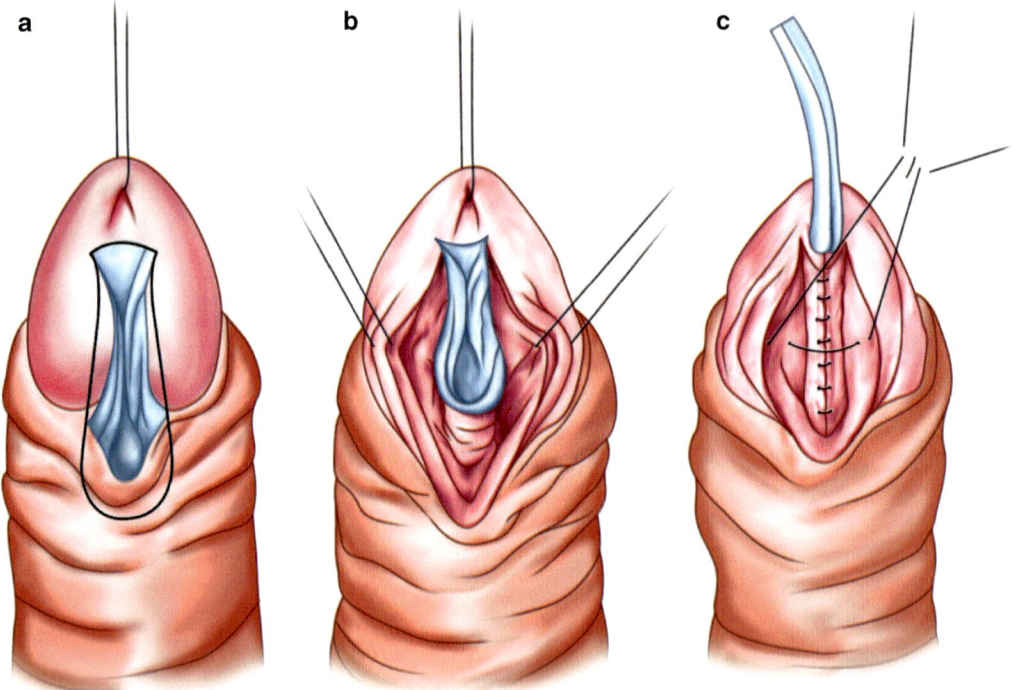

Fig. 17.6 Showing the Pyramid procedure in Megameatus Intact Prepuce. (**a**) U-shape incision around the urethral plate. (**b**) Raising the Glanular wings. (c) Tubularization of urethral plate and glansplasty started

17.5 Surgical Techniques

The surgical techniques for management of megameatus intact prepuce are:

17.5.1 Pyramid Procedure (Fig. 17.6)

1. A tennis racket shape incision is given around the margins of the urethral plate beside the groove of the glans down to the corona level (Fig. 17.6a).
2. The mobilization of the urethra is done up to the apex of the pyramid.
3. Then, the incision deepened proximally to create the glanular wings keeping the distal urethral plate intact dorsally (Fig. 17.6b).
4. Then, a small wedge is taken from the ventral tissue, and the distal urethra is sutured in continuity with the urethral plate (Fig. 17.6c).
5. In the next step urethra and the glanular wings are Tubularized over a stent to form the neourethra.
6. Then the glanuloplasty is done.

17.5.2 Modified Granular Approximation Procedure GAP (Fig. 17.7)

1. A U-Shaped incision is given around the Megameatus and the urethral plate.
2. Partial penile degloving is done.
3. Then, the glans wings are raised to assess the urethral width better (Fig. 17.1a).
4. The excess redundant urethral plate is trimmed to make the diameter of the urethra the same as that of the proximal urethra (Fig. 17.7b, c).
5. The urethral plate is Tubularized with 4–6/ Vicryl/PDS urethral tube according to the size of the urethra (Fig. 17.7d).

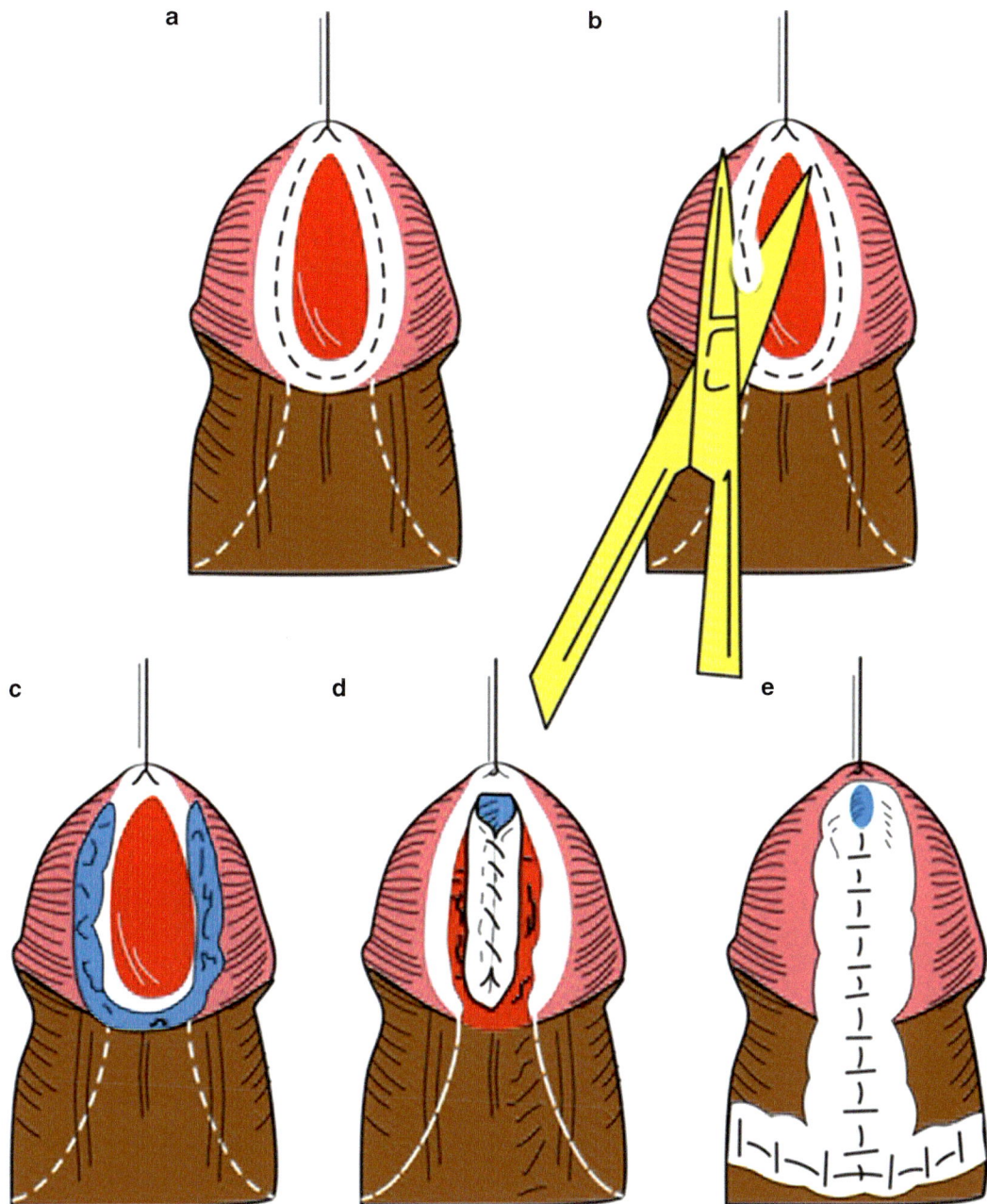

Fig. 17.7 Showing the GAP procedure in Megameatus Intact Prepuce. (**a**) The incision in the glans and distal penile shaft. (**b**) Excision of glanular margins. (**c**) Raising the glanular wing. (**d**) Closure of a urethral plate in the glans. (**e**) Closure of skin and Glans

6. Dorsal dartos or ventral dartos is harvested to cover the Neo-urethra as an intermediate layer (Fig. 17.7e).
7. Glanular wings are sutures over it to complete the urethroplasty and glansplasty followed by skin closure.

17.5.3 The Mathieu Technique

1. The vertical incisions are given on either side of the glans parallel to the urethral plate.
2. Same length and skin incision marked on the ventral surface of the shaft.
3. The glanular wings are dissected, ensuring the preservation of the urethral mucosa.
4. The excess mucosa is trimmed.
5. Parameatal based skin flap is raised.
6. The margins of the flap are sutured to the margins of the urethral plate after putting in the stent.
7. The glanular wings are sutured over the neo-urethra having an adequate meatus to complete the glanuloplasty followed by skin closure.

17.5.4 Tubularized Incised Plate Urethroplasty (TIP)

1. A circumscribing incision is given around the Mega meatus, and penile degloving is done.
2. Parallel longitudinal incisions are given approximately 6–8 mm apart to separate the glans from the lateral margins of the plate. The wings of the glans are developed and mobilized for subsequent tension-free glans closure.
3. After which, the urethral plate is deeply incised from the meatus to the end of the plate, just below the tip of the glans penis. Next, the incised urethral plate is tubularized over a catheter as a stent; the epithelium of the urethral plate is inverted toward the lumen to avoid fistula formation.
4. A vascularized dartos fascia flap covers the urethroplasty as a second layer; then, the prepuce is divided and rotated on both sides to cover the second layer.
5. Glanular wings are closed over neo-urethra to complete glansplasty, and skin closure is completed.

17.5.5 Tubularized Urethral Plate Urethroplasty (TUPU)

The prepuce is retracted, and a U-shape incision is given encircling the meatus, and only inner prepucial skin is incised (Fig. 17.8a, b, c). Dissection plane is created just proximal to the meatus at the level of tunica albuginea, and the urethral plate with spongiosum is mobilized up to mid-glans, and glanular flaps are raised (Fig. 17.8d). The margin of the urethral plate is trimmed in case of wider urethral plate than required. The tubularization of the urethral plate is done, keeping a wide urethral meatus (Fig. 17.8e). Spongiosum is sutured over the neourethra to complete the spongioplasty; glanular flaps are sutured for glansplasty (Fig. 17.8f, g). Inner prepucial skin closure reconstructs the frenulum creating normal meatus and intact prepuce (Fig. 17.8h, i). The following modifications in the classical Thiersch–Duplay technique are done for TUPU. The neourethra is covered with spongiosum in place of the dorsal dartos flap to preserve the prepuce, and frenuloplasty is done to create a normal-appearing penis and prepuce. Patients are followed at 1, 3, 6, 9, and 12 months. Postoperative results are excellent, with a wide slit-like meatus at the tip, well-formed prepuce, and frenulum.

17.5.6 TUPU in MIP with Chordee or Torque

Circum-coronal circumferential incision is given in cases with mild to moderate chordee or torsion, and complete penile de-gloving is done (Fig. 17.9a, b, c). The Gittes test is done to see the chordee correction (Fig. 17.9d). Then the urethral plate with spongiosum and proximal

17 Management of Megmeatus Intact Prepuce/Concealed Hypospadias

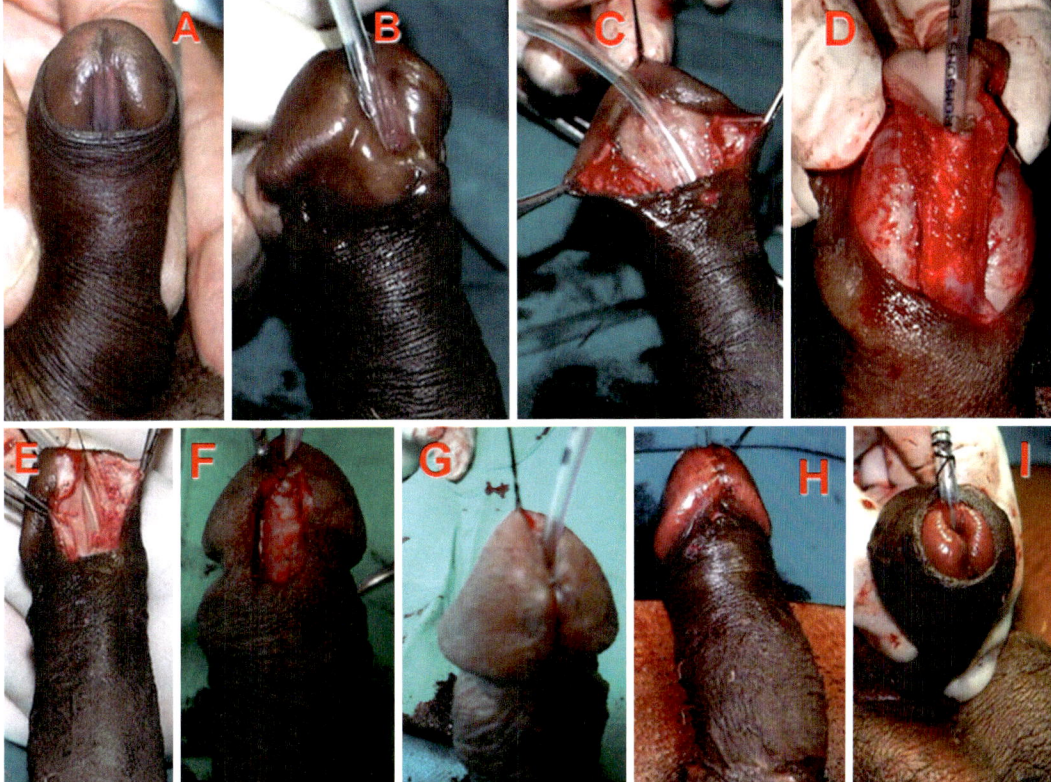

Fig. 17.8 Showing the Tubularized Urethral Plate Urethroplasty in Megameatus Intact Prepuce. (**a**) Sub-coronal Megameatus Intact prepuce. (**b**) Urethral stent inserted after the injection of 1:100,000 solution of adrenaline at the site of incision. (**c**) Inverted U-shaped incision given. (**d**) Urethral plate and spongiosum Mobilization. (**e**) Urethral plate tubularization started. (**f**) Spongioplasty. (**g**) Glanuloplasty. (**h** and **i**) Frenuloplasty and skin closure with intact prepuce

urethra is mobilized, and chordee/torque correction (Fig. 17.9e, f). If chordee/torque still persists, the urethral plate with spongiosum is mobilized into the glans. The Gittes test is repeated to confirm the chordee/torque correction. (Fig. 17.9g, h, i). Then the urethral plate is tubularized, and spongioplasty is done (Fig. 17.9j, k). The glanuloplasty is done to create a conical glans with the slit-like opening at the tip and Gittes test is done to confirm chordee/torsion correction (Fig. 17.9l, m, n). Then frenuloplasty & skin closure is done to create a normal frenulum and prepuce (Fig. 17.9l, m, n). A urethral catheter is put in and removed in 7–10 days and is followed up 1, 3, 6, 9, and 12 months. Patients/parents are asked to start retracting the prepuce after 4–6 weeks.

17.5.7 The Subcutaneous Frenulum Flap (Scuff)

1. A circum-meatal incision is given, and degloving of the penis is done.
2. Then glanular wings are raised.
3. The redundant mucosa trimmed and tubularization of the urethral plate is done over a stent.
4. Then, a well-vascularized inferior-based frenulum flap is developed.
5. The skin is de-epithelialized and advanced over the neourethra.
6. Then, the glanular wings are sutured to complete the glanuloplasty, and skin closure is done.

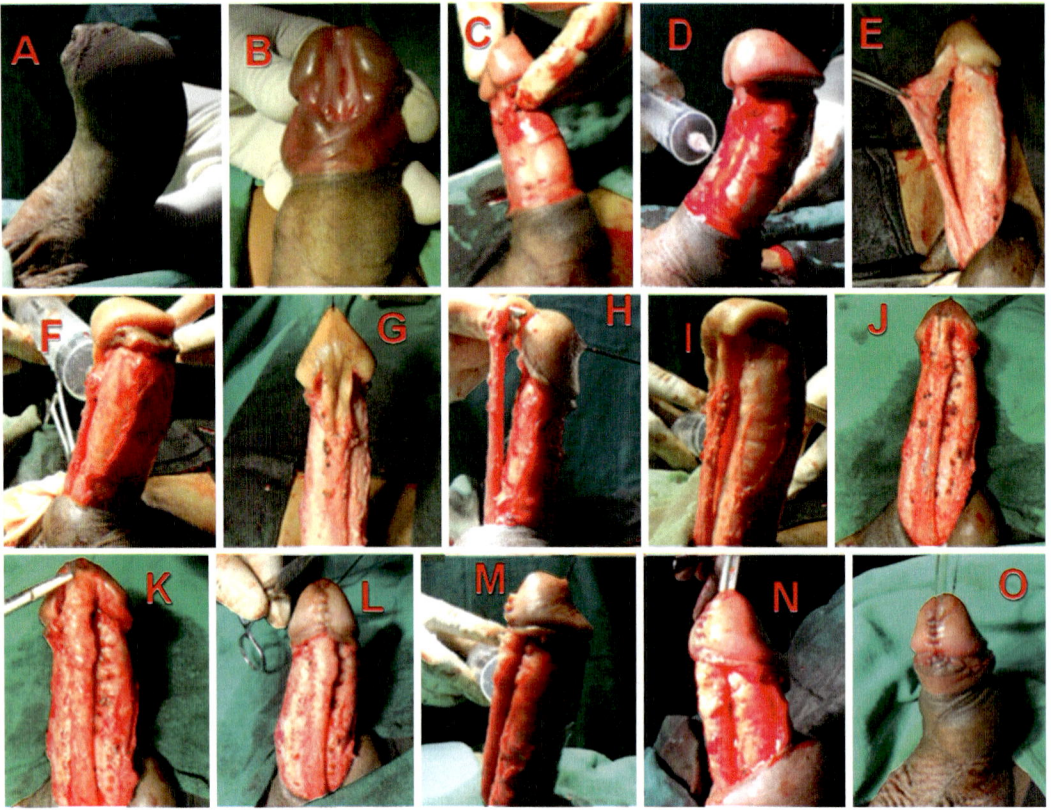

Fig. 17.9 Showing the Tubularized Urethral Plate Urethroplasty in Megameatus Intact Prepuce with ventral chordee. (**a** and **b**) Distal penile Megameatus Intact prepuce with moderate chordee. (**c**) De-gloving of the Penile skin. (**d**) Gittes test showing persistence of Chordee. (**e**) Urethral plate with spongiosum and proximal urethral mobilization and Lateral mobilization of Buck's Fascia. (**f**) Gittes test showing persistence of Chordee. (**g** and **h**) Urethral plate with spongiosum mobilization up to the mid-glans. (**i**) Gittes test showing correction of Chordee with glanular tilt. (**j**) Tubularization of the urethral plate. (**k**) Spongioplasty. (**l**) Glanuloplasty. (**m** and **n**) Gittes test showing correction of Chordee and glanular tilt corrected. (**o**) Frenuloplasty and skin closure

17.6 Choice of Technique

In a case report, a 41-year-old male was the only case managed conservatively, and authors advocated the patient participation in the surgical intervention decision [6]. But surgery is the treatment of choice in modern hypospadiology, giving excellent results in functionality and cosmesis in MIP patients. The good results of the Mathieu and the MAGPI are acceptable in distal hypospadias. Still, the techniques being not ideal for Mega meatus intact prepuce led to the development of techniques specifically to be used for the MIP. However, GAP is technically less demanding and achieves good results in glanular defects but has limitations. These are the unequal size of neo-urethra due to non-mobilization of glanular wings and superimposition of glanular suture lines without an interposing tissue layer which may lead to fistula. Dissatisfied with the results, people have modified the glanular approximation procedure by mobilizing glanular wings equal to the size of neo-urethra with that of the normal urethra for tension-free urethroplasty and added interposing a dorsal dartos layer. Though the cutaneous advancement techniques have also been used for megameatus intact prepuce, that may not be suitable for distal penile MIP, and also the glanular defect remains uncorrected.

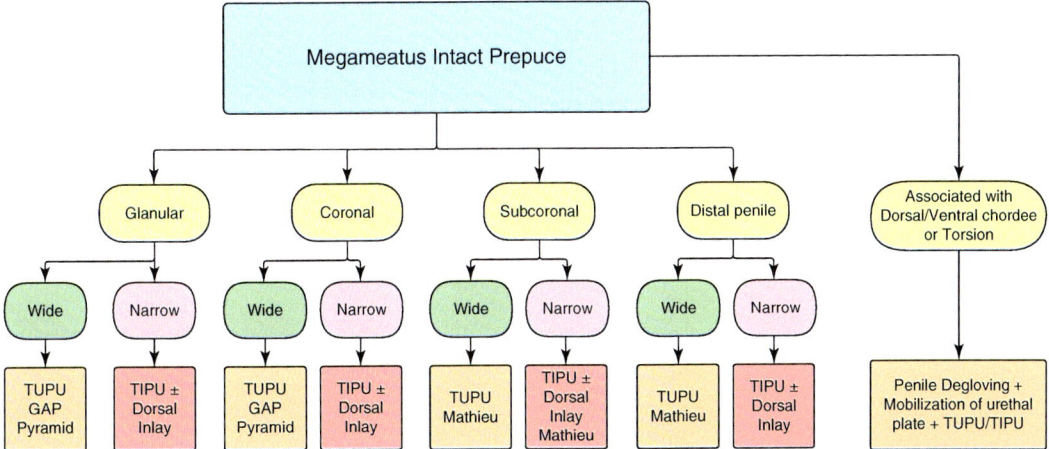

Fig. 17.10 Algorithm for management of Mega meatus Intact Prepuce

MIP is a surgical challenge in circumcised patients because the penile skin is usually thin and scarred and lacks the prepucial and dartos tissue. However, Snodgrass had good results in circumcised patients and narrated that circumcision does not affect the results of TIPU in MIP [11].

The anatomic characteristics of the MIP present a unique challenge to surgeons. The wide meatus and urethral plate dissection may create thin glanular wings more prone to dehiscence and urethral fistula formation. The TIP urethroplasty technique allows for better glanular wings and thicker glanular wings for glanular reconstruction. Because the lateral aspects of the urethral plate are not dissected as they are with the Pyramid and GAP. Nevertheless, the incision in the urethral plate is needed only in the narrow urethral plate, which is rare in MIP. So, we opted for tubularized urethral plate urethroplasty (TUPU) as it allows for more formal dissection of the glans wings on the expanse of the width of the urethral plate. Adding spongioplasty and frenuloplasty to tubularized urethral plate urethroplasty (TUPU) restores the normal urethral and penile anatomy. Based on the type of MIP and width of the urethral plate, an algorithm is proposed to manage MIP (Fig. 17.10). All kinds of MIP can be managed with TUPU or TIPU and GAP. Even minor to moderate curvature and torsion can also be corrected by mobilization urethral plate with spongiosum and urethra. The procedure is feasible with a good surgical outcome even after circumcision.

17.7 Conclusion

Megameatus Intact Prepuce is likely to be missed frequently due to the preputial covering. Patients being asymptomatic may present late. Examination of meatus by retracting the prepuce before circumcision is helpful in the early diagnosis and management of MIP. Surgical correction of MIP in the current era of increased cosmetic awareness is justified. It is a variant of anterior hypospadias, and the repair is feasible by the techniques used for distal hypospadias repair. Excellent functional and cosmetic outcome is seen with tubularized urethral plate urethroplasty (TUPU) with a few modifications like spongioplasty, prepuce preservation, and frenuloplasty. A wide urethral plate and well-developed spongiosum are available. Therefore, it should be the procedure of choice in all cases of MIP. Incised urethral plate urethroplasty is suitable for cases with a narrow urethral plate. Mathieu or onlay flap urethroplasty are rarely required for correction of MIP.

References

1. Juskiewenski S, Vaysse P, Guitard J, Moscovici J. Treatment of anterior hypospadias. Place of balanoplasty. Chir Pediatr. 1983;24(1):75–9.
2. Duckett JW, Keating MA. The technical challenge of the megameatus intact prepuce hypospadias variant: the pyramid procedure. J Urol. 1989;141(6):1407–9.
3. Bar-Yosef Y, Binyamini J, Mullerad M, Matzkin H, Ben-Chaim J. Megameatus intact prepuce hypospadias variant: application of tubularized incised plate urethroplasty. Urology. 2005;66(4):861–4.
4. Hill GA, Wacksman J, Lewis AG, Sheldon CA. The modified pyramid hypospadias procedure: repair of megameatus and deep glanular groove variants. J Urol. 1993;150(4):1208–11.
5. Sanal M, Karadag E, Konca Y, Kocabasoglu U. Megameatus and intact prepuce (MIP) associated with meatal web-a case report. Acta Chirurgica Austriaca. 2000;32(1):35–6.
6. Bourdoumis A, Kapoor S, Bhanot S. Megameatus intact prepuce revisited. Br J Urol Int. 2012.
7. Duckett JW. MAGPI (meatoplasty and glanuloplasty): a procedure for subcoronal hypospadias. Urol Clin North Am. 1981;8(3):513–9.
8. Zaontz MR. The GAP (glans approximation procedure) for glanular/coronal hypospadias. J Urol. 1989;141(2):359–61.
9. Bhat A, Bhat M, Bhat A, Singh V. Results of tubularized urethral plate urethroplasty in megameatus intact prepuce. Indian J Urol. 2017;33(4):315.
10. Nonomura K, Kakizaki H, Shimoda N, Koyama T, Murakumo M, Koyanagi T. Surgical repair of anterior hypospadias with fish-mouth meatus and intact prepuce based on anatomical characteristics. Eur Urol. 1998;34(4):368–71. https://doi.org/10.1159/000019742.
11. Snodgrass WT, Khavari R. Prior circumcision does not complicate hypospadias repair with an intact prepuce. J Urol. 2006;176(1):296–8.

Management of Penile Torsion in Hypospadias and Isolated Penile Torsion

18

Amilal Bhat

18.1 Introduction

Penile torsion is a three-dimensional axial rotational defect of the distal corporal bodies of the penile shaft as the corporal bodies' proximal part remain fixed to the pubic rami by its attachment. The median raphe deviates from the penis base around the penile shaft in a spiral manner to terminate at the distal end of the foreskin on the lateral or dorsal aspect (depending on the severity of torsion). The urethral meatus is rotated in the direction of the torque. The torque is more common toward the left side (counterclockwise) [1–3]. Verneuil described the first case of Congenital penile torsion with hypospadias in 1857. It can also be identified by the direction of the urethral meatus [1]. The direction of the meatus differentiates the penile torsion from the ventral and lateral chordee as the urethral meatus rotates toward torsion and remains orientated vertically in the pure ventral or lateral chordee. Diagnosis of penile torque may be delayed in phimosis till circumcision is done, or the foreskin becomes retractable to access glans. It is yet to be known how much of a functional or sexual difficulty this malformation causes in adults. It is important to counsel the parents and families about the problem and its correction as children are asymptomatic. Many parents may wish to get corrected for cosmetic reasons [1]. The torsion associated with hypospadias should be managed with the correction of the hypospadiac deformity.

18.2 Incidence

Penile torque/torsion is a rare congenital anomaly, and its true incidence is unknown. The penile torsion is rarely symptomatic, so it is often passed unnoticed/unreported historically and changes the true incidence [3, 5, 6]. Penile torsion is more common and severe in distal hypospadias and chordee without hypospadias. At the same time, it is almost absent in perineal and perineoscrotal hypospadias. The incidence of isolated penile torsion is 1.7% to 27%, and more than 90° is seen in 0.7% only [1–3]. The penile torque is more common on the left side (up to 99%). Bhat et al. (2009) found a right-to-left ratio of 1:3, in which the right-sided torsion is reported higher than in the litera-

A. Bhat (✉)
Bhat's Hypospadias and Reconstructive Urology Hospital and Research Centre,
Jaipur, Rajasthan, India

Department of Urology, Jaipur National University Institute for Medical Sciences and Research Centre,
Jaipur, Rajasthan, India

Department of Urology, Dr. S.N. Medical College,
Jodhpur, Rajasthan, India

Department of Urology, S.P. Medical College,
Bikaner, Rajasthan, India

P.G. Committee Medical Council of India,
New Delhi, India

Academic and Research Council of RUHS,
Jaipur, Rajasthan, India

ture [7]. Shaeer O (2008) reported 12% penile torque in adults, 80% of them had a mild, and 5% had moderate (60°). Two percent of the cases requested corrective cosmetic surgery [8]. Sarkis and Sadasivam reported isolated penile torsion of more than 5° in 27% of neonatal circumcision patients, while Eroglu et al. found in 20% of neonates [3, 9]. Bhat et al. reported overall 1.97% isolated penile torque and severe in 1.01% neonates, left-to-right ratio was 3:1 while in moderate torque group it was 5:1 [10]. The incidence differences are because of the variations in populations surveyed, systems of classification, and inclusion criteria for minimum torsion [1, 3, 10].

18.3 Etiopathogenesis

The exact etiopathogenesis of penile torsion is unclear as there is minimal data available in the literature. Embryologically, the midline fusion of medial endodermal urethral folds ventrally forms the male urethra at 8 weeks of gestation while fusion of lateral ectodermal urethral folds over the developing urethra forms the penile shaft skin and the prepuce. The fusion of the folds occurs from posterior to anterior and lateral folds fusion forms the median raphe. Mesodermal proliferation between the endo and ectodermal folds forms the corpora and other fascial coverings of the penile shaft [1, 10]. Some authors have expressed their view on the primary defect that the disorientation and the penile shaft rotation around its longitudinal axis are because of the abnormal development, and dartos fascia's & skin attachment. At the same time, the others believe that the defect is because of the asymmetric development of corpus cavernosum or unilateral adhesions between the pubic bone and corpus cavernosum [3, 5, 9]. There are many theories proposed to explain torsion. Recently, Bhat et al. reported that the eccentric fusion of the endodermal and ectodermal folds rather than fusion in the midline causes penile torque. This lateral fusion distally to one side leads to misdirected mesodermal proliferation, attachment of coverings of the penis and spongiosum to one side, causing the torque and deviation of median raphe from midline [1, 7] (Fig. 18.1a–d). The median raphe deviation is a vital sign to diagnose torsion and know its degree in a newborn with unretracted skin [1–3]. The deviation of median raphe is between the corona and penoscrotal junction (Fig. 18.2a–d), which signifies the origin of eccentric fusion.

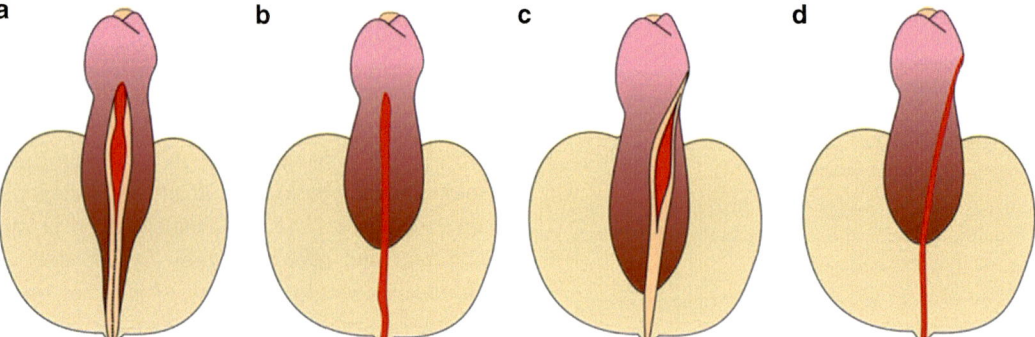

Fig. 18.1 Diagrammatic representation of Embryological explanation. (**a**) Showing the lateral Ectodermal and medial endodermal urethral folds. (**b**) Normal midline fusion from posterior to anterior and central median raphe. (**c**) Eccentric fusion of medial and lateral urethral folds causing torsion. (**d**) The shifted median raphe and penile torque

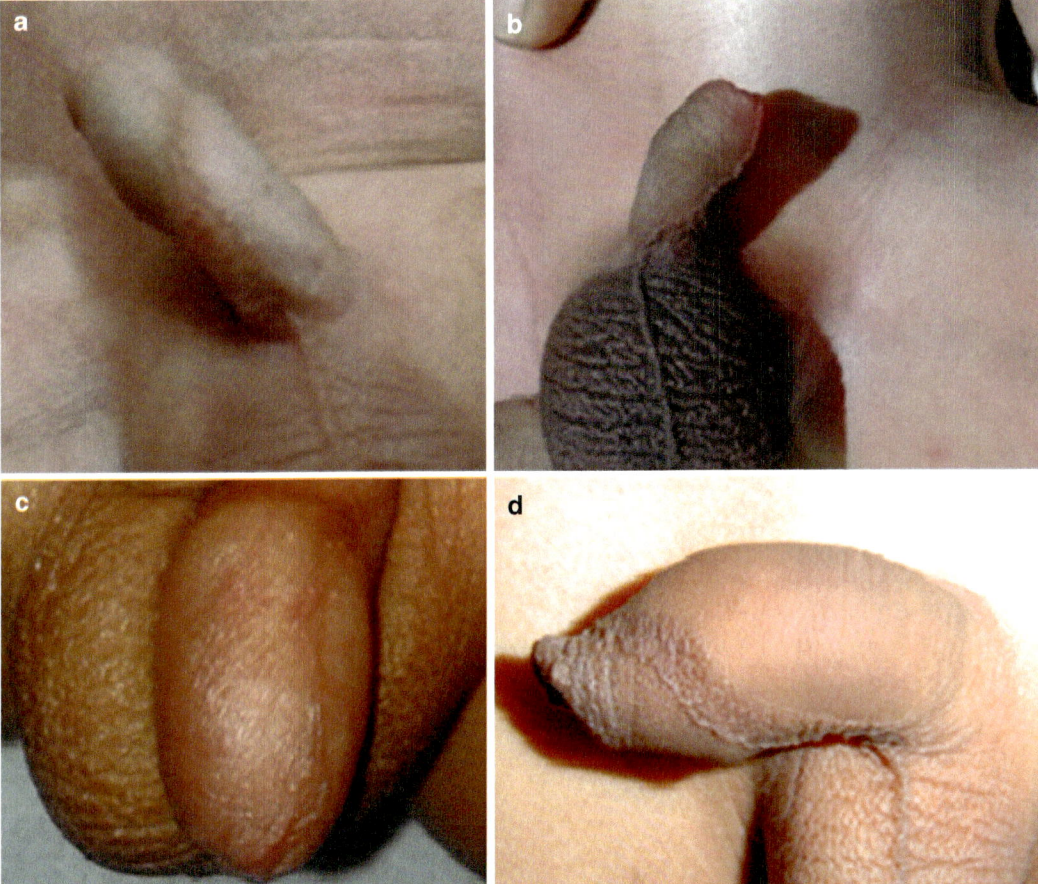

Fig. 18.2 Showing the deviance of Median Raphe at different levels (With permission from Bhat et al. [10] @ copyright Elsevier). (**a**) Showing Deviance of median raphe just proximal corona. (**b**) Deviance of median raphae at the penoscrotal junction; (**c** and **d**) Distal end of median raphae on the dorsal surface of prepuce

18.4 Classifications [1, 8, 9]

Types

A. Penile torsion can be classified according to etiology:
   1. *Congenital*: Congenital penile torsion may be an isolated deformity or may be associated with hypospadias, chordee without hypospadias and epispadias.
   2. *Acquired*: The torsion after surgery for trauma, circumcision, urethral reconstruction and hypospadias repair.
B. Penile torsion is classified according to the direction.
   1. Clockwise, i.e., right side.
   2. Counterclockwise direction toward the left side.
C. Depending on the degree of rotation from the midline, torsion may be classified as:
   1. Mild (<45°)
   2. Moderate (45–90°)
   3. Severe (>90°)

Shaeer et al. have classified

1. Mild 5–30°
2. Moderate 30–60 moderate
3. Severe >60

18.5 Measurement of Penile Torque

Sarkis and Sadasivam method is commonly used. A sterile small protractor is used to is measure the torsion by the urethral meatus deviation from the midline [1, 3, 4]. The measurements are done with meatus direction when meatus is visible with or without retraction of the prepuce (Fig. 18.3). But in cases of phimosis, the measurement is taken by the deviation of median raphe and the index points set is the ending of the median raphe at the tip of the preputium (Fig. 18.4). Another method described for measuring the torsion by the radiologist's software program for image analysis is to measure the rotation angle on a digital penile photograph. It applies to digital pictures pre- and postoperatively and can objectively evaluate torsion correction after surgery [7].

18.6 Corelation of Penile Torque with the Severity of Hypospadias and Chordee

Penile torsion associated with hypospadias is more common than reported. We should look at and note the torsion while examining patients with hypospadias preoperatively. Torsion is more common and severe in anterior hypospadias and chordee without hypospadias, but the chordee is severe and commoner in posterior hypospadias. On correlating, the severity of torsion is inversely proportional to the severity of chordee. The degree of rotation also correlates well with meatus direction toward the side of torsion and median raphe attachment to the dorsal hood toward the opposite side [1, 11]. We found the mean chordee 73.58° ± 32.96° in proximal penile hypospadias compared to 38° ± 18.55° in distal penile hypospadias, and it was statistically

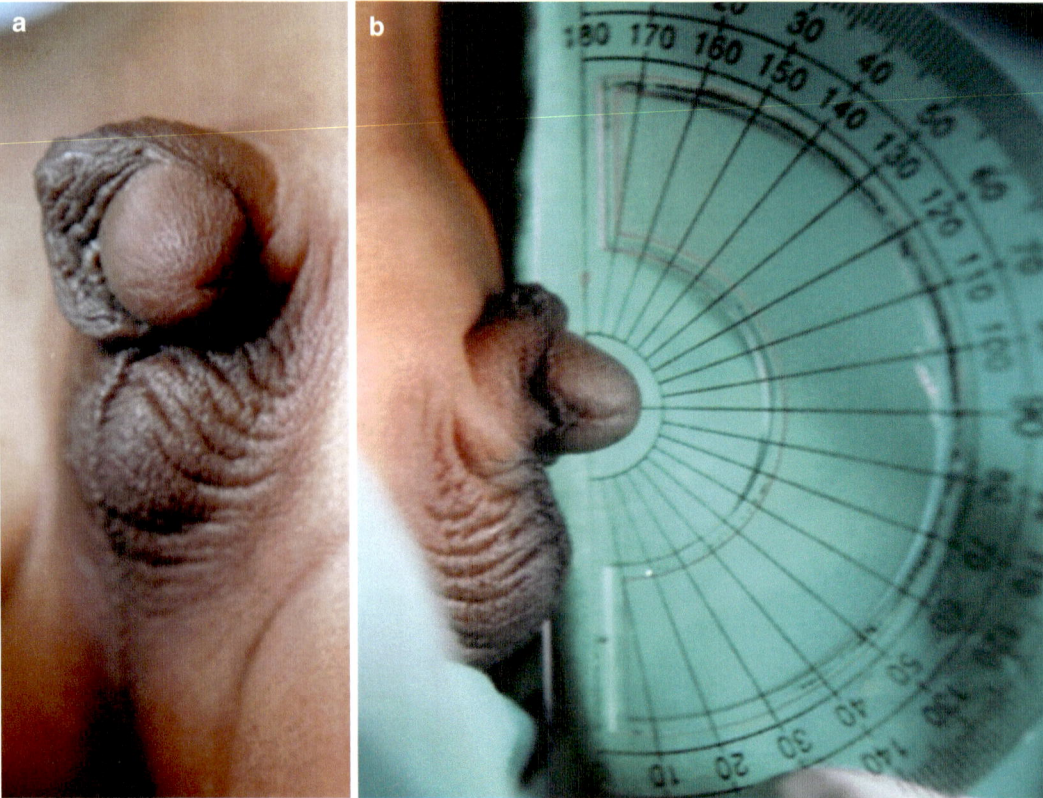

Fig. 18.3 The right torsion and measurement of torsion in hypospadias with torsion. (**a**) 90° right torsion. (**b**) Measurement of torsion by sterile small protractor

18 Management of Penile Torsion in Hypospadias and Isolated Penile Torsion

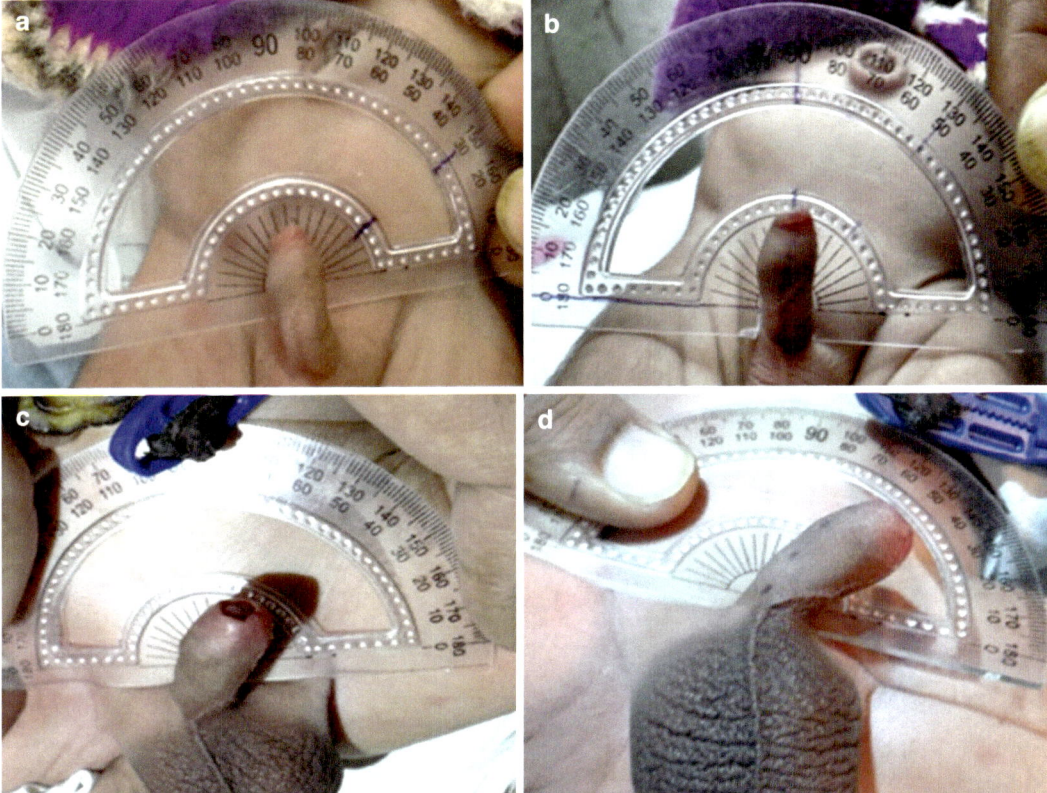

Fig. 18.4 Measurement of penile torsion in patients with phimosis measuring the (**a**) Deviance of median raphe from the midline. (**b**) Showing median raphe Deviance at the penoscrotal junction. (**c** and **d**) Median raphe ending on the dorsal surface of the prepuce (With permission Bhat et al. [10] @copyright Elsevier)

significant (P-value = 0.001). However, torsion was statistically significantly severe in distal hypospadias (62.38° ± 23.03°) than the mid penile (38.04° ± 18.50°) and proximal hypospadias vs. (18.25° ± 3.33°), ($P = 0.001$) (Table 18.1).

18.7 Management

Since the isolated penile torque/torsion is a benign condition and is asymptomatic except cosmetic disfigurement, surgical correction is not needed in less than 60-degree torsion [12]. Torsion correction associated with hypospadias or chordee without hypospadias is done with repairing these anomalies to achieve a cosmetically normal penis. So, the recognition of torsion is important before deciding the surgery and can be corrected by adding a simple maneuver such as penile degloving and reattaching.

18.8 Indication of Surgery

1. Torsion associated with Hypospadias or Chordee without Hypospadias.
2. More than 90° in isolated penile torsion.

18.9 Surgical Techniques

The common techniques described to correct penile torsion are penile degloving and reattaching the skin, plication procedures dorsal dartos wrap, and urethral plate and spongiosum. However, none of the techniques has been

Table 18.1 Correlation of type of hypospadias with severity of torsion and chordee

Hypospadias type	No. of cases (100)	Torsion range 15–110° (Mean 51.98°)[a], Range (Mean ± SD)	Correlation of torsion severity with hypospadias severity (total no. of Torsion 100)			Chordee Range 15–125° (Mean 46.58°)[b] Range (Mean± SD)	Correlation of severity of chordee with severity of hypospadias (Total no. of Cases-60; distal-34, mid-14, and proximal-12)		
			Total no. of mild degree	Total no. of moderate degree	Total no. of severe degree		Total no. of mild degree	Total no. of moderate degree	Total no. of severe degree
Distal	67 (67%)	25–110° (62.38 ± 23.03)	22 (32.83%)	36 (53.73%)	09 (13.43%)	15–90° (38.00 ± 18.55)	26 (76.48%)	08 (23.52%)	00 (0.00%)
Mid Penile	21 (21%)	25–90° (38.04 ± 18.50)	17 (80.95%)	04 (19.04%)	00 (0.00%)	15–90° (44.28 ± 21.11)	10 (71.43%)	04 (28.57%)	00 (0.00%)
Proximal	12 (12%)	15–25° (18.25 ± 3.33)	12 (100.00%)	00 (0.00%)	00 (0.00%)	25–125° (73.58 ± 32.96)	04 (33.3%)	03 (25.00%)	05 (41.66%)
Total	100		51 (51%)	40 (40%)	09 (9%)		40 (66.66%)	15 (25%)	05 (8.33%)
p value		0.001				0.001			

[a] Correlation of torsion severity with hypospadias type
Distal vs. mid penile: $t = 4.41$, $P = 0.001$
Distal vs. proximal: $t = 6.59$, $P = 0.001$
Mid penile vs. proximal: $t = 3.64$, $P = 0.001$
[b] Correlation chordee severity with hypospadias type
Distal vs. mid penile: $t = 1.30$, $P = 0.197$
Distal vs. proximal: $t = 5.34$, $P = 0.001$
Mid penile vs. proximal: $t = 3.12$, $P = 0.001$

accepted as the ideal one and accepted universally. The surgical procedures for correction of congenital penile torsion are as follows:

18.9.1 Penile Degloving and Skin Reattachment Technique

Azmy and Eckstein technique of penile degloving and reattaching the skin is straightforward [13]. The exact torsion measurement is taken after artificial penile erection, followed by penile degloving through a circumferential sub-coronal incision. Residual torsion is corrected re-suturing skin on glans at a 12-o'clock position to counter the residual torque, and loose ventral penile skin wedge is resected. The resultant skin tightening facilitates the proper alignment of the penis and better cosmesis, and then the rest of the circumferential incision is closed. The satisfactory results of 95% in isolated penile torsion were reported by penile degloving and realignment of the skin in a study by Bar-Yosef et al. (2007) [5]. Advantages of the technique are, it can easily be done even by beginners and has fewer chances of complication because of the limited dissection. The disadvantages are effective only in mild torsion, chances of recurrences in moderate and severe torsion, correction by an exact measurement being difficult, and may lead to under-correction.

18.9.2 Johnson's Technique

A circular incision is given at the base of the penis, and then the skin is re-sutured, adjusting the torsion correction. It again is an easy technique but effective only in mild torsion and having chances of the under-correction or recurrence of torque. The complication rates are high as it hampers the venous and lymphatic supply of penile skin. Tryfonas et al. had 25% keloid, 50% lymphedema, and 50% ugly scar at the base of the penis with this technique. The results were better when a circumcoronal incision was given [14, 15].

18.9.3 Nesbit Technique (Corporal Plication)

The plication technique is commonly used for the correction of ventral curvature. The same principle applied for the correction of penile torsion also. A circumferential circumcoronal coronal skin incision is given, and penile degloving is done. The site of maximal torsion is marked after creating artificial erection by injecting saline, and elliptical sections are marked on the elongated corpora. The orientation of the ellipses is determined by the degree of the torsion. These ellipses are excised at 45-degree angles to the longitudinal axis of the phallus. Varying the ellipses' angles will determine the proportion of corporeal shortening to corporeal de-rotation caused by each elliptical excision and primary closure. This creates a counter torque on the penis to fix the torsion. Traction sutures are placed along both borders of each marked ellipse. These sutures are then crossed and clamped to simulate the results obtained with actual excision and primary closure. In this manner, the correct combination of number, positioning, and angling of the segments to be excised can be determined after choosing the right combination for a given patient. The marked sections are excised with care to avoid the extension to the underlying erectile tissue. The defects in the tunica albuginea are then closed with 2-zero polyglycolic acid with interrupted sutures. The sutures are angled obliquely across the excised ellipse are tied to the de-torque of the shaft. After all, ellipses are closed and Gittes test is again done to confirm the adequacy of the correction. Further sections are excised if necessary. The skin closure is done by re-approximating the margins [16].

18.9.4 Diagonal Corporal Plication

The penile skin degloving is done up to the base of the penis and the Gittes is done to see the severity of chordee. The skin is over-rotated to allow the penis to be straight in the flaccid state and sutured to complete the repair; if the penile torsion is resolved with degloving of the shaft skin. If the artificial erection shows the persistence of the penile torsion, an inverted permanent braided 4–0 diagonal plicating suture is taken parallel to the neurovascular bundle on the maximal torsion site and the opposite half of the suture is taken parallel to the neurovascular bundle more proximally. These diagonal plicating sutures are then tied to protect the neurovascular bundle. The Gittes test is repeated to confirm the torsion correction. If the torsion persists, additional diagonal plicating sutures are taken. In case torsion continues, an incision in the tunica albuginea on each corpus beside the plicating sutures can be used to allow freshed cut edges to heal the plication if desired permanently [17].

18.9.5 Suturing Tunica Albuginea to the Pubic Periosteum [12]

The penile skin degloving is done, and all Buck's fascia attachments are dissected at the root of the penis. Next, the artificial erection test is done to see for torsion correction. If torsion persists, it is corrected by suturing the lateral edge of the corpus cavernosum to the pubic periosteum. Sutures are taken in tunica albuginea and passed through the pubic periosteum, and tied balancing torsion correction. The simple technique requires extensive dissection at the root of the penis, challenging to adjust correction and are chances of the bone infection.

Though Plication procedures are the most commonly used techniques with various modifications and variable results but are effective in mild to moderate torque.

Disadvantages of plication procedures are:

1. Against anatomical Principles
2. Shortens the penis
3. Recurrent torsion
4. Chances of nerve injury
5. Impotence
6. Numbness to glans and penile shaft
7. Penile pain
8. Can correct mild to moderate torque

These are not effective in severe torsion of more than 90°. In addition, the sutures may give way early or dissolve, causing the recurrence, and are against the anatomical surgical principles producing the counter torsion [1, 7, 11].

18.9.6 Dorsal Dartos Wrap Rotation Technique: [1, 18, 19]

The procedure starts with an exact measurement of torsion in degree and direction by the artificial erection test, and penile skin degloving is performed through a sub-coronal circumferential incision. Then a dartos flap is developed from the dorsal or dorsolateral penile skin and mobilized. The flap raised is wide-based and thick enough to assure vascularization and to maintain its integrity without compromising vascularity of the skin. The flap is then rotated across the dorsum of the penis to counter the torsion (clockwise or anticlockwise). Next, the flap's tip is sutured distally to the tunica albuginea's lateral aspect with sturdy inverted sutures. This counterrotation corrects torsion, and re-adjustment of the position of the flap's tip may be performed according to the desired degree of counterrotation.

Further adjustments can be made by plication or release of the proximal edge of the flap. The degloved skin is then sutured back to its original position. The final torsion correction is confirmed by the artificial erection (Gittes) test. Advantages are a simple technique that can be done by a beginner and can be done with hypospadias repair.

Disadvantages are ineffectiveness in severe torsion, chances of recurrence if sutures give way. It is difficult to adjust torsion's exact correction and produce the counter-torque rather than correcting the cause [1, 7, 11].

18.9.7 Urethral Mobilization Technique: [1, 7, 11, 20–23]

Bhat et al. reported urethral mobilization technique effective in correcting both penile torsion and chordee. Furthermore, the idea of torsion correction by urethral mobilization was perceived while reviewing the video recordings of chordee correction by the same technique.

Steps of the Technique

1. Penile skin degloving.
2. Mobilization of the divergent corpus spongiosum with urethral plate.
3. Proximal urethral mobilization up to the bulbar urethra.
4. Urethral plate and spongiosum mobilization into glans.
5. Spongioplasty.
6. Glanuloplasty.

The severity of torsion is measured by the urethral meatus deviation from the midline and the median raphe deviation toward the dorsal hood or foreskin in cases of chordee without hypospadias (Fig. 18.5a, b, c). 1:100,000 adrenaline solution is injected at the proposed site of the incision. A U-shaped incision encircling the urethral plate and preserving it is given and extended to the circumferential circumcoronal site in the hypospadias cases. A circumcoronal circumferential incision is given in chordee without hypospadias cases. A dissection plane is created at Buck's fascia, and penile skin degloving is done up to the root of the penis (Fig. 18.5d). An artificial erec-

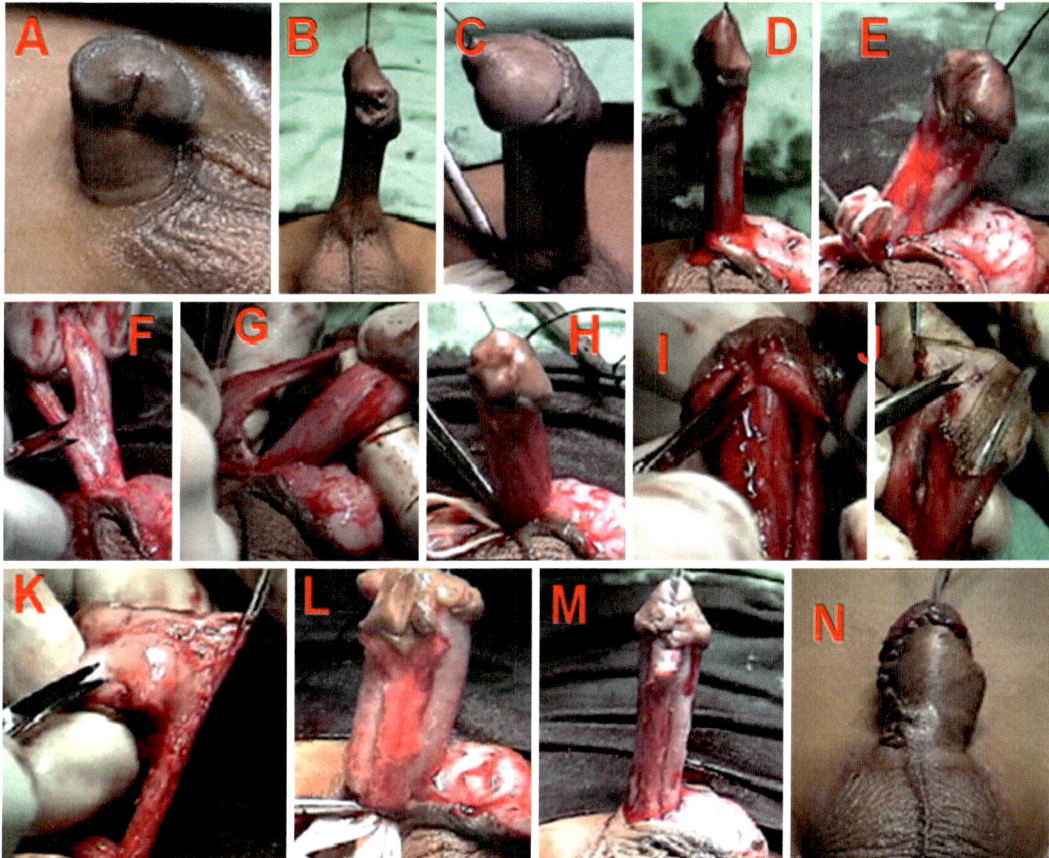

Fig. 18.5 All steps of correction of penile torsion by mobilization of urethral plate and urethra with spongiosum (With permission from Bhat et al. [7] @copyright Elsevier). (**a** and **b**) More than 90° right torsion. (**c**) Gittes test penile torsion more than 90°. (**d**) Persisting Penile torsion after penile skin degloving. (**e**) Confirming the torsion by Gittes test. (**f** and **g**) Urethral plate with corpus spongiosum and proximal urethral mobilization. (**h**) Gittes test showing torsion still persisting. (**i**, **j**, and **k**) Urethral plate with corpus spongiosum mobilization into the glans. (**l**) Artificial erection (Gittes) test showing torsion corrected. (**m**) Penile torsion corrected after urethroplasty and glanuloplasty seen on Gittes test. (**n**) Skin closure with fully corrected torsion

tion (Gittes) test is done to confirm the degree of torsion (Fig. 18.5e). Mobilization of the urethral plate and corpus spongiosum is done from just proximal to the meatus to the corona in hypospadias cases (Fig. 18.5g, h). And the diverting corpus spongiosum and hypoplastic urethra are mobilized up to the glans' corona in chordee without hypospadias (Fig. 18.6e, f). An artificial penile erection test again checks the correction of torsion.

Then the proximal urethral mobilization is done according to need, and torsion correction is confirmed by the Gittes test (Fig. 18.5i). The corpus spongiosum with urethral plate mobilization is carried out into the future meatus in the glans as a next step, and torsion correction is confirmed (Fig. 18.5j, k, l, m). Next, Tubularized Incise Plate Urethroplasty with Spongioplasty and glanuloplasty is carried out in hypospadias patients, and spongioplasty with glanuloplasty in chordee cases without hypospadias is done, keeping per urethral catheter in situ (Fig. 18.5m). The final adjustment of residual torque can be made during skin closure if required (Fig. 18.5n). The torsion mechanism by the attachment of the spongiosum and its correction by mobilization is shown in Fig. 18.6a–d. Mobilization of the urethral plate and spongiosum from the meatus into the glans corrected torsion in 75% of cases, and so this is proposed as a third step in the algorithm (Fig. 18.7).

Based on the etiology, torsion causes are an eccentric attachment facial covering and the attachment of spongiosum to corporal bodies and glans. The technique corrects torsion's etiological factors rather than countering the torque to the opposite side and confirms surgery's anatomical principles. The correction of the torsion is possible with the single-step or combining the further steps as per need.

1. The torsion can be corrected according to the factors in a particular case, like by simple penile degloving (Fig. 18.8a–g), which eliminates the factor of skin and dartos fascia.
2. The penile skin degloving and urethral plate/hypoplastic urethral with spongiosum mobilization (Fig. 18.9a–d) which corrects the factors in Buck's fascia.
3. The combination of penile skin degloving, mobilization of urethral plate/hypoplastic urethra with the spongiosum, and proximal ure-

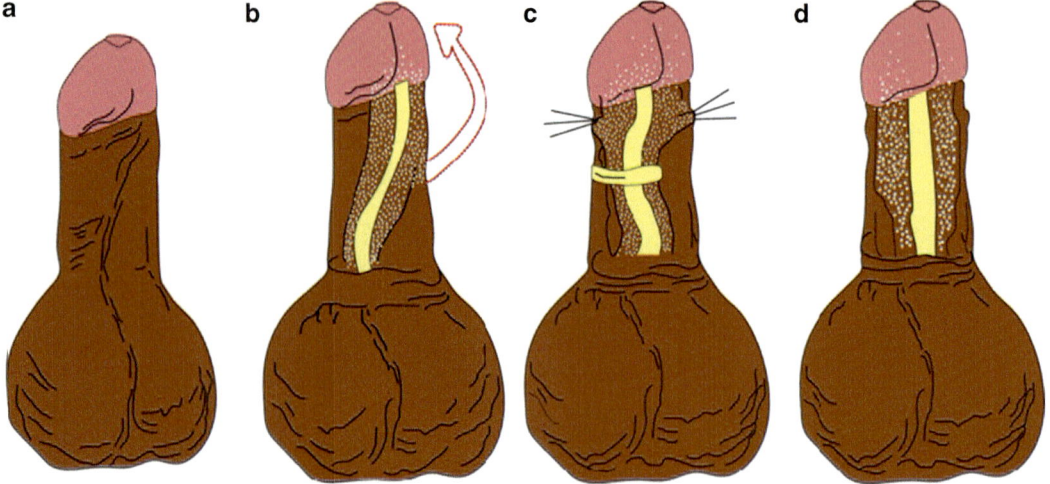

Fig. 18.6 Diagrammatic representation of torsion mechanism by attachment of hypoplastic urethra and spongiosum and correction by mobilizing the hypoplastic urethra with spongiosum. (**a**) Torsion in Chordee without hypospadias. (**b**) Torsion due to attachment of hypoplastic urethra and spongiosum to corpora and glans causing torsion. (**c**) Hypoplastic urethra and spongiosum mobilization. (**d**) Mobilization of urethra and spongiosum corrected, leading to release of the torsion

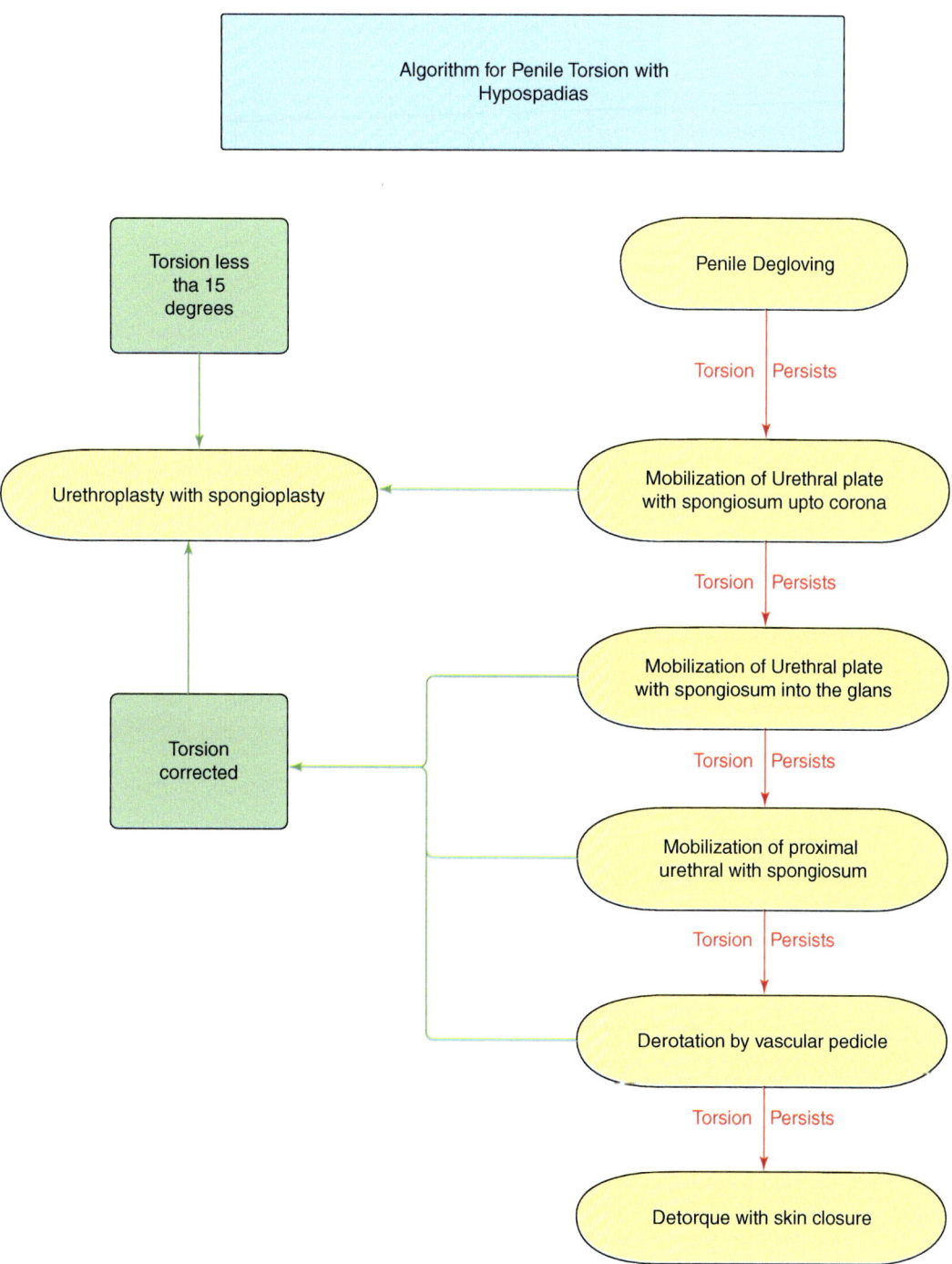

Fig. 18.7 Algorithm for correction torsion with hypospadias

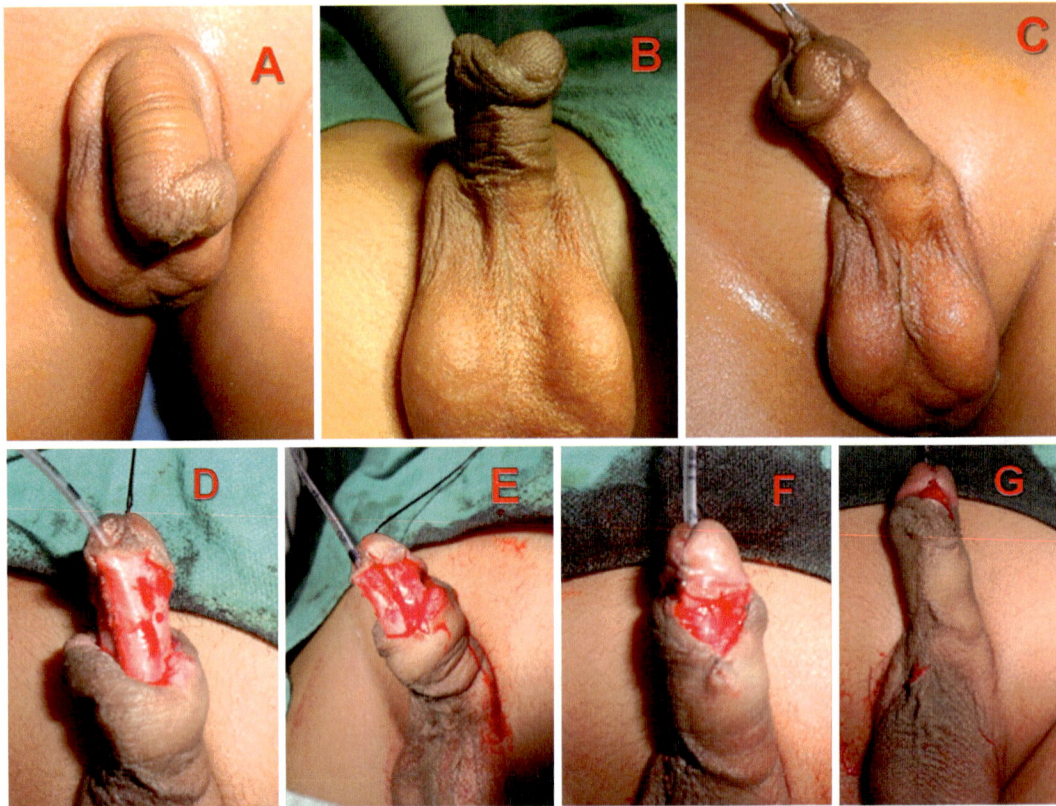

Fig. 18.8 Correction of torsion by penile degloving. (**a, b, c**) Glanular hypospadias 90 left degree torsion. (**d, e**) Torsion corrected after Penile skin degloving. (**f**) Glanuloplasty. (**g**) skin closure

thral mobilization (Fig. 18.10a–f) corrects the factor of attachment of spongiosum to the corporal bodies.
4. The combination of penile skin degloving, urethral plate with spongiosum, proximal urethral mobilization, and mobilization of urethral plate/hypoplastic urethra with spongiosum into glans (Fig. 18.5a–n) deals with factors of spongiosal attachment to the corporal bodies and glans.
5. Even isolated congenital penile torsion of 180° can be corrected by this technique (Fig. 18.11a, b).

Advantages
1. Simple, easy, safe, effective technique, and short learning curve.
2. Corrects the etiological factor and follows the anatomical principles of surgery.
3. Fewer chances of over or under rection.
4. An additional advantage of chordee correction simultaneously.
5. The spongiosum mobilization allows tension-free suturing of the spongiosum for spongioplasty.
6. The reconstructed urethra after spongioplasty is a near-normal one and also helps prevent the fistula.
7. The hypoplastic urethra is salvaged and eliminates the fistula risk in cases of chordee without hypospadias.

18.10 Correction Both Torsion and Chordee in Chordee Without Hypospadias [1, 21–23]

Chordee without hypospadias is a variant of hypospadias, and the incidence is around 9.5% of the hypospadiacs. The chordee without hypospadias

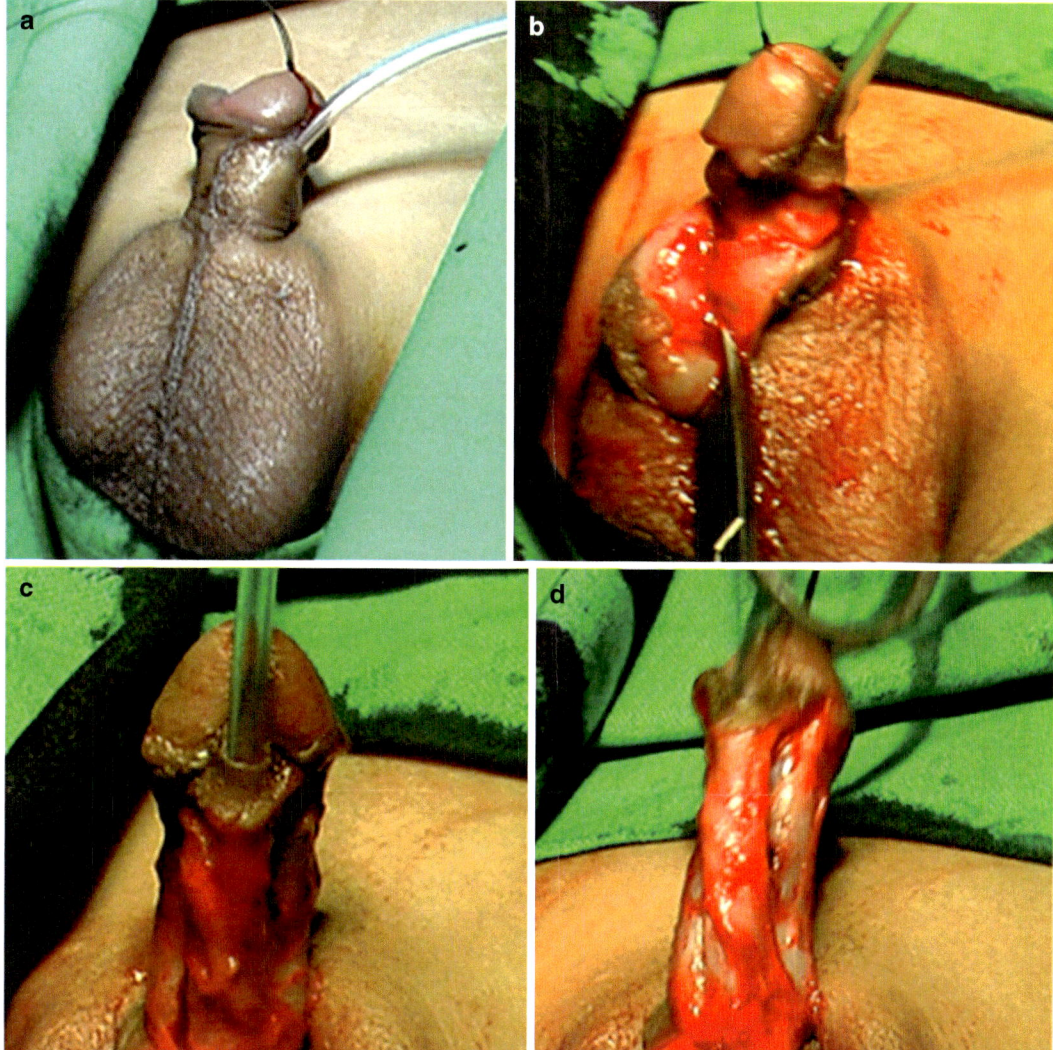

Fig. 18.9 Correction of torsion by penile skin degloving and urethral plate with spongiosum mobilization. (**a**) 70° Left torsion. (**b**) Penile torsion persisting after penile degloving. (**c**) The torsion correction after mobilization of the urethral plate with corpus spongiosum and urethra up to the penoscrotal junction. (**d**) Correction of torsion

associated with torsion is less common, and the incidence is 3.5%. Ours is the only published article on the management of both torsion and chordee by a single technique in the chordee without hypospadias with torsion. The ratio of chordee without hypospadias with torsion and hypospadias alone was 1:2.71, while the incidence of torsion in the cases of chordee without hypospadias was 37.0%. Though plication procedures and corporal rotation can also correct chordee and torque, these procedures are against surgery's anatomical principles. The corpora's dorsal normal surface is rendered abnormal rather than remedying the abnormal ventral surface. Other disadvantages of plication and corporeal rotation techniques are they are likely to produce fibrosis and shorten the penis. Replacement urethroplasty after resection of the hypoplastic urethra is extensive and carries the risk of fistula, stricture, meatal stenosis & diverticulum, and often requires redo surgeries. Corporoplasty with grafts can only be used for small defects, has a chance of graft contracture, unstable penile erections, may disturb the corporal structures, and hamper penile growth. The mobili-

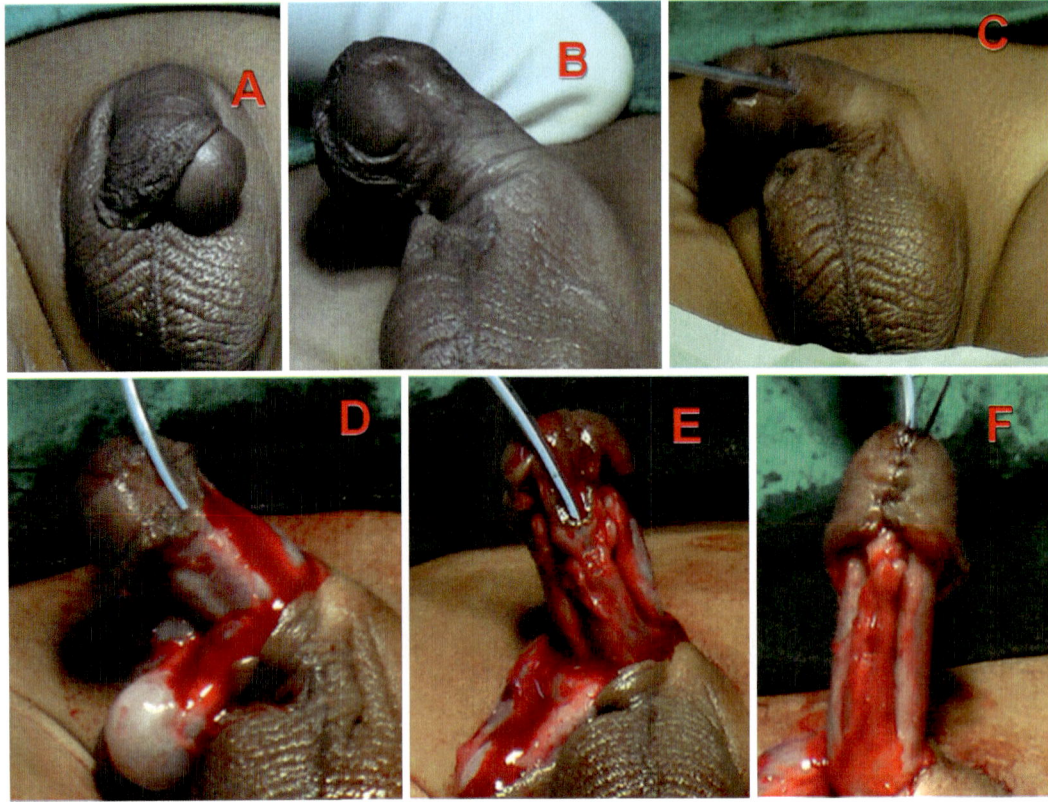

Fig. 18.10 Torsion correction by the urethral plate with spongiosum and urethral mobilization. (**a, b, c**) More than 90° left torsion. (**d**) Persisting Penile torsion after penile degloving. (**e**) Torsion correction by the urethral plate with corpus spongiosum into glans and proximal urethra beyond the penoscrotal junction mobilization. (**f**) Urethroplasty and glanuloplasty and torsion corrected

zation of hypoplastic urethra and spongiosum correct both torsion and chordee and is suitable in these cases.

18.11 Surgical Technique

An infant feeding tube is passed in the urethra, and a stay suture is applied. A circumcoronal circumferential incision is given at corona after subcutaneous injection of 1 in 1,00,000 solution of adrenaline. An artificial erection test (Gittes) is done to assess the torsion and chordee (Fig. 18.12a, b). A dissection plane is then created at Buck's fascia level, and penile skin degloving is done. The Gittes test is done again to observe the correction of chordee and torsion (Fig. 18.12c). The hypoplastic urethra with spongiosum mobilization is started proximal to the corpus spongiosum divergence and mobilized from the corpora distally up to the corona. The dissection is done carefully not to injure the hypoplastic urethra, underlying corpora and spongiosum. If ventral curvature or torsion persists, the urethra is mobilized into the glans (Fig. 18.12d). Mobilization of the urethra is done proximally up a bulb of the urethra to manage the remaining chordee or torsion. The artificial erection(Gittes) test is done again to confirm penile torsion and chordee correction (Fig. 18.12e, g). A single stitch dorsal plication is done if required to correct persistent chordee <30 degrees. Penile lengthening by ventral transverse superficial corporotomies or Corporoplasty is the last step on chordee persistence of more than 30 degrees. Spongioplasty over the hypoplastic urethra is done by suturing the mobilized divergent (Y-shaped) corpus spongiosum into I. Thus, a

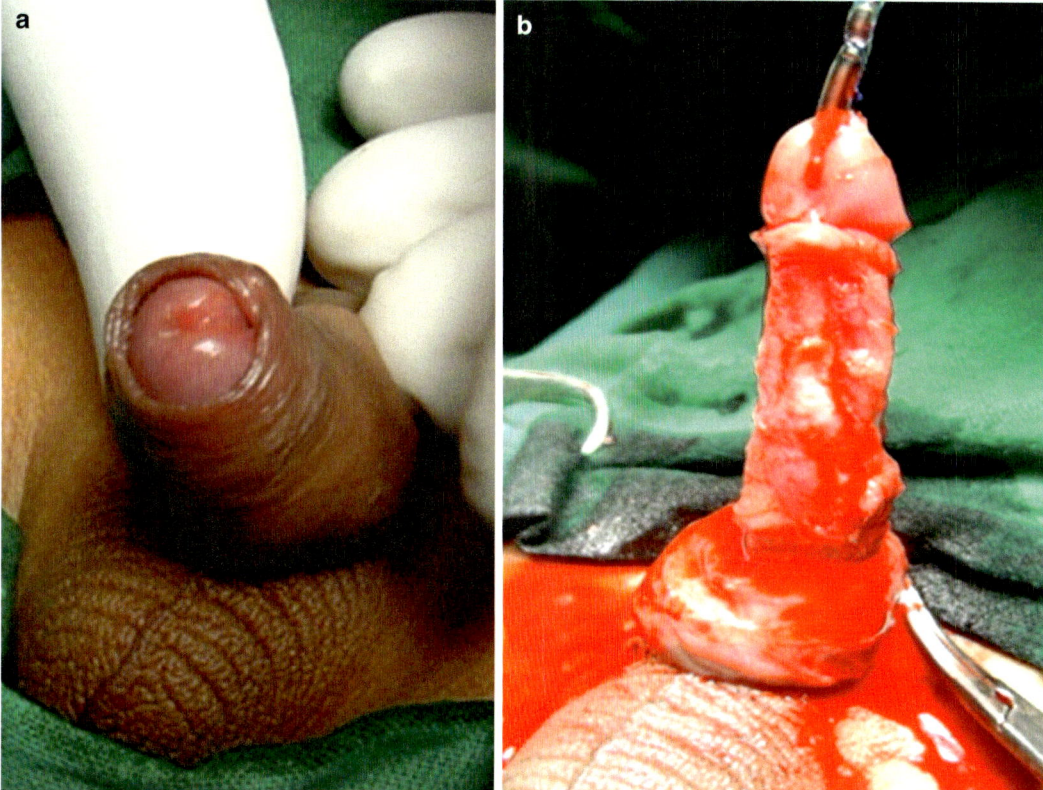

Fig. 18.11 Isolated congenital penile torsion correction by mobilization technique. (**a**) Isolated penile torsion of 180°. (**b**) Corrected after penile degloving and partial mobilization of the spongiosum

near-normal urethra is reconstructed after spongioplasty. Glanular flaps are approximated to reshape the glans as conical and bring the meatus to the tip to complete the glansplasty (Fig. 18.12h, i). Prepucioplasty is done whenever it is feasible and patient demands. The skin closure is done by adjusting the flaps to correct the remaining torque if any. A pressure dressing is done keeping the per urethral catheter. The dressing and catheter are removed after 3–5 days. Patients/parents are asked to observe for residual curvature or torque during erection, and examination of an erect penis is performed in follow-up visits.

18.12 Discussion

The etiology of both ventral curvature and penile torsion in chordee without hypospadias is overlapping. The etiological factors lie in the penile fascial coverings and spongiosum with the urethral plate. So, the simultaneous correction of torsion and chordee is feasible in a stepwise manner. The steps are mobilizing the spongiosum with hypoplastic urethra from the corporal bodies proximally up to the bulbar region and distally into the glans according to the severity. The technique is safe, reproducible, efficacious, and provides excellent cosmesis. This stepwise correction of torsion and curvature defines the type of chordee without hypospadias and probable etiological factors of the same, too (Fig. 18.13).

There is no universal agreement on the management techniques of penile torsion correction, and remains yet to be decided, which method is best. In a minireview, we found about 335 cases managed by different techniques: 63.58% cases were isolated penile torsion, 28.96% torsion with hypospadias, and 7.46% with chordee without hypospadias (Table 18.2). Eroglu et al. in a series of 200 cases among the newborns, found the incidence of isolated penile torsion to be 20%, but

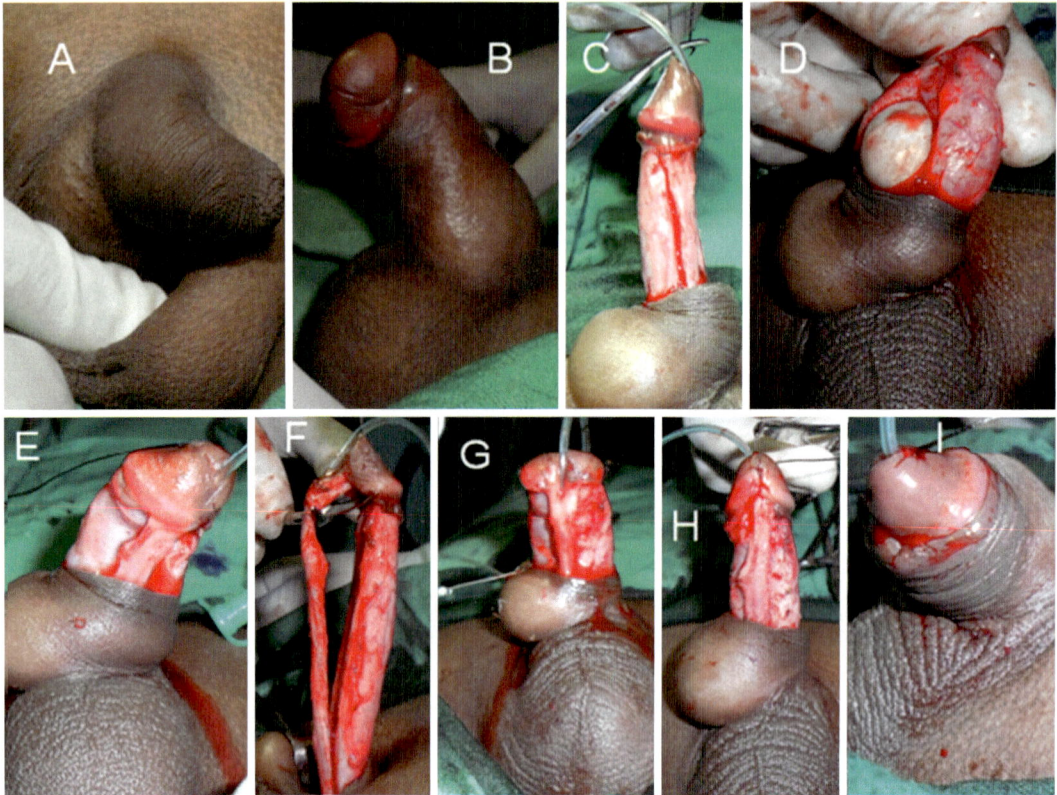

Fig. 18.12 The steps of torsion and chordee correction in chordee without hypospadias (with permission from Bhat et al. [21] @ Copyright Elsevier). (**a**) More than 90° left-sided torsion with moderate chordee. (**b**) Left torsion of more than 90° and moderate ventral curvature on Gittes test. (**c**) Persistence of torsion and ventral curvature after penile skin degloving. (**d**) Mobilization of the spongiosum with the hypoplastic urethra. (**e**) Partially correction of torsion and ventral curvature is seen on Gittes test. (**f**) Mobilization of urethra proximally up to the penoscrotal junction and distally into the glans. (**g**) Confirmation of correction of both torsion and chordee by Gittes test. (**h**) Glanuloplasty. (**i**) Final picture after skin closure showing torsion and chordee correction

only 4.3% of patients needed treatment [9]. This explains how this anomaly is overlooked. Though the overall incidence of penile torsion is high but severe forms requiring treatment are less frequent. Commonly used techniques are penile degloving and reattaching the skin, penile degloving, and dissection of Buck's fascia, dorsal dartos wrap, mobilization of spongiosum and urethra, and tunica plication. Dorsal dartos wrap is more frequently used to correct torque, and others have used fixing the corpora to the pubic ostium. Complications reported were residual torsion, fistula, lymphoedema, and keloid. Zeid A and Soliman H had a high residual torsion rate with penile degloving and reattaching of the skin (66.66%) and dorsal dartos wrap (20%) (Table 18.2). The correction penile torsion was possible in 89% of cases by the urethral plate, divergent corpus spongiosum, proximal urethra, and the urethral plate mobilization into the glans. The remaining 11% required adjustment during skin closure. We could correct the penile torsion with the mobilization technique in all cases without the need for plication or detorque by dorsal dartos. We were able to fix the severe torsion and moderate torsion in all cases. It is logical to use the step by step technique, which helps correct the chordee and torsion together, correct the etiological factors, and simultaneously facilitates hypospadias repair. Mobilizing the urethra and spongiosum is a better technique with a rational approach to correct the etiological factors [1, 7, 21].

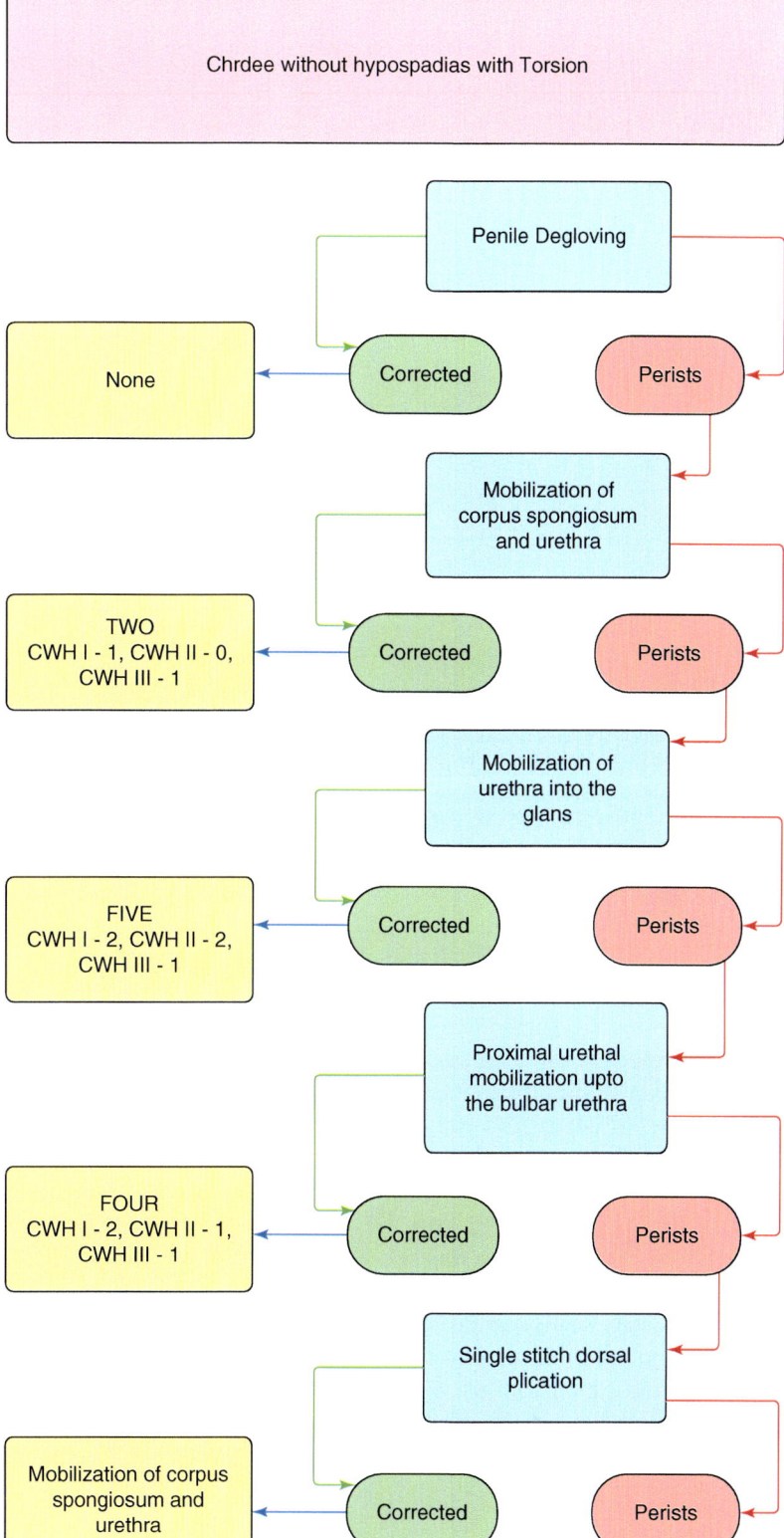

Fig. 18.13 Algorithm for management of chordee without hypospadias with torsion (with permission from Bhat et al. [21] @ Copyright Elsevier)

Table 18.2 The salient features of the reported cases and their management

Authors	Total cases	Hypospadias Type	No of cases	Degree of torsion	Chordee	Method of correction	Results
Mebley JE 1973 [24]	1	Coronal hypospadias	1	180	Severe	Penile de-gloving and reattaching skin	Corrected
Corriere Jr JN 1981 [27]	2	Chordee without hypospadias	2	90	Mild	Mobilization of Buck,s fascia	Corrected torsion in one, Improved in another
Azami A Eckstein HB 1981 [13]	3	Glanular hypospadias Isolated Penile torsion	1 2	90	---	Detorque by mobilization of skin and dartos	Corrected
Redman JF 1983[25]	15	Glanular Coronal Distal penile Chordee without hypospadias	3 8 1 3	45-90 45-90 45 >90	-- --	Dartos reflection 6 Buck,s reflection 2 Skin re attaching 7	Complete correction achieved
Tryfonas GI et al 1995 [14]	16	Minor degree hypospadias Isolated Penile torsion	9 7	45-90	----	Penile de-gloving, dissection of Buck's fascia and re-suturing 3 Skin Incision at base and mobilization of Buck's fascia --- 6	Torsion Corrected Keloid 2 Lymphedema 6 Scar at base 6
Fisher and Park 2004 [18]	8	Chordee Without hypospadias Hypospadias Isolated Penile torsion	4 2 2	45-180	--	Penile de-gloving and dorsal dartos wrap	Torsion corrected, no complications
Bhat et al 2009 [7]	27	Hypospadias Chordee without hypospadias Isolated penile torsion	18 7 2	45-180	-	Penile degloving 3.7% of cases mobilization of urethral plate and corpus spongiosum,- 25.29% mobilization of urethral plate and corpus spongiosum, 22.22% Mobilizing the urethral plate into the glans. 48.14%	Torsion corrected Fistula in one
Ismail M.A, Amin M. 2010[30]	1	Isolated penile torsion		180	-	Penile de-gloving and reattaching the skin	Torsion corrected
Zeid A, Soliman H 2010[28]	28	Anterior hypospadias Posterior hypospadias	19 9		-	Degloving and repositioning the penile skin 9 Dorsal dartos flap 10	Residual torsion 6, Residual torsion 2
Eroglu E and Gundogdu G 2015 [9]	200	Isolated penile torsion		<45 --157 45-90- 39 >90- 4	---	Circumcision -- 165 Penile degloving and reattaching 15 Dorsal dartos pedicle - 4 Lost in follow up 16	Torsion corrected
Aykaçet A al 2016 [29]	5	Isolated penile torsion	5	30-70	---	Penile Degloving 3 Dorsal dartos detorque 2	Residual curvature 1 degree 10
Elbakry et al 2013 [22]	19	Hypospadias with torsion		94.7 (75–160)	-	Penile degloving, Mobilization of urethral plate and urethra, Plication of tunica albuginea to Periosteum	Torsion corrected
Zvizdic Z et al 2020 [26]	1	Isolated penile Torsion		>90	-	Dorsal dartos flap	Torsion corrected
Bhat A et al 2014[21]	9	Trosion with chordee without hypospadias		30-120	45-100	Penile degloving, mobilization of hypoplastic urethra into 5, proximal urethral mobilization 4	Both chordee and torsion corrected
Total	335	Hypospadias-97, Chordee Without hypospadias-25, Isolated Penile torsion 213					

18.13 Conclusions

Penile torsion with hypospadias and its variants is more common than reported in the literature. Chordee is more common and severe in proximal hypospadias, while torsion is more severe and common in distal hypospadias and chordee without hypospadias. The deviation extent of the urethral meatus toward the side of torsion and the median raphe to the opposite side correlates well with the degree of torsion. Correction of the penile torsion should be planned along with hypospadias repair to achieve a cosmetically normal penis. The theory of eccentric fusion of urethral folds and mesodermal proliferation with the attachment spongiosum to corpora and glans explains the embryological development of torsion. However, the most commonly done procedure is dorsal dartos wrap.

In most cases, the step-by-step approach of mobilizing the urethral plate and diverting the corpus spongiosum into the glans corrects torsion. This approach corrects the etiological factors rather than producing counter-torque as in other techniques and is therefore better. Both torsion and chordee in chordee without hypospadias can be corrected by the mobilization technique simultaneously. The technique of urethral plate and spongiosum mobilization or hypoplastic urethra with spongiosum mobilization is simple, safe, and effective and per anatomical surgery principles and provides excellent results with minimal complications.

References

1. Bhat A, Singh V, Bhat M. Penile torsion. In: Surgical techniques in pediatric and adult urology. 1st ed. New Delhi: Jaypee Brothers Medical publishers; 2020. p. 207–22.
2. Ben-Ari J, Merlob P, Mimouni F, Reisner SH. Characteristics of the male genitalia in the newborn: penis. J Urol. 1985;134(3):521–2.
3. Sarkis PE, Sadasivam M. Incidence and predictive factors of isolated neonatal penile glanular torsion. J Pediatr Urol. 2007;3(6):495–9.
4. Hsieh J-T, Wong W-Y, Chen J, Chang H-J, Liu S-P. Congenital isolated penile torsion in adults: untwist with plication. Urology. 2002;59(3):438–40.
5. Bar-Yosef Y, Binyamini J, Matzkin H, Ben-Chaim J. Degloving and realignment—simple repair of isolated penile torsion. Urology. 2007;69(2):369–71.
6. Zeid A, Soliman H. Penile torsion: an overlooked anomaly with distal hypospadias. Ann Pediatric Surg. 2010;6(2):93–7.
7. Bhat A, Bhat MP, Saxena G. Correction of penile torsion by urethral plate and urethra mobilisation. J Pediatr Urol. 2009;5(6):451–7.
8. Shaeer O. Torsion of the penis in adults: prevalence and surgical correction. J Sex Med. 2008;5(3):735–9.
9. Eroglu E, Gundogdu G. Isolated penile torsion in newborns. Can Urol Assoc J. 2015;9(11–12):E805.
10. Bhat A, Bhat M, Kumar V, Goyal S, Bhat A, Patni M. The incidence of isolated penile torsion in North India: a study of 5,018 male neonates. J Pediatr Urol. 2017;13(5):e491–6.
11. Bhat A, Sabharwala K, Bhat M, Singla M, Upadhayaa R, Kumara V. Correlation of severity of penile torsion with the type of hypospadias & ventral penile curvature and their management. Afr J Urol. 2015;21(2):111–8.
12. Zhou L, Mei H, Hwang AH, Xie H-w, Hardy BE. Penile torsion repair by suturing tunica albuginea to the pubic periosteum. J Pediatr Surg. 2006;41(1):e7–9.
13. Azmy A, Eckstein H. Surgical correction of torsion of the penis. Br J Urol. 1981;53(4):378–9.
14. Tryfonas G, Klokkaris A, Sveronis M, Gavopoulos S, Violaki A, Limas C. Torsion of the penis. Pediatr Surg Int. 1995;10(5–6):359–36.
15. Hussein A, Nagib I, Wilson AM. Penile degloving and skin reattachment technique for repair of penile torsion, our experience. Egypt J Plast Reconstr Surg. 2007;31(1):19–23.
16. Slawin KM, Nagler HM. Treatment of congenital penile curvature with penile torsion: a new twist. J Urol. 1992;147(1):152–4.
17. Snow BW. Penile torsion correction by diagonal corporal plication sutures. Int Braz J Urol. 2009;35(1):56–9.
18. Fisher PC, Park JM. Penile torsion repair using dorsal dartos flap rotation. J Urol. 2004;171(5):1903–4.
19. Bauer R, Kogan BA. Modern technique for penile torsion repair. J Urol. 2009;182(1):286–91.
20. Bhat A. Extended urethral mobilization in incised plate urethroplasty for severe hypospadias: a variation in technique to improve chordee correction. J Urol. 2007;178(3):1031–5.
21. Bhat A, Sabharwal K, Bhat M, Singla M, Kumar V, Upadhyay R. Correction of penile torsion and chordee by mobilization of the urethra and spongiosum in chordee without hypospadias. J Pediatr Urol. 2014;10(6):1238–43. https://doi.org/10.1016/j.jpurol.2014.06.016.
22. Elbakry A, Zakaria A, Matar A, El Nashar A. The management of moderate and severe congenital penile torsion associated with hypospadias: urethral mobilisation is not a panacea against torsion. Arab J Urol. 2013;11(1):1–7. https://doi.org/10.1016/j.aju.2012.12.004.
23. Bhat A, Sabharwal K. The management of moderate and severe congenital penile torsion associated with hypospadias: urethral mobilisation is not a panacea against torsion. Arab J Urol. 2014;12(2):127–9. https://doi.org/10.1016/j.aju.2013.10.003.
24. Mobley JE. Congenital torsion of the penis. J Urol. 1973;109:517–9.
25. Redman JF, Bissada NK. One-stage correction of chordee and 180-degree penile torsion. Urology. 1976;7:632–3.
26. Zvizdic Z, Milisic E, Vranic S. Acta Medica Penile degloving and dorsal dartos flap rotation in the management of severe isolated penile torsion in a −6 years old boy. Hradec Kralove. 2020;63(1):52–4. https://doi.org/10.14712/18059694.2020.16.
27. Corriere JN Jr. Involvement of Buck's fascia in congenital torsion of the penis. J Urol. 1981;126:410e1.
28. Zeid A, Suleman H. An overlooked anomaly in distal hypospadias. Ann Surg. 2010;6:93–7.
29. Aykaç A, Baran O, Yapici O, Ayugan AB, Aydin C, Cakan M. Penile degloving and dorsal dartos flap rotation approach for the management of isolated penile torsion. Turk J Urol. 2016;42(1):27–31. https://doi.org/10.5152/tud.2015.34651.
30. Ismail MA, Amin M. Correction of a 180 degree (upside down) penile torsion in a 55-year-old patient with severe erectile dysfunction. UroToday Int J. 2010;3(6). https://doi.org/10.3834/in.1944-5784.2010.12.03.

Management of Iatrogenic Hypospadias

19

Amilal Bhat, Nikhil Khandelwal, and Akshita Bhat

19.1 Introduction

Iatrogenic hypospadias is defined as "the ventral opening of the urethra following a ventral urethra's injury". Other synonyms used for the condition are "penis cleft," "penile injury," "unknown penile condition," "Broken urethra." This injury is commonly caused by long-term catheterization or injury during circumcision [1]. Inadvertent glans injury during circumcision may lead to iatrogenic hypospadias. It may be associated with glans injury and is more common when a Mogel clamp is used for circumcision [2]. Though the injury is rare, the incidence increases because of the increasing age, associated comorbidities like neurological lesions and heart diseases requiring long-term catheterization. The catheter is the commonly used tool by the urologist and medical practitioners with its inherent chances of complications. Various Catheter induced complications are:

1. Mechanical: Bladder and Peritoneal perforation, Bladder spasm [3, 4]
2. Infectious—Cystitis, Prostatitis, Epididymitis, Urethritis, and Periurethral Abscess, Pyelonephritis [5, 6]
3. Calculi and encrustations [7, 8]
4. The catheter—knotting [9] and penile fracture [10]
5. Paraphimosis
6. Stricture formation and urethral damage [11, 12]
7. Urethral erosion
8. Bladder Malignancy associated with catheters [13]

The timely change of catheter and proper catheter care can minimize urethral erosion and other complications. Complications are to be identified early and treated as early as possible for a better outcome. The urethral injury's extent may vary from ventral meatal cleavage as the minor manifestation to complete penoscrotal tear

A. Bhat
Bhat's Hypospadias and Reconstructive Urology Hospital and Research Centre, Jaipur, Rajasthan, India

Department of Urology, Jaipur National University Institute for Medical Sciences and Research Centre, Jaipur, Rajasthan, India

Department of Urology, Dr. S.N. Medical College, Jodhpur, Rajasthan, India

Department of Urology, S.P. Medical College, Bikaner, Rajasthan, India

P.G. Committee Medical Council of India, New Delhi, India

Academic and Research Council of RUHS, Jaipur, Rajasthan, India

N. Khandelwal (✉)
Department of Urology, Vijayanagar Institute of Medical Sciences, Bellary, Karnataka, India

A. Bhat
Department of Surgery, Sawai Man Singh Medical College, Jaipur, Rajasthan, India

as the most major one [1]. The chapter describes all problems in iatrogenic hypospadias and their management.

19.2 Etiopathogenesis

Inadvertent glanulo-urethral injury during circumcision may lead to iatrogenic hypospadias. Neonatal circumcision is the most routine surgery conducted by the pediatric urologist, pediatric surgeon, and other medical practitioners. In ceremonial and neonatal elective circumcision, the most commonly used clamp is Mogen. The advantage is that the circumcision can be rapid and leaves no foreign body at the site of circumcision. However, it has the disadvantage of not directly protecting the glans during the procedure. There is a high risk of ventral glans injury because the ventral preputial adhesions with subsequent glans entrapment do not allow the complete skin release [2] and an oblique injury ventrolateral aspect. The urethra may consistently be involved causing iatrogenic hypospadias. Even partial damage to the urethra and infection with sloughing may lead to iatrogenic hypospadias.

Most commonly, urethral erosion is caused by long-term catheterization. The predisposing factors are loss of penile sensation in neurological patients, low resistance, and more chances of infection due to comorbidities like diabetes and heart diseases. Hanging catheter, large size catheter, or catheter fixed on thigh may lead to pressure necrosis and pent-up urethral discharge, increasing the chances of infection. Catheter fixation on the thigh with the leg bag will prevent the free movement of the catheter, which leads the indwelling catheter to act as a bowstring and urethral erosion during erections. Downward directed pressure of the transurethral catheter leads to compression of the ventral urethra and pressure necrosis. The weak ventral corpus spongiosum support increases the chances of urethral injury. At the same time, thick stronger corpora cavernosa support dorsally protects the urethra. Fixing the catheter to one side may lead to erosion of the urethra on that side.

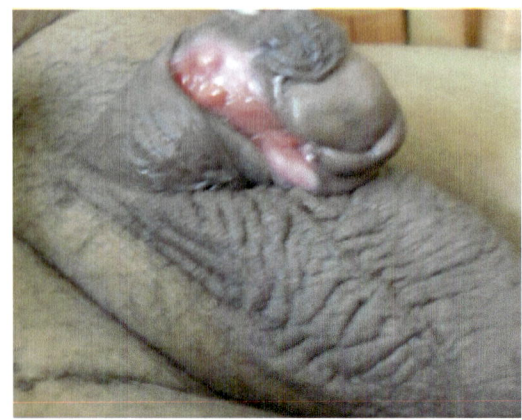

Fig. 19.1 Urethra Erosion and torsion of the penis

Fibrosis on the fixed side and fixation of urethral mucosa on that side may lead to torsion of the penis (Fig. 19.1). Mary Bell et al. reported a substantial role of the catheter material and its securing in urethral trophic ulcers and suggested using soft silicone catheters and securing these on the body's fixed part (abdominal wall) to decrease the complications. They noted that using unsecured Silicon-coated catheters rather than the soft silicone catheter increased the chances of urethral erosion [14].

19.3 Grading the Injury in Iatrogenic Hypospadias

19.3.1 In Males

19.3.1.1 Grading
The injury can be graded according to the extent of the erosion of the shaft of the penis [15] (Fig. 19.2)

Grade 1: Peno-urethral cleavage from the urethral meatus to the proximal part of the glans corona (Fig. 19.2a)
Grade 2: Peno-urethral from the urethral meatus to the distal part of the penis. (Fig. 19.2b)
Grade 3: Penile cleavage from the urethral meatus to the scrotum (Fig. 19.2c)
Grade 4: The meatus is unaffected, but pressure necrosis is seen along the penis shaft (Fig. 19.2d)

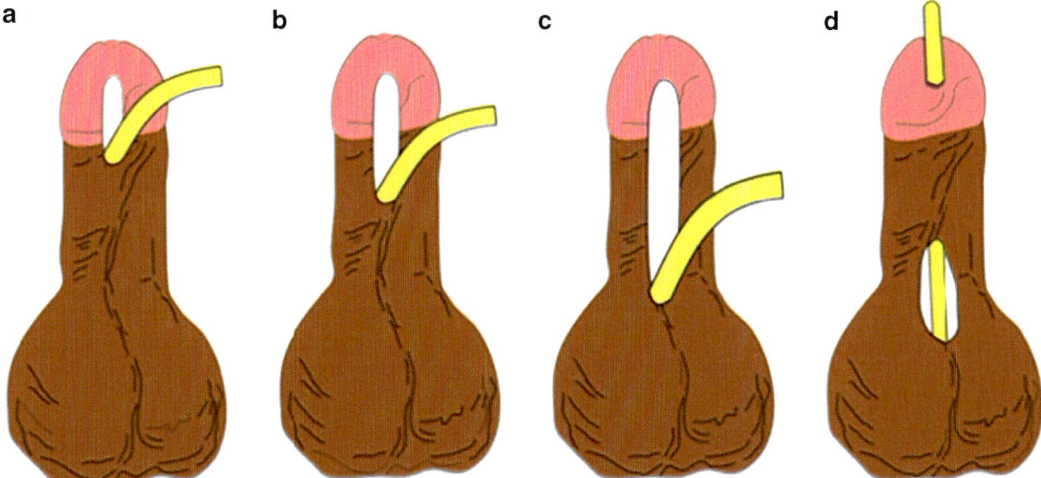

Fig. 19.2 Showing the classification of Iatrogenic hypospadias

19.3.1.2 Classification

Hypospadias may be classified according to the extent of meatus & urethral erosion.

1. Glanular 2. Coronal 3. Sub-coronal 4. Distal penile 5. Mid-Penile 6. Proximal penile 7. Penoscrotal

19.3.2 In Females

Female genital mutilation is still practiced in West Africa. Iatrogenic female hypospadias has been reported following female genital circumcision practiced in west Africa. However, the overall prevalence is decreasing, and up to 50% of females are circumcised, and 25% are young girls. A prolonged catheterization in females for neurogenic bladder in an elderly lady with comorbid cardiac condition and diabetes mellitus may also lead to urethral erosion and may be graded as:

Grade 1. minor erosion of the urethra (Figs. 19.3a and 19.4)
Grade 2. Erosion of the urethra up to the mid urethra (Fig. 19.3a)
Grade 3. Erosion of almost whole urethra (Fig. 19.3a)
Grade 4. Erosion of the urethra with laceration of labia minora (Figs. 19.3a and 19.5)

19.4 Management

19.4.1 Prevention of Injury

The ventral glans have a high risk of injury due to incompletely released ventral preputial adhesions with subsequent glans entrapment, as seen in the type and pattern of circumcision-induced injuries. Therefore, the ventral adhesions should be removed before applying the Mogen clamp to prevent this complication.

19.4.2 Preventing Urethral Erosion

1. Avoiding indwelling catheterization by using clean intermittent self-catheterization or supra-pubic catheterization.
2. Urinary incontinence is managed conservatively by incontinence containment disposable briefs or pads. There is a risk of developing maceration, dermatitis, bacterial infections and fungal, and skin breakdown. A toileting program, proven behaviors treatment plan should be considered for incontinent elderly with slight to moderate cognitive impairment.
3. Preferably, a silicon soft catheter is used and secured on the abdominal wall to prevent urethral erosion/injury.

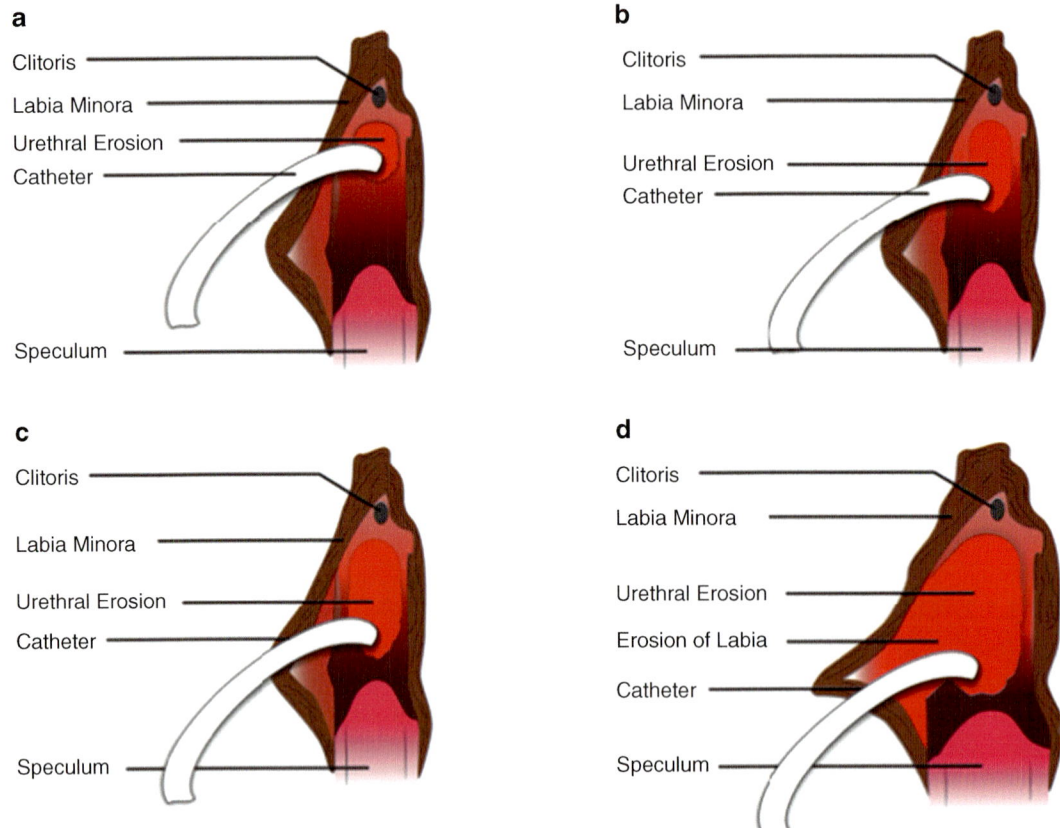

Fig. 19.3 Showing the erosion or urethra in Females (**a**) Erosion of meatus (**b**) Erosion up to mid urethra (**c**) Erosion beyond Mid-urethra (**d**) Erosion beyond mid-urethra and erosion of labia

19.5 Repair of Iatrogenic Hypospadias

19.5.1 Children

Sloughing and infection may cause meatal stenosis, which may require meatoplasty for correction. In children post circumcision iatrogenic hypospadias, a circumferential circumcoronal incision is given and extended around the urethral meatus encircling the opened urethra, and the penile skin is degloved. Gittes test is done to see the tunica's leakage or bulging to rule out the shaft injury. The urethral meatus and urethra up to 1 cm is mobilized and spatulated dorsally to prepare for Buccal mucosal graft. A buccal mucosal graft of adequate length is taken, fenestrated and designed for covering the distal part of the penile shaft and creating the neo-meatus. The graft is anastomosed with the urethral mucosa and penile skin with 5/0/6/0 PDS/Vicryl interrupted sutures and quilted over the distal end shaft to restore natural symmetry and cosmesis of the meatus and glans. Adequate size of the catheter is placed according to the child's age, and dressing is done. The catheter is removed about a week later. The patient is followed up with uroflowmetry at 1, 3, 6, and 12 months to evaluate for metal stenosis.

19.5.2 Female

The repair of iatrogenic hypospadias after female genital mutilation is more difficult for females because very short urethra with infection and conservative treatment may be reasonable. Iatrogenic hypospadias in females may be associ-

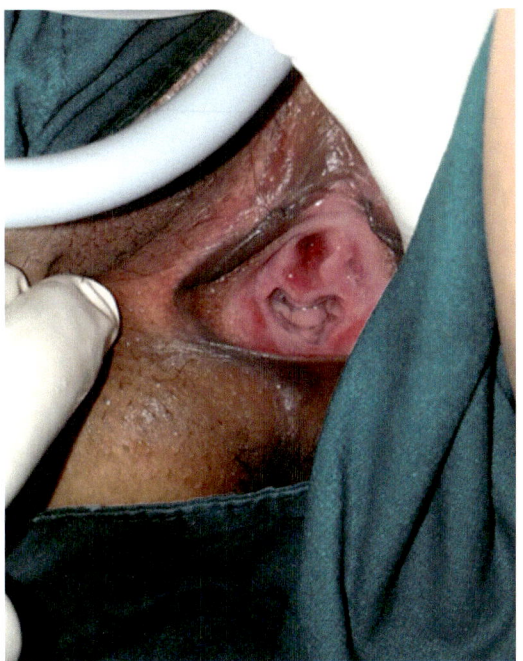

Fig. 19.4 Showing the erosion of meatus. Grade I Injury in a case of Neurogenic bladder

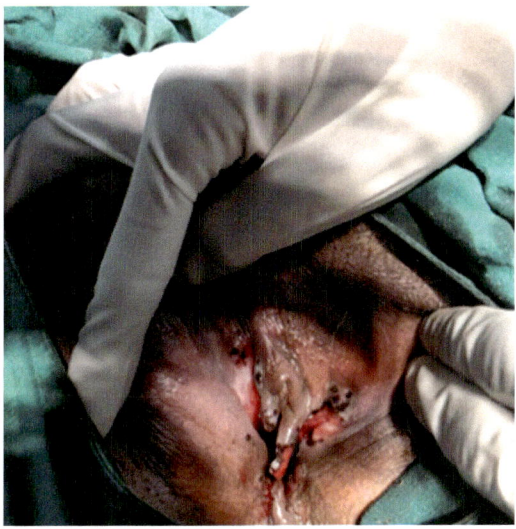

Fig. 19.5 Showing the erosion of urethra and Labia Grade IV Injury in a case of Neurogenic bladder

ated with urethral stricture or meatal stenosis and is more complicated, as the stricture would further shorten the already short hypospadiac urethra. Reconstruction may involve a combination of uretherolysis, urethral transposition, urethroplasty, or another cumbersome amalgam of procedures like urethral mobilization and transposition vaginal flap urethroplasty and/or dorsal/ventral buccal mucosal urethroplasty. Vaginal flap urethroplasty in female hypospadias is described in Chap. 16. Another more straightforward and reasonable alternative in meatal stenosis is urethral dilatation with long-term clean intermittent self-catheterization.

19.5.3 Male Adults

The repair results of iatrogenic hypospadias are very gratifying because the deformed penis is reconstructed to its normal appearance. The reconstructed urethra can be covered by the dartos or tunica vaginalis flap as an interposing layer to support the neourethra. The laid-open urethra can be tubularized in most cases. A substitution for urethroplasty is recommended when there is a narrow and scarred urethral plate for primary closure. The urethral plate is augmented for tension-free tubularization, with Buccal mucosal graft, penile skin graft, or non-hair bearing skin. Inner preputial flap or flap skin tube urethroplasty is an alternative when preputial skin is available. To have an infection-free, well-healed lesion for repair, patients should be put on suprapubic diversion before undergoing urethroplasty.

19.6 Tubularized Urethral Plate Urethroplasty

1:100,000 Adrenaline solution is injected at the site of the incision, and an inverted U-shaped incision was given encircling the laid open urethra and extended circumferential circumcoronal (Fig. 19.6a, b). The urethra plate of the opened-up urethra and spongiosum is mobilized off the corporal bodies from the penoscrotal junction and into the glans up to the meatus distally (Fig. 19.6c, d). This corrects the torsion or chordee is corrected if present. Tubularization of the urethral plate is done after freshening the margins, followed by the spongioplasty (Fig. 19.6e). Then meatal reconstruction, with glanuloplasty is undertaken and a urethral catheter is put in (Fig. 19.6f, g). Skin flaps

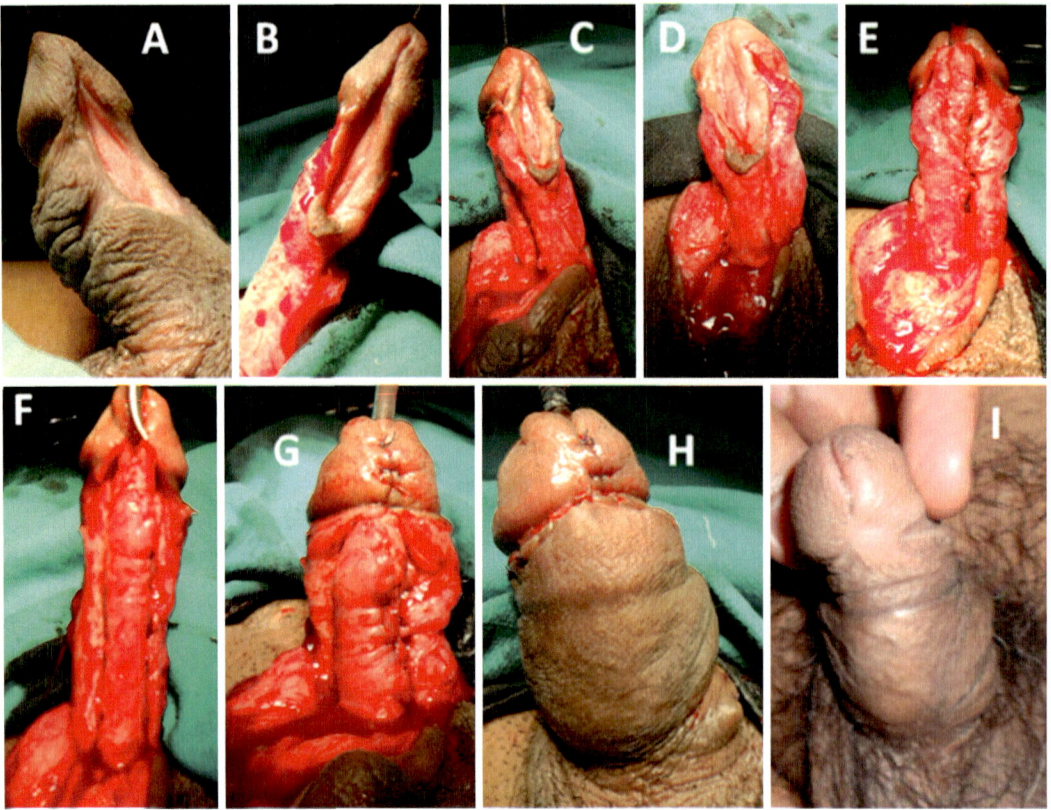

Fig. 19.6 Showing tubularized urethral plate urethroplasty. (**a**) An adult with iatrogenic Hypospadias (**b**) Penile skin degloving (**c** and **d**) Urethral Plate and Spongiosum Mobilization (**e**) Urethral Plate Tubularization (**f**) Spongioplasty (**g**) Glansplasty (**h**) Final Skin Closure (**i**) Postoperative picture with normal meatus and straight phallus (with permission Bhat A et al. [1] Copyright@ Springer Nature)

are adjusted to correct the torsion if there is residual torque, and skin closure is done (Fig. 19.6h). The urethral catheter is removed in 5–7 days. Patients are followed at 1, 3, and 6 months with uroflowmetry and the urethrogram at 6 months. Many of the patients with lower motor neuron bladder are asked to do clean self-intermittent catheterization after removing the catheter.

19.7 Our Experience and Discussion

We had 12 males, with catheter-induced urethral injury. Seven (5 spinal pathologies and one each of diabetes and coronary artery) had urethral reconstruction, and the rest had grade I injury and were treated conservatively. We had three female patients of grade I, III, and IV injuries each. Most of the cases reported in the literature are of the neurogenic bladder following the spinal trauma. We had seven cases of the neurogenic bladder due to spinal cord injury, one of quada equina syndrome, two patients with diabetes mellitus and cerebrovascular accident, three with diabetes mellitus and cardiovascular disease, and one each of them had diabetes mellitus and benign hyperplasia of the prostate. The mean duration of catheterization before the injury was seen as 10.9 months (Range 6–24 months). The majority of the patients and their attendants are often unaware of the urethral injury but get the attention during

Table 19.1 Showing Salient features of cases of urethral erosion and their management

S.N.	Sex	Age in years	Duration of Catheterication	Catheter secured or not	Referral Department	Co-morbidities	Extent of urethral erosion and grading	Reconstruction Urethroplasty	SPC
1.	Male	55	6 Months	Not	Neurology	Cauda Equina Syndrome, CAD	Penoscrodtal junction, with 110° Right torque Grade III	Yes	Yes
2.	Male	65	8 Months	Not	Neurology	Diabetes, Hypertension, Stroke	Mid penis, with 90° clockwise penile torque, Grade II	No	Yes
3.	Male	45	12 Months	Not	Physiotherapy and Rehabilitation	Traumatic Quadriplegin	Penoscrotal junction with 80° articlockwise penile torque Grade III	Yes	Yes
4.	Male	34	7 Months	Not	Neurocurgery	Traumatic Paraplegia	Glacular, Proximal penile urethrocetancoes fistula Grade IV	Yes	Yes
5.	Male	95	6 Months	Not	..	Hypertension, CAD	Glacular Grade I	No	Yes
6.	Male	42	14 Months	Not	Oreleopodies	Traumatic Paraplegia	Glacular Grade I	No	Yes
7.	Male	92	2 Years	Not	Medicine	Diabetes, Hypertension, CAD	Mid penis with 90° anticlockwise penile torque Grade III	Yes	Yes
8.	Male	63	11 Months	Not	..	Diabetes, Benign Prostatic Hyperplasia	Ventral urethral erosion till Distal penis Grade II	Yes	Yes
9.	Male	71	7 Months	Not	Medicine	CAD, Depression (on treatment	Gacular crosion till coroen Grade I	No	Yes
10.	Male	84	12 Months	Not	Medicine	Traumatic Paraplegia	Meatal crosion Grade I.	No	Yes
11.	Male	34	9 Months	Not	Orthopedics	Traumatic Paraplegia	Mid penis Grade II	Yes	Yes
12.	Male	55	15 Months	Not	Medicine	Hypertension, Coronary Artery Disease	Glacular Grade I	No	Yes
13.	Female	36	2 Years	Yes	Orthopedic	Traumatic Paraplegia	Grade I Injury, Meatal erosion Grade I	No	No
14.	Female	72	6 Years	No	Medicine	Traumatic Paraplegia	erosion mid urethral Grade III	No	No
15.	Female	75	5 Years	No	Orthopacdic	Traumatic Paraplegia	Grade IV Mid urethral with erosion of Labia Mirtora	No	Yes

CAD Coronary Artery Disease, SPC Suprapubic Cystostomy

difficult catheterization. Long duration of catheterization may cause distal urethral erosion and bladder stone. One patient had a bladder stone who presented with irritative symptoms (Table 19.1). Most of the patients with urethral erosion have underlying neurological dysfunction [12, 16, 17]. The impaired penile sensation may aggravate the injury, but it is not a prerequisite for the urethral injury [18].

Eight of the patients had one or more co-morbidities in our study. Old age with diabetes mellitus, a vascular disease with prolonged catheterization, and periurethral infection are the crucial factors in urethra erosion. Ventral erosion is more common because of weak ventral support of the corpus spongiosum to the urethra. Therefore, Supra-pubic cystostomy or Self-Intermittent catheterization is preferred to prevent urethral erosion in the patients requiring longer catheterization [1].Elderly patients with high-risk co-morbidities are poor candidates for reconstructing urethral surgery. Secrest et al. reported poor results in 17 patients of the neurogenic bladder who had reconstruction urethra; eleven of spinal cord injury underwent the second operation and ultimately required urinary diversion in all [16]. Andrews et al. reported successful outcome urethral reconstruction in six patients (6/16) of iatrogenic hypospadias [17].Tubularization of laid open urethra is feasible in most cases. Urethral erosion is a preventable complication of a long indwelling catheter. Patients and their attendants should be counseled and educated about the intricacies of catheterization and its prevention. Patients with neurogenic bladders could be best put on self-calibration. Patients requiring long term catheterization should be counseled for supra-pubic diversion of urine [1, 17].

19.8 Conclusion

Iatrogenic hypospadias in infants and children following circumcision is better prevented by the adequate release of ventral preputial adhesions or alternative circumcision clamp to Mogen clamp. Meatoplasty and glansplasty with buccal mucosa yield good results in this iatrogenic hypospadias. Neglected and poor catheter care in the elderly with prolonged catheterization may lead to severe complications of urethral erosion and iatrogenic hypospadias. The urethral erosion can be prevented by securing the catheter to the abdominal wall and ensuring the drainage system support without traction. The neurogenic bladder requiring prolonged catheterization should either be put on clean intermittent catheterization or suprapubic diversion. Tubularized Urethral Plate Urethroplasty results are excellent in such male iatrogenic hypospadias patients and severe cases may require augmented or replacement urethroplasty. Female iatrogenic hypospadias can be managed by uretherolysis and urethral transposition or vaginal flap urethroplasty.

References

1. Bhat AL, Bhat M, Khandelwal N, et al. Catheter-induced urethral injury and tubularized urethral plate urethroplasty in such iatrogenic hypospadias. Afr J Urol. 2020;26:17. https://doi.org/10.1186/s12301-020-00030-z.
2. Pippi Salle JL, Jesus LE, Lorenzo AJ, et al. Glans amputation during routine neonatal circumcision: mechanism of injury and prevention strategy. J Pediatr Urol. 2013;9(6, Part A):763–8.
3. Aymerich RJ, Morote RJ, de Torres MJ, Malet CJ. Intraperitoneal bladder perforation by a permanent bladder catheter. Actas Urol Esp. 1985;9(3):277.
4. Merguerian P, Erturk E, Hulbert W Jr, Davis R, May A, Cockett A. Peritonitis and abdominal free air due to intraperitoneal bladder perforation associated with indwelling urethral catheter drainage. J Urol. 1985;134(4):747–50.
5. Elhilali MM, Hassouna M, Abdel-Hakim A, Teijeira J. Urethral stricture following cardiovascular surgery: role of urethral ischemia. J Urol. 1986;135(2):275–7.
6. Weiss BD. Chronic indwelling bladder catheterization. Am Fam Physician. 1984;30(3):161–6.
7. Michael J, Fine PR, Cutter GR, Maetz HM. The risk of bladder calculi in patients with spinal cord injuries. Arch Intern Med. 1985;145(3):428–30.
8. Hukins D, Hickey D, Kennedy AP. Catheter encrustation by struvite. Br J Urol. 1983;55(3):304–5.
9. Anderson MH. Urethral catheter knots. Pediatrics. 1990;85(5):852–4.
10. Harland RW, DeGroot DL, Dewire DM. The "fractured Foley": an unusual complication of chronic indwelling urinary catheterization. J Am Geriatr Soc. 1992;40(8):827–8.
11. Barnes-Snow E, Luchi RJ, Doig R. Penile laceration from a Foley catheter. J Am Geriatr Soc. 1985;33(10):712–4.
12. Larsen T, Hansen BJ. Longitudinal cleavage of the penis, a rare catheter complication seen in paraplegic patients. Int Urol Nephrol. 1989;21(3):313–6.
13. Goble N, Clarke T, Teasdale C. Signet ring cell adenocarcinoma of bladder secondary to long-term catheterization. Urology. 1990;35(3):279–81.
14. Bell MA. Severe indwelling urinary catheter-associated urethral erosion in four elderly men. Ostomy Wound Manage. 2010;56(12):36–9.
15. Becker B, Witte M, Gross AJ, Netsch C. Iatrogenic hypospadias classification: a new way to classify hypospadias caused by long-term catheterization. Inter J Urol Notes. 2018;980–1. https://doi.org/10.1111/iju.13791.
16. Secrest CL, Madjar S, Sharma AK, Covington-Nichols C. Urethral reconstruction in spinal cord injury patients. J Urol. 2003;170(4):1217–21.
17. Andrews H, Nauth-Misir R, Shah P. Iatrogenic hypospadias–a preventable injury? Spinal Cord. 1998;36(3):177–80.
18. Bycroft J, Hamid R, Shah P. Penile erosion in spinal cord injury–an important lesson. Spinal Cord. 2003;41(11):643–4.

Acute Postoperative Complications of Hypospadias Repair

20

Amilal Bhat

20.1 Introduction

Complications in surgical procedures are inevitable, which holds specially true in hypospadias repair with a higher incidence than other reconstructive surgeries. Acute complications occur within the first 7–10 days after the primary surgery. The reported incidence varies from 6 to 30%. The complications correlates with the hypospadias severity, the surgical technique chosen, the penis size, child's age, and the operating surgeon's experience. Common errors are in the initial evaluation of the patient, choice of the technique and peri- and postoperative care [1, 2]. Complication rates are higher in replacement urethroplasties such as skin flap/graft tube or inner prepucial tube than the plate preservation procedures like tubularized urethral plate urethroplasty [3] and a single-stage repair as compared to two-staged procedures. Plate preservation procedures like TIPU and onlay flap are the commonly chosen procedure for distal hypospadias. Fistula and flap necrosis are seen less frequently. The surgery is convenient and has a better cosmetic result in tubularized urethral plate urethroplasty than Mathieu repair [4]. The tubularized incised plate urethroplasty is feasible even in re-do cases with a supple urethral plate. Though the incision in the urethral plate during previous surgery is not a contraindication, but redo TIPU repair is better avoided in patients with a scarred or resected urethral plate [5]. The inner prepucial tube repair is technically more demanding, and complications are higher than onlay flap repair [6, 7]. The most critical risk factor for complications is the severity of the hypospadias, because a severe malformation is often more challenging to treat and requires a long reconstruction. Additionally, the curvature, shortage of tissue, and extensive surgery generally require a staged reconstruction in these cases. Other factors are of lesser importance [8]. Though the results reported in both pediatric age and adulthood are similar. But a few of them have reported variation in wound healing, infection, complication rates, and overall success in cases operated in adult age. The patient undergoing surgery in adulthood should be informed regarding all of these variables to avoid unreasonable expectations [9, 10]. There is a significant learning curve in surgical repair of hypospadias, and results improve with the surgeon's experience [11, 12]. Results are poor in re-operative cases [13] and free graft [3]. Type of

A. Bhat (✉)
Bhat's Hypospadias and Reconstructive Urology Hospital and Research Centre,
Jaipur, Rajasthan, India

Department of Urology, Jaipur National University Institute for Medical Sciences and Research Centre, Jaipur, Rajasthan, India

Department of Urology, Dr. S.N. Medical College, Jodhpur, Rajasthan, India

Department of Urology, S.P. Medical College, Bikaner, Rajasthan, India

P.G. Committee Medical Council of India, New Delhi, India

Academic and Research Council of RUHS, Jaipur, Rajasthan, India

urinary diversion, the period of urinary diversion, type of dressing, catheter size, and the anesthetic regime did not influence the outcome significantly. Proper preoperative assessment and planning are essential for good results. An erroneous attempt to apply a minor hypospadias repair to a major deformity would lead to complications and failure. To provide insight into the learning curve for hypospadias repair among fellowship-trained pediatric urologists in the United States, Horowitz and Salzhauer examined complications rates in 231 consecutive patients over 5 years [14]. These investigators demonstrated a significant decrease in fistula rates in each year following completion of fellowship training. Titley and Bracka studied the hypospadias complication rates among plastic surgery trainees and found that the likelihood of complication decreased as the experience was accrued [15]. In a single-institution study, Snyder and associates found a marked discrepancy in success rates between pediatric urologists and other surgical specialists in repairing hypospadias complications (87% vs 33%) [16]. Frimberger and colleagues concluded that among fellowship-trained pediatric urologists in practice for <3 years, fistula rates of <3% should be achievable for distal hypospadias defects [17]. These data imply that the likelihood of success after hypospadias repair is more closely related to the surgical experience of the surgeon than to the specific technique employed. Although this statement is intuitive, technical expertise, training, and judgment play pivotal roles in determining the outcome. Moreover, a better understanding of the factors predisposing to complications helps in their prevention.

20.2 Common Early Postoperative Complications

Common early complications occurring within 7 days of surgery are:

Per operative Bleeding and hematoma, edema

Perioperative Hematoma wound infection, wound dehiscence, fistula, penile torsion, penile erections, skin necrosis, flap necrosis

Catheter-related Inadvertent urethral stent removal, bladder spasms, catheter blockade, catheter knot, and urinary retention.

In order of frequency, immediate postoperative fistula is the commonest complication, followed by edema and penile torsion. Though wound dehiscence is rare & disastrous, only a few cases are reported [1].

20.2.1 Bleeding and Hematoma

Bleeding during hypospadias surgery is inevitable, but sometimes it may occur in the immediate postoperative period. A significant big hematoma is hazardous and may cause wound infection and/or flap and graft devascularization and destroy the repair [18]. There are only a few cases reports in the literature, so hematoma's exact incidence is unavailable. Bleeding and hematoma are more common in adults than in the pediatric age group because of frequent penile erections. Various causes of bleeding are an improper plane of dissection, bleeding from damage to corpus spongiosum and cavernosum or resection of spongiosum for chordee correction, inadequate hemostasis, and rarely bleeding diathesis/dyscrasia. A bloodless operative field is required during hypospadias repair to have a better cosmetic outcome and decrease the failure of the surgery. It remains a challenge to the surgeon to create and maintain a proper plane of dissection and to prevent injury to the corpus spongiosum and cavernosum [1].

Bleeding can be minimized by applying a tourniquet, local injection of adrenaline, using adrenaline-soaked gauze pieces, and bipolar pinpoint cauterization preventing tissue damage. Very fine and least reactive sutures are used for ligating the bleeding vessels. Longer tourniquet and higher pressure to achieve a bloodless surgical field may lead to ischemia and/or reperfusion injury of the urethral wall. Injection of epinephrine may result in more prominent cellular changes as compared to tourniquet techniques [1]. Kajbafzadeh et al. reported that the ultrastructural injuries, apoptotic damages, tissue fibrosis, and cellular damage in the urethral wall were more prominent following epinephrine hemostasis in a rabbit model of hypospadias repair [19]. Cakmak et al. documented the effect of tourniquet application and epinephrine injection on penile skin. They concluded the epinephrine injection to penile skin exerts a deleterious effect on wound healing [20].

Treatment Fibrin sealants are the useful hemostatic agent and wound healing promoters in urethral reconstructive procedures [21]. Hafez and colleagues reported a fibrin sealant layer with angiogenesis and cellular infiltrate at 2 weeks and the regeneration of normal tunica albuginea without scarring at 6 and 12 weeks on histopathologic examination. In addition, they found no hematomas, no evidence of corporal narrowing, and no venous leakage on cavernosography [22].

Lahoti et al. in 2010 also reported that feracrylum is an effective and safe topical hemostatic agent which reduces the frequency of cauterization and tissue damage, blood loss during surgery, postoperative hematoma, wound edema, and post-surgical complications [23]. In addition, it significantly minimizes diffuse capillary oozing and surface bleeding and thus obtains a clear field during surgery of hypospadias. These agents are not in routine use.

Effective compression dressing and putting in a small drain helps in preventing the hematoma. The sustained and significant bleeding may require exploration to remove the hematoma and coagulate; if any, the bleeding point is identified and ligated or cauterized. A few skin sutures are removed if recognized late to allow the hematoma evacuation and hydrogen peroxide dressing to dissolve adherent clots [1]. Such cases should be evaluated for bleeding diathesis/dyscrasias [24]. Excessive use of cautery or ligature and residual clots may lead to excessive fibrosis and postoperative chordee. Extreme pressure in dressing and hematoma may lead to skin/flap necrosis [1].

20.2.2 Edema

Dartos is commonly used to cover the repair. Dartos is loose, fragile tissue and is susceptible to edema and infection. Neuropeptide's release from the skin nerve sensory endings influences wound healing, and hypospadiac prepuce has less sensory innervations compared to the normal. Nazir et al. found hypo-innervated for PGP 9.5 & CGRP positive nerves compared with the normal prepuce immunohistochemistry results ($P < 0.05$). SP-positive nerves were increased in the prepuce, but the increase was not found to be statistically significant ($P = 0.06$, confidence interval >95%). These differences in the tissue environment partially explain postoperative edema, poor wound healing leading to complications such as urethrocutaneous fistula (UF), and increased analgesia requirement in patients undergoing hypospadias surgery [25]. Postoperative edema reported in the literature is about 11.11% [26]. Edema due to inflammatory response may involve the penis and the scrotum. Typically, edema is seen after the removal of a pressure dressing. Prepucial edema is more common in hypospadias repair with prepucioplasty (Fig. 20.1). The swelling may be aggravated by hematoma or urinary extravasation due to bladder spasm or accidental urethral stent removal. Meatus involvement may lead to splaying of the urinary stream but is rarely of long-term significance [1].

Edema can be prevented by minimal tissue handling using microsurgical instruments and stay sutures, avoiding the lymphatic disconnection, utilizing the suction drain, compressive dressing, and anti-inflammatory drugs.

Isolated edema settles with time unless associated with infection or hematoma and does not cause permanent damage. The dressing plays a crucial role in postoperative edema prevention. Inadequate pressure may cause hematoma, edema, infection and increase the incidence of complications. However, excessive pressure may compromise the blood supply of the flap and skin, which may lead to tissue necrosis [1, 27].

20.2.3 Wound Infection

Mild and localized infections may be due to the decreased vascularity, humidity, high temperature, and proximity to a potentially contaminated area, and serious sepsis is rare after hypospadias repair. Sanders C et al. found a very high 90.90% infection in the swabs from the foreskin but cleared in 82% cases after local

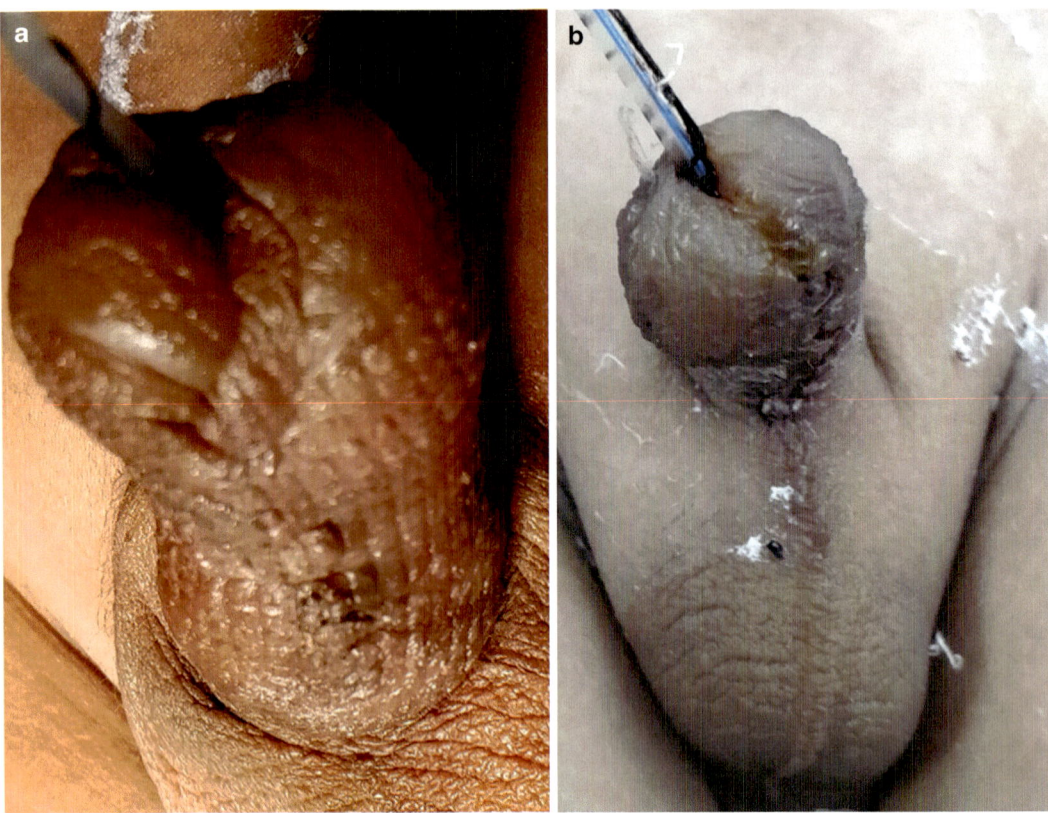

Fig. 20.1 (a, b) Showing the prepucial edema

preparations swabs. The most commonly grown organisms were Coliforms, and Staphylococcus aureus; was sensitive to cephalosporins and aminoglycosides. Preoperatively taken peri meatal swabs help to choose postoperative antibiotic therapy awaiting hypospadias repair [28]. Bacterial colonization was commonly seen before and after surgery in hypospadias surgery with prepucioplasty. Prepucial hood and glans cleansing at the time of surgery reduces pathogens under the foreskin. Usually, bacterial presence did not impact wound healing, but sometimes the wound infection can be a potential disaster to the repair [1].

Infection is better prevented by prophylactic antibiotics, antibiotic solution use during surgery, povidone-iodine scrubbing, prevention of hematoma, and the Mercurochrome local application [29]. Gentle tissue handling, using skin hooks and stay sutures are helpful in infection prevention. Suprapubic diversion is preferable to intubated perineal urethrostomies in cases of urinary and wound infection [1].

Treatment of infection Obvious sepsis (Fig. 20.2) requires to be treated vigorously with the opening of sutures to let out suppuration drain, irrigation with antibiotic solution, debridement of necrotic tissue, and supplementing with local and systemic antibiotics. Suprapubic urinary diversion is preferred in severe infection, wound disruption, and urinary leak from the open wound. Urethral stent seen through open wound better be removed. However, it can be left in situ if there is a little breakdown in healthy tissue coverings. A rapidly progressive infection in the skin, subcutaneous tissue, and superficial fascia (Necrotizing fasciitis) are rare in hypospadias surgery, and only one such case is reported [30]. Prophylactic antibiotics are advisable to reduce infective complications [31, 32]. Urinary tract infection after hypospadias surgery is not very

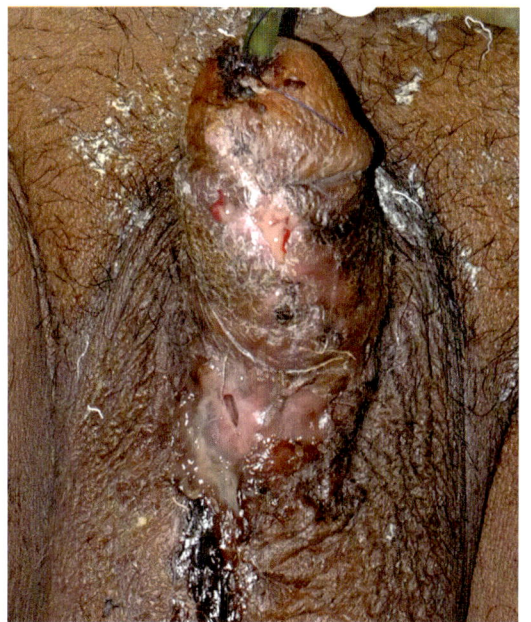

Fig. 20.2 Wound infection with fistula trickling the pus from the wound

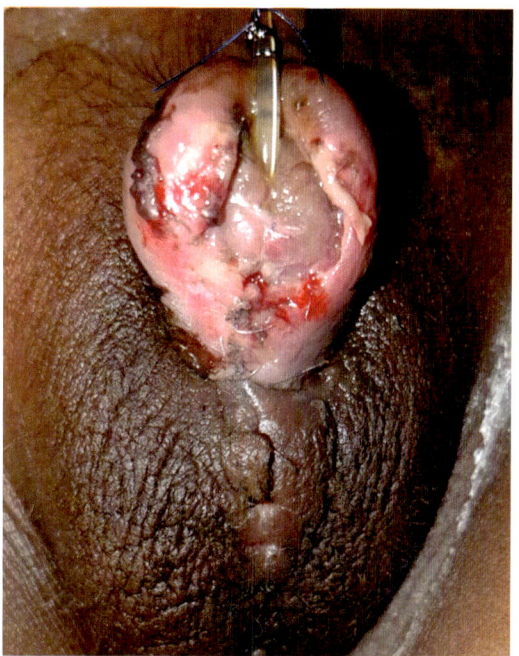

Fig. 20.3 Prepucial dehiscence

common. and antibiotics are rarely required beyond 7–10 days. The persistence, recurrent and chronic urinary tract infection may be due to urine stagnation in the urethra. It may be because of Urethral diverticula, enlarged prostatic utricle, urethral stone, and dilated urethra in skin tube urethroplasty.

Urethrogram and endoscopy are done in suspected cases to confirm the diagnosis and resection of the utricle, remove urethral stones, and reduction urethroplasty is needed to control the infection [1].

20.2.4 Wound Dehiscence

Wound dehiscence is a rare complication, and the reported incidence is 3.28% [5, 33]. But Lee et al. reported a high incidence (26%) of wound dehiscence [32]. Glans dehiscence is more common in TIP than Mathieu, but flap necrosis is more common in Mathieu [5]. The causes of wound dehiscence are edema, hematoma, infection, erections, diminished blood supply, tension at suture line, weakened suture material, and vigorous removal of dressing [33]. Such type of wound dehiscence may lead to complete failure of the repair. Partial wound dehiscence is noted in cases of prepucioplasty (Fig. 20.3). Wound dehiscence can be prevented by choosing the right technique with its systematic application, dartos fascia cover the urethroplasty, everting the skin edges, and proper postoperative management. Immediate treatment includes removing the devitalized, necrotic tissue, suprapubic urinary diversion, and dressings with antibiotic ointment.

Steristrips approximation of the skin margins will encourage wound closure and minimize scarring in large defects. Secondary suturing of the wound is not advisable. A small raw area is likely to granulate and re-epithelize, but large defects require second surgery after 6 months to 1 year [1].

20.2.5 Skin and Flap Necrosis

The flap or graft devascularization is a crucial complication of hypospadias surgery, and the incidence reported is 7% [7, 34]. Flap necrosis is seen less frequently in pediatric hypospadias repair than in adult hypospadias repair. The causes of skin and flap necrosis are damage to vascular supply while raising the flap, hematoma, infection, edema, vascular spasm, and tight pressure dressing leading to the loss blood supply of the flap and skin. Most of the time, the necrosis is superficial and dermal (Figs. 20.4a and 20.5b) and heals without permanent damage to the repair (Figs. 20.4b and 20.5b). In double island urethroplasty, the viability of the neourethra can be evaluated by only looking at the outer face of the flap. The skin and flap necrosis can be prevented by applying a proper surgical technique, maintaining the dissection plane, suitable graft design, adequate hemostasis to avoid hematoma by using pinpoint cautery and broad-spectrum antibiotics to prevent infection [1]. If suspected, the local application of nitroglycerin ointment may prevent vasospasm, and excessive pressure during dressing is avoided.

Treatment of skin and flap necrosis requires debridement of the devitalized part of the graft or flap judiciously. A satisfactory result can still be obtained without re-operating in a small area of devascularization and intact flap pedicle. But the major dehiscence, glanular wing & prepucial dehiscence will need further operative intervention [1].

20.2.6 Urethrocutaneous Fistula

Fistula formation is the most common complication of hypospadias repair, and the incidence varies from 0 [35] to 23% [7]. The fistula rate is lower in TIPU, augmented urethral plate urethroplasty (Snodgraft or onlay flap) than the inner prepucial flap and tube urethroplasty [12]. The commonest fistula site is the coronal

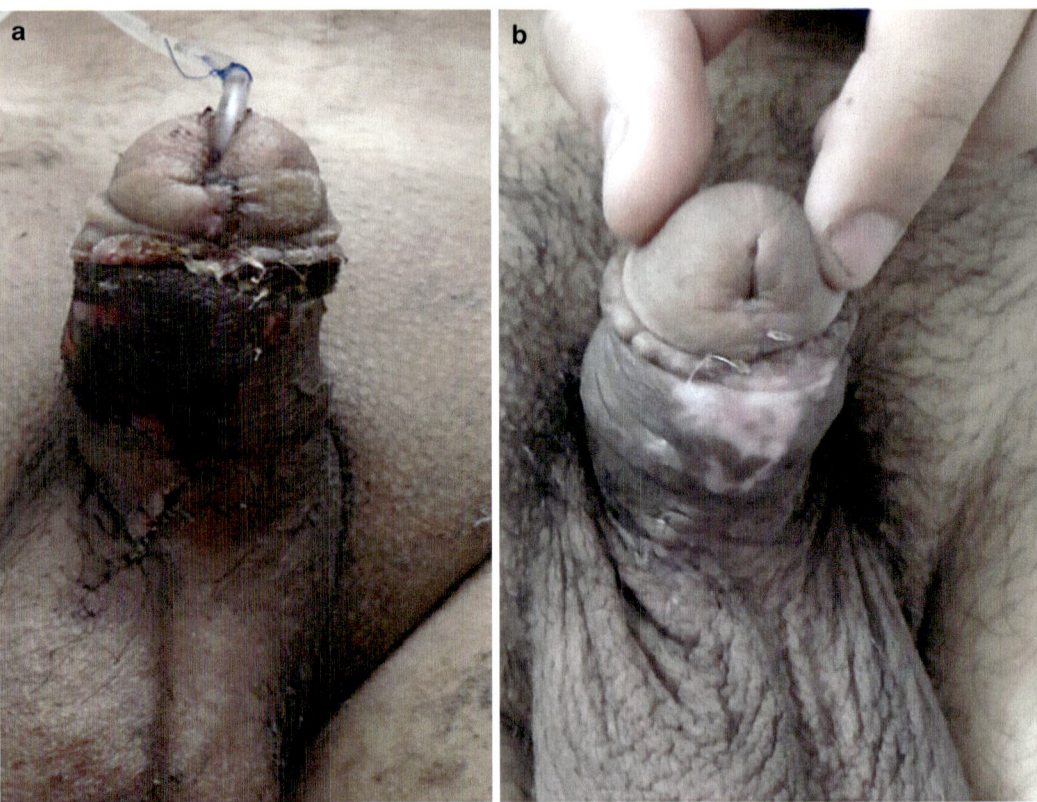

Fig. 20.4 (a) Showing superficial skin necrosis. (b) Healed with discoloration of the skin

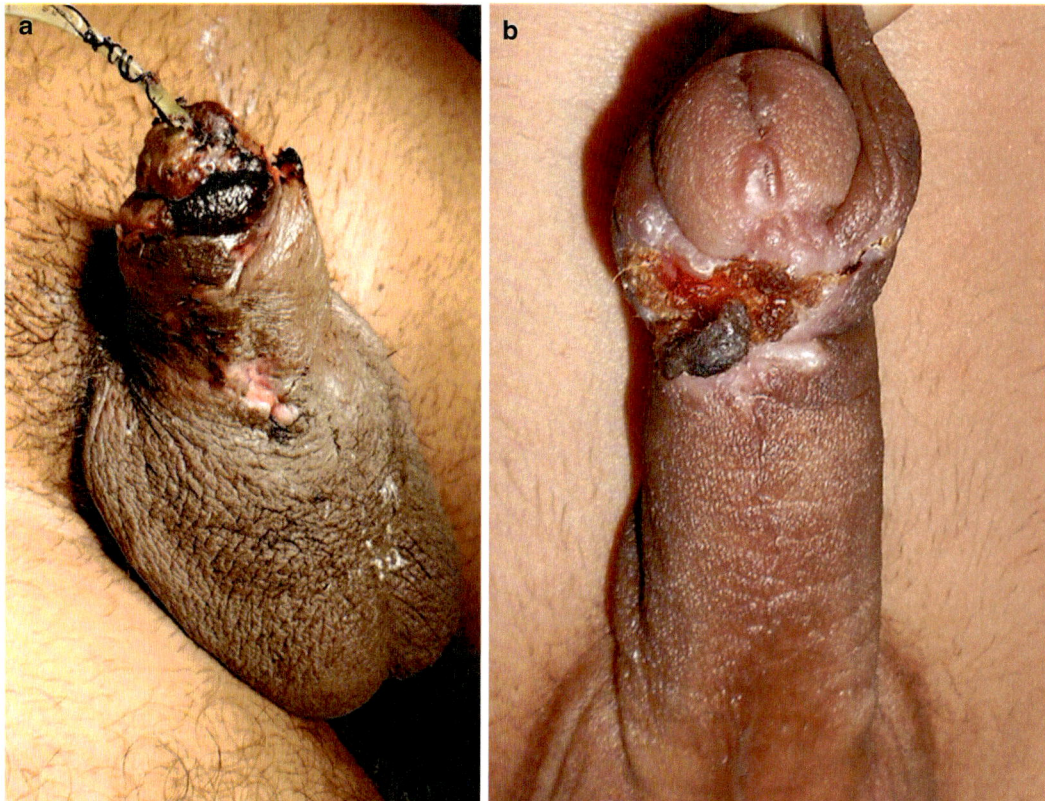

Fig. 20.5 (**a**) Superficial skin necrosis. (**b**) Encrustation

sulcus in incised plate tubularization urethroplasty and anastomosis in flap urethroplasty. But it may occur anywhere in the reconstructed urethra.

Pathophysiology Exact cause of fistulae remains unknown, but it is likely to be a combination of multiple factors, improper technique selection, local ischemia, infection, poor tissue healing, and distal obstruction due to meatal stenosis/encrustation. Fistula formation starts early in the healing process after ventral urethral repair. The incorporation of urethral mucosa in the ventral repair is an epicenter for the formation of the fistula with rapid migration of urethral mucosa and skin epithelium into the suture tracts. The mucosal or dermal migration along suture tracts can be attenuated or prevented by changing the biochemical environment remains to be investigated [36]. Various factor-like hypospadias and chordee severity, urethral plate and spongiosum development, and the surgeon's experience, contribute to the outcome of the surgery. Urine leakage is a strong risk factor, and local infection is moderate when applying stepwise binary logistic regression [37]. Suture material also has an impact on the fistula rate. The fistula was seen significantly higher with 6/0 polyglactin (Vicryl) in a single layer, full-thickness, and uninterrupted fashion (16.6%) compared to 7/0 PDS in subcuticular and uninterrupted fashion (4.9%, $P < 0.01$). Subcutaneous suturing with PDS is preferred in hypospadias repair [38]. However, Chung et al. (2012) reported that hypospadias repair type, suture materials, and surgical technique have no significant effect on the urinary fistula [39]. Dorsal dartos is the most commonly used interposing tissue, and double dartos reduces fistula by almost 50%. Spongiosum is very vascular, and spongioplasty reduces the chances of fistula (details are described in Chap. 21 on late complications).

Treatment Prevention of the fistula is of paramount importance to reduce the overall complications of hypospadias repair. Besides technical excellence and proper technique selection, people have tried fibrin sealant and Bio-glue surgical adhesive. Fibrin sealant has a unique characteristic of being a tissue adhesive, a hemostatic agent, and sealant, and its injection over the anastomosis prevents urinary leakage and promotes healing, thus helping in the prevention of urinary fistula. Kinahan and Johnson reported lower fistula rate with fibrin in hypospadias 9% ($n = 78$) vs. 28% ($n = 97$) [40]. But Kocherov (2013) did not find BioGlue's benefits in decreasing fistula rate and reconstruction breakdowns [41]. Sometimes supra-pubic urinary diversion may help in spontaneous closure of the fistula. The small fistulae are likely to heal in 2–3 weeks after urinary diversion provided there is no meatal stenosis or inflammation. Spontaneous fistula closure was reported in up to 30% [42]. Application n-butyl cyanoacrylate is also used for the repair of early fistula after hypospadias surgery [43]. The use of it does not affect subsequent fistula surgery adversely. Meanwhile, the meatus can be dilated with an ophthalmic ointment tube tip to ensure a satisfactory meatal caliber. Any attempt of fistula closure immediately is likely to fail and should be undertaken only after 3–6 months. Management of established fistula is discussed in Chap. 21 on late complications of hypospadias repair.

20.2.7 Penile Torsion

Penile torsion after the hypospadias may be either due to the uncorrected congenital torsion associated with the hypospadias or traction on the dartos vascular pedicle due to inadequate mobilization. Penile torque is seen in patients of inner prepucial flap/tube repair, the interposition of dorsal dartos healthy tissue cover, and unequal skin flaps during the closure of skin flaps. Penile torsion is more severe in a single dartos flap (mild glanular torsion 90.7% and moderate glanular torsion 9.3%) interposing tissue than double dartos flap (0%) [44]. It can be prevented by adequate mobilization of vascular pedicle/dartos flap up to the root of the penis, bringing the dartos flap ventrally by making a hole in the flap and proper adjustment of skin flaps at the time of skin closure. Mild torsion of <30° does not require any corrective treatment. But moderate to severe torsion should be corrected at least six months after the initial surgery. The techniques of torsion correction are penile degloving and realignment [45]. Plication/suturing the tunica albuginea to pubic periosteum [46, 47], and de-torque by suturing dorsal dartos opposite to torque in primary cases [48].

20.2.8 Penile Erections

Three to eight nocturnal erections during REM sleep are observed in prepubertal boys and adults. Penile erections after hypospadias surgery are more common in adults than the pediatric age group and may lead to a local hematoma, predispose to infection, subsequent devascularization, and increase the chances of complications, especially the urethral fistula. Many methods are used to prevent, but no single treatment method is useful to prevent nocturnal erections postoperatively. The methods used for erection prevention are compressive penile dressing, estrogens, antiandrogens, continuous noradrenaline infusion, chlorpromazine, dorsal nerve block, and patient-controlled epidural analgesia (PCEA). Diazepam is used in doses of 0.1 mg/kg body weight for 7 days postoperatively; have a sedative effect, but still, patients have erections [1]. Estrogens may hinder erections but are less acceptable because of their possible thromboembolic effects. Ketoconazole 400 mg orally three times daily starting on the day of surgery and cyproterone acetate 300 mg daily, started at least 10 days preoperatively, have been reported to help prevent postoperative erections. Johansen et al. reported effective use of a continuous intra-cavernous injection by a micro-infusion pump in 20 patients [49]. However, most of the above-mentioned methods can have side effects related to drugs. In authors view anti-erotics do not have much role in pediatric age but may reduce the erections in adolescents and adults.

20.2.9 Urethral Stent-Related Problems and Bladder Spasms

The urethral catheter is likely to kink, block or knot and occasionally may slip out or removed inadvertently. Bleeding and inadequate hydration may block the catheter. The urethral catheter irrigation with sterile normal saline usually solves the problem. Rarely the urethral catheter may be removed inadvertently prematurely, leading to catastrophic complications. The problem becomes twofold as the repositioning of the urethral stent may disrupt the neourethra. It is better to put in suprapubic catheter drainage, especially in patients of flap urethroplasty or proximal hypospadias repair if inadvertent auto-removal of the stent occur within 48 h of repair. But accidental removal of the stent after 5 days in well-done TIP in distal hypospadias may be left as such after a single gentle trial of repositioning the stent fails. Catheter Knotting (Fig. 20.6) is an infrequent complication of the urethral stent [50]. Catheter knotting is suspected at the time of catheter removal if the urethral stent is stuck up and requires force for removal. Forceful removal of the stent with a knot should not be done as it will damage the neourethra. Knotting may result from the coiling of the intravesical catheter. During bladder decompression, the catheter tip can migrate through a coil leading to a knot, or postoperative bladder spasms may aggravate the knotting during longer catheterization [51]. Proper placement of the catheter and optimum duration of catheterization may prevent knotting. The tricks in catheter placement are that the urethral tube is introduced into the bladder, withdrawn slowly till the urine stops dribbling. Now the tip of the feeding tube lies just distal to the bladder neck and then pass the tube slowly in again till urine starts draining (the end is just proximal to the bladder neck); push the tube in a further 2–3 cm and anchor it at this position with the glans traction suture. The maneuver not only prevents knotting but troublesome bladder spasms also. The

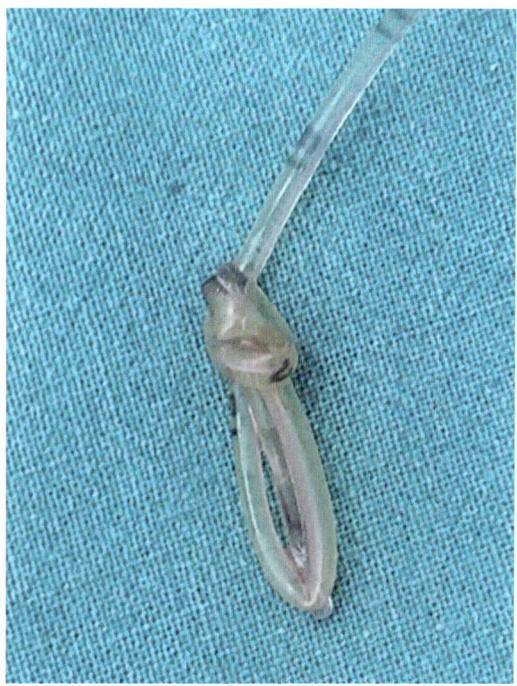

Fig. 20.6 Knotting of the urethral stent

percutaneous suprapubic route should be preferred to remove knotted stents. In pediatric cases, knotting of suprapubic catheters has been reported in longer catheterization, bladder decompression and spasms [52, 53]. Despite all, bladder spasms still may be troublesome and require anticholinergics like oxybutynin. Rotation of urosac is likely to kink the urethral stent; this can be prevented by adequately fixing the stent and urine collection bag and educating the mother to avoid tube kinking. Meatal encrustations after removal of the stent may require regular cleaning and application of ointment locally [1].

20.3 Conclusions

1. Complications are higher in severe hypospadias and flap/graft procedures in adults than in childhood plate preservation procedures.
2. Overall, most of the early complications can better be prevented to avoid disasters.
3. Most common complication of hypospadias repair is a fistula, and healing is spontaneous

in about one-third of cases in the absence of distal obstruction.
4. Hypospadias surgery has a long learning curve, and outcomes become better with the surgeon's experience.
5. Surgery should be avoided in acute complications, except exploration for bleeding, infection, or debridement.
6. Preoperative planning can minimize complications (<5% in distal hypospadias and <10% in proximal hypospadias) by choosing an appropriate surgical technique, surgical expertise, operating in childhood, using magnification, fine suture material and judicious postoperative management.

References

1. Bhat A, Mandal AK. Acute postoperative complications of hypospadias repair. Indian J Urol IJU: J Urol Soc India. 2008;24(2):241.
2. Beuke M, Fisch M. Salvage strategies after complications of hypospadias repair. Der Urologe Ausg A. 2007;46(12):1670–5.
3. Powell CR, Mcaleer I, Alagiri M, Kaplan GW. Comparison of flaps versus grafts in proximal hypospadias surgery. J Urol. 2000;163(4):1286–9.
4. Snodgrass W, Lorenzo A. Tubularized incised-plate urethroplasty for hypospadias reoperation. BJU Int. 2002;89(1):98–100.
5. Guo Y, Ma G, Ge Z. Comparison of the Mathieu and the Snodgrass urethroplasty in distal hypospadias repair. Zhonghua nan ke xue=Natl J Androl. 2004;10(12):916–8.
6. Njinou B, Terryn F, Lorge F, Opsomer R, De PG, Veyckemans F, et al. Correction of severe median hypospadias. Review of 77 cases treated by the onlay island flap technic. Acta Urol Belg. 1998;66(1):7–11.
7. Elbakry A. Complications of the preputial island flap-tube urethroplasty. BJU Int. 1999;84:89–94.
8. Hansson E, Becker M, Åberg M, Svensson H. Analysis of complications after repair of hypospadias. Scand J Plast Reconstr Surg Hand Surg. 2007;41(3):120–4.
9. Hensle TW, Tennenbaum SY, Reiley EA, Pollard J. Hypospadias repair in adults: adventures and misadventures. J Urol. 2001;165(1):77–9.
10. Dodson JL, Baird AD, Baker LA, Docimo SG, Mathews RI. Outcomes of delayed hypospadias repair: implications for decision making. J Urol. 2007;178(1):278–81.
11. Castañón García-Alix M, Martín Hortigüela ME, Rodó Salas J, Morales FL. Complications in hypospadias repair: 20 years of experience. Cirugia pediatrica: organo oficial de la Sociedad Espanola de Cirugia Pediatrica. 1995;8(3):118–22.
12. Uygur MC, Ünal D, Tan MÖ, Germiyanoğlu C, Erol D. Factors affecting the outcome of one-stage anterior hypospadias repair: analysis of 422 cases. Pediatr Surg Int. 2002;18(2-3):142–6.
13. Emir L, Germiyanoglu C, Erol D. Onlay island flap urethroplasty: a comparative analysis of primary versus reoperative cases. Urology. 2003;61(1):216–9.
14. Horowitz M, Salzhauer E. The learning curve in hypospadias surgery. BJU Int. 2006;97(3):593–6.
15. Titley OG, Bracka A. A 5-year audit of trainees experience and outcomes with two-stage hypospadias surgery. Br J Plast Surg. 1998;51(5):370–5.
16. Snyder CL, Evangelidis A, Hansen G, Peter SDS, Ostlie DJ, Gatti JM, et al. Management of complications after hypospadias repair. Urology. 2005;65(4):782–5.
17. Frimberger D, Campbell J, Kropp BP. Hypospadias outcome in the first three years after completing a pediatric urology fellowship. J Pediatr Urol. 2008;4(4):270–4.
18. Grobbelaar A, Laing J, Harrison D, Sanders R. Hypospadias repair: the influence of postoperative care and a patient factor on surgical morbidity. Ann Plast Surg. 1996;37(6):612–7.
19. Kajbafzadeh A-M, Payabvash S, Tavangar SM, Salmasi AH, Sadeghi Z, Elmi A, et al. Comparison of different techniques for hemostasis in a rabbit model of hypospadias repair. J Urol. 2007;178(6):2555–60.
20. Cakmak M, Caglayan F, Kisa U, Bozdogan O, Saray A, Caglayan O. Tourniquet application and epinephrine injection to penile skin: is it safe? Urol Res. 2002;30(4):268–72.
21. Hick EJ, Morey AF. Initial experience with fibrin sealant in pendulous urethral reconstruction. Is early catheter removal possible? J Urol. 2004;171(4):1547–9.
22. Hafez AT, El-Assmy A, El-Hamid MA. Fibrin glue for the suture-less correction of penile chordee: a pilot study in a rabbit model. BJU Int. 2004;94(3):433–6.
23. Lahoti BK, Aggarwal G, Diwaker A, Sharma SS, Laddha A. Hemostasis during hypospadias surgery via topical application of feracrylum citrate: a randomized prospective study. J Indian Assoc Pediatr Surgeons. 2010;15(3):87.
24. Horton CE Jr, Horton CE. Complications of hypospadias surgery. Clin Plast Surg. 1988;15(3):371–9.
25. Nazir Z, Masood R, Rehman R. Sensory innervation of normal and hypospadiac prepuce: possible

implications in hypospadiology. Pediatr Surg Int. 2004;20(8):623–7.
26. Nonomura K, Kakizaki H, Shimoda N, Koyama T, Murakumo M, Koyanagi T. Surgical repair of anterior hypospadias with fish-mouth meatus and intact prepuce based on anatomical characteristics. Eur Urol. 1998;34(4):368–71.
27. Gangopadhyay A, Sharma S. Brief Report-Peha-haft bandage as a new dressing for pediatric hypospadias repair. Indian J Plast Surg. 2005;38(2):162–4.
28. Ratan S, Sen A, Ratan J. Pattern of bacterial flora in local genital skin and surgical wounds in children undergoing hypospadias repair: a preliminary study. Int J Clin Pract. 2002;56(5):349–52.
29. Ratan S, Sen A, Ratan J, Pandey R. Mercurochrome as an adjunct to local preoperative preparation in children undergoing hypospadias repair. BJU Int. 2001;88(3):259–62.
30. Luo C-C, Chao HC, Chiu CH. Necrotizing fasciitis: a rare complication of hypospadias surgery in a child. J Pediatr Surg. 2005;40(4):E29–31.
31. Meir DB, Livne PM. Is prophylactic antimicrobial treatment necessary after hypospadias repair? J Urol. 2004;171(6 Part 2):2621–2.
32. Lee Y-C, Huang C-H, Chou Y-H, Wu W-J, Lin C-Y. The outcome of hypospadias reoperation based on preoperative antimicrobial prophylaxis. Kaohsiung J Med Sci. 2005;21(8):351–7.
33. İmamoğlu MA, Bakırtaş H. Comparison of two methods–Mathieu and Snodgrass–in hypospadias repair. Urol Int. 2003;71(3):251–4.
34. Chin T, Liu C, Wei C. Hypospadias repair using a double onlay preputial flap. Pediatr Surg Int. 2001;17(5–6):496–8.
35. Kass EJ, Bolong D. Single-stage hypospadias reconstruction without fistula. J Urol. 1990;144(2 Part 2):520–2.
36. Edney MT, Lopes JF, Schned A, Ellsworth PI, Cendron M. Time course and histology of urethrocutaneous fistula formation in a porcine model of urethral healing. Eur Urol. 2004;45(6):806–10.
37. Ratan S, Sen A, Pandey R, Hans C, Roychaudhary S, Ratan J. Lesser evaluated determinants of fistula formation in children with hypospadias. Int J Clin Pract. 2001;55(2):96–9.
38. Ulman I, Erikci V, Avanoğlu A, Gökdemir A. The effect of suturing technique and material on complication rate following hypospadias repair. Eur J Pediatr Surg. 1997;7(03):156–7.
39. Chung J-W, Choi SH, Kim BS, Chung SK. Risk factors for the development of urethrocutaneous fistula after hypospadias repair: a retrospective study. Korean J Urol. 2012;53(10):711–5.
40. Kinahan T, Johnson H. Tisseel in hypospadias repair. Can J Surg/Journal Canadien de Chirurgie. 1992;35(1):75–7.
41. Kocherov S, Lev G, Chertin B. Use of bioglue surgical adhesive in hypospadias repair. Curr Urol. 2013;7(3):132–5.
42. Lay L, Zamboni WA, Texter JH, Zook EG. Analysis of hypospadias and fistula repair. Am Surg. 1995;61(6):537–8.
43. Ambriz-Gonzalez G, Velazquez-Ramirez GA, Garcia-Gonzalez JL, de León-Gómez JMG, Mucino-Hernandez MI, Gonzalez-Ojeda A, et al. Use of fibrin sealant in hypospadias surgical repair reduces the frequency of postoperative complications. Urol Int. 2007;78(1):37–41.
44. Kamal BA. Double dartos flaps in tubularized incised plate hypospadias repair. Urology. 2005;66(5):1095–8.
45. Bar-Yosef Y, Binyamini J, Matzkin H, Ben-Chaim J. Degloving and realignment—simple repair of isolated penile torsion. Urology. 2007;69(2):369–71.
46. Hsieh J-T, Liu S-P, Chen Y, Chang H-C, Yu H-J, Chen C-H. Correction of congenital penile curvature using modified tunical plication with absorbable sutures: the long-term outcome and patient satisfaction. Eur Urol. 2007;52(1):261–7.
47. Zhou L, Mei H, Hwang AH, Xie H-w, Hardy BE. Penile torsion repair by suturing tunica albuginea to the pubic periosteum. J Pediatr Surg. 2006;41(1):e7–9.
48. Fisher PC, Park JM. Penile torsion repair using dorsal dartos flap rotation. J Urol. 2004;171(5):1903–4.
49. Johansen L, Kirkeby H, Kiil J. Prevention of erection after penile surgery. Urol Res. 1989;17(6):393–5.
50. Singh R, Pavithran NM, Parameswaran RM. The knotting of the feeding tube is used for bladder drainage in hypospadias repair. 2005.
51. Mayer E, Ankem MK, Hartanto VH, Barone JG. Management of urethral catheter knot in a neonate. Can J Urol. 2002;9(5):1649–50.
52. Arda İS, Özyaylali İ. An unusual complication of suprapubic catheterization with Cystofix: catheter knotting within the bladder. Int J Urol. 2001;8(4):188–9.
53. Gardikis S, Soultanidis C, Deftereos S, Kambouri K, Vaos CG, Touloupidis S, et al. Suprapubic catheter knotting: an unusual complication. Int Urol Nephrol. 2004;36(4):537–9.

21

Late Postoperative Complications of Hypospadias Repair

Amilal Bhat

21.1 Introduction

Though there has been much advancement in Hypospadialogy, and the results of hypospadias repair have improved significantly, however still, complications are inevitable regardless of surgical experience and technique used to repair hypospadias. High success rates have been reported in childhood, but the follow-up has been short in most studies. Available information about these patients at adolescence and sexual maturity are less. Some childhood hypospadias repair complications like urethral stricture and chordee may develop after many years and may present late. The complications may be as high as 54% in long-term follow-up even in experienced hands. The first complication may appear even after five years, and the most prolonged interval documented has been 14 years. Patients/parents of these children are asked to follow-up until their transition to adolescence and adulthood. So, the urination problems, cosmetic appearance, sexual dysfunction, infertility, and psychological issues can be addressed [1]. Primary hypospadias repair patients older than six years at the time of surgery are less satisfied than their younger counterparts. These problems become of more of a concern to the patients after puberty due to the changes in physical appearance, more awareness and interest in sexual activity. The patient requires rectification of urethral stricture, fistula and diverticula, meatal stenosis, residual/persistent chordee, urethral hairs and stones and recurrent UTI. The complications are likely to involve a single compartment of the male genitalia (urethra, corpora cavernosa, glans, or penile or scrotal skin) or a combination. Surgical therapy of the patients is challenging, as the available tissue for the construction of neo-urethra has already been utilized. The most crucial issue in complications of hypospadias repair to be addressed is why hypospadias surgery failed. Some of these may be due to the inexperience of the operating surgeon or improper application of the procedure and others from the tissues' failure to heal properly. Complications are more significant in proximal hypospadias than distal one, flap repair than TIPU, urethral plate resection than preservation, severe versus minimal chordee, and healthy tissue cover versus no cover [2].

A. Bhat (✉)
Bhat's Hypospadias and Reconstructive Urology Hospital and Research Centre,
Jaipur, Rajasthan, India

Department of Urology, Jaipur National University Institute for Medical Sciences and Research Centre,
Jaipur, Rajasthan, India

Department of Urology, Dr. S.N. Medical College,
Jodhpur, Rajasthan, India

Department of Urology, S.P. Medical College,
Bikaner, Rajasthan, India

P.G. Committee Medical Council of India,
New Delhi, India

Academic and Research Council of RUHS,
Jaipur, Rajasthan, India

21.2 Common Postoperative Complications

These late complications can be divided as follows:

1. External urinary meatus and glans—Meatal stenosis, retrusive meatus and glans dehiscence, glanular scars
2. Urethra—Fistula, stricture, and diverticulum, laid-open neo-urethra, hairy urethra, urethral stones
3. Penile shaft—Chordee, torsion, and aesthetic deformity, inclusion dermoid, granuloma
4. Psychosocial and psychosexual

21.3 External Urinary Meatus and Glans

21.3.1 Meatal Stenosis

There are no strict criteria defined for meatal stenosis. Snodgrass defined a meatal calibre of less than 8 French is to be considered as meatal stenosis. Incidence varies from 0.7% to 21% [3]. It may be due to technical issues during the surgery, like fashioning a narrow urethral meatus or suturing the glans wings too tight. Glanular wrap and urethral tunnelling are surgical techniques to position the meatus at the tip of the glans. Performing either of the techniques erroneously may result in meatal stenosis. Meatal stenosis can be prevented in the glanular wrap technique by generously incising ventrally up to the corpora and laterally along both sides of the site proposed for neo-urethral placement. An adequate plane between the corpora and glans tissue tips is created to prevent unwanted tension, which risks the collapse of the underlying neo-urethra. Deepening the glanular incision is mandatory if the approximation of the glans cannot be accomplished without tension.

An adequate size sound for the age is interposed between the neo-urethra with its indwelling stent and the glanular wrap when the glans is approximated (Fig. 21.1). Suturing of the glans wings is done up to mid-glans to have conical meatus and avoid the meatal narrowing. The glans tunnelling technique is an acceptable alternative in the well-formed glans with a normal-appearing meatal cleft. The scissors are passed deep through the glans, and an ellipse of the deeper tissue along with epithelium at the meatal cleft is excised to create a tunnel. The completed tunnel must allow the easy passage of an 18 French sound.

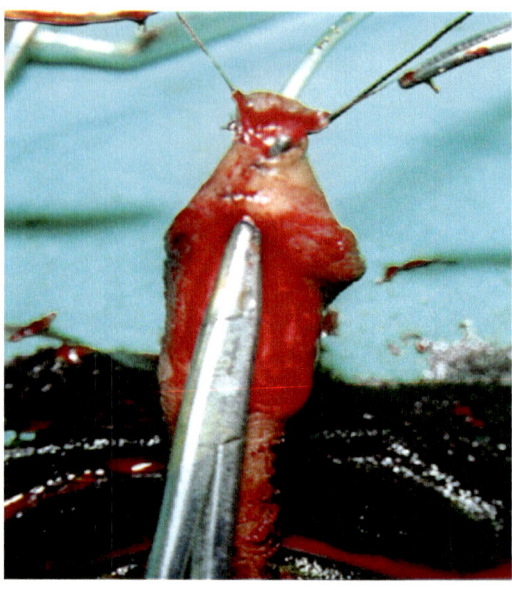

Fig. 21.1 Diagram showing adequacy of glanular wings

21.3.1.1 Treatment of Meatal Stenosis
1. Meatal dilatation
2. Meatotomy
3. Meatoplasty
4. Redo repair

Meatal narrowing at a one-month visit may be due to glanular oedema, and meatal calibration is sufficient, but if it persists at the 3-month visit, then meatal dilation is indicated. A meatotomy may be required for persistent stenosis. The scarred meatus is incised dorsally or ventrally, depending on the position of the meatus, and the skin is re-approximated to urethral mucosa, horizontally opening the urethra in a Y–V fashion. In more severe cases, an extensive glanular meatoplasty may be required. In these situations, a ventral transverse onlay island flap or a tubularized incised urethroplasty may be used and covered with glans wings, or a ventral flap is developed and folded into the split glans. Severe meatal stenosis with proximal extension or BXO may require a redo repair with a buccal mucosal graft. No studies were found reporting the results of meatal dilatation.

21.3.2 Retrusion of Meatus

Meatal retrusion is occasionally encountered after the meatal advancement with glanuloplasty incorporated (MAGPI) technique and the Mathieu hypospadias repair in which the glansplasty sutures have given way. Incidence varies from 1.2% to 26% [4, 5]. Now incidence has come down because most of these patients are treated with TIP repair. Meatal regression is caused by the selection of the wrong repair for the patient's anatomic features. The urethra, which is immobile or the meatus that is non-compliant, results in retrusion of the neo-urethra to its original position. In the Mathieu repair, an inadequate ventral skin flap may lead to the glansplasty sutures' premature dissolution with the same result. The consequences of this complication are predominantly cosmetic rather than functional. However, if significant splaying or deflection of the stream occurs, revision of the meatus is advisable. Revision of urethroplasty with TIP repair (Fig. 21.2a–f) yields good results in such cases.

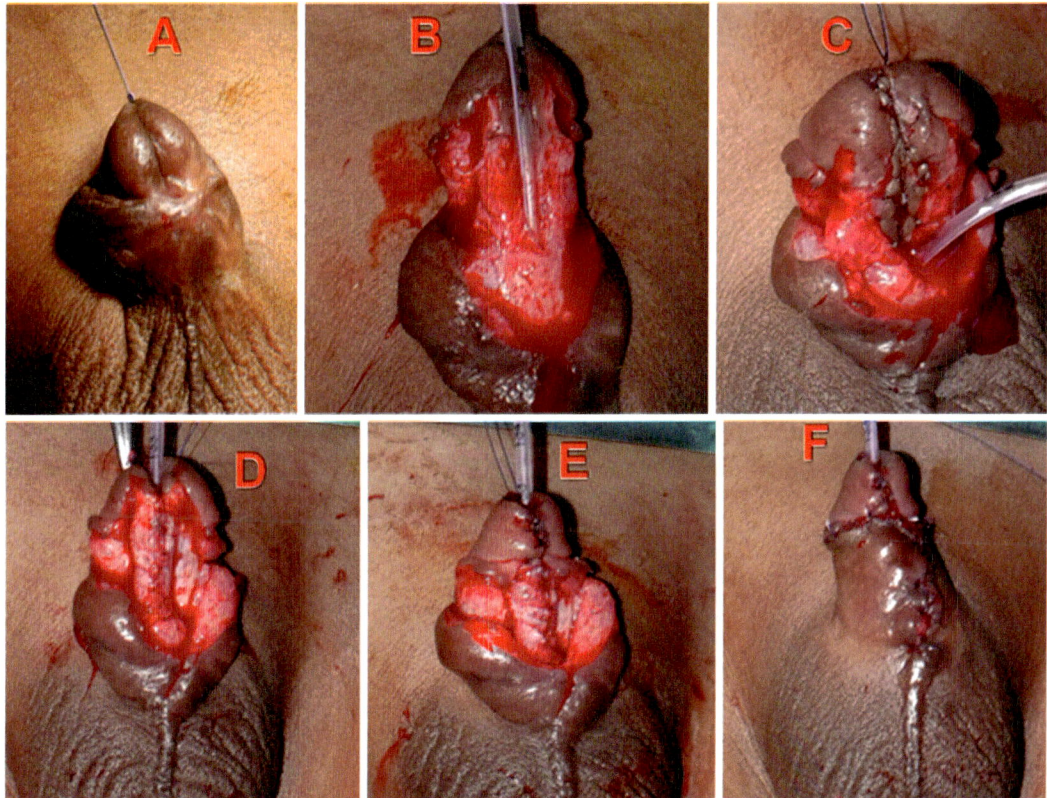

Fig. 21.2 Tubularized urethral plate urethroplasty in a case of fistula and retrusive meatus. (**a**). Two-year-old male with retrusive meatus after TIP. (**b**). Penile skin degloving and spongiosum mobilization. (**c**). Dorsal inlay graft of residual prepucial skin. (**d**). The urethral plate tubularization. (**e**). Spongioplasty and glanuloplasty. (**f**). Final picture after skin closure

21.3.3 Glans Dehiscence

Complete or partial separation of glanular wing is defined as glans dehiscence. The incidence of glanular dehiscence varies from 1.7% to 6.6%. Glans size is a crucial variable in glans dehiscence. Glanular size of less than 14 mm has more chances of dehiscence. Snodgrass reported a 3.5 fold increase in dehiscence in cases with glans size less than 14 mm [6]. Glans dehiscence is more in proximal and re-operative TIPU than the distal one. Incomplete mobilization of granular wings contributes significantly to dehiscence. Extended mobilization of glanular wings deep up to corporal bodies' tip creates wide glanular wings for tension-free closure of glans wing to reduce the glans dehiscence. Few studies have reported increased glans dehiscence when the interposing dartos high up under the glans wings [7], but others have not found it. According to the urethral plate's size and glans wings, glans dehiscence requires second surgery as re-operative TIPU with or without dorsal inlay graft (Figs. 21.3a–f, 21.5a–h). The results of redo surgery are usually good.

21.3.4 Glans Scars

Scars on the glans are rarely discussed as a hypospadias repair complication, but this is of cosmetic concern to the parents and patients. The scars are usually seen at the stay suture site dorsally (Fig. 21.4a–f), ventrally when the glanular sutures are taken through and through and/or mattress sutures are applied, and partial dehiscence of the distal-most sutures. The causes of scar formation are the needle's calibre, the type and size of the suture material, duration of suturing, infection, or an abnormality in tissue healing. If anchoring is required, it can be done using tapes or thinner materials other than silk or

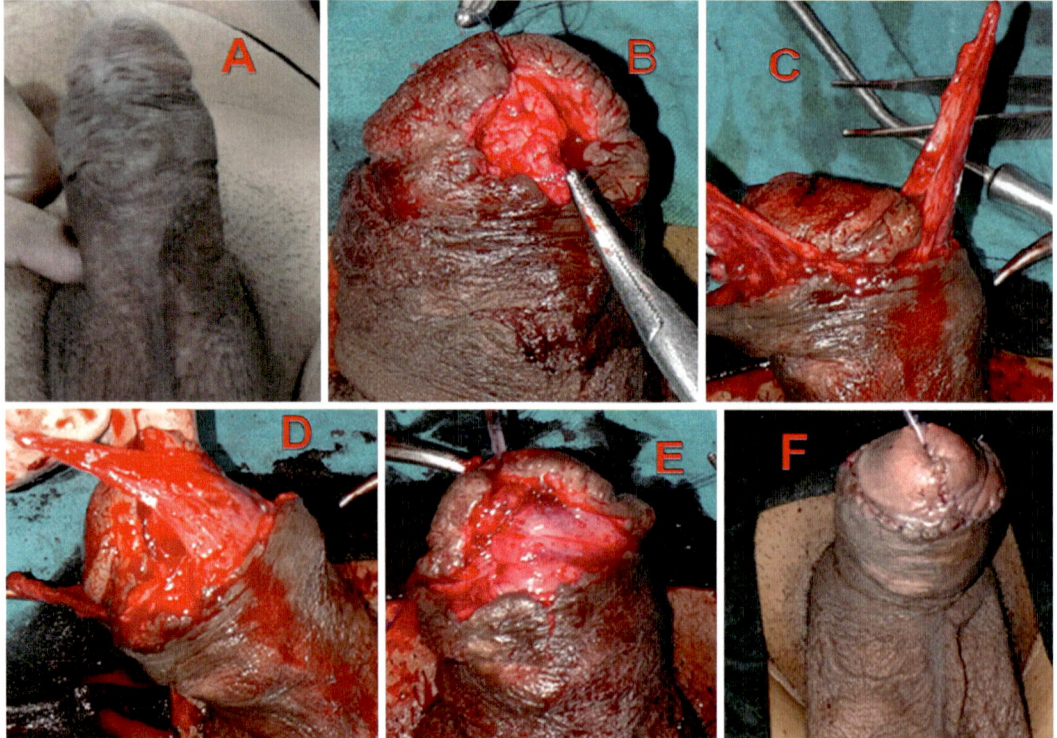

Fig. 21.3 TIPU and spongioplasty in glans dehiscence. (**a**). Glans dehiscence. (**b**). Tubularization of urethral plate and spongioplasty. (**c, d**). Double dartos flaps raised for covering of neo-urethra. (**e**). Covering the neo-urethra with double dartos. (**f**). Final picture after skin closure

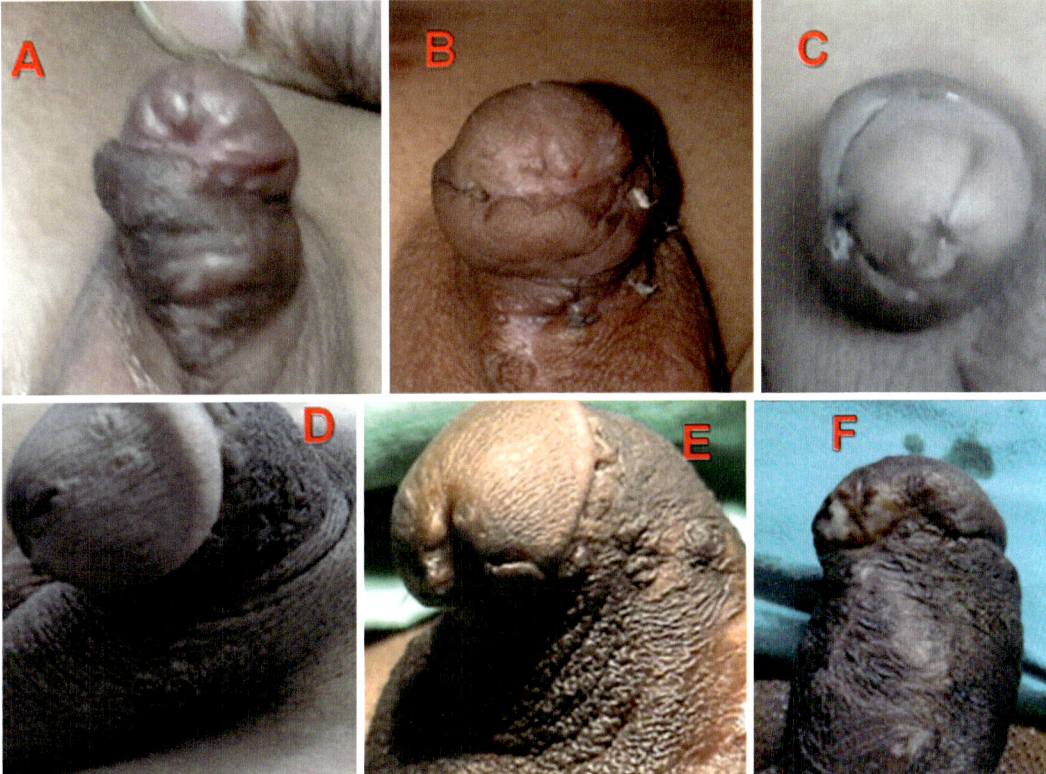

Fig. 21.4 Glans scarring after hypospadias repair. (**a, b, c**). Isolated glans scarring. (**d, e**). Glans scarring associated with chordee. (**f**). Glans scarring with penile scarring

anchoring through preputium. Sub-epithelial sutures for glans closure prevent these scars. Ugly scars can be repaired by excision of the epithelium and suturing it again by sub-cuticular sutures. A scar associated with partial dehiscence of glans requires the revision of TIPU and glansplasty (Fig. 21.5a–h).

21.4 Urethra

21.4.1 Urethrocutaneous Fistula

Urethrocutaneous fistula is the most common and major hypospadias repair complication. The more extensive the urethroplasty, the higher is the frequency of this complication. Though fistula incidence has been steadily decreasing with microsurgical equipment and improved operative technique, it is still the most troublesome complication. The urethral fistula incidence varies from 4% to 28% [8]. The development of the fistula is multifactorial. Oedema-attenuated vascular supply, infection, and haematoma may impair healing of the newly reconstructed urethra. In addition, urethral obstruction distal to repair from meatal crusting or stenosis may lead to high-pressure voiding and disrupt a proximal suture line. Finally, technical factors such as overlapping suture lines, inadequate inversion of the epithelium, or poorly absorbable suture material have been implicated. Detailed pathophysiology is discussed in Chap. 20 on acute complications of hypospadias repair.

The site of the fistula may be according to the type of hypospadias and previous surgical technique (Fig. 21.6a–i). Sub-coronal fistulae are most common in distal hypospadias repair. Urethral fistula management depends on location, size, and time interval from the surgical procedure. A urine leak usually becomes apparent in the first few days after initiation of voiding, and most are noticed in the first six months, but some cases may appear after many years. Small fistulae

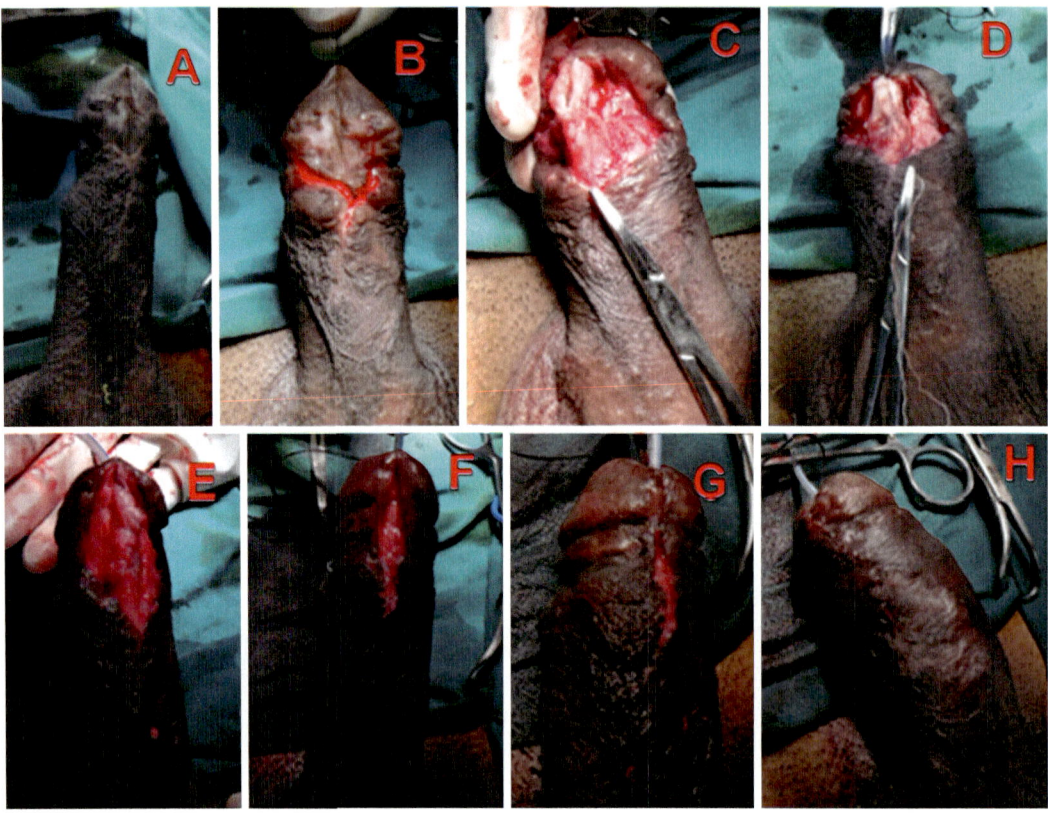

Fig. 21.5 TIPU in glans scar and dehiscence. (**a**). Deformed glans with scarring and dehiscence. (**b**). Skin incision marking the urethral plate. (**c, d**). The urethral plate tubularization. (**e**). Spongioplasty. (**f**). Dartos cover over spongioplasty. (**g**). Glanuloplasty. (**h**). Final appearance after skin closure

noted perioperatively, without concomitant inflammation or meatal stenosis, occasionally may close. Larger fistulae and those persisting beyond several weeks invariably require operative intervention. This intervention must be delayed until tissues have thoroughly healed from the previous operation. Six months is generally adequate time to allow ingrowth of blood vessels and resolution of inflammation and oedema. So, fistula repair should be done 6–12 months after the surgery.

21.4.1.1 Prevention
Fistula can be prevented by using inverting sutures with fine suture material. The interposition of a healthy tissue layer plays a vital role in the prevention of fistula. Various interposing healthy tissues to cover the neo-urethra described in the literature are transverse island dorsal subcutaneous flap, dorsal, lateral, ventral, or scrotal dartos flap, single or double dartos flaps, de-epithelized local penile skin, preputial flap, paraurethral tissue, tunica vaginalis flaps, and spongioplasty.

21.4.1.2 Dorsal Dartos
The dorsal dartos flap is the most commonly used as healthy interposing tissue. However, nil fistula was reported by Djordjevic et al. with single dartos flaps [10], while others have reported fistula rates of 13% and 26% [11]. Few studies reported having a better outcome in reduction of fistula formation with the double dartos flaps. But the statistically significant difference was reported only by Appignani et al. [12]. Maarouf A M. et al. (2012) found a higher fistula rate (8%) in the urethroplasties covered with a single layer than with a double layer (none) [7]. However, the difference was not statistically significant ($P = 0.1$). Elsayed et al. had no significant difference in ure-

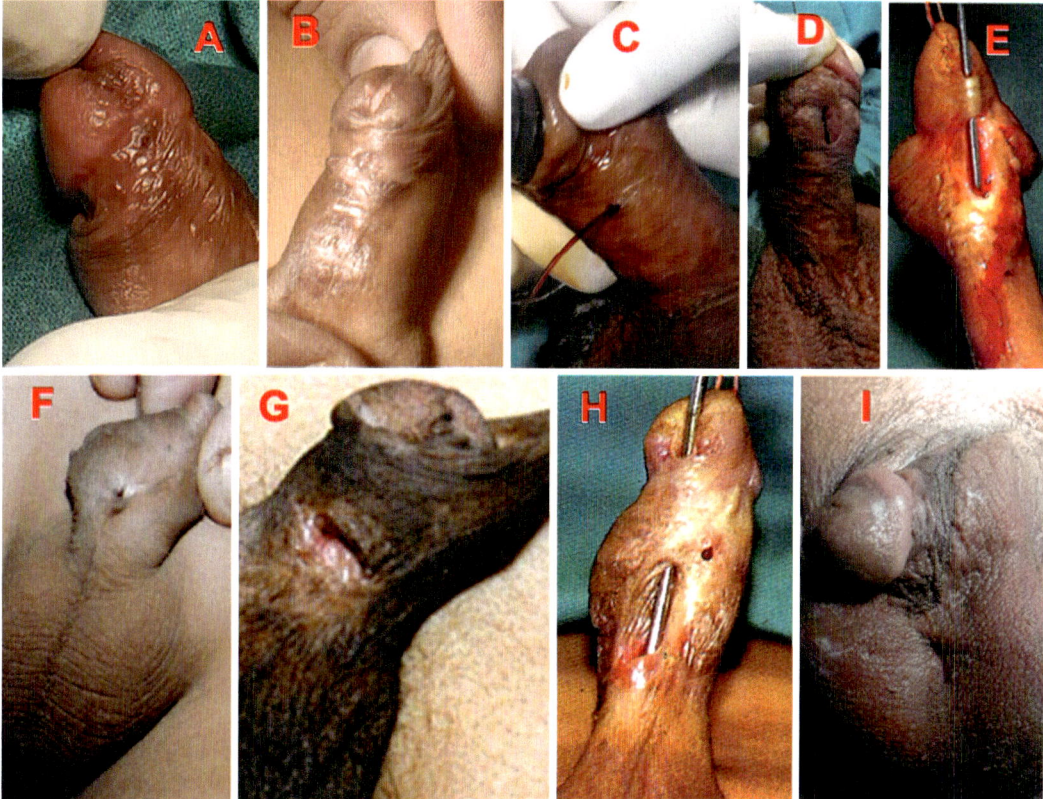

Fig. 21.6 The site and size of fistula. (**a**). Small sub–coronal, (**b** & **c**). Small mid-penile, (**d** & **e**). Large mid-penile, (**f**). Small proximal penile, (**g** & **h**). Large proximal penile, (**i**). Scrotal

throcutaneous fistula between a double-layered dorsal dartos flap and a single layer covering the urethra as a part of TIP urethroplasty [13]. These dartos flaps can be used as a second heathy tissue cover after spongioplasty to reduce the fistula rate.

21.4.1.3 Spongiosum

The results of spongioplasty and spongioplasty with dartos cover are almost similar in both groups of our study. But Bilici et al. (2011) compared the neo-urethra cover with the dartos alone (75 patients) and spongioplasty with the dartos flap (86 patients). They reported 8% fistula formation with dartos alone while no fistula in spongioplasty with dartos cover [14]. They recommended using the corpus spongiosum with the dartos flap as healthy interposing tissue, as it can be applied easily and effectively to prevent fistulae formation. We also found a reduced fistula formation rate, even in proximal hypospadias repair, when combined with spongioplasty [15]. We compared the complication rate of spongioplasty alone vs spongioplasty and a dorsal dartos flap and did not find a significant difference between the two groups [16]. Thus, spongioplasty, when feasible, is adequate as an interposing layer and may be combined with a dorsal dartos flap or other healthy interposing tissue.

21.4.1.4 De-epithelialized Skin Flap

Durham Smith (1973) first described the de-epithelialized overlap flap in second-stage hypospadias and fistula reported only in 2% of cases [17]. Belman (1988) used the de-epithelialized preputial skin flap as a vascular cover for hypospadias repairs [18]. The same was reported later by many surgeons and Snodgrass himself in TIP procedure. Belman reported a fistula rate of 3.5% after covering the neo-urethra with a de-epithelialized preputial skin flap wrap [18].

21.4.1.5 Tunica Vaginalis

Tunica vaginalis is an excellent interposing tissue and is the first choice in cases of fistula repair, re-operative surgery, and proximal hypospadias repair. Snow et al. (1995) first described the use of tunica vaginalis as an interposition graft and reported a 9% fistula rate in their series [19]. Shankar et al. and Handoo reported similar results in their study [20, 21]. Snodgrass et al. could reduce the fistula rate to 0% using tunica vaginalis flap in their recent study [22].

21.4.1.6 Evaluation and Investigation

Effective management demands a careful assessment of associated urethral disorders such as chordee, stricture, and diverticula. The penile shaft must be evaluated for the presence of other unrecognized fistulas. Distension of urethra with saline mixed Betadine will delineate the hidden fistulae. The fistula tract can be cannulated with a lacrimal probe to determine the site of entrance into the urethra. This manoeuvre is useful in planning the orientation of skin flaps for coverage of the fistula. The lacrimal probe can also be a valuable aid for the dissection of the fistula tract. A micturating cystourethrogram is advisable to delineate the number of fistulas, stricture urethra, proximal dilatation of the urethra, and diverticula. Cystoscopy may help see the size of the urethra and healing after previous surgery, especially to see any hair growth in the cases of prior skin flap surgeries, location and status of urethral diverticula.

21.4.1.7 Treatment

Once the fistula's origin is appreciated, it can be closed with a delicate 7–0 or finer absorbable suture. Small-calibre fistulas can be closed primarily without compromising the diameter of the urethral lumen. An ideal fistula repair should have:

1. Delicate tissue handling
2. Fistulous tract excision
3. Inversion of urethral mucosa
4. Needlepoint cautery
5. Use of magnification
6. Late-absorbable proper suture material
7. Avoiding overlapping of suture line
8. Multilayer closure with well-vascularized tissue

The fistula's closure involves three critical steps: excision of the fistulous tract and closure of the fistula with fine sutures, covering the repair with a healthy interposing tissue layer and skin closure, avoiding superimposition suture line.

A small coronal fistula is excised, and penile shaft skin is advanced to cover the defect. If retrusive meatus with fistula, the ledge between meatus and fistula is excised, and TIPU with spongioplasty (Fig. 21.7a–i) is done. If the urethral plate is not wide, then dorsal inlay skin graft/buccal mucosal graft (Fig. 21.8a–g) or onlay flap urethroplasty is done to avoid the stricture and tension-free closure. Larger fistulas may require coverage with a trap-door or island flap of penile shaft skin. Multiple fistulae can be combined, and closure is done with or without the dorsal inlay. If the defect is larger after connecting all fistulae, then onlay flap urethroplasty is done. In general, better results can be achieved when a second layer or flap coverage is possible, especially in recurrent urethral fistula cases. Skin coverage can be obtained by several methods to avoid overlap of urethral and skin suture lines. Despite a well-performed repair, 4–30% or more of fistulas will recur. Sunay M et al. (2007) reported fistulas at the distal penile in 43.2%, mid in 37.5%, and 31 19.2% in the proximal penile region [9]. There was no statistically significant relationship between the fistula site, size and number of the fistula with success rate.

Snodgrass (2015) et al. had only 5% recurrence after simple fistula and interposing dartos flap [22]. This recurrence rate can be decreased by interposing a non-epithelialized layer between the urethral closure and the skin. Various investigators advocate the use of a scrotal based tunica vaginalis flap, scrotal dartos tissue and de-epithelialized flap. There is no need to divert the urine for simple repairs, but it is advisable to divert the urine for 7 to 10 days with a silicone urethral stent for more extensive repairs. Finally, in cases of severe fistula problems, buccal mucosa grafts have been used with some success.

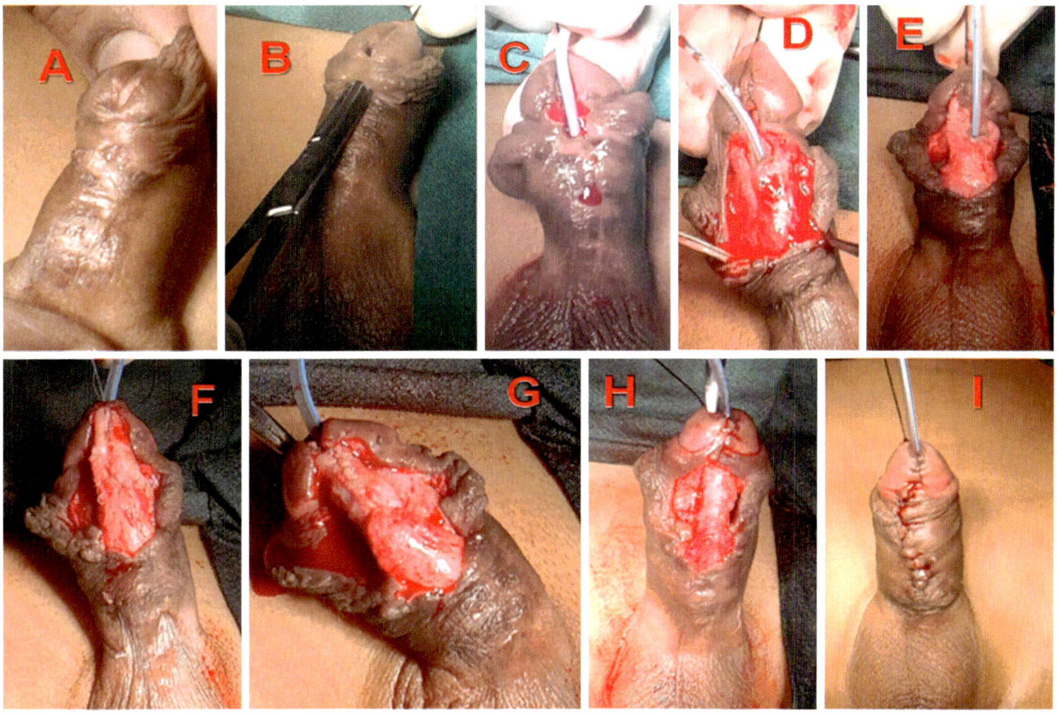

Fig. 21.7 TIPU with spongioplasty in retrusive meatus with fistula. (**a**). Retrusive meatus with urethrocutaneous fistula and glanular chordee. (**b**). Haemostat in the fistula showing skin ledge. (**c**). Laid-open distal urethra after incising the skin ledge. (**d**). Urethral plate and spongiosum mobilization. (**e**). Urethral plate mobilization into the glans. (**f**). Urethral plate tubularization. (**g**). Spongioplasty. (**h**). Glansplasty. (**i**). Skin closure

21.4.2 Stricture Urethra

Stricture of the urethra is the second most frequently reported complication after fistula in hypospadias surgery. Strictures are likely to form at anastomotic suture lines of the urethra and neo-urethra, sub-meatal sutures of the glans closure, or incision site of the urethral plate. Three months after the surgery, the strictures become apparent with the decreased urinary stream force, straining during voiding, or urinary tract infection. Sometimes the patient may present with splaying of the urinary stream, urethrocutaneous fistula, or rarely urinary retention. There are several factors implicated in the formation of neo-urethral stricture. Poor design of the neo-urethra, insufficient calibre, tension on suture lines, and inadequate spatulation of the urethra at the anastomosis are important factors. Trauma, infection, and tissue ischaemia can result in inflammation and concentric scarring of the lumen. In tubularized pedicle flaps, a stricture may be functional, secondary to a redundant neo-urethra kinking at the proximal anastomosis. Although there were initial concerns that TIP's relaxing incision would create strictures, it is rarely encountered. Diagnosis of the stricture with accurate length and location is done by urethrogram and is confirmed by cystoscopic examination with a 0-degree lens under anaesthesia. Proximal dilation of the urethra (Fig. 21.9a, b) may be delineated in the urethrogram and help plan the treatment.

Others favour diagnosis with symptomatology only, and preoperative cystoscopy without urethrogram [23]. We prefer a urethrogram for better planning of the treatment. As long as stricture with the narrow urethra, it may not be possible to see the stricture's proximal extent.

Management of Stricture Methods applied for the management of stricture are

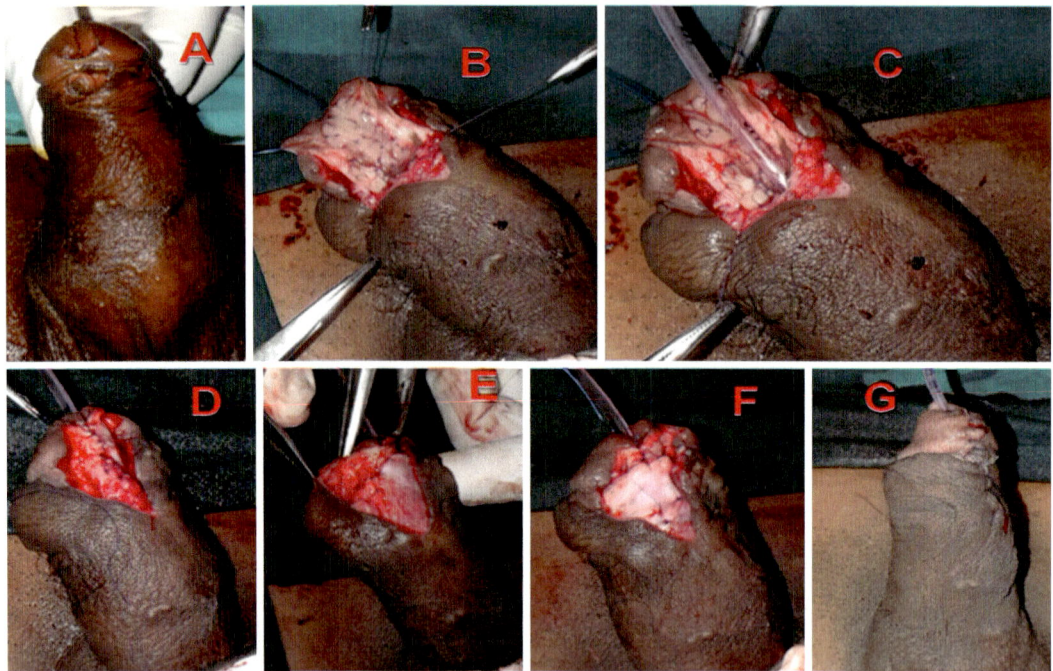

Fig. 21.8 TIPU with dorsal buccal mucosal inlay double dartos flap cover in fistula repair. (**a**). An adult patient with glans dehiscence and sub-coronal fistula. (**b**, **c**). Urethral plate mobilization and placing the buccal mucosa inlay graft. (**d**). Urethral plate tubularization. (**e**). Spongioplasty and raising the double dartos flap. (**f**). Sutured double dartos flaps covering the neo-urethra. (**g**). Final appearance after glansplasty and skin closure

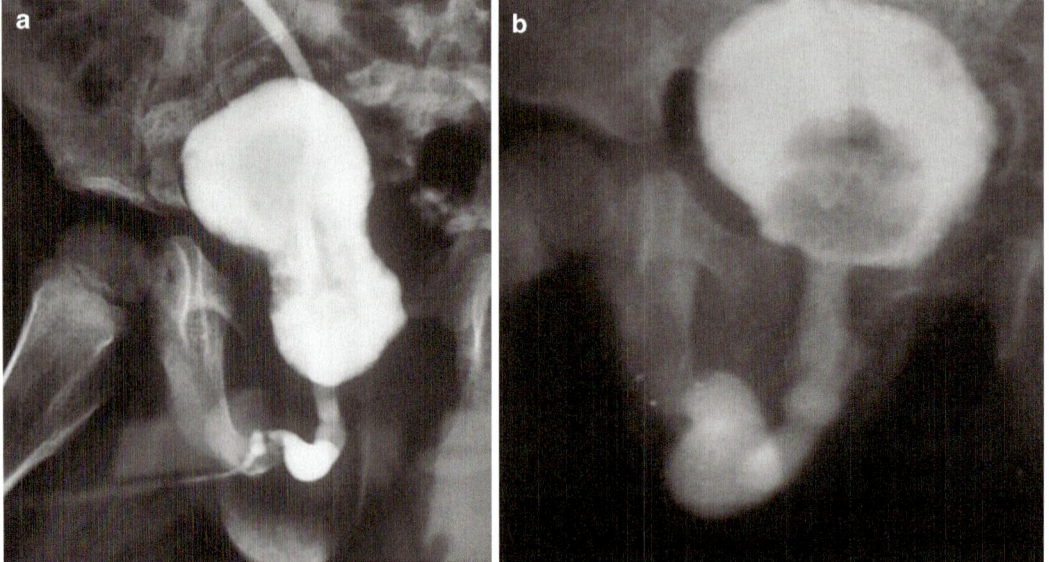

Fig. 21.9 RGU and MCU in post hypospadias stricture. (**a**). Retrograde urethrogram showing short segment urethral stricture with proximal dilatation. (**b**). Micturating cystourethrogram showing blind-ending urethra with proximal dilatation

1. Urethral dilatation
2. VIU
3. Excision & primary anastomosis
4. Replacement urethroplasty—Adjacent skin flaps, pedicle flaps, and tube grafts, buccal mucosa grafts—single/two stage

These strictures are amenable to dilatation or visual internal urethrotomy. Husmann and Rathbun showed success rates of 22%–24% with urethrotomy for stricture disease after hypospadias repair, whether clean intermittent catheterization was employed or not. Success rates of 72% and 63% have been reported for onlay flap urethroplasty strictures and post TIPU strictures, respectively [24]. Visual internal urethrotomy is more effective in TIPU strictures and short anastomotic than tubed grafts or tubed flaps repairs strictures. Repeated dilation or urethrotomy in such patients may worsen the existing fibrosis, better be avoided. Failed dilatation or VIU and a long, complicated stricture is an indication of revision urethroplasty. Choice of urethroplasty is end to end in a small segment stricture but has more recurrence chances. Most of the cases are suitable for dorsal inlay. Recently Saavedra and Rourke (2019) coined the term HAUS (Hypospadias Associated Urethral Strictures), grouped the patients in four, and advised the treatment modalities as single-stage, two-stage urethroplasty, and perineal urethrostomy according to the group [25]. In our opinion, most hypospadias strictures can be managed in one- or two-stage using buccal or labial graft. An algorithm is proposed for the management of post hypospadias strictures (Fig. 21.10).

21.4.3 Urethral Diverticulum

Diverticula are diffuse dilation of either the neo-urethra or the native urethra. Proximal dilation of the native urethra occurs secondary to a stricture in the neo-urethra or otherwise in flap repairs after six months. They present with recurrent urinary tract infections, dribbling of urine, weak stream, and ballooning of the undersurface of the penis with lateral displacement of the penile shaft during micturition. The patient or parents have to milk the urethra to empty the collected urine in the urethra. The diverticula are more frequently observed in patients with onlay flaps and two-stage repairs because of the lack of spongiosum and a longer urethroplasty. The reported incidence of urethral diverticula in tube and flap urethroplasties is 7–12% [26, 27]. The urethral diverticula rarely occur in TIPU; Snodgrass reported in only three patients (0.33%) of 885 cases of TIPU and 1.43% in two-stage graft repairs [28]. Various factors for diverticula are lack of supporting tissue, turbulence due to poor fixity of urethra, distal resistance at the glans with or without metal stenosis or stricture urethra, and a sudden step-off in diameter at the level of the neo-urethral anastomosis. Surprisingly, distal obstruction is not so commonly associated with post hypospadias surgery diverticula. Snyder et al. found stricture only in one out of thirteen cases [29]. Snodgrass reported diverticula in 5 patients out of nine who underwent Byars flap repair in proximal hypospadias, but none had distal obstruction [22].

Retrograde and micturating urethrogram helps delineate the urethra for distal obstruction, size of the diverticula, and any associated fistula. Cystoscopy before a repair will make the surgeon wiser about the status of the urethra, diverticula, stones in diverticula, prostatic utricle, and any secondary changes in the bladder. The urethra and diverticula's distension with saline on the operating table will show the diverticula's size and leakage to locate the fistula. A localized diverticulum is usually excised and sutured longitudinally to prevent narrowing of the urethra. In large diverticula cases, the tissue is typically elastic and well-vascularized, making it suitable for repair. Repair is done by excising the excessive part of the diverticular skin wall. A portion of it is denuded to cover the suture line and neo-urethra, creating a pseudo spongiosum (Fig. 21.11a–f). The technique is called pseudospongioplasty. A tunica vaginalis flap cover over the repair

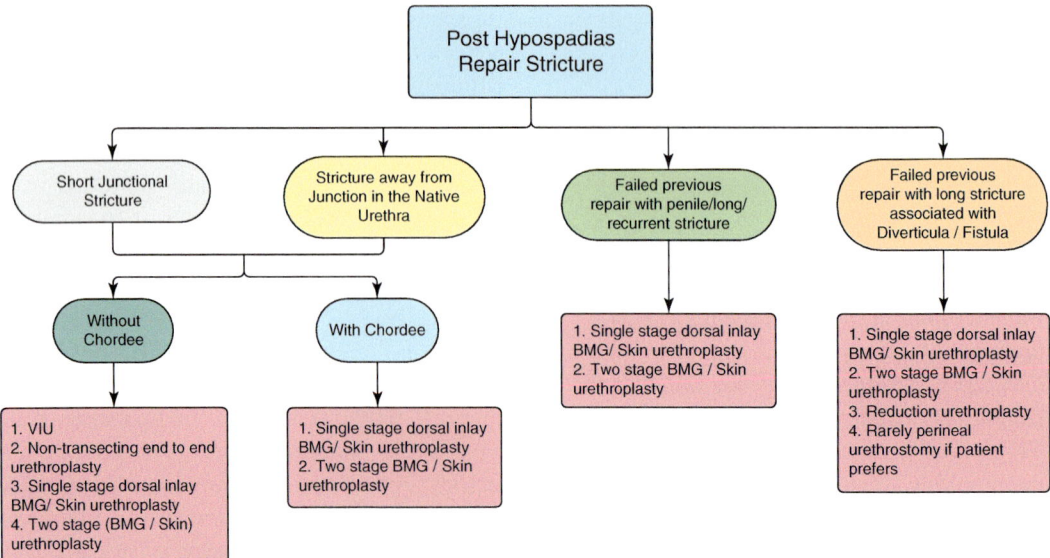

Fig. 21.10 Algorithm for post hypospadias repair strictures

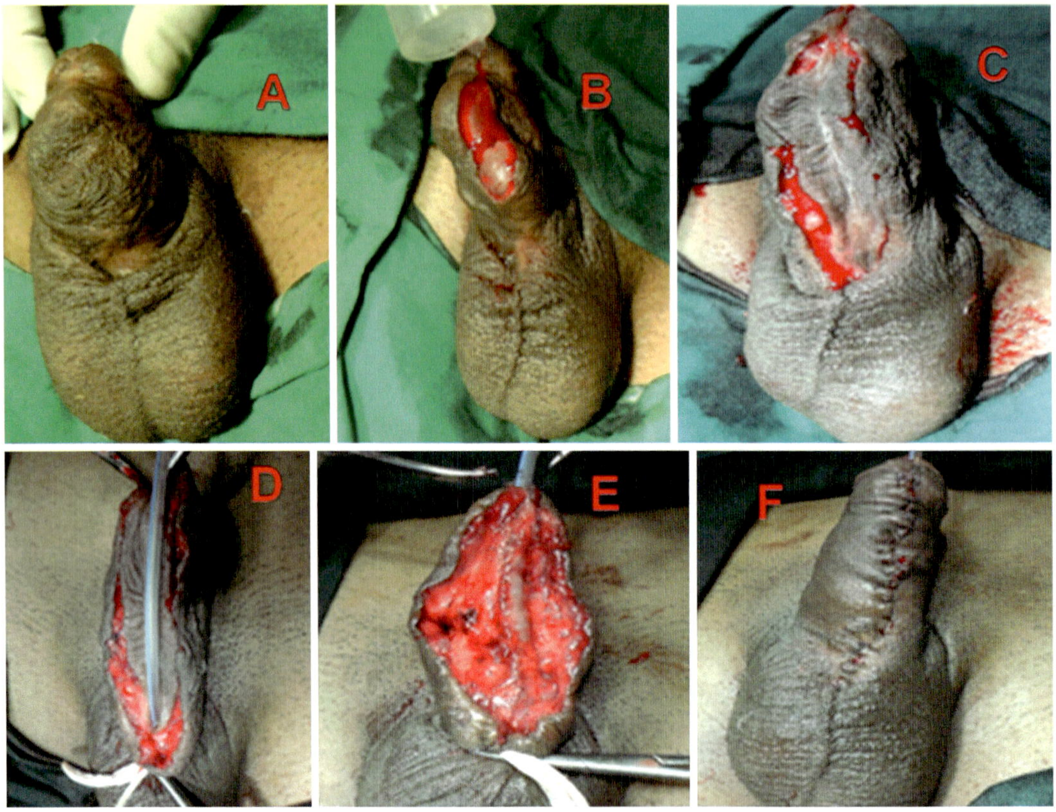

Fig. 21.11 Reduction urethroplasty in urethral diverticula. (**a**). An adult patient with a urethral diverticulum. (**b**). Skin incision showing saline-filled diverticulum. (**c**). Laid-open diverticula. (**d**). Urethral skin trimmed to create the urethral plate of adequate size. (**e**). Urethral plate tubularization and covering it with dartos. (**f**). Skin closure

effectively decreases the urethrocutaneous fistula rate. Alternatively, a dartos flap or a de-epithelialized flap may be employed. Results of diverticula repair are good, but there are chances of fistula and recurrence of the diverticula. Snyder et al. repaired the diverticula in 13 cases with a success rate of 76.23% [30].

21.4.4 Hairy Urethra

This complication is seen in flap procedures where hair-bearing skin is used and incidence rate as high as 5–15% [8]. The hirsute graft may cause dysuria, infection, urethral calculi, urethral moustache, and hair bezoars. Hairy urethras are most commonly seen in older patients with multiple staged procedures. In modern hypospadiology, a hairy urethra is rare, as hair-bearing skin is used less frequently, but the Koyanagi procedure may have this [31]. The best solution to the problem is to avoid using the hairy urethra. The best replacement hairy skin is the inner prepuce, which most closely resembles the urethra and other substitutes include non-hair-bearing skin of the inner arm or upper thigh, bladder mucosa, and buccal mucosa when prepuce is not available.

Treatment

1. **Chemical Epilation**: Singh and Hemal instilled a Thioglycolate dilute solution into the neo-urethra three monthly to ensure complete tricholysis and prevention recurrence of hair growth in future [32]. But this modality fails, and recurrence has been documented.
2. **Electro-epilation**: Local measures are to remove the hair and calculi endoscopically and fulguration of the follicles at the same time. Usually, the stone associated with hair can be removed, but it is challenging to fulgurate all hair follicles.
3. **LASER (CO_2 YAG)**: Cohen S et al. used CO_2 laser desiccation with reasonably good results. They recommended it as the choice of modality for a hairy urethra, especially in cases of the failure of electrolysis, but long-term results are not available [33]. Beiko D. et al. reported the urethroscopic Holmium YAG laser epilation in urethral diverticular hair follicles following hypospadias repair in one case [34]. Unfortunately, data on long-term success is not available.
4. **Replacement urethroplasty**: Replacement urethroplasty is the option after the failure of chemical and electro-epilation and CO_2/YAG laser ablation. The replacement of urethroplasty with buccal or bladder mucosa in one stage or two stage is the choice in these cases.

21.4.5 Urethral Stones

Urethral calculi are a rare but troublesome complication and are seen in the hair-bearing scrotal skin urethroplasties. It may also form in the urethral diverticula or secondary to stricture urethra in hypospadiacs. The exact incidence is not known, but there are case reports. Somerville et al. reported urethral calculi in two patients (8%) among 24 patients of second-stage urethroplasty [35]. Barbagli et al. reported 1 in 60 patients with failed hypospadias surgery [36]. The largest series of 5 cases was reported by Hayashi et al. [37]. Four of the patients had previously undergone Thiersch-Duplay repair, and the type of repair was not known in the fifth case. Diagnosis is easy as stones may be visible on the skin surface because of minimal tissue support without spongiosum after hypospadias repair (Fig. 21.12a, b) and can be palpated in the urethra on clinical examination. A plain radiograph may delineate the number of stones, size, and location (Fig. 21.12c). If needed, ultrasonography clinches the diagnosis. Small stones can be removed endoscopically, and energy used for breaking the larger stone is lithoclast and laser. Holmium: YAG laser is an excellent option for removing stones and hair in the urethra. Recurrence is common unless complete epilation of hairs is done. A large stone, multiple stones, and stones in diverticula require urethrotomy and/or redo urethroplasty. We had six such patients with urethral stones, two of them were with impacted urethral stones and required the urethrotomy, and four were managed endoscopically.

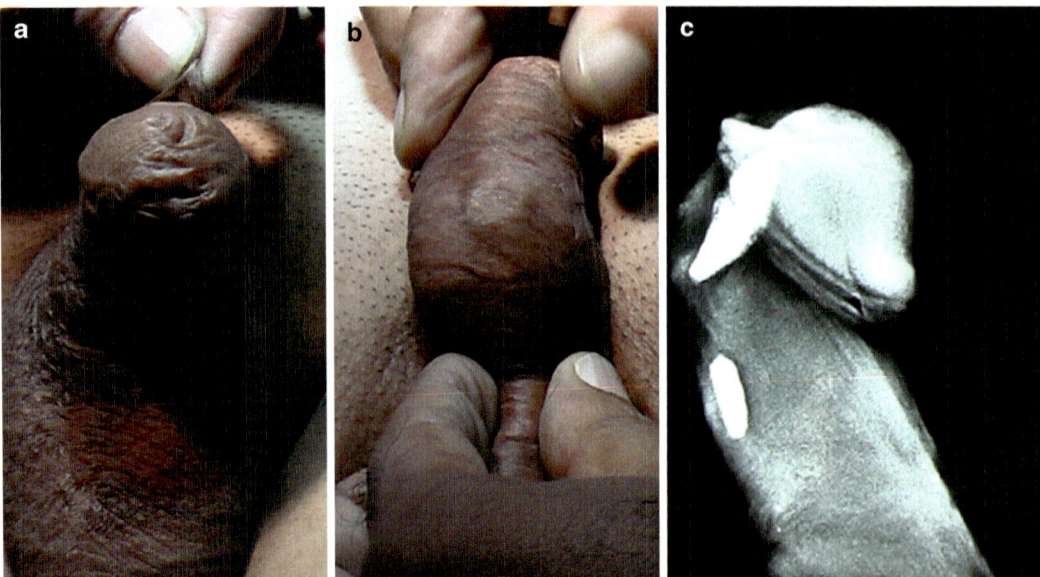

Fig. 21.12 Showing impacted urethral stones and fistula. (**a**). Sub-meatal stenosis and glans fistula. (**b**). Stone is visible on the ventral aspect of the penis on stretching. (**c**). Penile soft tissue X-ray showing impacted stones in the urethra

21.4.6 Recurrent/Chronic Urinary Tract Infections

Recurrent UTI may be seen in a few cases after hypospadias surgery. The causes are diverticula, stricture, an enlarged prostatic utricle, and a hairy urethra. Urethrogram and cystoscopy are done to confirm the diagnosis and delineate the urethral anatomy. Prostatic utricle should be suspected in patients of severe hypospadias repair with chronic or recurrent UTI, and very rarely, they might require excision to control the infection.

21.5 Penile Shaft

21.5.1 Chordee

Residual/persistent chordee is the third most common complication of hypospadias repair after fistula and stricture. With the use of intra-operative erection, it can be prevented in most cases. The occurrence of persistent chordee is primarily because of the misinterpretation of intra-operative chordee correction. Although rare, this complication may result from corporeal disproportion or extensive urethral fibrosis. The residual or persistent chordee may cause sexual dysfunction and requires correction. Significant chordee of more than 30 degrees needs surgical correction. The definitive evaluation is performed in the operating room under general anaesthesia at the time of repair. The penile skin is de-gloved in a circumferential fashion. The urethra/urethral plate with spongiosum is mobilized from corpora cavernosa, any remaining chordee or fibrous tissue is resected from the ventral aspect of corpora (Fig. 21.13a–f).

Even after these steps, the persistence of chordee is confirmed by the Gittes test, and if the urethra is bowstringing; it is divided. Fibrous and scar tissue present on the penile shaft requires excision. Mild chordee of less than 30 degrees can be managed with dorsal plication in patients with an adequate length of the penis. And severe chordee or patients with a smaller penis, the correction is done by superficial corporotomy or corporoplasty by a dermal or tunica vaginalis graft. First, dermal or tunica vaginalis grafts are performed by making a ventral transverse incision in the tunica albuginea at the point of maximal penile curvature. This incision may allow the

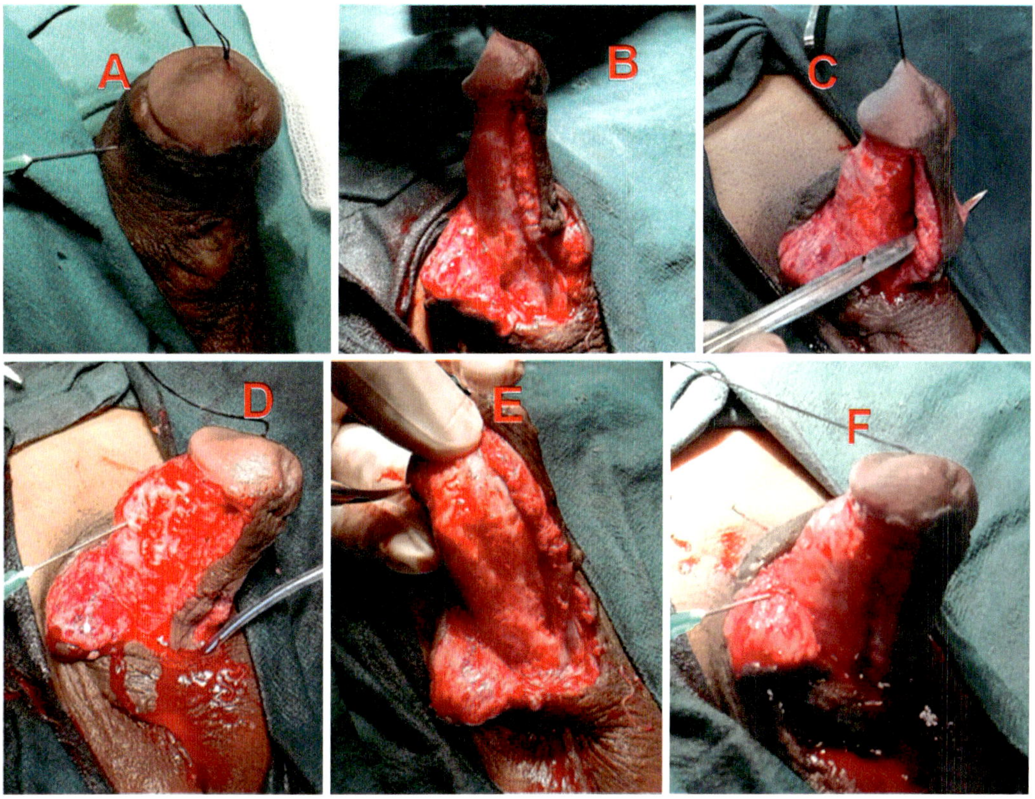

21 Late Postoperative Complications of Hypospadias Repair

Fig. 21.13 Showing correction of residual chordee by mobilization of spongiosum. (**a**). Gittes test showing mild to moderate chordee. (**b, c**). Penile skin degloving and urethral plate mobilization. (**d**). Gitte's test showing mild curvature. (**e**). Midline dissection and excision of fibrous tissue for chordee correction. (**f**). Gitte's test showing correction of curvature

edges of the tunica to spring apart and to straighten the corporal bodies. Next, a dermal or tunica vaginalis graft is interposed and secured with a running, interlocking, fine suture. The correction of the curvature is finally confirmed on the table. Then urethroplasty is done with the available tissue in a one- or two-stage buccal mucosal urethroplasty.

21.5.2 Penile Torsion

The second common complication seen in patients of inner prepucial flap urethroplasty (Fig. 21.14). The traction on dorsal dartos as interposing tissue or uncorrected torsion associated with hypospadias may be the cause in plate preserving procedures. In cases with dorsal dar-

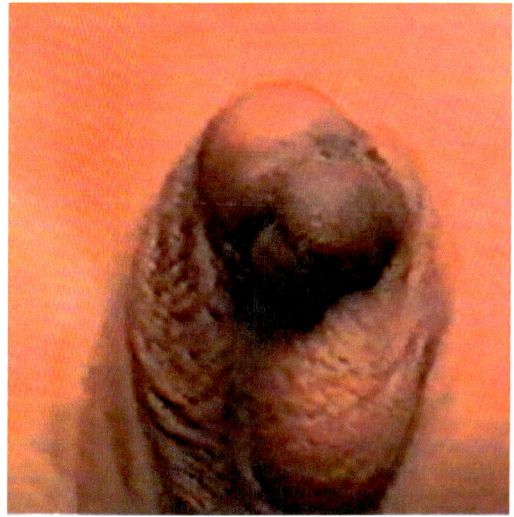

Fig. 21.14 Showing right torsion of 90-degree with diverticula, and retrusive meatus

tos cover, single dartos flap has higher chances (mild glanular torsion 90.7% and moderate glanular torsion 9.3%) than the double dartos flap (0%) [38]. The causative factor is an inadequate mobilization of the vascular pedicle and traction on the pedicle.

The torsion can be prevented by adequate vascular pedicle/dartos flap to the root of the penis and proper adjustment of skin flaps during skin closure. A mild torsion of <30° does not require treatment, but moderate to severe torsion requires corrective repair after six months. The treatment modalities are releasing the dorsal dartos pedicle, de torque by penile degloving and realignment, tunica albuginea plication sutures the tunica albuginea to pubic periosteum and sutures dorsal dartos opposite to torque in primary cases. The techniques for the management of torsion are described in Chap. 18 on torsion.

21.5.3 Inclusion Dermoid and Granuloma

Penile dermoid cyst may be congenital and acquired. Congenital occurs in the midline and may also be associated with hypospadias (Fig. 21.15a). Acquired inclusion dermoid cyst is an infrequent complication. We came across such three cases presented with swelling on the penis and mild torsion of the penis. Clinical examination showed a firm, well-defined swelling free from the skin. We did excision of the cyst in a daycare surgery (Fig. 21.15d–f) and

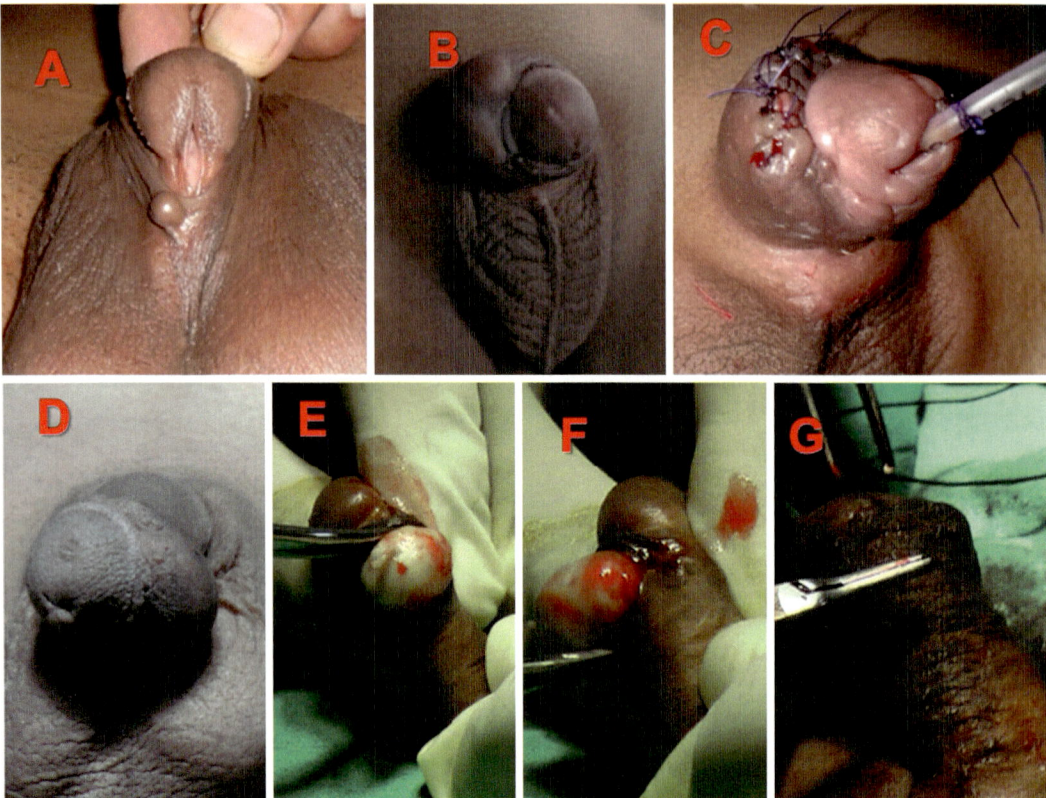

Fig. 21.15 Showing dermoid cyst and granuloma. (**a**). Dermoid cyst with hypospadias. (**b**). Post hypospadias male child showing swelling on the right side of the inner prepucial skin after hypospadias repair. (**c**). Excision of the granuloma and skin sutures. (**d**). Post hypospadias repair left-sided penile shaft swelling. (**e, f, g**). Excision of dermoid cyst

biopsy confirmed the dermoid cyst. Another rare complication is granuloma; because of the impregnated smegma or any other foreign material like late absorbing sutures. Excision of granuloma and re-suturing of the skin resolves the issue (Fig. 21.15b, c).

21.5.4 Balanitis Xerotica Obliterans

BXO is a chronic inflammatory process of unknown aetiology, and it affects the glans, prepuce, or urethral meatus and may extend into the urethra. The cause of BXO in hypospadiacs is not iatrogenic, and many cases are reported even before surgery. BXO is sometimes seen in patients after hypospadias repair and may affect the meatus, prepuce, glans, and the fossa navicularis. The clinical appearance is that of a sharply marginated white patch on the glans. Occasionally a rough, lichen-type scab is present. Patients are treated according to the stage of the disease. Early cases can be treated with topical steroids and Tacrolimus, a highly selective immune modulator.

Surgical repair is required for most of these patients. This involves relieving the meatal stenosis, initially by meatotomy, followed by more extensive resection and finally two-stage buccal mucosal urethroplasty. There are rare reports of malignant degeneration. Therefore, BXO lesions require periodic follow-up, and biopsy is indicated whenever a change in clinical appearance is observed.

21.5.5 Cosmesis

The shape of glans, glans dehiscence, chordee, penile torsion, and skin may contribute to an ugly appearance of the penis post-operatively. Mureau and colleagues reported that many children and adolescents of hypospadias (39%) desired functional and/or cosmetic penile improvement but were reluctant to seek advice. Similarly, adult hypospadias patients reported a more negative genital appraisal than comparison subjects and 37% desired functional or cosmetic penile improvement [39].

21.6 Psychosocial and Psychosexual

Psychosexual issues are more in hypospadias patients (32.8%) than in comparison subjects (12.8%) and are inhibited from seeking sexual contact. The variables affecting sexual function are the severity of hypospadias, patient age at final operation, and sociosexual development. The majority of patients experienced a normal adult sex life but were reluctant to seek advice for sexual problems. Bubanj and coworkers (2004) concluded that the sexual function of patients who underwent surgery for hypospadias, in general, is not affected [40]. However, a difference in certain aspects of sexual behaviour was noted. Patients with hypospadias were less sexually active and had a smaller total number of sexual partners than control subjects, and control subjects were significantly more delighted with their sexual life. A detailed description is available in Chap. 27.

21.7 Conclusions

Patients of hypospadias surgery should be followed for long-term to adolescence and adulthood as late complications may present years after surgery. Fistula, stricture, meatal stenosis, and diverticula are common complications. Non-responder to meatal dilatation cases require meatoplasty. Visual internal urethrotomy is indicated in short, simple anastomotic stricture, but complex strictures must be dealt with buccal mucosal urethroplasty in a single or two stage. Reduction urethroplasty with pseudospongioplasty and or tunica vaginalis cover is the choice of treatment. Single fistula is closed after freshening of margins with healthy tissue cover dartos or tunica vaginalis, and multiple fistulae are combined together, and onlay/inlay flap urethroplasty is done. Residual curvature or persistent curvature of more than 30 degrees requires treatment with ventral lengthening in small penises. The psychosexual problems are dealt with by the teamwork of psychiatrists, urologists, and andrologists. The multiple chronic complications can be managed by correcting chordee/penile torsion, reconstructing the urethra, healthy tissue cover, and skin resurfacing of the skin in one or two stages.

References

1. Nuininga JE, De Gier RP, Verschuren R, Feitz WF. Long-term outcome of different types of 1-stage hypospadias repair. J Urol. 2005;174(4 Part 2):1544–8.
2. Uygur MC, Ünal D, Tan MÖ, Germiyanoğlu C, Erol D. Factors affecting the outcome of one-stage anterior hypospadias repair: analysis of 422 cases. Pediatr Surg Int. 2002;18(2–3):142–6.
3. Jayanthi VR. The modified Snodgrass hypospadias repair: reducing the risk of fistula and meatal stenosis. J Urol. 2003;170(4 Part 2):1603–5.
4. Duckett JW, Snyder H 3rd. The MAGPI hypospadias repair in 1111 patients. Ann Surg. 1991;213(6):620.
5. Hastie K, Deshpande S, Moisey C. Long-term follow-up of the MAGPI operation for distal hypospadias. Br J Urol. 1989;63(3):320–2.
6. Snodgrass W, Cost N, Nakonezny PA, Bush N. Analysis of risk factors for glans dehiscence after tubularized incised plate hypospadias repair. J Urol. 2011;185(5):1845–51.
7. Maarouf AM, Shalaby EA, Khalil SA, Shahin AM. Single vs double dartos layers for preventing fistula in a tubularised incised-plate repair of distal hypospadias. Arab J Urol. 2012;10(4):408–13.
8. Cimador M, Vallasciani S, Manzoni G, Rigamonti W, De Grazia E, Castagnetti M. Failed hypospadias in paediatric patients. Nat Rev Urol. 2013;10(11):657.
9. Sunay M, Dadalı M, Karabulut A, Emir L, Erol D. Our 23-year experience in urethrocutaneous fistulas developing after hypospadias surgery. Urology. 2007;69(2):366–8.
10. Djordjevic ML, Perovic SV, Slavkovic Z, Djakovic N. Longitudinal dorsal dartos flap to prevent fistula after a Snodgrass hypospadias procedure. Eur Urol. 2006;50(1):53–7.
11. Muruganandham K, Ansari M, Dubey D, Mandhani A, Srivastava A, Kapoor R, Kumar A. Urethrocutaneous fistula after hypospadias repair: outcome of three types of closure techniques. Pediatr Surg Int. 2010;26(3):305–8.
12. Appignani A, Prestipino M, Bertozzi M, Nardi N, Falcone F. Double-cross flap protection: a new technique for coverage of neourethra in hypospadias repair. J Urol. 2009;182(4):1521–7.
13. Elsayed ER, Zayed AM, El Sayed D, El Adl M. Interposition of dartos flaps to prevent fistula after tubularized incised-plate repair of hypospadias. Arab J Urol. 2011;9(2):123–6.
14. Bilici S, Sekmenli T, Gunes M, Gecit I, Bakan V, Isik D. Comparison of dartos flap and dartos flap plus spongioplasty to prevent the formation of fistulae in the Snodgrass technique. Int Urol Nephrol. 2011;43(4):943–8.
15. Bhat A. Extended urethral mobilization in incised plate urethroplasty for severe hypospadias: a variation in technique to improve chordee correction. J Urol. 2007;178(3):1031–5.
16. Bhat A, Singla M, Bhat M, Sabharwal K, Kumar V, Upadhayay R, Saran RK. Comparison of results of TIPU repair for hypospadias with "Spongioplasty alone" and "Spongioplasty with dorsal dartos flap". Open J Urol. 2014;4(5):41–8.
17. Smith D. A de-epithelialised overlap flap technique in the repair of hypospadias. Br J Plast Surg. 1973;26(2):106–14.
18. Belman AB. De-epithelialized skin flap coverage in hypospadias repair. J Urol. 1988;140(5):1273–6.
19. Snow BW. Use of tunica vaginalis to prevent fistulas in hypospadias surgery. J Urol. 1986;136(4):861–3.
20. Shankar K, Losty P, Hopper M, Wong L, Rickwood A. Outcome of hypospadias fistula repair. BJU Int. 2002;89(1):103–5.
21. Handoo YR. Role of tunica vaginalis interposition layer in hypospadias surgery. Indian J Plast Surg. 2006;39(2):152–7.
22. Snodgrass W, Grimsby G, Bush NC. Coronal fistula repair under the glans without reoperative hypospadias glansplasty or urinary diversion. J Pediatr Urol. 2015;11(1):39.e31–4.
23. Snodgrass WT, Bush NC. Management of urethral strictures after hypospadias repair. Urol Clin North Am. 2017;44(1):105–11. https://doi.org/10.1016/j.ucl.2016.08.014.
24. Husmann D, Rathbun S. Long-term followup of visual internal urethrotomy to manage short (less than 1 cm) penile urethral strictures following hypospadias repair. J Urol. 2006;176(4):1738–41.
25. Saavedra AA, Rourke KF. Characterization and outcomes of urethroplasty for hypospadias-associated urethral strictures in adults. Can Urol Assoc J. 2019;13(11):E335–40.
26. Vallasciani S, Berrettini A, Nanni L, Manzoni G, Marrocco G. Observational retrospective study on acquired megalourethra after primary proximal hypospadias repair and its recurrence after tapering. J Pediatr Urol. 2013;9(3):364–7.
27. Wiener JS, Sutherland RW, Roth DR, Gonzales ETJ. Comparison of Onlay and tubularized island flaps of inner preputial skin for the repair of proximal hypospadias. J Urol. 1997;158(3):1172–4.

28. Snodgrass W, Villanueva C, Bush NC. Duration of follow-up to diagnose hypospadias urethroplasty complications. J Pediatr Urol. 2014;10(2):208–11.
29. Snyder CL, Evangelidis A, Hansen G, Peter SDS, Ostlie DJ, Gatti JM, Gittes GK, Sharp RJ, Murphy JP. Management of complications after hypospadias repair. Urology. 2005;65(4):782–5.
30. Snyder CL, Evangelidis A, Snyder RP, Ostlie DJ, Gatti JM, Murphy JP. Management of urethral diverticulum complicating hypospadias repair. J Pediatr Urol. 2005;1(2):81–3.
31. Catti M, Lottmann H, Babloyan S, Lortat-Jacob S, Mouriquand P. Original Koyanagi urethroplasty versus modified Hayashi technique: outcome in 57 patients. J Pediatr Urol. 2009;5(4):300–6.
32. Singh I, Hemal A. Recurrent urethral hairball and stone in a hypospadiac: management and prevention. J Endourol. 2001;15(6):645–7.
33. Cohen S, Livne PM, Ad-El D, Lapidoth M. CO2 laser desiccation of urethral hair post-penoscrotal hypospadias repair. J Cosmet Laser Ther. 2007;9(4):241–3.
34. Beiko D, Pierre SA, Leonard MP. Urethroscopic holmium: YAG laser epilation of urethral diverticular hair follicles following hypospadias repair. J Pediatr Urol. 2011;7(2):231–2.
35. Somerville J, Adeyemi O, Clark P. Long-term results of two-stage urethroplasty. Br J Urol. 1985;57(6):742–5.
36. Barbagli G, De Angelis M, Palminteri E, Lazzeri M. Failed hypospadias repair presenting in adults. Eur Urol. 2006;49(5):887–95.
37. Hayashi Y, Yasui T, Kojima Y, Maruyama T, Tozawa K, Kohri K. Management of urethral calculi associated with hairballs after urethroplasty for severe hypospadias. Int J Urol. 2007;14(2):161–3.
38. Kamal BA. Double dartos flaps in tubularized incised plate hypospadias repair. Urology. 2005;66(5):1095–8.
39. Mureau MA, Slijper FM, van der Meulen JC, Verhulst FC, Slob KA. Psychosexual adjustment of men who underwent hypospadias repair: norm-related study. J Urol. 1995;154(4):1351–5.
40. Bubanj TB, Perovic SV, Milicevic RM, Jovcic SB, Marjanovic ZO, Djordjevic MM. Sexual behaviour and sexual function of adults after hypospadias surgery: a comparative study. J Urol. 2004;171(5):1876–9.

Management of Hypospadias Cripple

22

Amilal Bhat

22.1 Introduction

The complications are inevitable in any surgery. The hypospadias surgery is a complex one, having more chances of complications, and requires multiple surgeries. The repair goals are to reconstruct an adequate size & straight penis for successful intercourse with a forward-directed projectile urinary stream. These can be achieved by chordee correction, urethroplasty, meatoplasty/glansplasty, scrotal transposition repair, and skin coverage. Choosing an inappropriate and poor surgical technique, postoperative infection, wound dehiscence, urine extravasations, hematoma, ischemia, and necrosis of the flap or graft are responsible for increasing the complications [1]. These factors lead to poor healing of the reconstructed tissue. The theory is that the neourethra (a man-made tube) likely fails to grow adequately compared to the rest of the genital tissues during puberty and may create a narrow or short tube. The complications may appear during puberty due to rapid genital growth. It is also assumed that the neourethra's congenital lack of spongiosal cover may not provide adequate vascular support to the urethra during puberty growth. Urethra without spongiosum cover support is unlikely to tolerate the trauma sustained during erections and sexual activity [2]. The exact extent, number, nature, and range of complications seen in adulthood after childhood hypospadias surgery remain poorly defined. When multiple surgeries fail, it will lead to functional loss of the penis, landing in the problem of "hypospadias cripple" [3]. In 1981, Stecker et al. first used the term "hypospadias cripples" to emphasize the complexity of the deformities faced during the repair of difficult hypospadias cases [4]. Horton and Devine used the term hypospadias cripple for the patient who had undergone multiple unsuccessful hypospadias repairs [5]. Multiple attempts for repair in such patients result in significant resultant penile deformity. Therefore, surgical repair in these complicated cases is less likely to succeed. The exact prevalence of the hypospadias cripple is unknown, but the best available estimate shows it occurs in 5–7% of patients after multiple failed attempts of repair [6, 7].

A. Bhat (✉)
Bhat's Hypospadias and Reconstructive Urology Hospital and Research Centre,
Jaipur, Rajasthan, India

Department of Urology, Jaipur National University Institute for Medical Sciences and Research Centre,
Jaipur, Rajasthan, India

Department of Urology, Dr. S.N. Medical College,
Jodhpur, Rajasthan, India

Department of Urology, S.P. Medical College,
Bikaner, Rajasthan, India

P.G. Committee Medical Council of India,
New Delhi, India

Academic and Research Council of RUHS,
Jaipur, Rajasthan, India

Hensle et al. reported the adulthood complications 37.5% in the patients without previous hypospadias surgery, 41.67% in the patients who had one or more surgical procedures in childhood but local tissue was relatively intact, and 63.6% in the patients who underwent multiple unsuccessful hypospadias repairs with various degrees of penile deformity and loss of local tissue [8]. Others have opined that although the number of surgeries for the correction of primary hypospadias is a risk factor, the stricture length is more significant than the number of surgeries [9]. Complications after the hypospadias repair are a difficult population to treat. They are likely left with deformities significantly worse than the primary disease itself [2]. The complications are considerably more significant for re-operations as compared to primary repairs using the same surgical procedure. These facts guide us to careful patient selection, modification of methods for re-operation, and consideration of novel procedures not commonly used for primary repair. Redo-surgery in patients with hypospadias crippled has very high complication rates. Multiple surgeries are often required to have improved and successful outcomes, even in the best of hands. Multiple studies have noted that 24–32%, 7–12%, and 3–4% of patients needed approximately two, three, and even four repairs, respectively [7, 10, 11]. Whether this can be achieved in a single surgery or multiple depends on the severity of problems, availability of tissue and experience of the operating surgeon.

22.2 Assessment of the Patient

Patients with hypospadias cripple may present to the hospital with complaints of penile deformity, complex psychosexual problems, and urinary or ejaculatory problems [12]. Though the detailed history of previous surgery, previous surgery records, and reasons for the surgery's failure are to be sought and are very important for surgical planning. But many a time, these are not available with the patients. Careful and systematic evaluation is an essential step in the workup of the crippled hypospadias. The penile and glans size, location and size of the meatus are noted. Multiple openings suggestive of fistulae, presence of scars, the flexibility of the tissue, chordee, torsion, prepucial hood or residual prepucial skin, palpable thickening of the urethra, ballooning of ventral side during micturition are recorded. The meatus is calibrated for the size of the meatus. If the stricture and diverticula are suspected, then the urethrogram is done to locate the stricture and diverticula's site, size, and length. Patient/parents may be asked to take a photograph in erection position in all directions to understand the residual curvature/recurrence of curvature or torsion. Clinical examination and an artificial erection with pharmacological agents and curvature measurement may help decide the plan plication procedure or ventral lengthening procedures. In the patient with urinary complaints, history of hematuria, and repeated urinary tract infection; cystoscopy is done to evaluate for stricture, prostatic utricle, diverticula, urethral hairs, and urethral stones. The patient should be counseled before surgery, considering their aspirations and realistic expectations about the penile size and shape, urinary and sexual functions. Other issues are frequently seen in seemingly simple cases, such as fistulae, scarring, recurrent chordee, and an abnormal meatus, often related to a small glans and nearly always with a deficiency of the dartos layer often with underlying associated psychosexual problems [2]. The assessment helps in the planning of the surgery and alternatives in the surgical approach.

22.3 Management

Depending on the type of previous surgeries, hypospadias cripple are likely to have multiple issues to be solved. Pre-decided protocols may have to be changed to manage these patients. Management has to be tailored to the individual patient. The problems of hypospadias cripples can be categorized into five major groups, and treatment is tailored accordingly in one stage or multiple:

1. Correction of Residual Chordee/Penile Torsion
2. Reconstruction of the urethra

3. Adjuncts to urethroplasty/Healthy tissue cover.
4. Resurfacing of the skin
5. Reconstruction of penile part loss

22.3.1 Chordee Correction

Recurrent curvature in hypospadias cripple is likely to be due to the peri-urethral and skin fibrosis, shortening of the reconstructed urethra and disproportionate ventral corpora by the relatively poor growth of the hypoplastic ventral corporal wall. The causes may be single or combination in the individual case. The surgical correction of chordee either by ventral lengthening or dorsal shortening procedures will depend on the severity of chordee after penile skin degloving. Chordee due to skin fibrosis is likely to be corrected after penile skin degloving itself, but it is to be confirmed by Gittes test before proceeding further. The urethra/urethral plate is examined to see whether it is healthy or fibrotic. If the urethra/urethral plate is healthy, then the urethra/urethral plate is mobilized to correct the chordee and confirmed by the Gittes test. The urethra/urethral plate is utilized for urethral reconstruction (Fig. 22.1a–f). A fibrotic urethra/tethered urethral plate causing the chordee to be transected or resected to correct the ventral curvature. The corporal disproportion is managed by dorsal plication if the penile length is adequate and the chordee is less than 30 degrees. In cases with a short penis with chordee of less than 30 degrees, and the patient wants a penile lengthening procedure, superficial corporotomy is done. If the chordee is more than 30 degrees, then corporoplasty is done. The urethral plate is reconstructed by the Buccal mucosal or skin graft to be tubularized in the second stage. If needed, ventral shortening of the skin can be covered by Z plasty, double Z plasty, or multiple Z plasties. This may lengthen ventral skin up to 2–5 cm as required according to the patient's age: will help correct

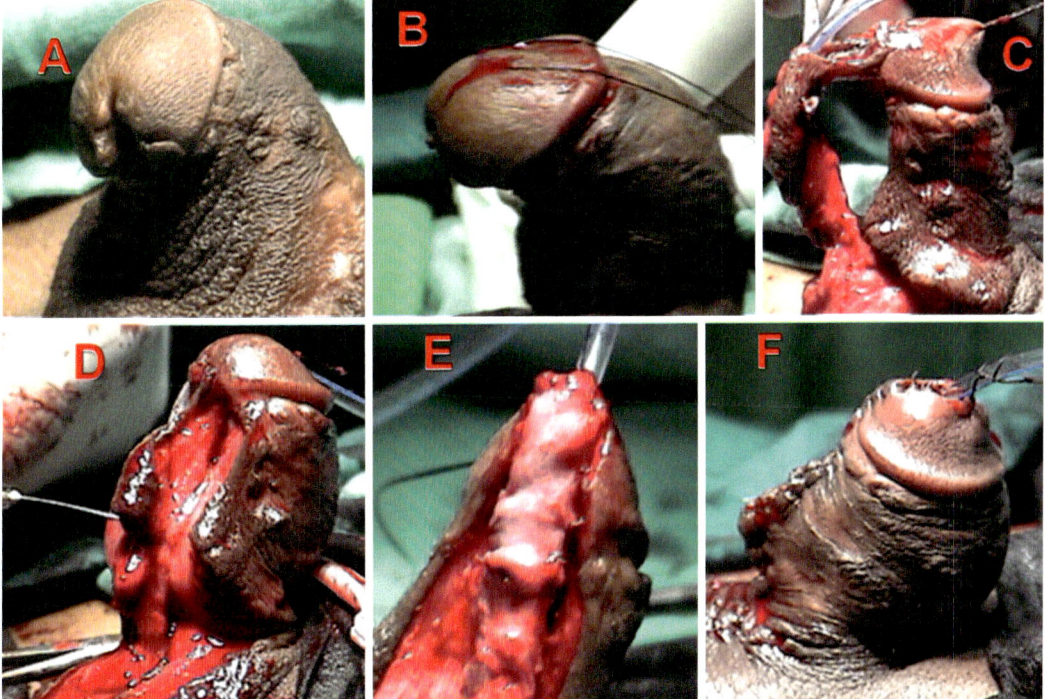

Fig. 22.1 Showing correction of chordee by urethral plate and urethra mobilization. (**a**) Hypospadias cripple after three previous surgery having chordee, glans scar, distal laid open urethra. (**b**) Gittes test Showing chordee. (**c**) Urethral plate with spongiosum and urethra mobilization up to the penoscrotal junction. (**d**) Gittes test showing correction of chordee. (**e**) Tubularized urethral plate perimeatal dartos cover. (**f**) Glanuloplasty and skin closure

the chordee and prevent the recurrence chordee. Hana et al. (2017) reported correction of ventral curvature in 59 cases of recurrent chordee. The correction was done with single-stage skin detethering and dorsal plication in 32, one-stage by mobilization of the urethra and corporal/dermal grafts in 12 patients, staged corporal/dermal graft and skin coverage followed by urethroplasty 8–12 months later in 15 patients [13].

22.3.2 Penile Torsion

Penile torsion is likely because of traction on the vascular pedicle of the inner prepucial flap, traction on the tunica flap used for interposing healthy tissue during previous surgery, or intrinsic corporal shortening. Unequal skin flap closure may also be responsible for penile torsion. Torsion is corrected by penile degloving and again assessed for the torsion (Fig. 22.2a–h). If there is traction on the vascular pedicle, that is released by mobilization of the pedicle. Still, it persists, then counter traction by dartos wrap, plication procedures, and final adjustment with skin closure is done [14].

22.3.3 Reconstruction of the Urethra

Urethroplasty in hypospadiac cripple is a real challenge to the surgeon as the patient had repeated surgery leading to fibrosis starting from the skin to corpora. Depending upon the available tissue, chordee, torsion, stricture, fistula, diverticula, the feasibility of chordee correction one-

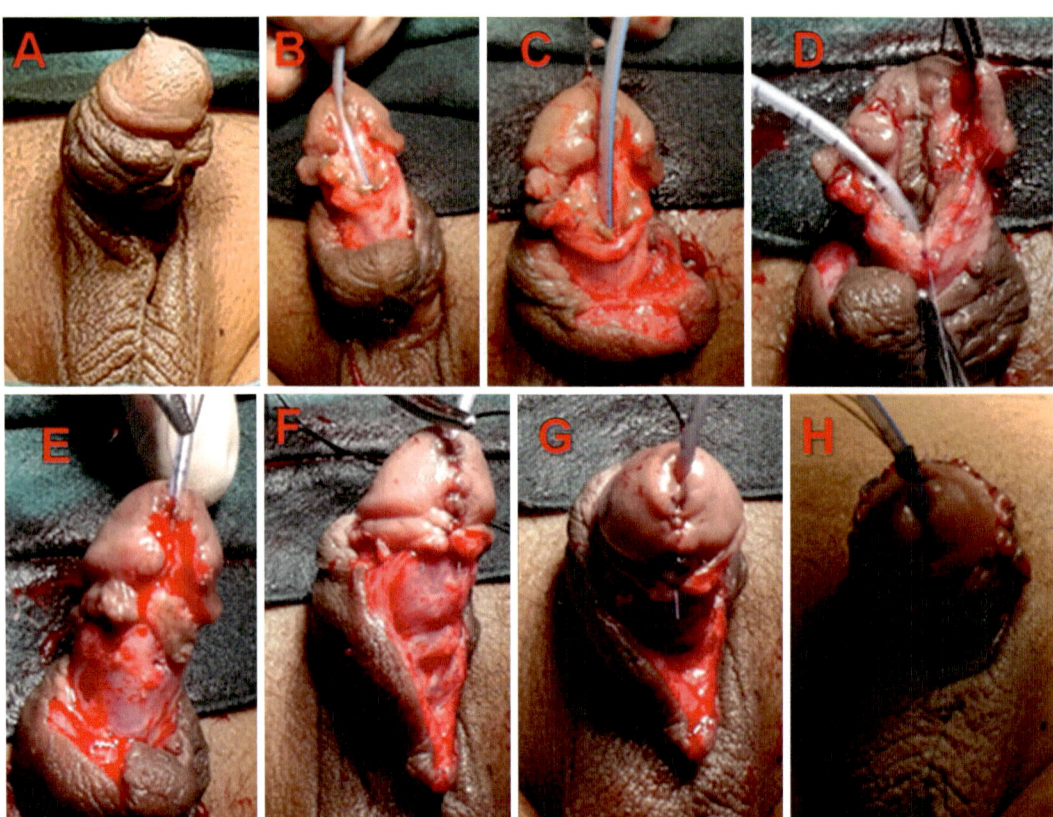

Fig. 22.2 Showing torsion correction in a 3-year male child with distal laid open urethra with TIPU and dartos cover. (**a**) Failed hypospadias repair showing torque. (**b**, **c**) Correction of torque after penile degloving. (**d**) Urethral plate tubularization started. (**e**) Urethral plate tubularization and spongioplasty. (**f**, **g**) Coverage with dartos flap and glansplasty. (**h**) Skin closure

stage or two-stage urethroplasty is planned [15]. The final decision about the single-stage or two-stage is taken on the operating table. The majority of the cases will need two-stage surgery. Strictures in hypospadias cripple are rarely amenable to visual internal urethrotomy [16]. The available options in stricture urethra management are excision and primary anastomosis, preputial skin flap, single-stage Buccal graft repair, and two-stage repair with buccal/Lingual mucosal graft, skin graft, bladder mucosal graft, and allografts. Small Strictures can be dealt with the end-to-end urethroplasty, but long and or multiple strictures require replacement urethroplasty. Suppose the segment is small and other associated problems like chordee or torsion have been corrected by the penile degloving and the urethral mobilization. In that case, one-stage repair may be an option (Figs. 22.1a–f and 22.2a–h), but the two-stage repair is preferable in most cases. Barbagli 2010 reported a success rate with single-stage urethroplasty in 90% in a largely failed hypospadias repair from Europe. 20% of the patients were done in the single-stage urethroplasty by a penile skin flap [11]. Myers (2012) has found that the utilization of either local penile

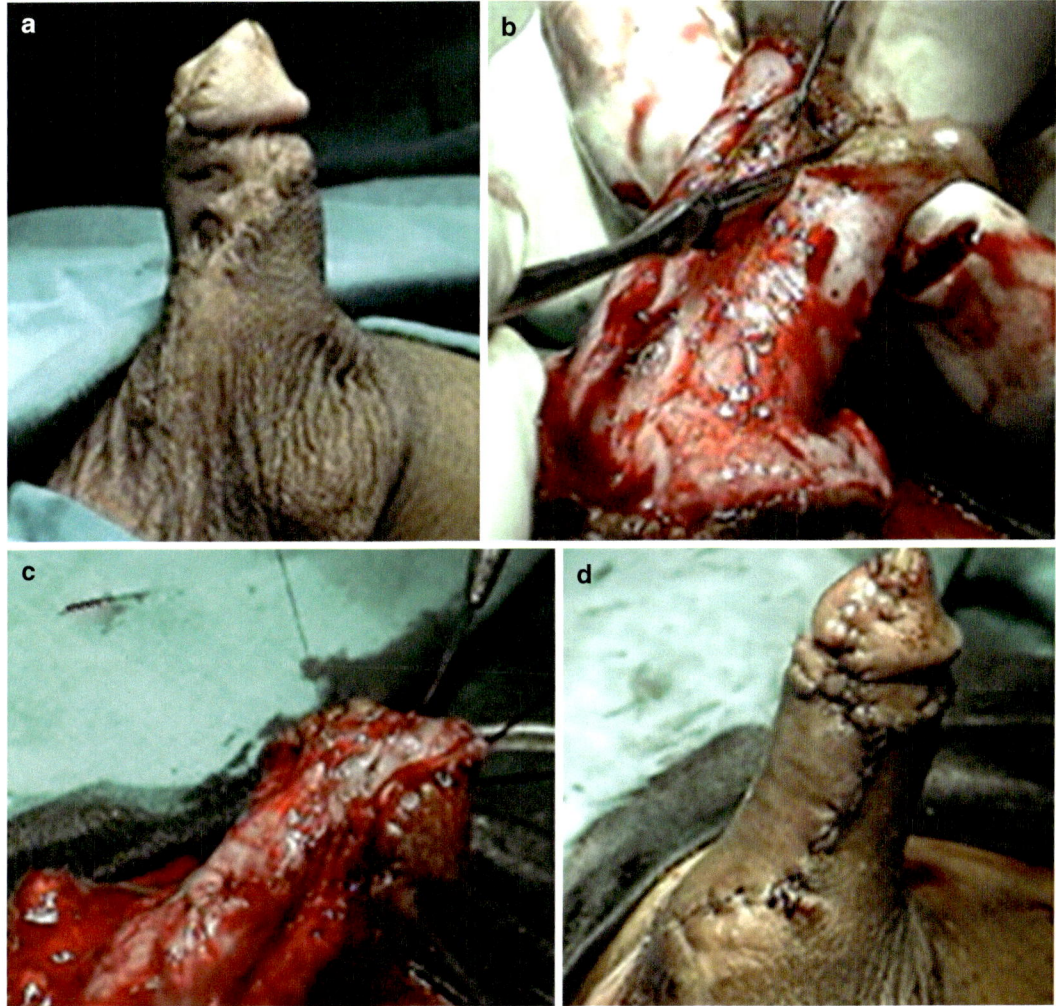

Fig. 22.3 Showing after five surgeries, multiple fistulae, glans dehiscence and glans scar. (**a**) Multiple fistulae with glans scar and dehiscence. (**b**) Penile degloving, laying open fistula create a urethral plate. (**c**) Urethral plate tubularization and dartos cover. (**d**) Glansplasty and skin closure

flaps or penile circular fascia-cutaneous flaps have a failure rate of 42% in the long-term follow-up [10].

If the available urethral plate is healthy or laid open multiple fistulae gives a healthy urethral plate (Fig. 22.3a–d). Then it either can be tubularized with or without augmentation of the urethral plate. The width of the urethral plate is narrow then can be supplemented with the dorsal Buccal graft or prepucial/penile skin available and tubularized tension free. Next, Neo-urethra should be covered with tunica vaginalis as an interposing healthy tissue (Fig. 22.4a–g). Another option is if partial/complete dorsal hood is available, then onlay flap urethroplasty can be done (Fig. 22.5a–f).

Most of the time, a group of patients who had diverticula with other associated complications can be managed in a single stage. The diverticula usually occur following flap repairs and two-stage repairs. Etiology and causes are discussed in Chap. 21 of chronic complications. The diverticula maybe with a narrow neck or dilation of the reconstructed urethra as a whole. These cases may be associated with other complications like urethral stone due to stagnation of urine. Diverticular neck excision and supporting the urethral with dartos will suffice in arrow neck cases, but others require reduction urethroplasty with pseudospongioplasty [17, 18] (Fig. 22.6a–g). It is often feasible to deal with multiple problems diverticula, fistula, and torsion in a single stage (Fig. 22.7a–k).

Sometimes patients with multiple problems like chordee, torsion, fistula urethral stones can be repaired in a single stage (Fig. 22.8a–f). But most of the time, multi-staged surgery remains the only choice.

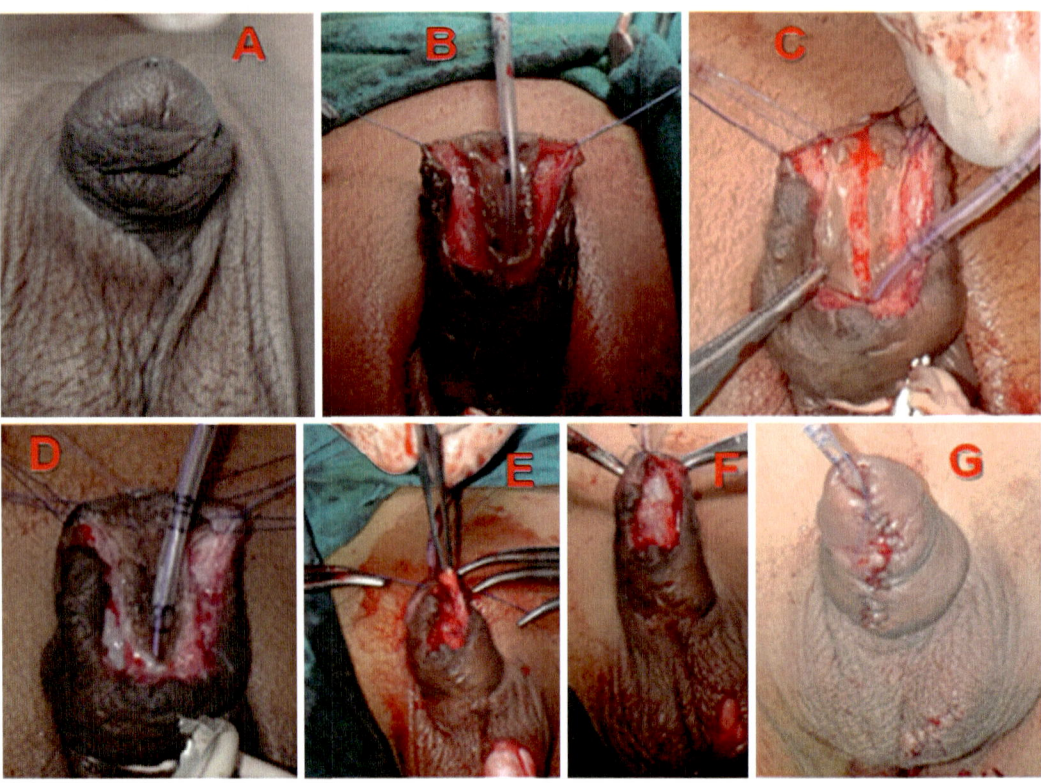

Fig. 22.4 TIPU with Spongioplasty in retrusive meatus with fistula. (**a**) A large fistula with glans dehiscence. (**b**) Urethral plate and spongiosum mobilization after incising the skin ledge. (**c**) Incising the urethral plate. (**d**) Dorsal inlay graft placed. (**e**) Tubularization of the urethral plate and mobilized tunica vaginalis flap tunneled to the site. (**f**) Covering neourethra with tunica vaginalis flap. (**g**) Glansplasty and skin closure

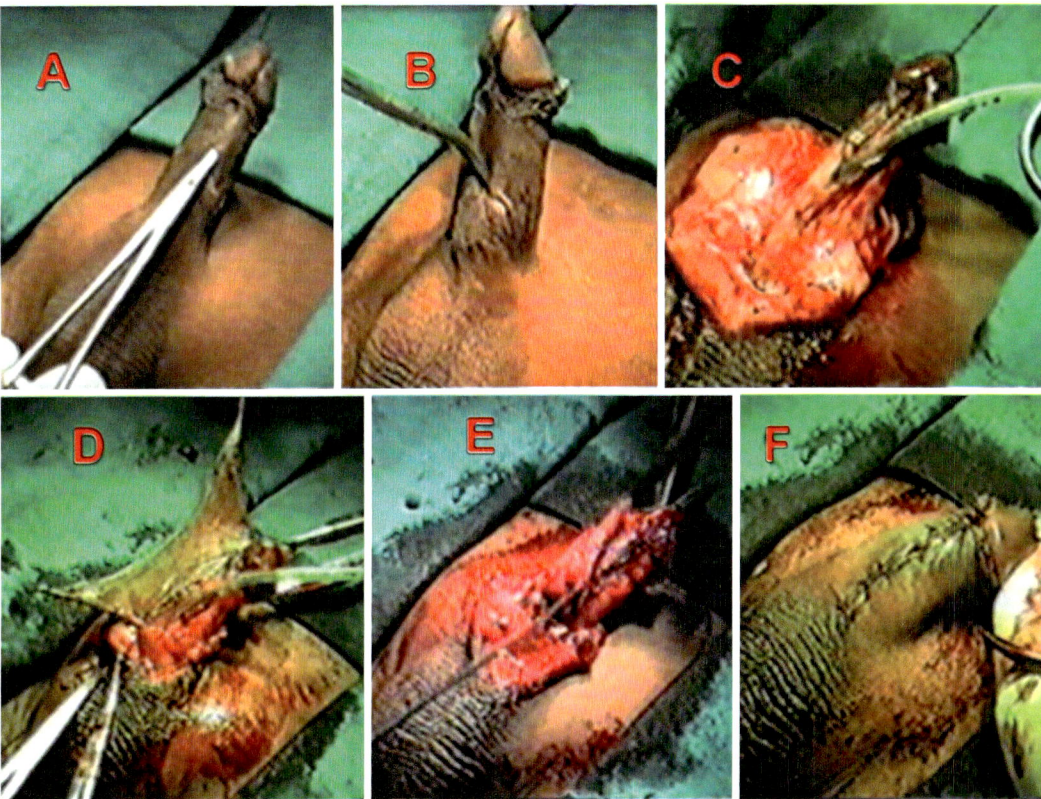

Fig. 22.5 (**a**, **b**) Multiple fistulae and distal laid open urethra. (**c**) Penile degloving and creating urethral plate by combining all fistula. (**d**) Onlay flap urethroplasty. (**e**) Dartos cover over neo-urethra. (**f**) Glansplasty and skin closure

Two-stage repair in hypospadias cripples the standard of care in modern Hypospadiology. Bracka popularized it as a potential solution to high-risk cases [6]. In staged repair, the most important consideration is the complete removal of the scarred and diseased tissue, correction of chordee, and placement of the tissue to be used for urethral substitution. The most commonly used substitution tissues are Buccal mucosa, non-hair-bearing abdominal skin, and Bladder mucosa. The attractive part of the abdominal skin is its availability and ease of harvesting with low morbidity, but the long-term durability of a skin-based urethroplasty is questionable. The Buccal mucosa graft is preferred for urethral replacement in hypospadias salvage surgery, and our choice is also the same. The graft is taken wider than required to compensate for the estimated 15% contracture in graft width and extend distally into the glans (Fig. 22.9a–c). The graft is supported by tunica vaginalis flaps affixed to the corporal bodies where the graft the bed is unsuitable. Other important points are the proper placement of the graft and quilting the graft to the underlying corpora with the tunica dartos or soft tissue to support the graft material's lateral edges. This will help ensure an adequate blood supply during mobilization of the edges of the graft for tubularization. A bolster dressing is sewn to the graft's underside with the Foley catheter running through the dressing. In spite, all measure graft contracture is inevitable in quite a number of patients (19–22%) who require revision or replacement of the graft [7].

Usually, second stage urethroplasty is done 6–12 months later. We prefer to wait up to 12 months before closure. The size of the neo-urethra is decided by proximal urethral calibration with a sound, and the urethral plate is mobilized. Care is taken to mobilize the urethral

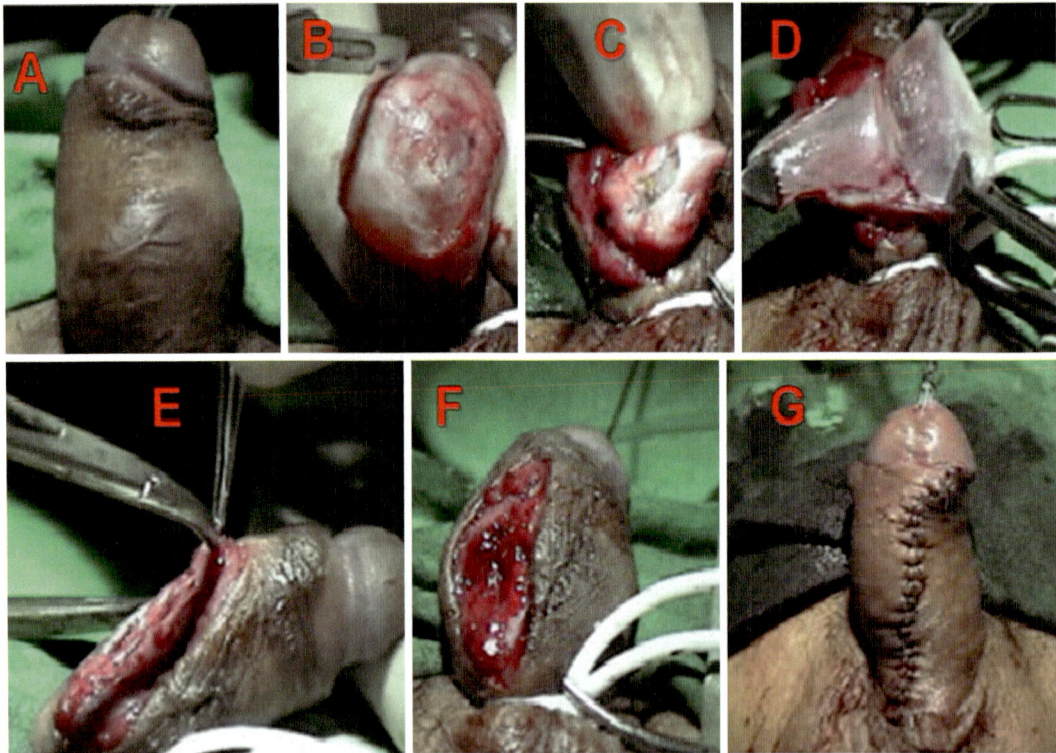

Fig. 22.6 Showing diverticula, torsion, and urethral stones. (**a**) Deformed shaft, torsion, and ballooning of ventral surface of the shaft. (**b**) Mobilized urethral diverticula. (**c**) Urethral stones in opened diverticula. (**d**) Excision of urethral diverticula closure of the neck of diverticula. (**e, f**) Supporting the urethra with dartos. (**g**) Skin closure and final picture

edges as little as possible to prevent the devascularization of the graft material. In cases with less than 25% contracture (Fig. 22.10), it may be augmented with a dorsal Buccal mucosal graft to prevent the re-stricture. But where almost the whole graft is lost or there is severe contracture, then the graft procedure has to be done again (Fig. 22.11). Lingual or lip mucosal graft may be used or supplemented in cases contracture after Buccal mucosal graft (Fig. 22.12).

The tubularization is done in two layers and is supported by the available dartos. We prefer to cover it with tunica vaginalis in all cases to prevent fistula, which is a commonest complication. The per-urethral catheter is placed and kept for 2–3 weeks postoperatively. A few prefer a suprapubic catheter for 3–4 weeks to avoid the ventral pressure on the incision from a full urinary drainage bag pulling on the catheter.

Cheritin B et al. 2007 [19] reported the results of 28 patients of hypospadias cripple who had undergone 2–5 surgeries earlier. Twenty-three cases were managed by a single-stage (penile skin flap repair 21+ bladder mucosa graft 2) in whom the meatus was located in the proximal part in 19 patients and mid-penile 4 cases. Fourteen patients had chordee, which was corrected by excision of scar tissue and dorsal plication. Five cases were managed in a staged manner. The complication rates were very high (46.3%), and 14.2% needed revision. They had placed the local penile skin flap with an adequate vascular supply to treat hypospadias cripples. Snodgrass and Elmore repaired 25 cases of failed hypospa-

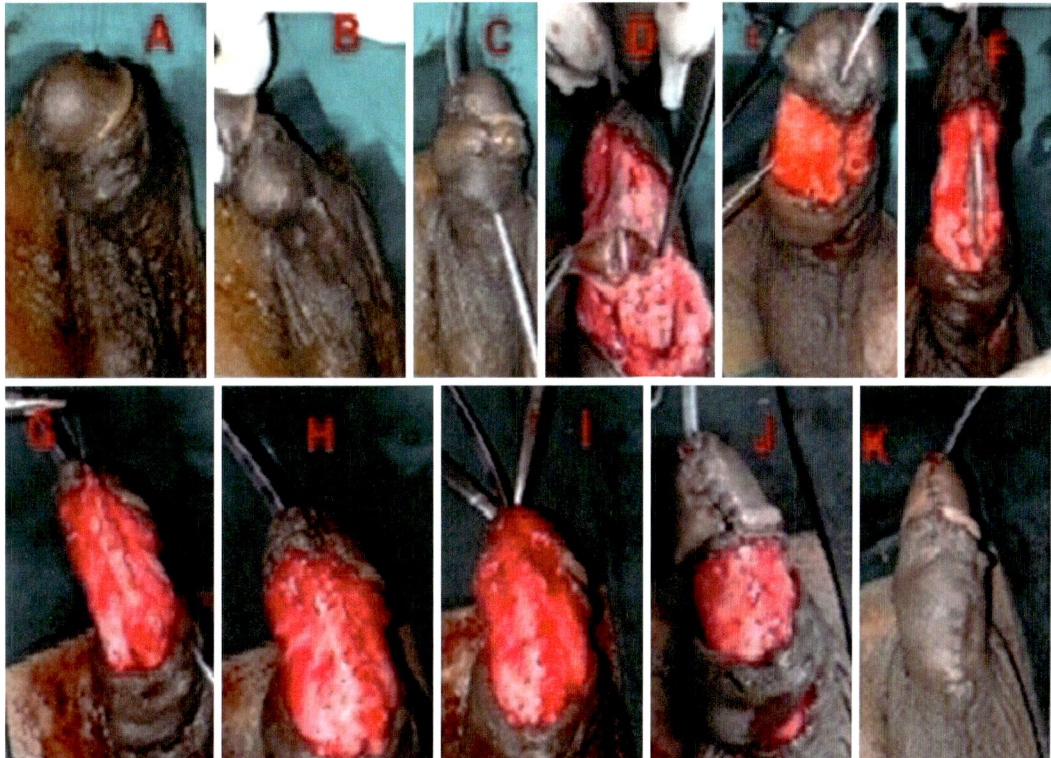

Fig. 22.7 Showing hypospadias cripple after four surgeries. Penile torsion urethral fistula and diverticula. (**a**) Right torsion, mild chordee, urethral fistula, retrusive meatus, and diverticula. (**b**) Inflated diverticula with xylocaine jelly, retrusive meatus, and fistula. (**c**) Infant feeding tube in fistula. (**d**) Penile Degloving & Laid-open diverticula. (**e**) Gittes test torsion corrected and mild glanular chordee. (**f**) Reduction of urethral diverticula and urethral plate prepared. (**g**) Urethral plate tubularization. (**h**) Dartos cover. (**i**) Glanular flaps raised. (**j**) Glansplasty. (**k**) Final picture. Skin closure torsion and chordee corrected

dias using Buccal mucosal grafts in multi-stage repairs having a success rate of 78% [20]. Barbagli et al., in 408 patients, found a correlation of the length of stricture and the presence of lichen sclerosis with a higher risk of treatment failure [21]. Bladder mucosa graft in hypospadias repair is feasible, but it is not popular, and long-term follow-up data are lacking. Li et al. reported their experience using a free bladder mucosa graft in failed hypospadias in adolescents and adults with a complication rate of 12.4% after a follow-up ranging from 3 months to 2 years. Bladder mucosa for urethroplasty after hypospadias repair did not achieve the same results in both studies [22, 23].

22.3.4 Adjuncts to Urethroplasty and Healthy Tissue Cover

Use of biologically based glue All measures should be taken to prevent the surgery failure of hypospadias cripple, who has already undergone two or more surgeries. Fibrin glue has the quality of sealing the suture line, making it waterproof, and also helps in hemostasis [24, 25]. Barbagli in 2006 used fibrin and reported significantly better graft take up, graft adherence, healing, and reduction in hematoma formation [3]. We use the fibrin sealant in selected cases of urethroplasty in these hypospadias cripples. But it is difficult to analyze

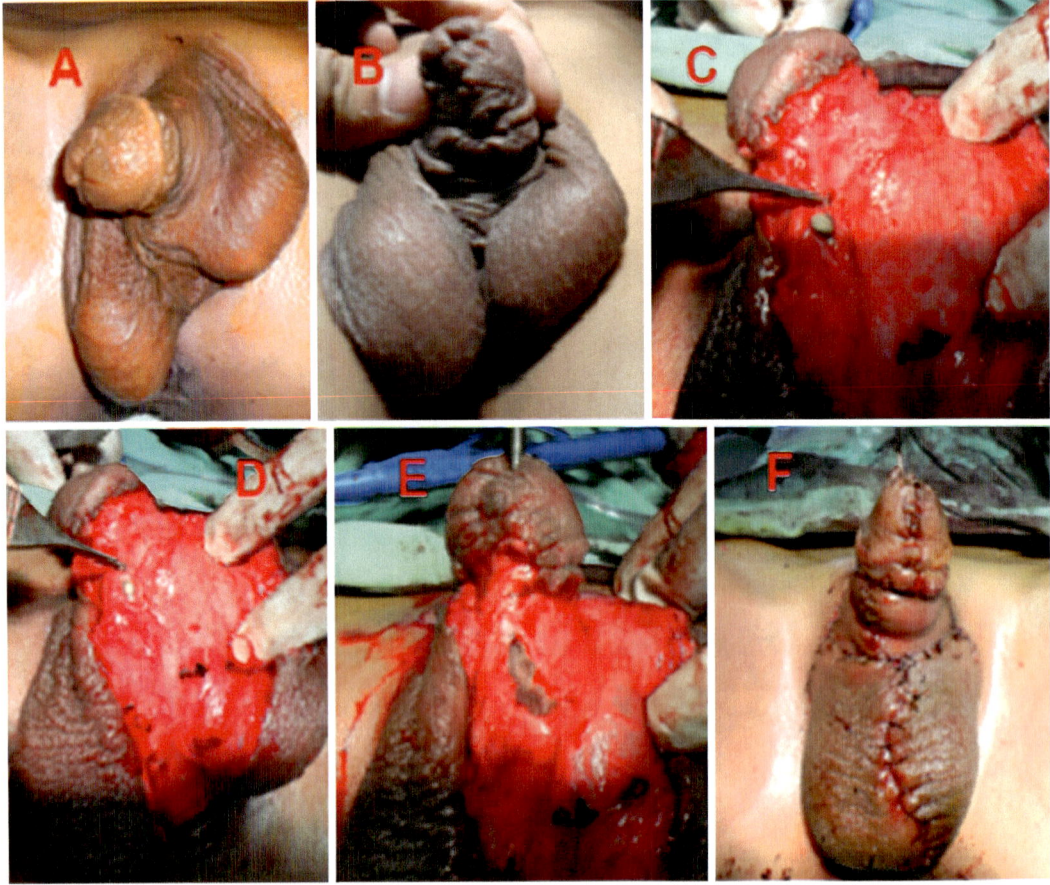

Fig. 22.8 Failed multiple hypospadias problem torsion, Glans scars, unsupple shaft skin, urethral stones, and bifid scrotum. (**a**, **b**) Right-sided torsion of the penis, rough skin on the ventral aspect of the penis, scarred glans, bifid scrotum, and penoscrotal transposition. (**c**, **d**) Penile degloving and incised the urethra showing urethral calculi. (**e**) Removal of stone and excision of excess skin to prepare the urethral plate for tubularization. (**f**) Scrotoplasty and skin closure

how useful it is until we exclude all other variables responsible for redo surgeries' failure.

Spongioplasty It is mandatory to cover the neo-urethra with healthy tissue. Availability of the tissue depends on the type and number of previous surgeries. In cases of previously urethral plate preservation procedures, if spongiosum is available, then the spongioplasty with dartos/tunica gives a better outcome. The residual urethral plate can be tubularized, covered with spongiosum (Fig. 22.13a–g), or created a urethral plate with skin (Fig. 22.14a–g), and supported with dartos or tunica vaginalis flap.

Ventral or Scrotal dartos Reconstructed neo-urethra with the available urethral plate or by tubularization of neo-urethral plate second stage of two-stage procedures are covered by ventral dartos/scrotal dartos to support the repair. Hayashi et al. (2005) used scrotal dartos wrap after urethral fistula closure with no recurrence of fistula. The scrotal dartos wrapping technique was recommended to cover the neourethra with a well-vascularized flap [26].

Tunica vaginalis flap The local penile tissue vascularity is being compromised because of the multiple surgeries and scaring. So revasculariza-

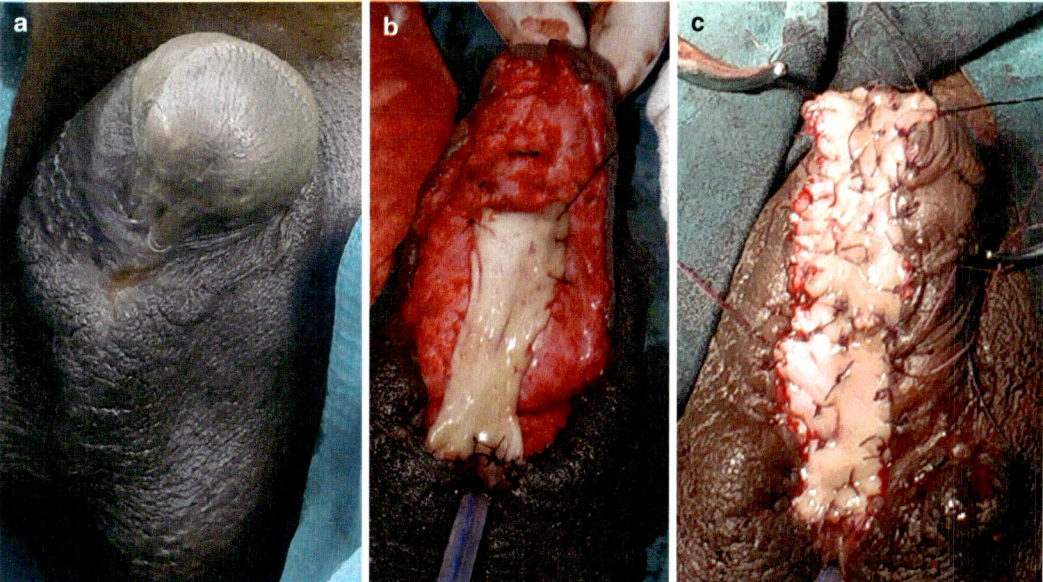

Fig. 22.9 Failed hypospadias in first stage chordee correction and Buccal Mucosal graft. (**a**) Failed hypospadias repair with scrotal meatus, chordee, and unhealthy ventral skin. (**b**) Buccal mucosa graft placement after penile degloving and chordee correction. (**c**) Graft Quilting on the ventral aspect of the penis up to the glans' tip

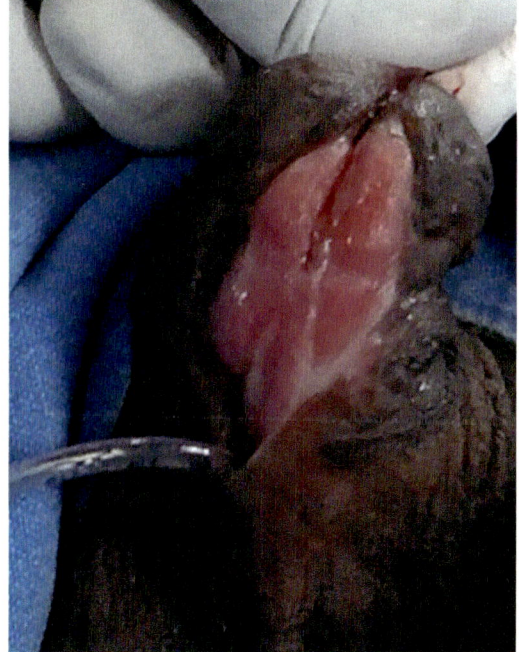

Fig. 22.10 Showing contracture of the graft near the meatus and corona

tion of the newly reconstructed neo-urethra is of paramount importance. The blood supply of the tunica is separate from the local tissue and remains preserved even after repeated surgeries. Thus, tunica vaginalis is the most commonly used interposing healthy tissue cover, and its results are better than the dartos wrap [27, 28]. We use the tunica vaginalis flaps to cover a lengthy or marginal ventral suture line in all cases of redo surgeries.

22.3.5 Resurfacing the Skin

Primary skin closure is difficult if the penile skin has been used to reconstruct the urethra. The dorsal releasing incision may help cover the skin; if not, then a free skin graft. Dorsal transposition flap of preputial the prepucial skin after penile degloving may be designed to cover the ventral skin defect, avoiding the suture line's superimposition. Dorsal dartos-based prepucial skin flap

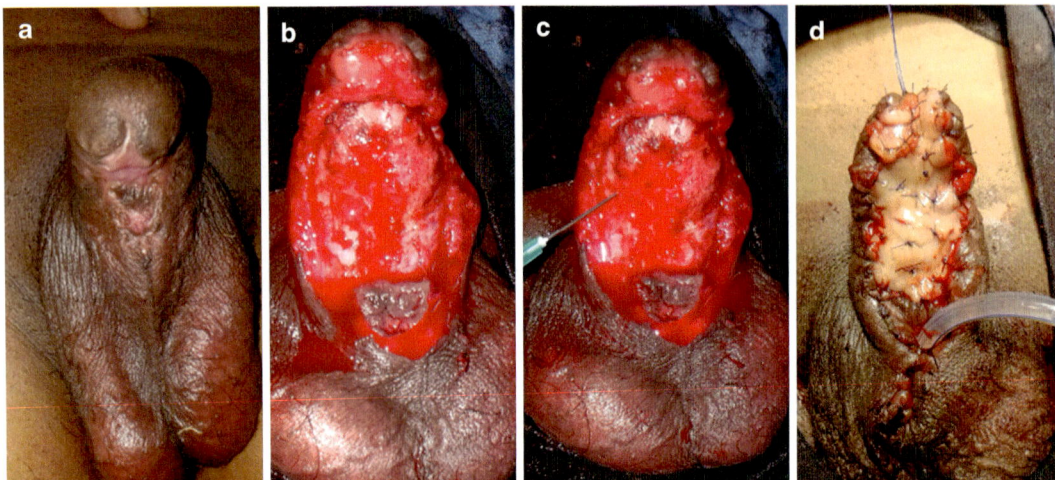

Fig. 22.11 Hypospadias cripple operated five times failed Buccal Mucosal graft. (**a**) Failed hypospadias repair with proximal meatus, chordee, contracture and loos Buccal graft and unhealthy ventral skin. (**b**) Chordee correction done with excising the fibrous tissue after. (**c**) Gittes test to confirm chordee correction. (**d**) Buccal mucosal graft and Quilting on the ventral aspect of the penis up to the glans' tip

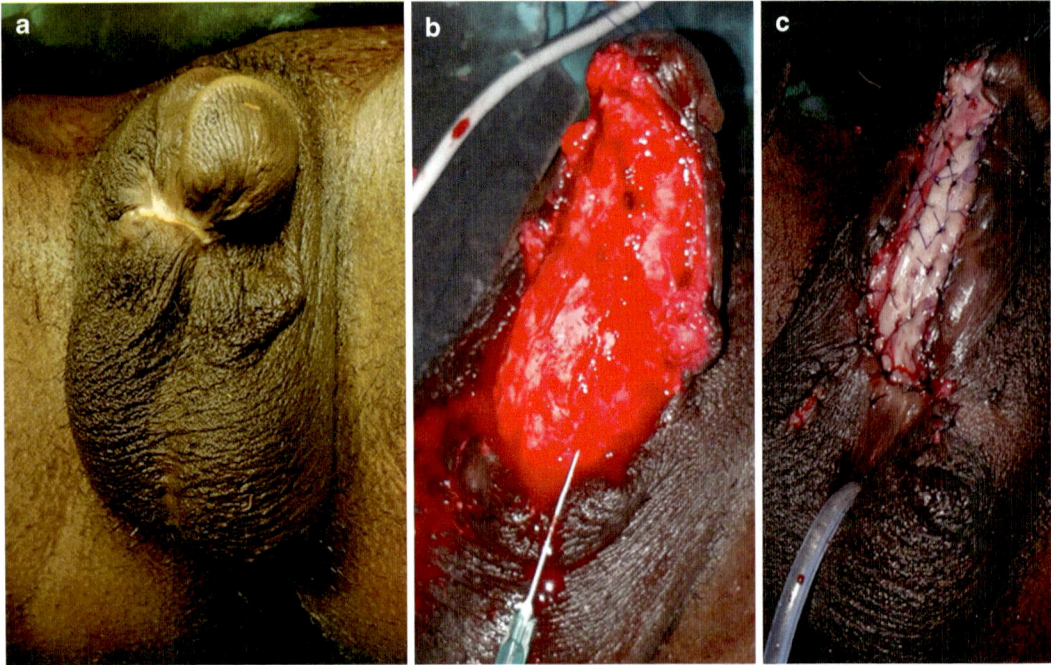

Fig. 22.12 (**a**) Hypospadias cripple had surgery five times with severe chordee and penile torsion correction and graft contracture. (**b**) Chordee correction done with excising the fibrous tissue and Gittes test to confirm chordee correction. (**c**) Buccal and lower lip Graft fixed to the ventral aspect of the penis up to the glans tip

may be brought ventrally to cover the skin if the partial dorsal hood is available. Single or double Z plasties at the penoscrotal junction to cover the skin on the ventral surface are good options (Fig. 22.15a–f). This will not only cover the ventral surface but also will prevent the recurrence of

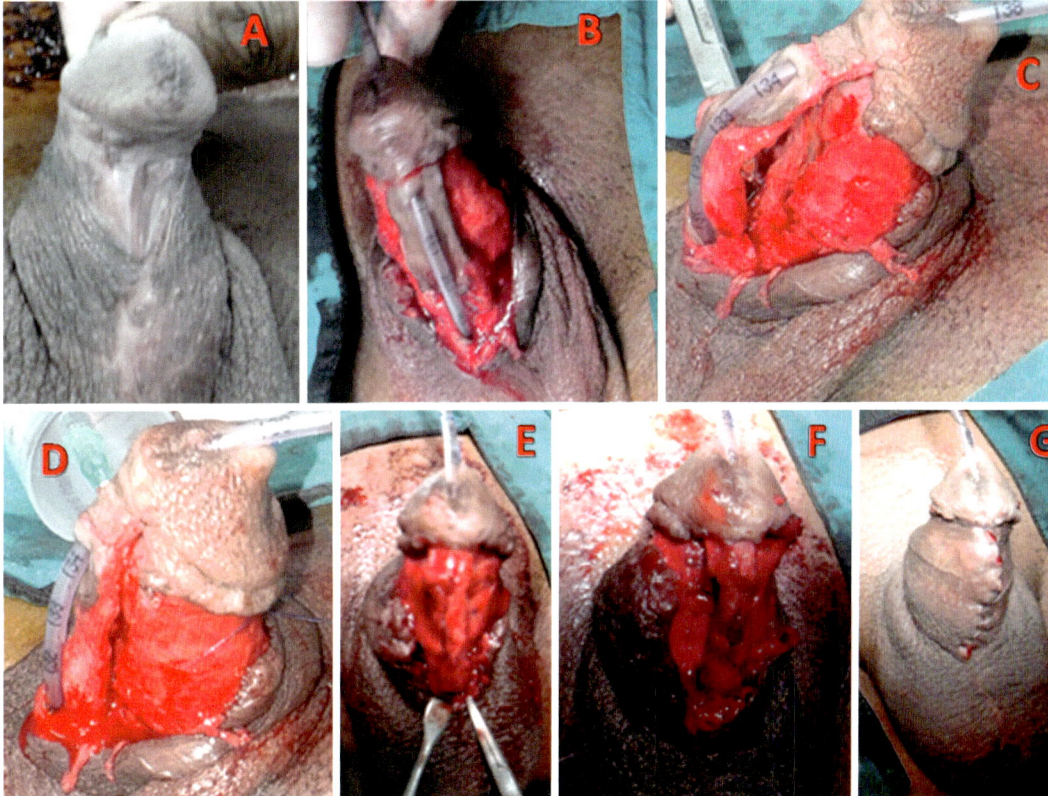

Fig. 22.13 Hypospadias cripple after multiple surgeries. (**a**) Chordee, fistula, Scared ventral skin. (**b**) Penile degloving. (**c**) Residual urethral plate and spongiosum mobilization. (**d**) Gittes test to confirm the Chordee Correction. (**e**) Urethral plate tubularization for fistula closure. (**f**) Spongioplasty. (**g**) Skin closure and final picture

chordee. Scrotal flaps may be a useful alternative in such extreme cases (Fig. 22.16a, b) but hairs on the skin restrict its use. If these measures fail, then a tissue expander is a viable option to cover the skin deficit. The tissue expander is also utilized for penile reconstruction in hypospadias cripples [29]. Full-Thickness Skin Graft is used in the staged procedure to cover the ventral side of the penis and the bed of the neo-urethral plate after resection of all scar tissue and correcting the chordee. Hana et al. (2017) published the results of 85 out of the 215 patients who failed hypospadias who did not have local penile skin to resurface the penis after urethroplasty. Fifty-four patients were resurfaced with scrotal skin, 23 with full-thickness skin grafting, and 4 received a split-thickness skin graft. And six who had 5–8 failed surgeries required the tissue expansion of the dorsal penile skin during 12–16 weeks before the penile resurfacing. Tissue expansion was possible in all six, and they underwent penile skin flap reconstruction of their penises. One patient each had urethrocutaneous fistula and meatal stenosis, which were successfully corrected [13].

In large skin defects with exhausted resources, the old gold Cecil Culp principle is used to stage the urethroplasty and cover the deficiency in the second stage [30]. Weiss (2018) reported their good results, including 23 patients with hypospadias cripple, increasing the detachment of penis from scrotum 9–12 months. The modification of Ceil Culp repair by delaying 9–12 months before take-down enhanced the benefits of a robust vascular bed for wound healing and helped avoid the transfer of hair-bearing scrotal skin penile shaft [31]. Therefore, the procedures mentioned above should be seen as in the armamentarium or strategy to solve the problems seen with hypospadias

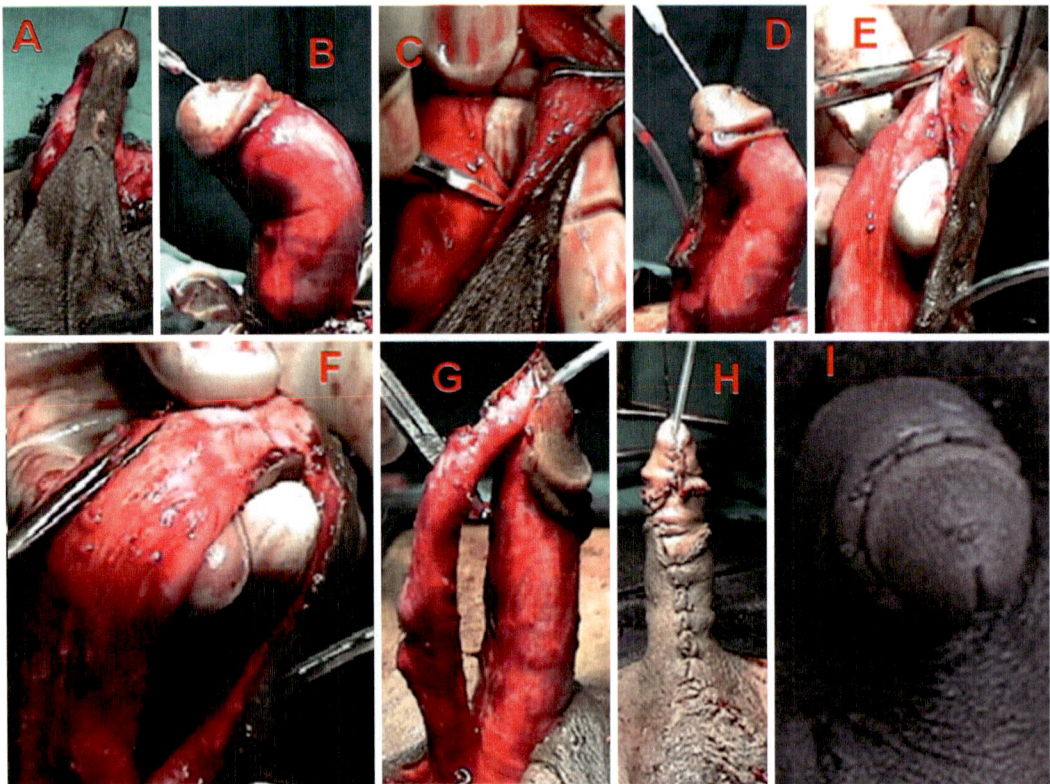

Fig. 22.14 Hypospadias cripple after multiple surgeries having laid-open urethra with significant chordee. (**a**) Penile degloving. (**b**) Gittes test showing severe chordee. (**c**) Midline skin urethral plate and spongiosum mobilization. (**d**) Gittes test showing chordee. (**e, f**) Resection of the tethering tissue from the ventral surface of corpora. (**g**) Midline skin Urethral plate and spongioplasty tubularization. (**h**) Skin closure and final picture. (**i**) Postoperative picture Meatus at the tip

crippled. When necessary, a combination of techniques is used in a single or staged repair.

22.3.6 Reconstruction Penile Part Loss

Ischaemic injury to the penis and glans by injection of epinephrine, tourniquet, and infection after corporotomy/corporoplasty is likely to occur and may cause partial or complete loss of penis and glans. Hana (2020) presented his results of hypospadias surgery's grievous complications in a web conference on controversies in hypospadias surgery. He had partial penile/glans loss in five, total glans loss in six, total penile loss in four and fibrotic corpora in one case [32].The penile enhancement surgery may increase 1–2-cm penile length and a 2.5-cm augmentation of penile girth. Penile length can be added by cutting the suspensory ligament. A tissue expander has also been used for increasing the penile length. But the frequent complications, like penile deformity, paradoxical penile shortening, disagreeable scarring, granuloma formation, migration of injected material, and sexual dys-

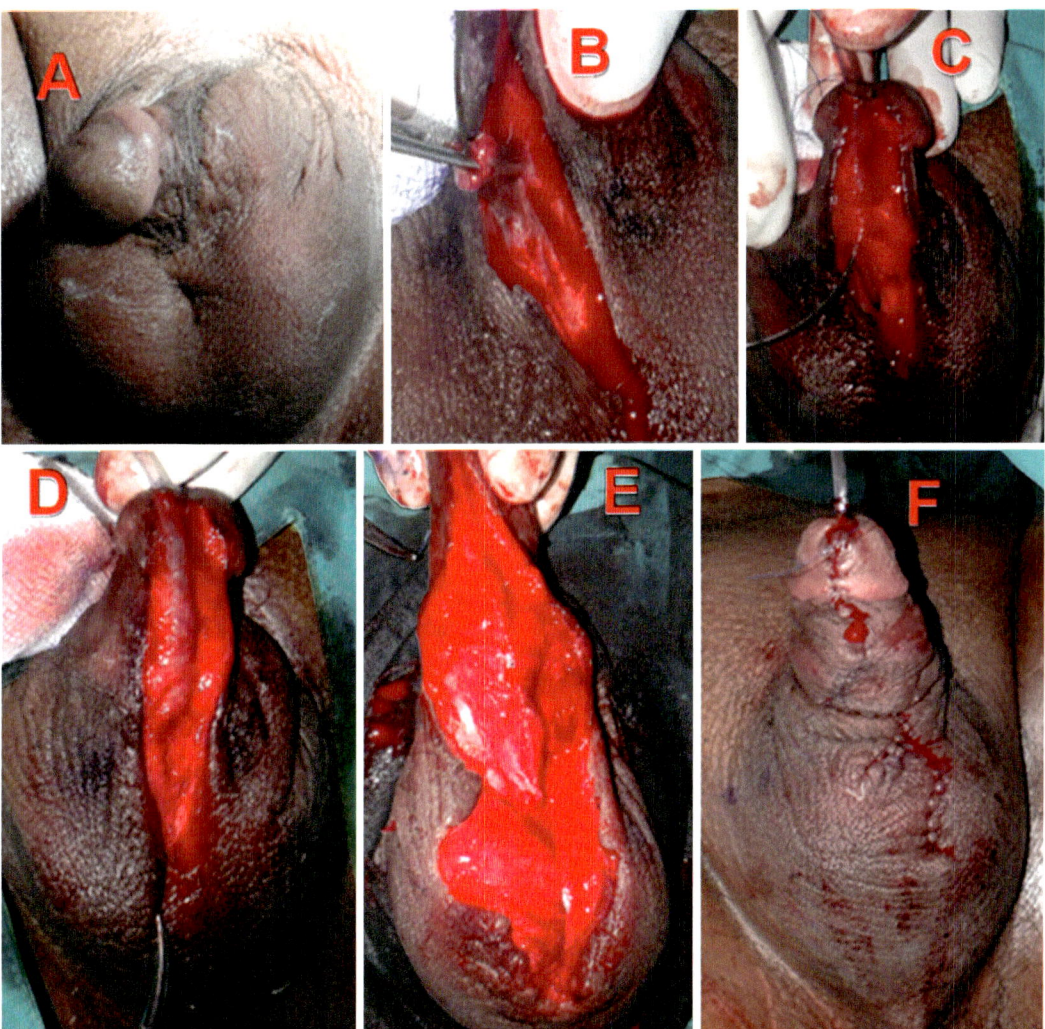

Fig. 22.15 Hypospadias cripple after five surgeries fistula, chordee, torsion, retrusive meatus, and skin scarring. (**a**) Fistula, chordee, torsion, and skin scarring. (**b**) Mobilization of the fistulous tract. (**c**) Excision of the fistulous tract. (**d**) Closure of fistula. (**e**) Dartos cover over the urethra and prepared skin flap for closure. (**f**) Final picture skin closure correction of chord and torsion

function, limits their routine use. Glans can be re-shaped by coronal sculpting with tubed graft/dermal graft placed subcutaneously in patients with a partial or total loss of the glans. Phalloplasty is recommended in complete loss of penis or fibrosis of corpora. The technique used for phalloplasty is Bevan and Decosto abdominal flap or forearm flap phalloplasty [33]. These viable options help reconstruct a functional penis. With good results, Hana used the abdominal flap phalloplasty in four cases and forearm flap phalloplasty in one patient.

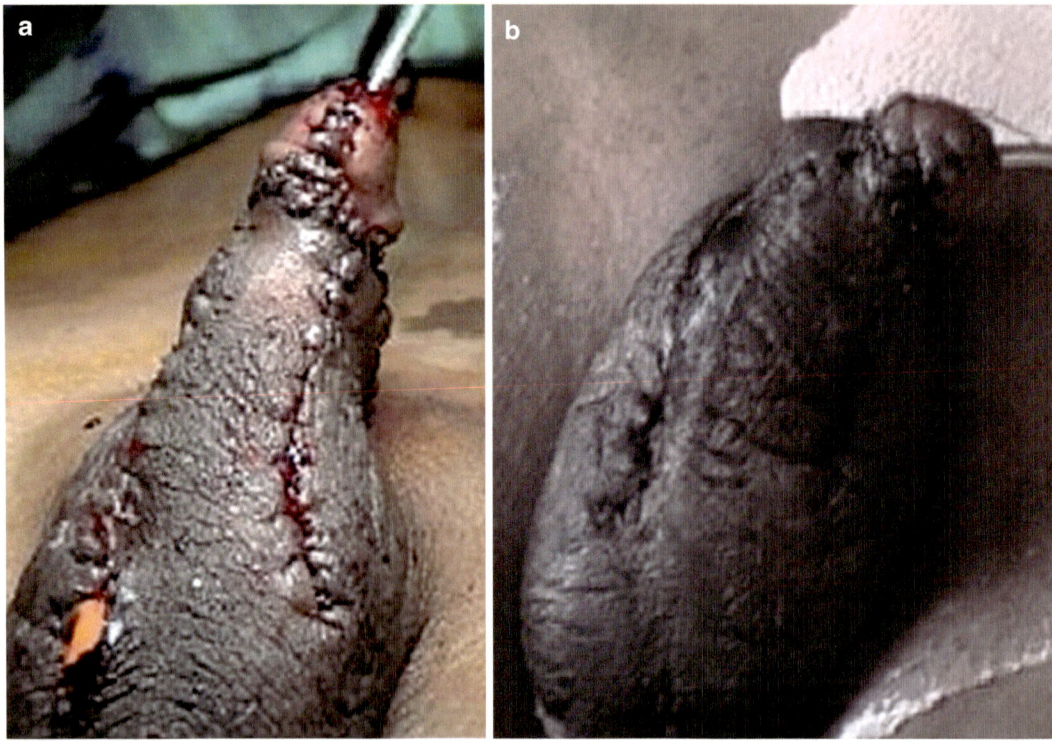

Fig. 22.16 Showing scrotal skin flap (**a**, **b**) for skin closure after failed hypospadias repair

22.4 Conclusions

No single technique is considered standard of care for crippled hypospadias repair; they have multiple problems of variable deformities and the consequent functional abnormality. Evaluation and treatment of each patient should be individualized. The surgeon's experience with all surgical techniques of hypospadias repair is an important factor in a successful outcome. Problems can be grouped in as and treated accordingly:

1. Residual Chordee/Penile Torsion—Penile degloving, urethra/urethral plate/Vascular pedicle mobilization, Plication procedures. Corporotomy/Corporoplasty.
2. Reconstruction of the urethra: In single or preferably two-stage urethroplasty; Previous urethra, Residual urethral plate, Peri fistula skin flap, penile skin flap, onlay flap, Bladder/Buccal mucosal graft
3. Healthy tissue cover: Dorsal, ventral, and scrotal Dartos/spongioplasty, Tunica vaginalis flap.
4. Resurfacing of the skin: Primary skin closure, dorsal releasing incision, dorsal skin flap, Scrotal flap, and free skin graft, tissue expanders, and Cecil Culp staged repair
5. Reconstruction of penile part loss: Glans supplementation. Penile implants and penile reconstruction.

Tissue expanders are safe and effective for acquiring genital skin for resurfacing in selected cases of hypospadias cripples and should have a place in the surgical armamentarium of complicated, redo-hypospadias and hypospadias cripple repair. Alternatively, penile skin graft, non-hair bearing skin grafts,

Buccal mucosal, or bladder mucosal grafts are used to reconstruct the neo-urethra. In severe cases, Cecil Culp urethroplasty may be used where either skin is unavailable to cover the penile shaft, and urethroplasty needs support.

References

1. Bhat A. General considerations in hypospadias surgery. Indian J Urol IJU: J Urol Soc India. 2008;24(2):188.
2. Aldamanhori R, Chapple CR (2017) Management of the patient with failed hypospadias surgery presenting in adulthood. F1000Research. 6.
3. Barbagli G, De Angelis M, Palminteri E, Lazzeri M. Failed hypospadias repair presenting in adults. Eur Urol. 2006;49(5):887–95.
4. Stecker JF Jr, Horton CE, Devine CJ Jr, McCraw JB. Hypospadias cripples. Urol Clin North Am. 1981;8(3):539–44.
5. Horton CE, Devine CJ Jr. A one-stage repair for hypospadias cripples. Plast Reconstr Surg. 1970;45(5):425–30.
6. Bracka A. Hypospadias repair: the two-stage alternative. Br J Urol. 1995;76(6):31–41.
7. Craig JR, Wallis C, Brant WO, Hotaling JM, Myers JB. Management of adults with prior failed hypospadias surgery. Transl Androl Urol. 2014;3(2):196.
8. Hensle TW, Tennenbaum SY, Reiley EA, Pollard J. Hypospadias repair in adults: adventures and misadventures. J Urol. 2001;165(1):77–9.
9. Barbagli G, Fossati N, Larcher A, Montorsi F, Sansalone S, Butnaru D, Lazzeri M. Pd60-04 predictive factors of success in adult patients treated for urethral stricture after primary hypospadias repair failure: a multivariable analysis of a single-surgeon series. J Urol. 2017;197(4S):e1184.
10. Myers JB, McAninch JW, Erickson BA, Breyer BN. Treatment of adults with complications from previous hypospadias surgery. J Urol. 2012;188(2):459–63.
11. Barbagli G, Perovic S, Djinovic R, Sansalone S, Lazzeri M. Retrospective descriptive analysis of 1,176 patients with failed hypospadias repair. J Urol. 2010;183(1):207–11.
12. Kiss A, Sulya B, Szász AM, Romics I, Kelemen Z, Tóth J, Merksz M, Kemény S, Nyírády P. Long-term psychological and sexual outcomes of severe penile hypospadias repair. J Sex Med. 2011;8(5):1529–39.
13. Fam MM, Hanna MK. Resurfacing the penis of complex hypospadias repair ("Hypospadias Cripples"). J Urol. 2017;197(3 Part 2):859–64.
14. Bhat A, Singh V, Bhat M. Penile torsion. In: Surgical techniques in pediatric and adult urology. 1st ed. New Delhi: Jaypee Brothers Medical Publishers; 2020. p. 207–22.
15. Snodgrass WT, Bush N, Cost N. Algorithm for a comprehensive approach to hypospadias reoperation using 3 techniques. J Urol. 2009;182(6):2885–92.
16. Soto-Aviles OE, Santucci RA. Management of recurrent urethral strictures. In: Practical tips in urology. Springer; 2017. p. 179–90.
17. Cordon BH, Zhao LC, Scott JF, Armenakas NA, Morey AF. Pseudospongioplasty using periurethral vascularized tissue to support ventral buccal mucosa grafts in the distal urethra. J Urol. 2014;192(3):804–7.
18. Radojicic ZI, Perovic SV, Djordjevic ML, Vukadinovic VM, Djakovic N. 'Pseudospongioplasty' in the repair of a urethral diverticulum. BJU Int. 2004;94(1):126–30.
19. Chertin B, Pollack A, Farkas A. Surgical management of hypospadias cripples. J Pediatr Urol. 2007;3: S53–4.
20. Snodgrass W, Elmore J. Initial experience with staged buccal graft (Bracka) hypospadias reoperations. J Urol. 2004;172(4 Part 2):1720–4.
21. Barbagli G, Fossati N, Larcher A, Montorsi F, Sansalone S, Butnaru D, Lazzeri M. Correlation between primary hypospadias repair and subsequent urethral strictures in a series of 408 adult patients. Eur Urol Focus. 2017;3(2–3):287–92.
22. Li L-C, Zhang X, Zhou S-W, Zhou X-C, Yang W-M, Zhang Y-S. Experience with the repair of hypospadias using bladder mucosa in adolescents and adults. J Urol. 1995;153(4):1117–9.
23. Fichtner J, Filipas D, Fisch M, Hohenfellner R, Thüroff JW. Long-term followup of buccal mucosa onlay graft for hypospadias repair: analysis of complications. J Urol. 2004;172(5):1970–2.
24. Mittermayr R, Wassermann E, Thurnher M, Simunek M, Redl H. Skin graft fixation by slow clotting fibrin sealant applied as a thin layer. Burns. 2006;32(3):305–11.
25. Foster K, Greenhalgh D, Gamelli RL, Mozingo D, Gibran N, Neumeister M, Abrams SZ, Hantak E, Grubbs L, Ploder B. Efficacy and safety of a fibrin sealant for adherence of autologous skin grafts to burn wounds: results of a phase 3 clinical study. J Burn Care Res. 2008;29(2):293–303.
26. Hayashi Y, Kojima Y, Kurokawa S, Mizuno K, Nakane A, Kohri K. Scrotal dartos flap to prevent the urethrocutaneous fistula on hypospadias urethroplasty. Int J Urol. 2005;12(3):280–3.
27. Ehrlich RM, Alter G. Split-thickness skin graft urethroplasty and tunica vaginalis flaps for failed hypospadias repairs. J Urol. 1996;155(1):131–4.
28. Sharma N, Bajpai M, Panda SS, Verma A, Sharma M. Tunica vaginalis flap cover in hypospadias cripples our experience in a tertiary care center in India. Nigerian J Surg Sci. 2014;24(1):7.
29. Mir T, Simpson RL, Hanna MK. The use of tissue expanders to resurface the penis for hypospadias cripples. Urology. 2011;78(6):1424–9.
30. Weiss DA, Smith ZL, Taylor JA, Canning DA. Old tools, old problems, new solution: the use of a

modified Cecil-Culp concept in the trauma setting. Urology. 2017;106:196–9.
31. Weiss D, Long C, Frazier J, Shukla A, Srinivasan A, Kolon T, DiCarlo H, Gearhart JP, Canning D. Back to the future: the Cecil-Culp technique for salvage penile reconstructive procedures. J Pediatr Urol. 2018;14(4):328.e321–7.
32. Chang C, White C, Katz A, Hanna MK. Management of ischemic tissues and skin flaps in re-operative and complex hypospadias repair using vasodilators and hyperbaric oxygen. J Pediatr Urol. 2020;16(5):672.e671–8.
33. Morrison SD, Shakir A, Vyas KS, Kirby J, Crane CN, Lee GK. Phalloplasty: a review of techniques and outcomes. Plast Reconstr Surg. 2016;138(3):594–615.

23

Management of Hypospadias in Patients with Disorders of Sexual Development (DSD)

P. Ashwin Shekar and Amilal Bhat

23.1 Introduction

Though most hypospadias cases occur as an isolated anatomical defect, in a small subset of patients, the hypospadias may be part of a more complex anomaly of a disorder of sex development (DSD) [1, 2]. The HP in this group of patients tends to be severe with a more proximal division of corpus spongiosum and prominent hypoplasia of ventral tissue distal to it, leading to a more proximal urethral opening and a higher incidence of penile curvature [2, 3]. Besides, the presence of other associated anomalies like a bifid scrotum, penoscrotal transposition, micro-penis, undescended testis (UDT), or a prostatic utricle in these patients that needed to be addressed along with HP repair necessitates the formulation of individualized surgical strategies on a case to case basis [4].

23.2 When to Suspect DSD in a Child with Hypospadias and How to Evaluate it?

One of the most important questions that arise in the mind of a treating surgeon when dealing with hypospadias is, "Should I evaluate for DSD in this patient of hypospadias?" Unfortunately, there is still no evidence-based consensus on the best answer for this perplexing question to date [3, 5]. Presently, recommendations are based mostly on the experience of individual surgeons or individual centers with marked heterogenicity in the diagnostic criteria and investigation protocols used, which make generalization of such recommendations difficult [2].

Generally, any patient with a proximally located urethral meatus and severe ventral curvature with an associated bifid scrotum and undescended testicle needs evaluation for DSD by a multidisciplinary team that includes the treating surgeon. Specifically, assessment of gonadal position is a crucial aspect of the initial assessment, which influences the direction of further investigations [6]. Additional useful clinical markers that may indicate the need for DSD eval-

P. Ashwin Shekar (✉)
Consultant Urologist, Department of Urology, Sri Sathya Sai Institute of Higher Medical Sciences, Puttaparthi, India

A. Bhat
Bhat's Hypospadias and Reconstructive Urology Hospital and Research Centre,
Jaipur, Rajasthan, India

Department of Urology, Jaipur National University Institute for Medical Sciences and Research Centre, Jaipur, Rajasthan, India

Department of Urology, Dr. S.N. Medical College, Jodhpur, Rajasthan, India

Department of Urology, S.P. Medical College, Bikaner, Rajasthan, India

P.G. Committee Medical Council of India, New Delhi, India

Academic and Research Council of RUHS, Jaipur, Rajasthan, India

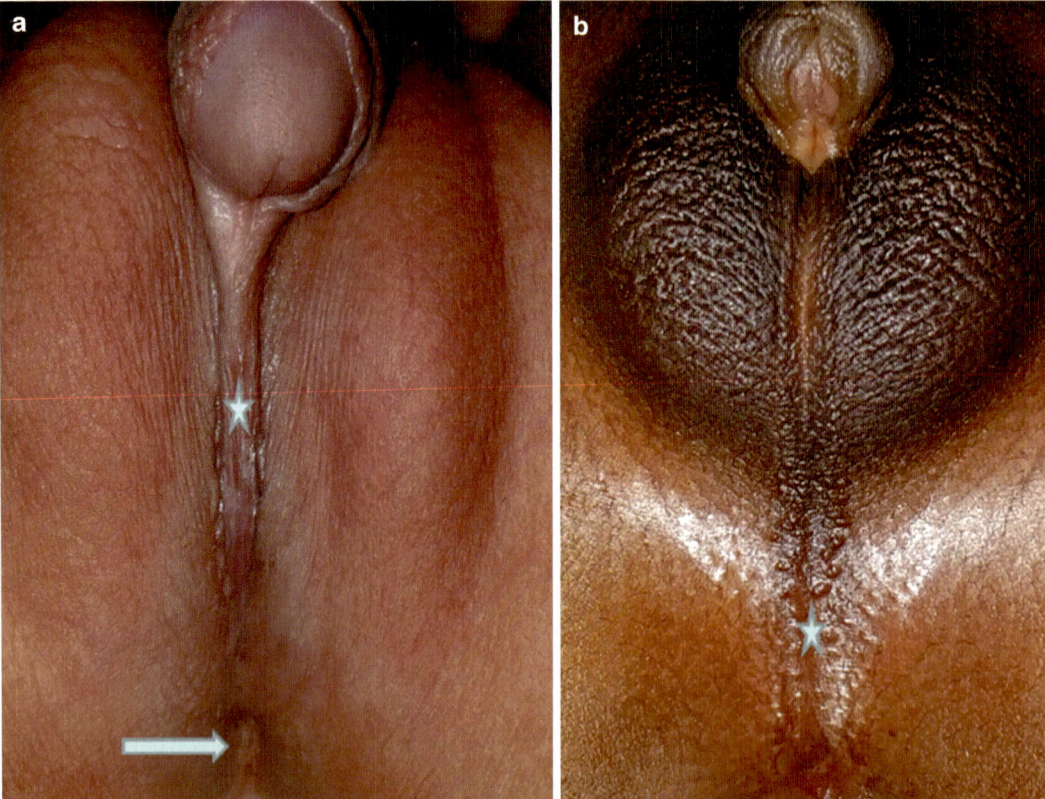

Fig. 23.1 (**a** and **b**) Clinical picture showing bifurcation of the median raphe (star) and a dimple in the perineum (arrow)

uation include an incomplete fusion of the median raphe and a dimple in the perineum (Fig. 23.1).

Investigations as part of the DSD workup would typically include

- Serum electrolytes immediately to rule out CAH
- Karyotype
- Pelvic ultrasound
- Hormonal studies
  - 17-OH progesterone
  - Serum testosterone, Dihydrotestosterone (if age <3 months or after HCG stimulation, if older).
  - Serum luteinizing hormone (LH) and follicle-stimulating hormone (FSH).
- Imaging studies (Ultrasound/MRI abdomen and pelvis)—to assess Mullerian structures/gonads, if impalpable.
- Genitogram
- Diagnostic laparoscopy—to assess gonadal status when impalpable.
- Cystourethroscopy
- Genetic studies—if available, for specific genetic defects.

If the investigations mentioned above are normal, the patient is considered to have idiopathic proximal hypospadias. If abnormalities in the chromosome or hormonal profile are identified, further study for a specific diagnosis should be done by a multidisciplinary DSD team. This would make it easier to give the family and caregivers the best information available that addresses specific concerns like the need for pubertal hormone supplementation, available surgical options, later fertility potential, cancer risk, and stability of sex of rearing with aging [7]. Also, identifying a specific diagnosis will help the clinicians better understand the associated pathophysiology and, more importantly, its correlation with surgical outcomes [7].

23.3 Gender Assignment Considerations

Another unique situation that the treating clinician will frequently face is the issue of gender assignment in babies born with ambiguous genitalia, where the hypospadias appears to be a part of the spectrum of DSD. Again, this is a sensitive issue and requires to be handled with the utmost care and gentleness. Most families are under considerable distress due to the atypical appearance of the patient's genitalia.

Some of the significant factors that have to be considered here are the external phenotype, the internal karyotype, ease of reconstruction, and parental expectations/attitudes. In the past, when the investigations were limited, the "nurture vs nature" approach was used commonly, leading to the assignment of female gender in many of these patients due to ease of reconstruction; however, the knowledge of brain imprinting in the last few decades and the incidence of gender dysphoria in these patients reared as females in later life, has made this approach questionable [6]. Nowadays, with better investigations, a multidisciplinary effort must be made to come to an accurate diagnosis in all these patients, which will help in offering the best possible advice on gender assignment. Due to this more scientific approach, over the past three decades, there has been a substantial increase in male gender assignment, especially in the group of under-virilized XY males with disorders of androgen synthesis or a partial androgen insensitivity syndrome (PAIS) profile who have both testicular and phallic tissue present and also demonstrates an adequate response to stimulation of the pituitary–gonadal axis [8–10].

23.4 Timing of Re-evaluation and Surgery for Hypospadias

Surgical intervention is not typically required in these children diagnosed at birth during the neonatal period since the proximal urethral opening does not usually cause any voiding symptoms; however, it is prudent to schedule a visit to the surgeon at around 3–6 months. This time period would allow the parents to process all information received in the postnatal period with respect to the further investigations required in DSD and also allow the parents to establish a strong bond with their child, which ultimately would lead to a more focused discussion on the further course of action including surgery [6]. Also, many of these patients will have associated undescended gonads, and this would give enough time for spontaneous descent to happen [11]. As per present guidelines since infants benefit from better wound healing and therefore decreased complications in comparison to older children, HP repairs irrespective of the association with DSD has been recommended between the ages of 6 and 18 months [12]. Another purported advantage of this approach is that early reversion to normal-appearing genitalia significantly relieves parental distress and improves parent–child attachment. However, strong evidence for this belief is lacking [12, 13].

However, over the last decade, the ideal timing of surgical intervention in patients with hypospadias has become a subject of debate from an ethical perspective, more so in children with associated DSD [14–16]. Though there are obvious benefits of early intervention with respect to functional improvement in voiding and positive adaption in these children, arguments against an early age of intervention have revolved around the issue of consent of patients with this condition, with child rights activists advocating that only the patient himself can give consent to surgical intervention on their genitalia and any intervention should be deferred until the patient has developed a stable gender identity, to avoid the possibility of gender dysphoria at adulthood leading to dissatisfaction and even necessitating a sex reversal [14–16].

It is clear now that this issue of timing and need for surgical intervention is a sensitive one. The treating clinician must present both sides of the argument to the parents and caregivers in a very unbiased way and assist in their decision-making process on whether to proceed with surgery or not [6]. Ultimately, both the patient's physical status and the parents' psychosocial preparedness have to be considered when deciding on the timing of surgery to ensure the best possible results for the child and the family [17, 18].

23.5 Preoperative Evaluation and Goals for Surgical Intervention

Thought the primary aim of a masculinizing genitoplasty done in childhood is the reconstruction of the external genitalia to better correspond with male sex of rearing and prevention of complications like infection and malignancy, a good reconstruction should also allow for future sexual activity and optimize the fertility potential [8, 19].

When preparing for a masculinizing genitoplasty in these children, the physical examination should focus on the dimensions of the phallus, including length and girth, urethral meatus location, and presence of an orifice suggestive of a potential vaginal cavity. Careful palpation for gonads that can be present in the inguinal region, labioscrotal folds or scrotum, is crucial for clinical examination, which cannot be overemphasized [1, 19]. Regarding the scrotal appearance, patients can present in a spectrum ranging from a normally formed scrotum to a bifid scrotum with separated labioscrotal folds or varying degrees of penoscrotal transposition, depending on the degree of under-virilization [19]. Another clinical finding which can be used as a surrogate marker of abnormal male reproductive tract masculinization and sexual dimorphism is a reduced anogenital distance (AGD) which, along with penile length, are now considered as accessible end-point markers for male reproductive health. An essential part of the workup which should be done in all cases of the suspected DSD is a genitogram, which will delineate the length of common confluence and presence of vagina, prostatic utricle, uterine and fallopian tubes, and their size, location, and relation with the urethra (Fig. 23.2a–b). Patients with a common perineal opening will also need an urethrocystoscopy to assess for a potential vaginal cavity/prostatic utricle (Fig. 23.3a–b).

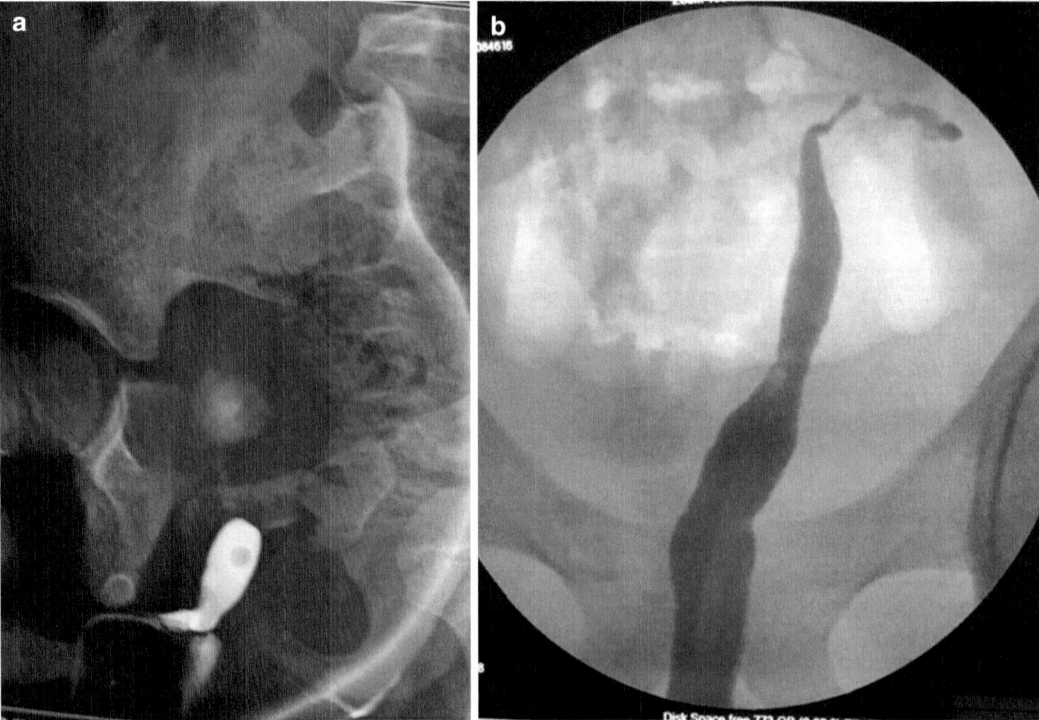

Fig. 23.2 Genitogram showing (**a**) Well-delineated vagina and common urethral canal, (**b**) Vagina, hypoplastic uterine cavity, and fallopian tube

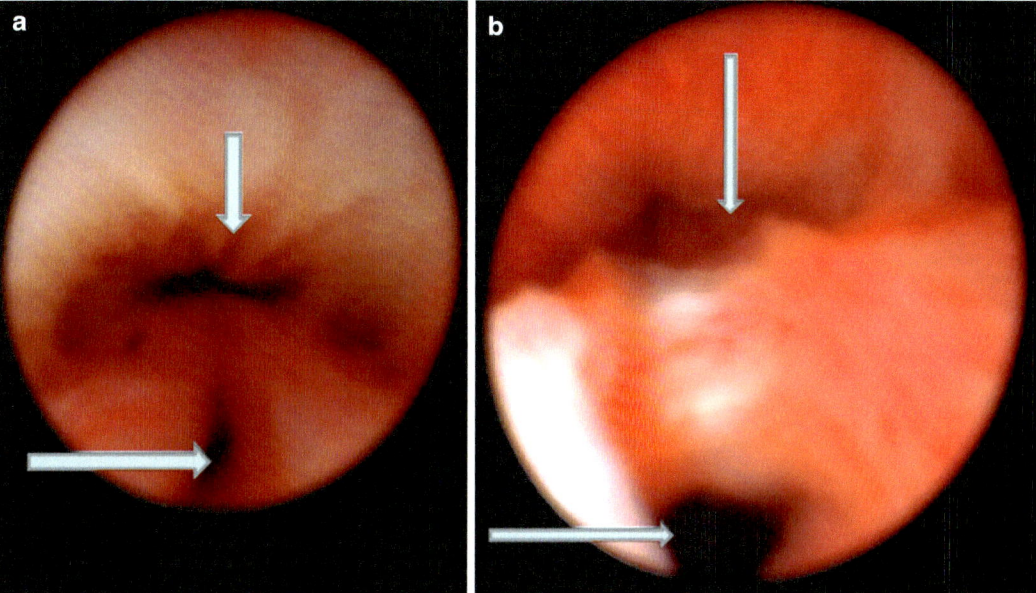

Fig. 23.3 (a and b) Cystoscopic view showing the double opening in the urethra (upper urethral and lower vaginal opening)

23.6 Preoperative Administration of Testosterone

Another controversial area in hypospadias surgery that has divided hypospadiologists over the years has been the role of preoperative testosterone administration before hypospadias surgery. The present consensus is that testosterone has a role in children with a small penis, more so in those children with small glans and severe curvature, where it can improve the surgical outcomes by making tissues more robust for surgical handling [6, 20]. However, there are marked variations among different surgeons and centers on the timing of testosterone administration, dose and route of administration (intramuscular vs topical application). In our center, we prefer the intramuscular route for testosterone administration given at a dose of 2 mg/kg/month for two consecutive months followed by surgery after a month of the second dose (Fig. 23.4a—pre- and, b—post-testosterone). It has to be noted that in children with significant androgen insensitivity, comparatively higher testosterone doses may be needed of testosterone to demonstrate the desired response [6].

23.7 Surgical Considerations

Hypospadias surgery in patients with concomitant DSD is no different from those without DSD in the surgical technique used. The basic principles of hypospadias surgery remain the same, which involves the following main steps.

23.7.1 Surgical Technique

Cysto-urethroscopy is done after inducing the general anesthesia. This helps assess the length of the common urethrovaginal canal, the orifice of the urethra and vagina (Fig. 23.3a and b), orifice of vaginal opening and length of the vaginal cavity, prostatic utricle, bladder size, and any other abnormality of ureteric orifice/bladder. Circumferential circumcoronal incision is given after injecting the 1:100000 solution of adrenaline, and penile degloving is done while dissecting at the level of Buck's fascia. Gittes test is done to assess chordee (Fig. 23.5b). If the chordee still persists, then the proximal urethra is mobilized (Fig. 23.5c and d, 23.6b). Mobilization of the urethra is done along with

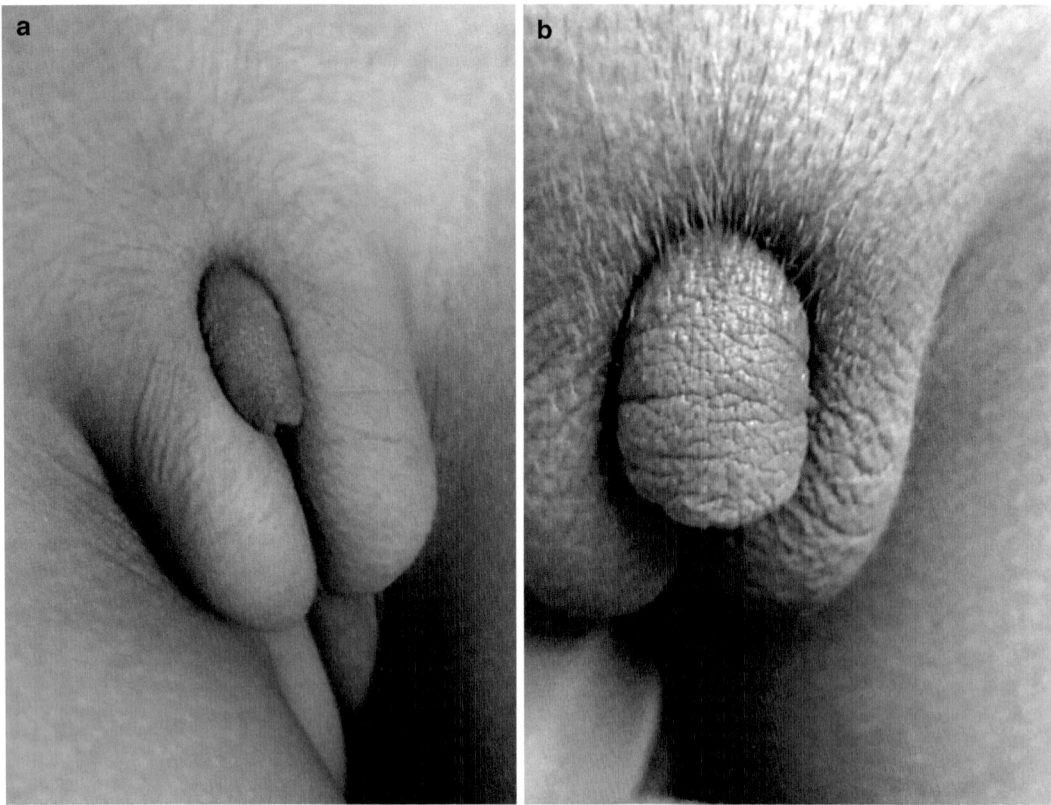

Fig. 23.4 (a) The appearance of phallus and scrotum before (**a**) and after (**b**) testosterone therapy

the mobilization of the vaginal cavity. Care is taken not to damage the urethra and bladder while mobilizing the vagina. This mobilization of the vagina releases the urethral attachments and adds length, which helps in the correction of chordee (Fig. 23.6c, d and e). The Gittes test is repeated again to confirm chordee correction (Fig. 23.5e). The vaginal cavity is closed in two to three layers according to the depth of the cavity after resection of the vagina (Fig. 23.6f). The urethral plate is tubularized with or without incision and dorsal inlay, followed by spongioplasty (Fig. 23.5f and g, 23.6g). Dorsal dartos flap flaps are mobilized and used to cover the urethra in a single or double-layer as an interposing healthy tissue (Fig. 23.5h). Glanuloplasty is done in two layers to bring the meatus to the tip, and a conical glans is refashioned. Midline scrotal tissue is mobilized, scrotoplasty is done in layers, and finally skin closure is done (Fig. 23.5i). If parents choose preputioplasty, the tunica vaginalis can be used to interpose healthy tissue, and the spared prepuce is utilized for preputioplasty (Fig. 23.6h).

In cases with severe curvature, the urethral plate is transected at the corona, and the urethral plate with spongiosum is mobilized at the level of tunica albuginea (Fig. 23.7a, b and c). Chordee correction is then confirmed. If the chordee persists still, then the proximal urethra alone or the urethra with the vagina is mobilized to correct the chordee (Fig. 23.7d). The mobilized urethra is then brought up to the penoscrotal junction. The prepuce is brought ventrally either as a flap by Byars technique or as a preputial graft and fixed to the shaft to create a urethral plate for second-stage urethroplasty followed by scrotoplasty (Fig. 23.7e).

The three main considerations in these hypospadias repairs are:
1. *Correction of ventral curvature/Chordee*
   This involves degloving of the penis to passively assess the severity of the hypospadias based on the level of division of the corpus spongio-

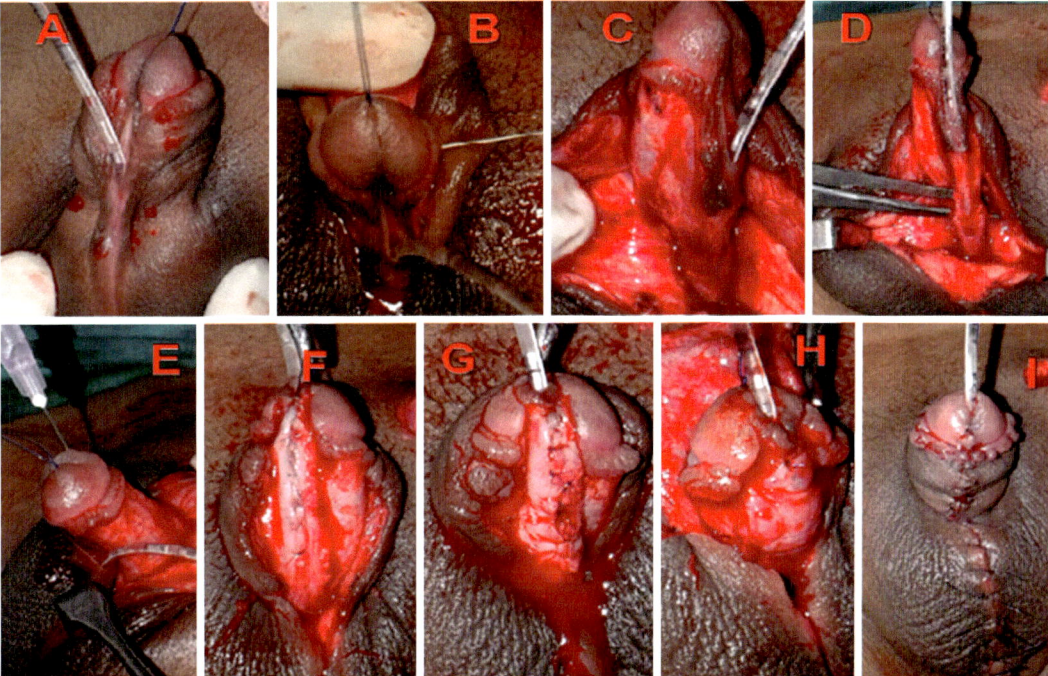

Fig. 23.5 Intraoperative pictures showing the steps of tubularized urethral plate urethroplasty. (**a**) Proximal penile hypospadiac opening. (**b**) Penile degloving and Gittes test showing chordee. (**c** and **d**) Proximal urethral mobilization. (**e**) Repeat Gittes test confirming chordee correction. (**f**) Tubularization of the urethral plate. (**g**) Spongioplasty. (**h**) Dorsal Dartos cover. (**i**) Glanuloplasty and skin closure

sum, the degree of hypoplasia of the ventral tissues, and the subsequent ventral curvature and then performing a Gitte's test by injecting saline into corpora to see for the extent and location of maximum ventral curvature [8]. Correction of chordee can be done by penile degloving, mobilization of urethral plate and spongiosum, dorsal plication, urethral transaction, ventral corporotomies with or without graft, or a combination of these depending on the severity and degree of curvature in individual circumstances. Caution must be exercised while using dorsal plication for chordee correction as though this has the advantage of leaving the urethral plate intact. But it can cause penile shortening, which can be quite significant in this group of patients who already have a shorter than average penile length. Hence, overzealous usage of dorsal plication to straighten the penis to allow a one-stage procedure should be avoided. This increases the chance of recurrent curvature in later life, which will necessitate a complete redo surgery [6].

2. *Refashioning of the missing urethra (urethroplasty)*

In cases with mild curvature, a one-stage urethroplasty is feasible if the chordee is correctable by penile degloving, mobilization of the urethral plate with spongiosum, with or without dorsal plication without the need to transact the urethral plate. The usage of the popular TIP (tubularized incised plate) repair or an onlay flap procedure for proximal hypospadias is possible in these cases [21]. Preputioplasty is also feasible in some of these cases where the patients or parents opt for foreskin preservation.

In cases with severe curvature that necessitate urethral transection for chordee correction, options include a single-stage repair using preputial based flaps or a staged repair with

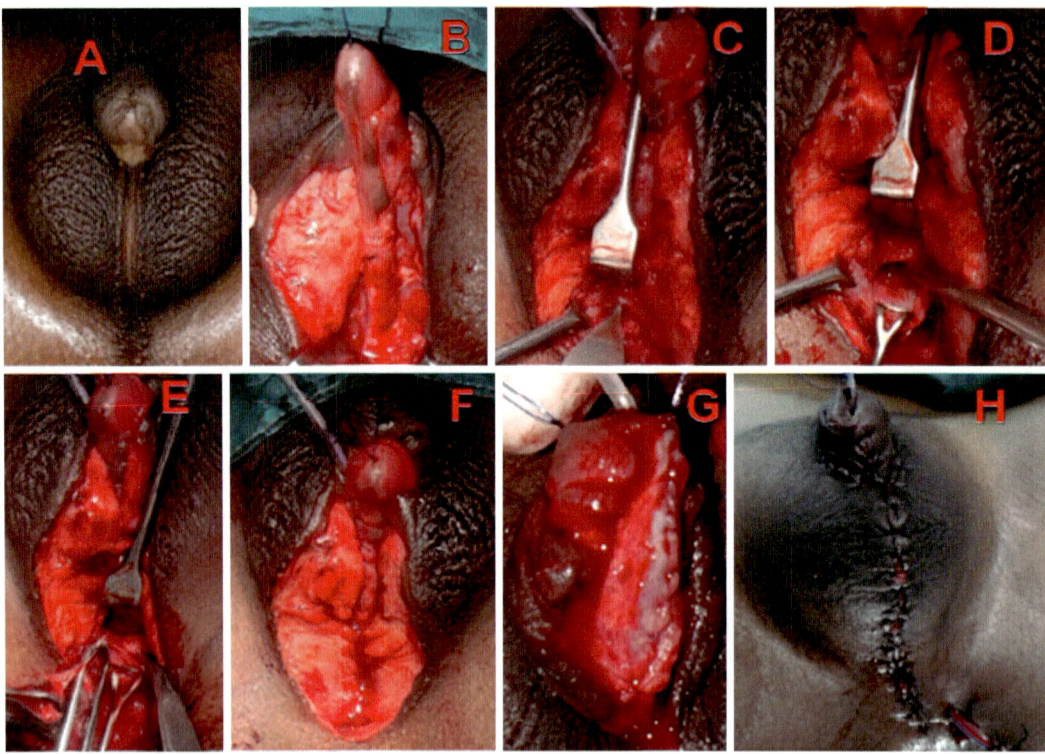

Fig. 23.6 Intraoperative pictures showing steps of tubularized urethral plate urethroplasty along with excision of the vagina. (**a**) Proximal penile hypospadias. (**b**) Penile degloving and proximal mobilization of common urethra canal. (**c**) Opening of vagina. (**d**) Mobilization of vagina. (**e**) Excision of vagina. (**f**) Closure of cavity after excision of the vagina. (**g**) Tubularization of the urethral plate. (**h**) Scrotoplasty, preputioplasty, and skin closure

preputial grafts, with the current trend towards choosing a staged approach as shown in Table 23.1 [4, 22–30]. In a staged approach, the technique is standard one as described by Bracka in redo hypospadias surgery where he used buccal mucosal grafts [31]. After transection of the urethral plate, a preputial graft is harvested from the dorsal hood, quilted to the ventral aspect of corpora and wrapped around the receded proximal urethral opening. Distally, glans is incised in the midline and opened in an open book fashion, and the graft is sutured to the wide-open glans to allow a tension-free glansplasty later on. If corporotomies were needed for chordee correction, the graft would act as a scaffold to promote the healing of the incised tunica albuginea of the corpora [6]. Following the grafting, a bolster dressing is applied, which is left undisturbed for a week to promote graft uptake. The second stage of the repair is usually done after six months. The graft is tubularized over a urethral stent, with a tunica vaginalis flap being commonly used as a second layer cover.

3. *Refashioning of skin*

Efficient management of skin is another important concern in these children, which directly correlates with cosmetic results, and this may be in the form of scrotoplasty or a correction for associated penoscrotal transposition. Depending on the degree of undervirilization, scrotoplasty can consist of simple mobilization of surrounding skin or complex mobilization and rotation of scrotal flaps to the midline [19]. Though this procedure can be safely performed simultaneously with urethroplasty, whenever there are concerns about the vascularity of the skin flaps, it is advisable to perform scrotoplasty as a separate procedure later.

In some patients, an associated penoscrotal transposition leads to additional complexity of the

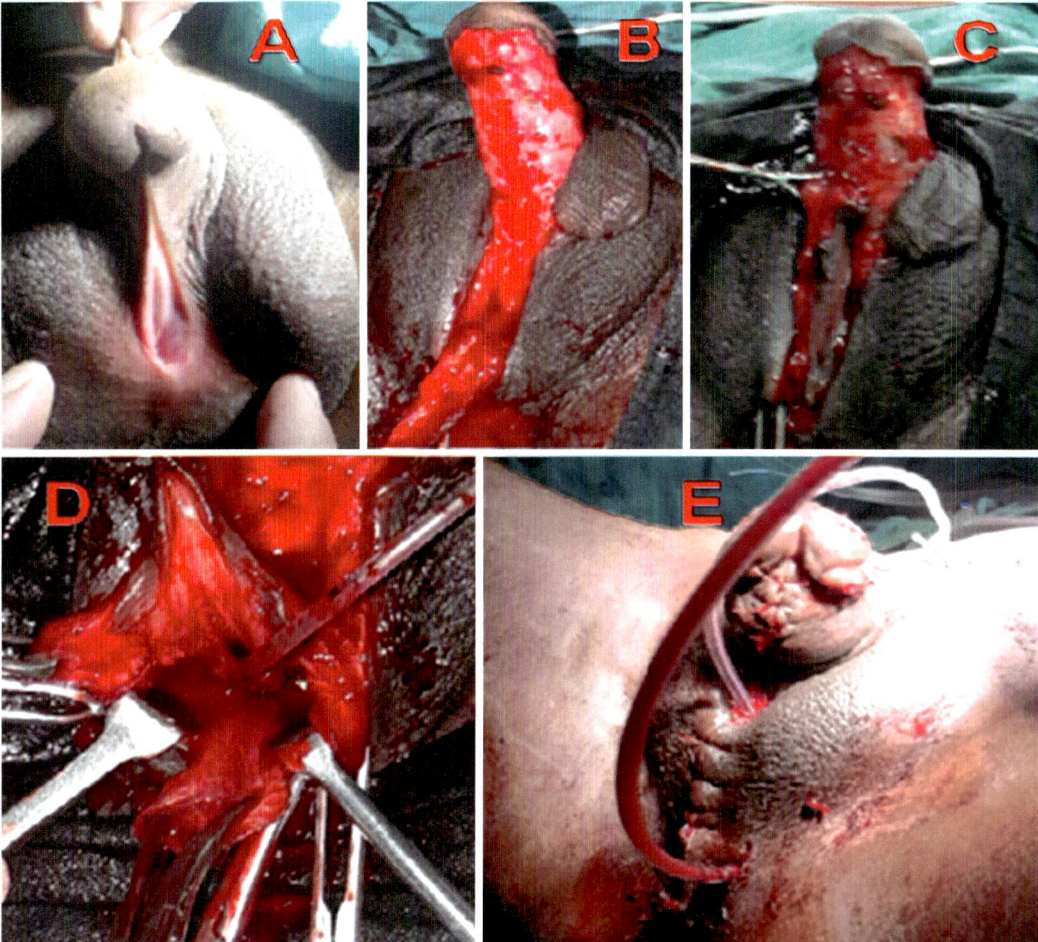

Fig. 23.7 Intraoperative pictures showing steps of two-stage repair including chordee correction, tubularization preserved urethral plate, and scrotoplasty. (**a**) Perineoscrotal hypospadias. (**b**) Transection and mobilization of the urethral plate with spongiosum to correct the chordee. (**c**) The mobilized urethral plate is preserved for later tubularization of the urethral plate. (**d**) Mobilization of proximal urethra and vagina. (**e**) Scrotoplasty and neo-urethral plate formation by Byars flap

repair, correction of which is usually achieved during the 1st or 2nd stage of the hypospadias repair; However, as mentioned above, in situations where the surgeon has doubts about vascular supply to the skin flaps due to extensive dissection during the hypospadias repair, it can be deferred to a later date and done as a stand-alone procedure [6].

4. A further important consideration in these children with DSD is that most of them will need additional procedures for the management of gonads and Mullerian structures.

   (a) *Management of gonads/testes*—Many of these children with hypospadias and DSD, especially those with partial gonadal dysgenesis, PAIS, or disorders of testosterone biosynthesis, will have associated undescended testis (UDT either unilateral or bilateral), which require to be managed along with the hypospadias. Orchidopexy in these patients can be done either before or during hypospadias repair, with the approach (open or laparoscopic) being decided by the position of the gonads [32]. In children with ovotesticular DSD, conservative gonadal surgery, with preservation of gonadal tissue that is concordant with the gender identity, is possible when

Table 23.1 Summary of the series of patients with hypospadias and DSD who underwent masculinizing genitoplasty

Series	No of patients, n	Types of DSD	Types of Hypospadias	Pre-op hormone treatment/mode of supplementation	Median age at first surgery, years	Procedure done	Auxiliary surgeries	Mean number of procedures n	No of complications, n (%)	Complications	Follow-up, years
Farkas [22] (1993)	16	46 XY=16	n.a	16/16, i.m injections	n.a	Primary=2 Staged=14	Orchidopexy=11 Testicular biopsy=5	n.a	6(37.5)	Meatal stenosis=2 UCF=3 Dehiscence=1	n.a
Chertin [23] (2005)	39	46 XY=25 46 XX=10 SC=4	Penoscrotal=30 Perineal=9	7/39, i.m injections	1.8	Primary=39	Gonadal biopsy=39 Gonadectomy=2 Transurethral incision of the utricle opening=1 Open removal of the utricle=1.	n.a	14(35.9)	Rec chordee=4 UCF=5 Dehiscence=3 Recurrent infection due to persistent vaginal pouch=2	6
Fekete [24] (2006)	25	46 XY=19 46 SC=6	n.a	n.a	n.a	n.a	n.a	n.a	5(20)	UCF=4 Penile deformity=1	n.a
Sharma [25] (2008)	356	46 XY=298 46 XX=7 SC=51	Penoscrotal=242 (68%) scrotal=61 (17%), perineal=53 (15%)	351/356, local application after first stage	23.6 months	Primary=5 Staged=351	n.a	n.a	83(23.3)	UCF=56 Stricture=12 Baggy urethra=8 Recurrent infection due to persistent vaginal pouch=5 Diverticula=3 Hair growth in urethra=5	n.a

Series	No of patients, n	Types of DSD	Types of Hypospadias	Pre-op hormone treatment/mode of supplementation	Median age at first surgery, years	Procedure done	Auxiliary surgeries	Mean number of procedures n	No of complications, n (%)	Complications	Follow-up, years
Sirçili [26] (2010)	59	46 XY=44 46 XX=7 45XY/45 X0=8	n.a	n.a	6	Staged=59	n.a	2	43(72.8)	UCF=30 Stricture=13	14.1± 9.2
Sharma [27] (2012)	6	46 XX=6	n.a	no	14.2	Staged=6	Mullerian structures removal=6 Bilateral mastectomy=6	4.9	1(16.7)	Rec UTI due to persistent vaginal pouch =1	9.2
Palmer [28] (2012)	17	46 XY=8 SC=7 Others=2	Proximal shaft=2 Penoscrotal=3 Perineal=12	n.a	2.37	Primary=7 Staged =10	Orchidopexy= 8 (47.1) Gonad biopsy= 4 (23.5) Gonadectomy= 6 (35.3)	2.06	5(29.4)	n.a	2.07
Saltzman [29] (2018)	30	46 XY=26 46 XX=2 Others=2	Midshaft=2 Penoscrotal=9 Perineal=19	7(24.1)	9 months	Primary=6 Staged =24	Orchidopexy= 18	n.a	24(80)	UCF=8 Stricture=1 Dehiscence=8 Skin issue=4 Graft issue=1 Diverticulum=1	35.1 months
Ochi [4] (2019)	58	46 XY=51 46 XX=1 SC =4 47XY +21=2	Perineal=26 Scrotal=16 Penoscrotal=15 Midshaft =1	n.a	n.a	Primary=6 Staged =52	Orchidopexy= 17(29.3)	n.a	8 (13.8)	Stenosis=3 Diverticulum=2 UCF=2 Rec curvature=1	5.16 ± 0.56

Key: *n.a.* not available, *DSD* Disorders of sex development, *SC* Sex chromosomal, *UCF* urethrocutaneous fistula guided by intraoperative frozen section analysis of gonadal tissues to define the margins between ovarian and testicular components [33]. Rarely, when there is a high risk of malignancy (dysgenetic gonads), gonadectomy is recommended, (Fig 23.8b) which can be combined with concurrent testicular prosthesis insertion in young adults [19, 34].

(b) *Mullerian structures*—In DSD patients, rudimentary Mullerian structures are not an unusual occurrence. Among these, a commonly encountered structure during hypospadias repairs is the prostatic utricle, a cystic structure that communicates with the urethra at the level of the verumontanum. Apart from causing some difficulty in catheterization during or after hypospadias repair in these patients, most utricles are asymptomatic and do not affect urethroplasty. Rarely, it can become symptomatic due to the stone formation or vasal efflux leading to recurrent episodes of epididymorchitis, which necessitates its removal either laparoscopically or through an open sagittal posterior approach [35–37]. Other Mullerian duct structures like vagina and hypoplastic uterus with fallopian tubes require excision (Figs. 23.8a and 23.6d). Resection of these structures may be combined with the hypospadias surgery or can be done separately.

23.7.2 Complications

In general, complications following HP repairs can be divided into anatomical (urethral healing failures (fistula, dehiscence), urine flow impairments (stenosis, diverticulum), persistent penile curvature) and functional (poor cosmetic results, sexual disorders) complications. The anatomical complications like urethrocutaneous fistulas, urethral strictures, meatal stenosis, and glans dehiscence usually present in the immediate postoperative period and will require surgical intervention, which may vary from a simple meatal dilatation to complete redo repair.

Being a more complex surgery than distal repairs, complication rates for proximal hypospadias repair are significant, and rates in excess of 50% have been historically reported [21, 38–40]. Unfortunately, very few studies have focused on the outcomes following HP repairs in patients with a definitive diagnosis of DSD [4, 22–29]. As shown in Table 23.1, among the few studies that have studied outcomes in this cohort of patients with DSD, the complication rate ranges between 13 and 72%. Regarding the question of whether there is a difference in outcomes in children with and without DSD diagnosis, Palmer et al. showed that though boys with a specific DSD diagnosis have significantly more atypical anatomy and are more likely to require procedures for the management of the gonads, they do not have an increased risk of complications or number of surgeries [28]. However, this observation has been refuted by Saltzman et al., who in a more recent study observed that proximal hypospadias repair on patients with DSD is associated with higher reoperation rates in the first two years than a standard proximal hypospadias repair (80 vs 45.9%), with staged repairs being a particular risk factor for reoperation [29]. A similar observation has been made by Lucas-Herald et al. also who, in their study on outcomes in partial androgen insensitivity syndrome, observed that young men with an AR mutation were more likely to have multiple procedures [41]. Ultimately, the bottom line is proximal hypospadias repair with or without DSD is still a challenging and humbling experience, even for the most experienced surgeons. This aspect should be truthfully informed to all the stakeholders involved [6]. More importantly, since many of these patients will need to undergo multiple genital surgeries to ensure good anatomical and functional results, including enabling optimal sexual functioning, all clinicians involved in managing this challenging condition should emphasize the need for long-term follow-up in these patients and caregivers.

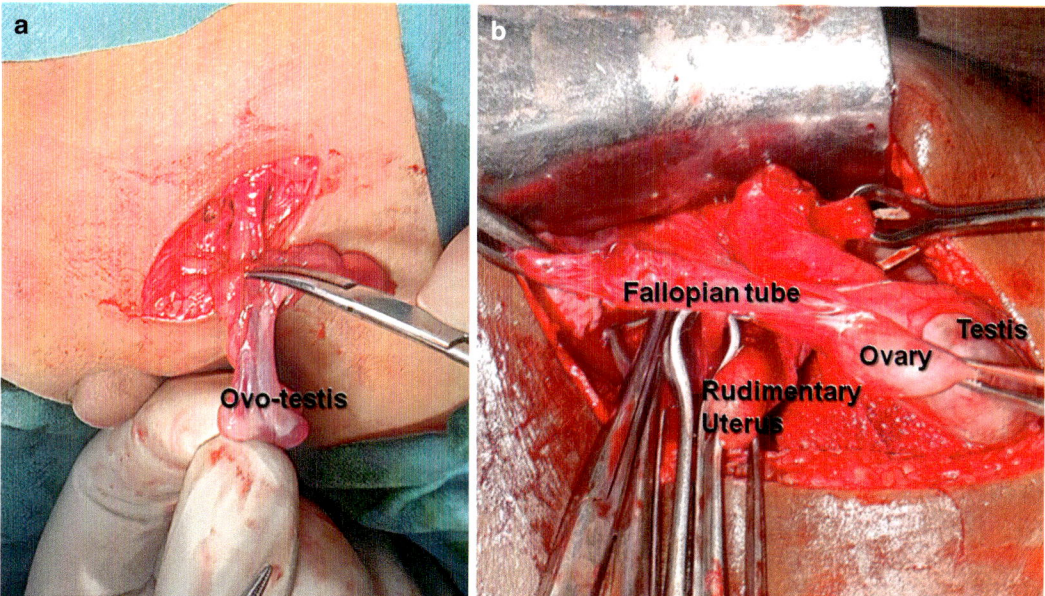

Fig. 23.8 Intra-operative picture showing Mullerian duct strictures. (**a**) Ovotestis in hernia sac of undescended testis. (**b**) Testis, Ovary, Fallopian tube, and rudimentary uterus

23.8 Long-term Follow-up and Outcomes

As mentioned earlier, an important aspect of hypospadias repair that has been stressed time and again has been the need for long-term follow-up to assess long-term functional outcomes. This is all the more important in this unique subgroup as, along with the anatomical results, the aspect of gender identity also comes into play as these children get older. Further, many patients, specifically those with 46 XY DSD, will need hormone supplementation in monthly intramuscular testosterone to induce puberty and maintain adequate hormone levels through adulthood [42, 43].

In recent years, validated instruments like the Pediatric Penile Perception Score (PPPS), the Penile Perception Score, Hypospadias Objective Scoring Evaluation (HOSE) have been developed to report patient perceptions of anatomical and functional outcomes hypospadias repair [6]. There have also been studies that have reported on the patient-reported urinary and sexual function outcomes in adults who had undergone masculinizing genitoplasty for DSD in childhood [42–47]. In the majority of these series, although specific complaints about reduced penile length, difficulties in voiding and sexual activity were frequently reported, patients were overall satisfied with the long-term results of masculinizing genitoplasty. In one of the earliest studies by Miller et al., men who underwent staged hypospadias repair for severe ambiguous genitalia with perineoscrotal hypospadias had continued difficulty with both ejaculation and micturition, but no major psychiatric or psychological disturbance [47]. Some of the common problems reported by adults, who had undergone masculinizing genitoplasty in childhood are dissatisfaction due to reduced penile length, poor or premature ejaculation, erectile dysfunction that sometimes translate into even fear of sexual contact. In general, good results may be expected if the initial phallus size is adequate (with or without testosterone supplementation); however, the results tend to be poor in cases with micropenis and minimal virilization [24, 27]. Interestingly, despite the problems, men with DSD are more likely to be satisfied than women with regard to their surgical outcomes and sexual function [19, 26, 45]. Presently, prospective collection of patient-centric data in this group of proximal hypospadias with DSD is an active area of research. This data is vital to improve care in this difficult condition further [6].

23.9 Conclusion

To summarize, patients with hypospadias and a diagnosis of DSD are a unique subpopulation of patients with proximal hypospadias where management includes both surgical and psychosexual care for promoting positive adaptation. Because of the predominantly proximal type of hypospadias seen in these patients, two-stage repair with a preoperative course of testosterone gives better anatomical and functional results in most of these patients [27]. An individualized approach with a focus on integrated communication between the multidisciplinary medical team and the patient's family, which continues beyond the initial post-surgical period to adulthood, is crucial for successful outcomes.

References

1. Kearsey I, Hutson JM. Disorders of sex development (DSD): not only babies with ambiguous genitalia. A practical guide for surgeons. Pediatr Surg Int. 2017;33(3):355–61.
2. Wong YS, Tam YH, Pang KKY, Yau HC. Incidence and diagnoses of disorders of sex development in proximal hypospadias. J Pediatr Surg. 2018 Dec;53(12):2498–2501. https://doi.org/10.1016/j.jpedsurg.2018.08.010. Epub 2018 Sep 1.
3. Snodgrass W, Macedo A, Hoebeke P, et al. Hypospadias dilemmas: a round table. J Pediatr Urol. 2011;7(2):145–57.
4. Ochi T, Ishiyama A, Yazaki Y, Murakami H, Takeda M, Seo S, et al. Surgical management of hypospadias in cases with concomitant disorders of sex development. Pediatr Surg Int. 2019;35(5):611–7.
5. Ahmed SF, Achermann JC, Arlt W, et al. Society for Endocrinology UK guidance on the initial evaluation of an infant or an adolescent with a suspected disorder of sex development (Revised 2015). Clin Endocrinol (Oxf). 2016 May;84(5):771–88.
6. Romao RL, Pippi Salle JL. Update on the surgical approach for reconstruction of the male genitalia. Semin Perinatol. 2017;41:218–26.
7. Palmer BW, Reiner W, Kropp BP. Proximal hypospadias repair outcomes in patients with a specific disorder of sexual development diagnosis. Adv Urol. 2012;2012:708301.
8. Mouriquand PD, Gorduza DB, Gay CL, Meyer Bahlburg HF, Baker L, Baskin LS. Surgery in disorders of sex development (DSD) with a gender issue: if (why), when, and how? J Pediatr Urol. 2016;12(3):139–49.
9. Houk CP, Lee PA. Approach to assigning gender in 46, XX Congenital adrenal hyperplasia with male external genitalia: replacing dogmatism with pragmatism. J Clin Endocrinol Metab. 2010;95(10):4501–8.
10. Kolesinska Z, Ahmed SF, Niedziela M, et al. Changes over time in sex assignment for disorders of sex development. Paediatrics. 2014;134(3):e710–5.
11. Kolon TF, Herndon CDA, Baker LA, et al. evaluation and treatment of cryptorchidism: AUA guideline. J Urol. 2014;192(2):337–45. https://doi.org/10.1016/j.juro.2014.05.005.
12. Timing of elective surgery on the genitalia of male children with particular reference to the risks, benefits, and psychological effects of surgery and anaesthesia. American Academy of Pediatrics. Paediatrics. 1996;97(4):590–4.
13. Hughes IA, Houk C, Ahmed SF, Lee PA, Lawson Wilkins Pediatric Endocrine Society/European Society for Paediatric Endocrinology Consensus Group. Consensus statement on management of intersex disorders. J Pediatr Urol. 2006;2(3):148–62.
14. Carmack A, Notini L, Earp BD. Should surgery for hypospadias be performed before an age of consent? J Sex Res. 2016 Oct;53(8):1047–58.
15. Harris RM, Chan YM. Ethical issues with early genitoplasty in children with disorders of sex development. Curr Opin Endocrinol Diabetes Obes. 2019 Feb;26(1):49–53.
16. Gillam LH, Hewitt JK, Warne GL. Ethical principles for the management of infants with disorders of sex development. Horm Res Paediatr. 2010;74(6):412–8.
17. Creighton S, Chernausek SD, Romao R, Ransley P, Salle JP. Timing and nature of reconstructive surgery for disorders of sex development - introduction. J Pediatr Urol. 2012 Dec;8(6):602–10.
18. Springer A, Baskin LS. Timing of hypospadias repair in patients with disorders of sex development. Endocr Dev. 2014;27:197–202.
19. Wisniewski AB, Migeon CJ. Long-term perspectives for 46, XY patients affected by complete androgen insensitivity syndrome or congenital micropenis. Semin Reprod Med. 2002;20(3):297–304.
20. Wright I, Cole E, Farrokhyar F, Pemberton J, Lorenzo AJ, Braga LH. Effect of preoperative hormonal stimulation on postoperative complication rates after proxi-

mal hypospadias repair: a systematic review. J Urol. 2013;190(2):652–9.
21. Pippi Salle JL, Sayed S, Salle A, Bagli D, Farhat W, Koyle M, Lorenzo AJ. Proximal hypospadias: a persistent challenge. Single institution outcome analysis of three surgical techniques over a 10-year period. J Pediatr Urol. 2016;12(1):28.e1–7.
22. Farkas A, Rosler A. Ten years experience with masculinizing genitoplasty in male pseudohermaphroditism due to 17 beta-hydroxysteroid dehydrogenase deficiency. Eur J Pediatr. 1993;152(Suppl 2):S88–90.
23. Chertin B, Koulikov D, Hadas-Halpern I, et al. Masculinizing genitoplasty in intersex patients. J Urol. 2005;174:1683–6.
24. Nihoul-Fekete C, Thibaud E, Lortat-Jacob S, Josso N. Long-term surgical results and patient satisfaction with male pseudohermaphroditism or true hermaphroditism: a cohort of 63 patients. J Urol. 2006;175:1878–84.
25. Sharma S, Gupta K, D. Male genitoplasty for intersex disorders. Adv Urol. 2008;2008:685897.
26. Sircili MH, Silva FA, Costa EM, et al. Long-term surgical outcome of masculinizing genitoplasty in a large cohort of patients with disorders of sex development. J Urol. 2010;184:1122–12.
27. Sharma S, Gupta DK. Male genitoplasty for 46 XX congenital adrenal hyperplasia patients presenting late and reared as males. Indian J Endocr Metab. 2012;16:935–8.
28. Palmer BW, Reiner W, Kropp BP. Proximal Hypospadias repair outcomes in patients with a specific disorder of sexual development diagnosis. Adv Urol. 2012;2012:1–4.
29. Saltzman AF, Carrasco A Jr, Colvin A, Campbell JB, Vemulakonda VM, Wilcox D. Patients with disorders of sex development and proximal hypospadias are at high risk for reoperation. World J Urol. 2018 Dec;36(12):2051–8.
30. Springer A, Krois W, Horcher E. Trends in hypospadias surgery: results of a worldwide survey. Eur Urol. 2011;60(6):1184–9.
31. Bracka A. The role of two-stage repair in modern hypospadiology. Indian J Urol. 2008;24(2):210–8.
32. Tack LJ, Maris E, Looijenga LH, Hannema SE, Audi L, Köhler B, et al. Management of gonads in adults with androgen insensitivity: an international survey. Horm Res Paediatr. 2018;90(4):236–46.
33. Sircili MHP, Denes FT, Costa EMF, Machado MG, Inacio M, Silva RB, et al. Long term follow up of a large cohort of patients with ovotesticular disorder of sex development. J Urol. 2014;191(5 Suppl):1532–6.
34. Cools M, Looijenga LHJ, Wolffenbuttel KP, T'Sjoen G. Managing the risk of germ cell tumourigenesis in disorders of sex development patients. Endocr De. 2014;27:185–96.
35. Wang W, Wang Y, Zhu D, Yan P, Dong B, Zhou H. The prostatic utricle cyst with huge calculus and hypospadias: a case report and are view of the literature. Can Urol Assoc J. 2015;9(5–6):E345–8.
36. Jiwane A, Soundappan SVS, Pitkin J, Cass DT. Successful treatment of recurrent epididymoorchitis: laparoscopic excision of the prostatic utricle. J Indian Assoc Pediatr Surg. 2009;14(1):29–30.
37. Keramidas DC. Posterior sagittal approach for excision of the prostatic utricle. Pediatr Surgery Int. 2001;17(7):586.
38. Castagnetti M, El-Ghoneimi A. Surgical management of primary severe hypospadias in children: systematic 20-year review. J Urol. 2010;184(4):1469–74.
39. McNamara ER, Schaeffer AJ, Logvinenko T, et al. Management of proximal hypospadias with 2-stage repair: 20-year experience. J Urol. 2015;194(4):1080–5.
40. Long CJ, Chu DI, Tenney RW, et al. Intermediate-term follow up of proximal hypospadias repair reveals a high complication rate. J Urol. 2017;197(3 Pt 2):852–8.
41. Lucas-Herald A, Bertelloni S, Juul A, et al. The long-term outcome of boys with partial androgen insensitivity syndrome and a mutation in the androgen receptor gene. J Clin Endocrinol Metab. 2016;101(11):3959–67.
42. Gupta D, Bhardwaj M, Sharma S, et al. Long-term psychosocial adjustments, satisfaction related to gender and the family equations in disorders of sexual differentiation with male sex assignment. Pediatr Surg Int. 2010;26:955–8.
43. Fisher AD, Ristori J, Fanni E, Castellini G, Forti G, Maggi M. Gender identity, gender assignment and reassignment in individuals with disorders of sex development: a major of dilemma. J Endocrinol Invest. 2016 Nov;39(11):1207–24.
44. Lee P, Schober J, Nordenström A, Hoebeke P, Houk C, Looijenga L, Manzoni G, Reiner W, Woodhouse C. Review of recent outcome data of disorders of sex development (DSD): emphasis on surgical and sexual outcomes. J Pediatr Urol. 2012 Dec;8(6):611–5.
45. Meyer-Bahlburg HF, Migeon CJ, Berkovitz GD, Gearhart JP, Dolezal C, Wisniewski AB. Attitudes of adult 46, XY intersex persons to clinical management policies. J Urol. 2004;171(4):1615–9.
46. Migeon CJ, Wisniewski AB, Gearhart JP, et al. Ambiguous genitalia with perineoscrotal hypospadias in 46, XY individuals: long-term medical, surgical, and psychosexual outcome. Pediatrics. 2002;110:e31.
47. Miller MA, Grant DB. Severe hypospadias with genital ambiguity: adult outcome after staged hypospadias repair. Br J Urol. 1997;80:485.

Management of Penoscrotal Transposition with or without Hypospadias

Amilal Bhat and Akshita Bhat

24.1 Introduction

The surgical strategy in severe hypospadias and penoscrotal transposition aims to achieve orthoplasty (correction of chordee), urethroplasty, spongioplasty, glanuloplasty, meatoplasty, scrotoplasty, and skin coverage with circumcision or prepucial reconstruction. Penoscrotal transposition is a rare anomaly. Broman described the first case of penoscrotal transposition in 1911 and the accurate description of the proper anatomical relationship between the penis and the scrotum. Classically, the scrotum is viewed as being improperly positioned in reference to the penis. The penis appears to arise from the centre of the scrotum or is enveloped by scrotal tissues in less severe forms. The penis is positioned behind the scrotum in the complete transposition. Many a times, it may be associated with severe hypospadias with varying degrees of transposition. The presentation can often be variable ranging from location of the penis through bifid scrotum to the most severe variant where the penis emerges through the perineum [1]. Scrotoplasty in these cases depends on the severity of its transposition. It can be done in a single stage or three stages with correction of hypospadias or as a separate surgical procedure [2].

24.1.1 Definitions

Scrotum is located in a cephalic/dorsal position with respect to the penis in complete penoscrotal transposition. A less severe form is defined by a bifid scrotum where the two halves of the scrotum meet above the penis. A minor degree of scrotal tissue transposition is called a shawl scrotum (doughnut scrotum). As scrotal tissue is above the root of the penis, it could be bilaterally symmetrical on both sides of the penile shaft or unilaterally. Regression of the scrotum caudally, ending with a vast distance between penis and scrotum, is a new entity described recently [3].

A. Bhat
Bhat's Hypospadias and Reconstructive Urology Hospital and Research Centre,
Jaipur, Rajasthan, India

Department of Urology, Jaipur National University Institute for Medical Sciences and Research Centre,
Jaipur, Rajasthan, India

Department of Urology, Dr. S.N. Medical College,
Jodhpur, Rajasthan, India

Department of Urology, S.P. Medical College,
Bikaner, Rajasthan, India

P.G. Committee Medical Council of India,
New Delhi, India

Academic and Research Council of RUHS,
Jaipur, Rajasthan, India

A. Bhat (✉)
Department of Surgery, Sawai Man Singh Medical College, Jaipur, Rajasthan, India

24.1.2 Incidence

True incidence is not known as significant transposition is reported as case reports only, and the less severe cases go unreported. National Institute of Health in the US reported less than 200,000 cases of major and minor cases in the office registry of rare congenital diseases. The recently reported incidence was about 0.7% in the patients referred for phimosis and other congenital diseases [3]. These reports show that more attention needs to be paid to diagnosis and reporting this anomaly to know the exact incidence.

24.2 Embryology

The embryological basis of penoscrotal transposition is not fully elucidated. The aspect of sexual differentiation and the mechanism controlling the position of genitalia are still poorly understood. The external position of male gonads represents one of the most important differences between both sexes. The labioscrotal swellings migrate inferiomedially and fuse in the midline caudal to the penis during normal development in a male embryo under the influence of dihydrotestosterone. The abnormal positioning of the genital tubercle in relation to the labioscrotal swellings may result in partially or wholly failed migration of labioscrotal folds caudally during the 4th–5th weeks of gestation. Intrinsically associated abnormality affects the development of the corporal bodies and the urethral groove and folds. That explains the frequent occurrence of the other genital abnormalities like hypospadias.

It has also been suggested that scrotal anomalies like penoscrotal transposition may result from early division and/or abnormal migration of the labioscrotal swelling. Labioscrotal folds fail to migrate caudally or migrate, and they remain fused anterior or lateral to the genital tubercle leading to a different grade of penoscrotal transposition. Lamm and Kaplan suggested that abnormal migration or unilateral failure might result in the ectopic scrotum or unilateral penoscrotal transposition. Early division of labioscrotal swelling and subsequent abnormal migration might also result in an accessory scrotum [4].

There is evidence of 5-alpha-reductase type 2 deficiency in penoscrotal transposition. The 5-alpha reductase type 2 deficiency being an autosomal recessive sex-limited condition, prevents conversion testosterone to dihydrotestosterone. Some of the authors believe that gubernaculum abnormality is the underlying cause for the development of this anomaly. A genetic basis for this abnormality with deletion of a critical region on chromosome 13 has been seen in these patients. A familial basis is reported in about 13% of cases, with an X-linked inheritance pattern in few cases [5]. Though the condition may present as an isolated anomaly, it is often associated with various genitourinary abnormalities like chordee, hypospadias, anorectal malformations, hernias, renal agenesis, or dysplasia. Hypospadias and chordee are seen in about 80% of cases [6]. Parida et al. had noted significant renal anomalies in the form of agenesis, horseshoe kidney, ectopic and dysplastic kidney, obstructive uropathy and hydronephrosis [7]. The penoscrotal transposition has been reported in association with VACTERL anomalies [8]. Gastrointestinal abnormalities, craniofacial, and central nervous system abnormalities are often seen in about 30% of cases. Mental retardation and growth deficiency have been noticed in 60% of patients. About 20% of patients have underlying cardiovascular abnormalities [8]. Sometimes the diagnosis can present a challenge, especially during intrauterine life when abnormal appearances of the external genitalia are diagnosed on routine prenatal ultrasonography. The appearance may also have superimposing features resembling pseudohermaphroditism, penoscrotal hypospadias, micropenis, and intrauterine penile amputation. Cases have been reported showing isolated renal dysplastic anomalies [1].

24.3 Classification

1. **Congenital**: Congenital disability with complete penoscrotal transposition to minor defect.

2. **Acquired** (secondary severe infection and scarring): Extensive scarring and debridement after Fournier's gangrene may pull the penis below the scrotum causing penoscrotal transposition. Repositioning of such scrotum is more complicated and challenging than congenital penoscrotal transposition.
3. **Iatrogenic**: Sometimes penis may have to be located below the scrotum to bridge the long urethral defect and achieve continuity of the urethra. Sometimes it is a post-circumcision webbed penis.

24.4 Congenital

Fahmy [9] proposed a new classification for these congenital penoscrotal transpositional anomalies:

Penoscrotal transportation is divided into.

1. (A)■ Incomplete.

■ Complete (extreme).
(B) Minor, which is subdivided into:
■ Bilateral (symmetrical).
* Unilateral.

2. Central scrotalization of the median raphe.
3. Wide penoscrotal distance or caudal penoscrotal transposition.

24.5 Central Scrotalization

The scrotum is attached to the penis by a longer-than-usual stretch of skin, and the webbing of the scrotum varies from mild scrotalization to a completely buried penis. The theory of penoscrotal transposition is the scrotal skin migration towards the ventral penile area. The penoscrotal angle loss may cause sexual problems during adulthood for these children. Abnormal genital appearance is the cause of anxiety in these children and their families. Usually, the diagnosis is made early, but sometimes it is delayed to adult age, and they present with urinary stream abnormalities or genital pain and dysfunction. This is classified as:

24.5.1 I. Primary Webbing [10]

A. Simple

Grade 1 web extends up to proximal 1/3 of shaft of the penis (Fig. 24.1a).

Grade 2 web extend sup to the middle 1/3 of the shaft of the penis (Fig. 24.1b).

Grade 3 web extends up to distal 1/3 of the shaft of the penis (Fig. 24.1c).

Grade 4 Buried penis when the penis remains hidden and embedded under the suprapubic area, this condition is called a buried penis (Fig. 24.1d).

B. Compound

Type 1. Web with pre-penile scrotum.
Type 2. Web with penile curvature.
Type 3. Broad web.

24.5.2 II. Secondary Webbed Penis

Post-circumcision in obese children or concealed penis.

24.6 New classification

We classified the penoscrotal transposition and graded it with scrotal location to the penis.

A. Cranial

This can be graded according to the severity into

Grade S. Scrotalization of penis mild, moderate, and severe (Fig. 24.1a–d).
Grade 1. The scrotum covers the penis superiorly, and only there is no bifurcation of the scrotum (Fig. 24.2a–c).
Grade 2. Scrotum covering of the penis with the partial bifurcation of the scrotum (Fig. 24.2d–h).
Grade 3. Complete bifurcation of the scrotum (Fig. 24.2i).

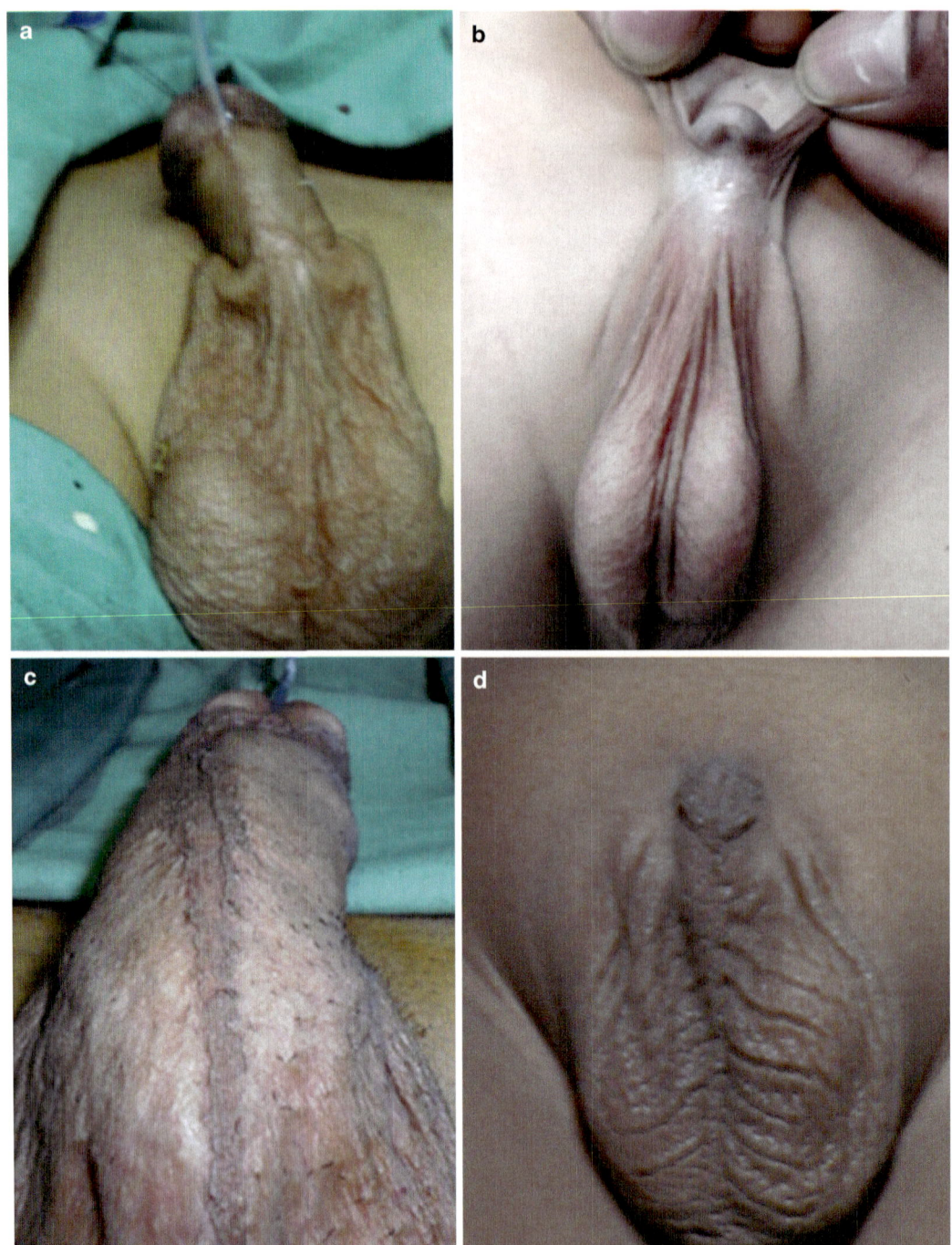

Fig. 24.1 Grading of penoscrotal webbing. (**a**) Grade 1. (**b**) Grade 2. (**c**) Grade 3. (**d**) Grade 4

Grade 4. Complete bifurcation of the scrotum with superiorization of the scrotum (Fig. 24.2j, k).

Grade 5. No bifurcation of the scrotum but complete superiorization of the scrotum (Fig. 24.2l–n).

B. Caudal

Grade 1 Fig. 24.3a.
Grade 2 Fig. 24.3b.
Grade 3 Fig. 24.3c, d.

24 Management of Penoscrotal Transposition with or without Hypospadias

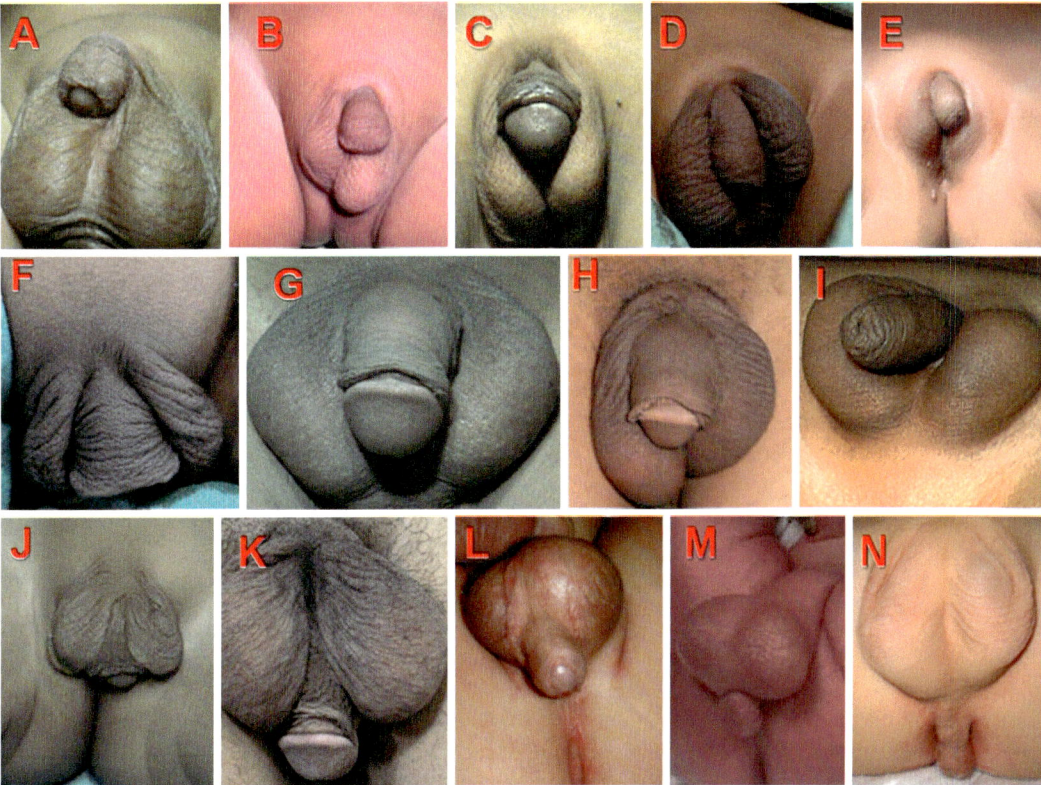

Fig. 24.2 Showing grading of penoscrotal transposition cranial. (**a**). mild to (**n**). most severe

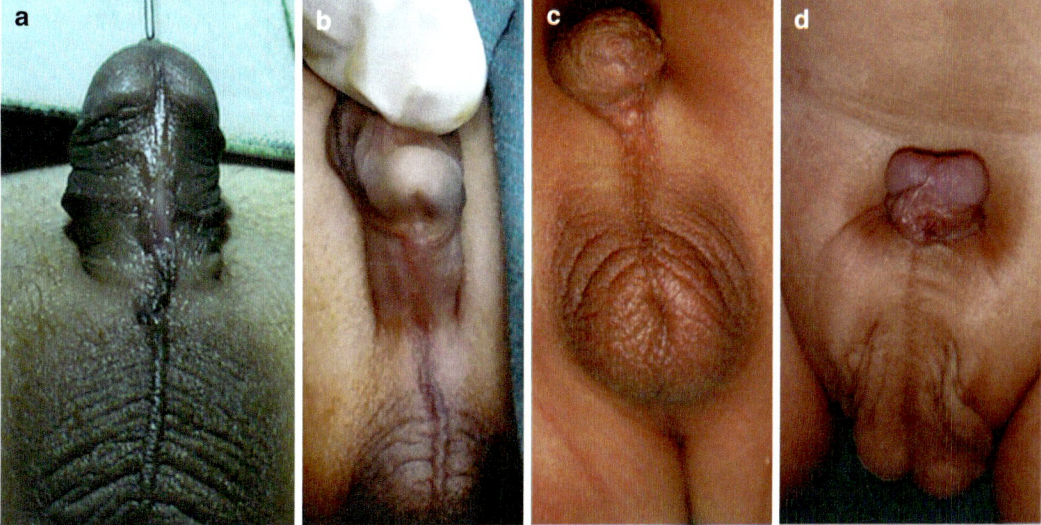

Fig. 24.3 Grading of penoscrotal transposition caudal

24.7 Management

The management of penoscrotal transposition may be divided into.

24.7.1 I. Surgery for Penoscrotal Web

Simple minor degree (Grade 1&2) of penile webbing may not require surgery. But severe and complex penoscrotal webbing may require surgery. Unfortunately, there is no uniform opinion and universal consensus on the timing of surgery. Still, it is crucial to perform reconstructive surgery for penoscrotal web before achieving gender identity, so surgery is recommended at the same age as hypospadias repair (6–18 months).

Surgical approach: The surgical correction objective is to reconstruct a normal-looking scrotum with an adequate penoscrotal angle in a single or two stage, depending on the severity. Various scrotoplasty to achieve these goals are:

Heineke–Mikulicz principle: A transverse incision is made centred at the expected penoscrotal angle. The horizontal incision must not be extended too laterally as it may cause a resultant narrowing at the base of the penis. Then the skin flaps are sutured a two-layer vertically, closing the defect, including subcutaneous sutures before the skin closure.

V-Y Scrotoplasty. The V-Y scrotoplasty technique allows tissues lengthening by an inverted V-shaped flap. The centre of the V should be located at the maximal skin tension on the ventral shaft, and the Y leg—ends at the new penoscrotal angle. Traction sutures and skin hooks are used to facilitate the design and raise of the skin flaps. The created defect is closed by forming a 'Y' configuration in two layers with a deep dermal plication stitch to relieve excess tension.

Z-Scrotoplasty: A vertical incision is given proximal to penoscrotal junction, and two wings of the Z are created, having the parallel angles 60 degrees on the proximal and distal ends of the incision. The two flaps created by these three incisions are approximated in such a way as to elongate the coverage over the ventral shaft and to create the penoscrotal angle. All three incisions lengths should be equal to avoid asymmetry from twisting penile skin. Wide based flaps are developed to maintain the blood supply of the flap and prevent flap necrosis. Multiple Z-plasty incisions may be needed sequentially to augment the repair in severe cases, and excess skin of the flaps raised may be resected along the median raphe.

Hanna and Bonitz [11] reported the results of these three techniques in different grades of the non-circumcised webbed penis with acceptable results. The complications rates were 5.3% in the Heineke–Mikulicz scrotoplasty, 7.8% in the V-Y technique, and 2.9% in Z-plasty patients while Negm and Nagla 2020 [12] had a complication rate of 4.54% in Heineke–Mikulicz patients and 11.1% in multiple Z-plasty. Another technique was described by Chen et al. [13] for webbed penis correction in adults using a longitudinal median incision and the separation of the scrotal and ventral penile dartos with longitudinal closure. However, the technique has a limitation in that it only corrects the web at the dartos fascia level, so it does not resolve the problem if there is deficient ventral skin.

24.7.2 II. Management of Penoscrotal Transposition (PST)

The management should start with a multidisciplinary approach taking care of other associated anomalies and parents' involvement in the treatment plan. Early treatment is ideal for preventing the psychological trauma to the child and parents, but this should not be done at the cost of evading through evaluation protocol. Patients with severe penoscrotal transposition should be evaluated for other associated VACTERL anomalies. A staged repair is often needed if the pathology is associated with hypospadias or other anorectal malformations. Objectives in complete PST management are locating the penis in normal position, chordee correction, urethroplasty, glanuloplasty, and scrotoplasty. There may not be hypospadias in the severe form of penoscrotal transposition, but the urethra is usually short, so these patients also require urethroplasty with scrotal correction transposition. Repair may be staged or can be done in a single stage, provided the goals mentioned above are achieved. The repair may be staged in two or three in perineal hypospadias and bifid scrotum cases. Orthoplasty is done in the first stage, followed by urethroplasty or scrotoplasty in the second, and scrotoplasty or urethroplasty in the third stage. In two-stage orthoplasty and/or scrotoplasty in the first stage, and urethroplasty glanuloplasty and scrotoplasty in the second stage. The principle to be followed in all types of scrotoplasty is to preserve the blood supply and lymphatics of the penis to prevent complications like penile skin necrosis and lymphoedema.

24.8 Surgical technique:

The common surgical method includes rotating two scrotal flaps, joining them in the midline, and vertical skin closure. Other complex surgical procedures require reorienting the scrotum inferiorly with limited rotation flaps, inguinal based groin flaps, and transposition of the penis superiorly in a planned two-stage approach. The urethroplasty and transposition of the scrotum can be done along with the Koyanagi procedure and tubularized incised plate urethroplasty in a single-stage procedure. The two-stage repair is preferred in severe proximal hypospadias with penoscrotal transposition due to its lower complication rates. Prior reconstruction of transposition may give more satisfying results since the scrotum is placed in its proper anatomical position before urethroplasty. The penile shaft also becomes more prominent with an acceptable appearance cosmetically that, in turn, affects the outcome after hypospadias surgery. Sometimes the dimpling of the skin in the midline of the scrotum may occur, resulting in suboptimal aesthetic results.

24.8.1 Modified Glenn–Anderson Technique

The incisions are given around the root of the penis on both sides to elevate the two halves of the rotational scrotal flaps keeping the dorsal penile skin connected to the mons pubis skin. It is ensured that the designed incisions do not meet in the midline, leaving a bridge of skin about 5–10 mm separating the two incisions and connecting the penile skin to the skin of mons pubis (Fig. 24.4a). No circular incision is given around the root of the penis as in other techniques, and penile skin remains connected and drained to the mons pubis skin. Dartos based two scrotal wings are thus created, mobilizing the flaps. The scrotal raphe is incised along approximately half its length, leaving the mobilized urethra entirely free. Tubularized incised plate urethroplasty/flap procedure is done for hypospadias (Fig. 24.4b). It is ensured to have a complete mobilization and fixation of the testes in all cases. The two scrotal wings are rotated inferior-medially and sutured with 4–0 absorbable sutures (Fig. 24.4c, d). A complete closure of the scrotum in layers, shows almost normal appearing scrotum (Fig. 24.4e).

The technique can be used even in two-stage urethroplasty. An inverted U-shaped incision is given, and skin is mobilized to prepare the midline skin urethral plate (Fig. 24.5a, b, c). The tubularization of the urethral plate is done to reconstruct the neourethra and then covered with dartos fascia. Scrotal flaps are raised sparing dorsal midline penile skin (Fig. 24.5d) and penile skin flaps are sutured together to complete the scrotoplasty, and penile skin closure is done (Fig. 24.5e, f). Continuity of the dorsal penile skin is maintained with the suprapubic skin to prevent oedema (Fig. 24.5f).

24.8.2 Single-stage Correction of Hypospadias and Scrotoplasty

Scrotoplasty is feasible with hypospadias repair in a single stage. Hypospadias repair is decided according to the hypospadias type, severity of the curvature, urethral plate, spongiosum development, and the urethral plate's width. The penoscrotal defect may be incomplete in penoscrotal and scrotal hypospadias and complete in perineal hypospadias (Figs. 24.6a and 24.8a). Scrotoplasty can be done after tubularized urethral plate urethroplasty in scrotal and perineal hypospadias and the penoscrotal defect. And in the skin

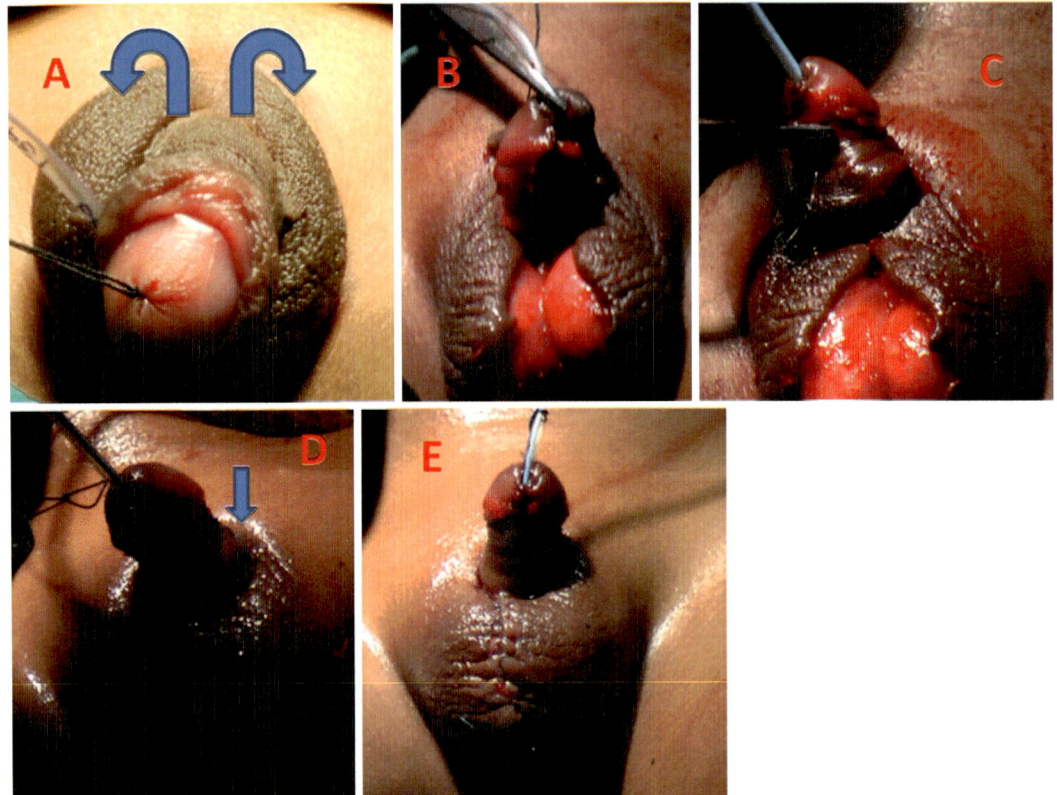

Fig. 24.4 Scrotoplasty in penoscrotal hypospadias. (**a**) Penoscrotal hypospadias lines showing the incision leaving midline skin attached to the penile shaft for raising the scrotal flaps; (**b**) Inner preputial flap urethroplasty completed; (**c**) Glanuloplasty and penile skin closure; and (**d** and **e**). Scrotoplasty completed and an arrow showing the continuity skin to the penile shaft

flap urethroplasty, penile degloving is done, and curvature is corrected (Fig. 24.6b, c). The inner preputial flap is marked with stay sutures, and the flap is mobilized (Fig. 24.6d, e). The inner preputial flap is tubularized to reconstruct the neourethra (Figs. 24.6f and 24.8b, c). Then the urethroplasty and glanuloplasty are done (Fig. 24.7a). After urethral plate tubularization with spongioplasty in TIPU and neourethral reconstruction in flap urethroplasty, scrotal wings are raised, and midline skin over the scrotum is excised. Both scrotal sacs are sutured in the midline to create the midline septum. Then skin closure is done starting from the perineum to the penoscrotal junction. The final reconstructed scrotum shows an almost normal appearance (Fig. 24.7b). Scrotoplasty is feasible even in perineal and perineoscrotal hypospadias (Fig. 24.8a–d). Scrotoplasty should be done in incised plate tubularized urethroplasty in scrotal or perineoscrotal hypospadias. Prepucioplasty can also be done with scrotoplasty in such cases (Fig. 24.9a, b). A partial or complete penoscrotal defect may often be seen in mid-penile hypospadias and proximal penile hypospadias. Scrotoplasty is feasible in single-stage flap urethroplasty in such cases (Fig. 24.10a, b).

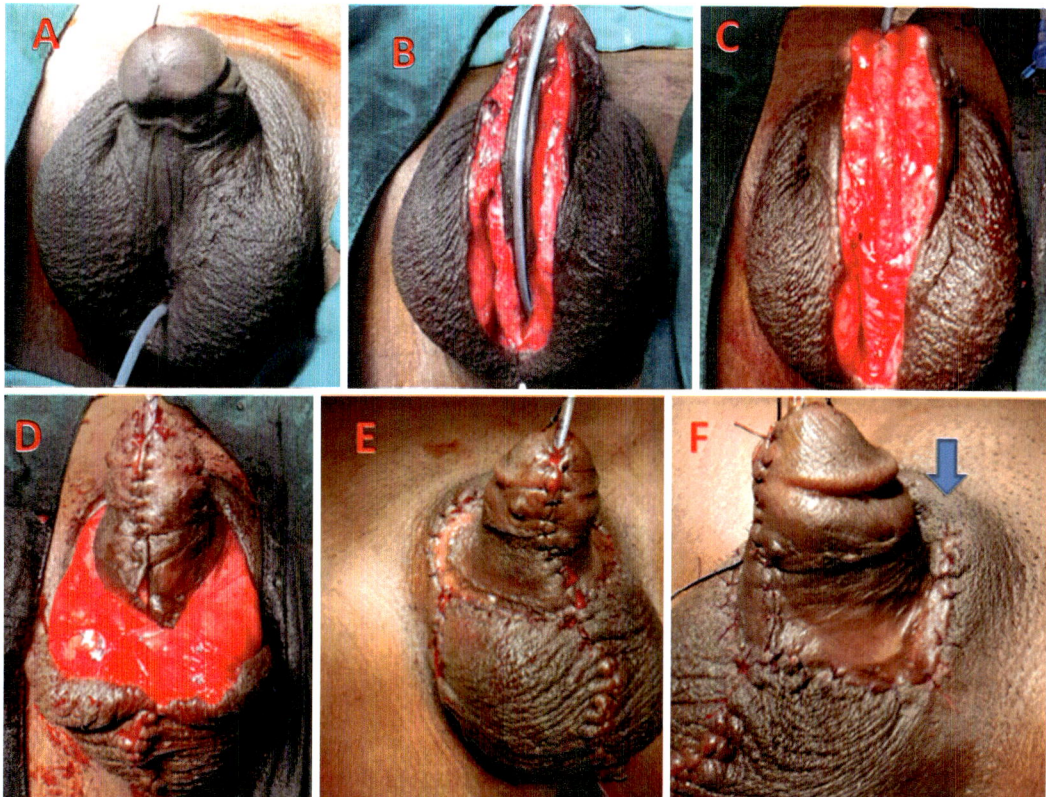

Fig. 24.5 Showing scrotoplasty in second-stage urethroplasty. (**a**). Perineoscrotal meatus. (**b** & **c**). Tubularization of the midline skin urethral plate. (**d**). Mobilization of the scrotal flaps. (**e** & **f**) Completed Scrotoplasty with arrow continuity of dorsal penile skin

24.9 Discussion

An ideal approach for proximal hypospadias and bifid scrotum still remains to be decided. Commonly such complex, severe cases are treated in a multistage repair. A few techniques are described in the literature for two-stage repair. The objective of managing penoscrotal transposition with hypospadias or de-novo is creating phallus in the normal position with the urethra at the tip of the glans. The aim of the techniques and their various modifications are to preserve the blood and lymphatics supply of the penis and closure of scrotum cosmetically in the midline. Surgical management has come a long way. Though Broman described the first case of penoscrotal transposition in 1911, details of the case were not mentioned. Appleby published the first detailed description of it in 1923 [14]. Initial repairs were based on creating scrotal-based rotational flaps. Mcilvoy and Harris [15] first performed surgery for scrotal transposition and moved the penis in more cranial position by creating a subcutaneous tunnel. This was followed by an era of scrotal-based flaps popularized by Forshall and Rickham [16], wherein scrotal flaps

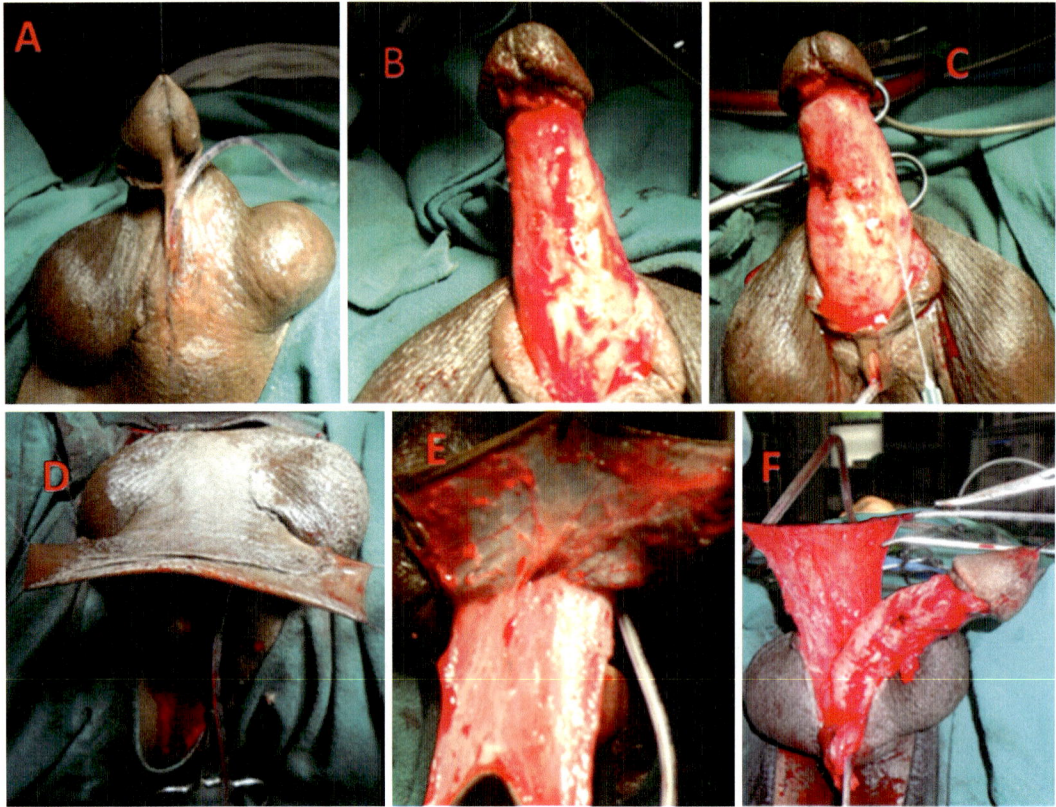

Fig. 24.6 (**a**–**f**) Scrotoplasty in scrotal hypospadias with bifid scrotum. (**a**) Scrotal hypospadias with bifid scrotum; (**b**) Degloving giving circumferential circumcoronal incision; (**c**) Complete correction of chordee on Gittes test; (**d, e**). Raising of the inner preputial flap; (**f**). Tubularized inner preputial flap to reconstruct the neourethra

are moved medially and caudally. Glenn and Anderson also used the same method. Dresner [17] later modified the technique in 1982 and is common in practice as modified Glenn and Anderson technique. Kolligian et al. [18] corrected it by transferring the penis after creating a buttonhole in the skin of the pubic area. However, the cosmetic results were suboptimal, as this correction was associated with chordee due to the non-releasing of soft tissue bands. Of late, based on the principle of preserving blood supply, various types of repairs based on release incisions have been in vogue like M-plasty or W-plasty with acceptable results in different reported case series. When associated with hypospadias, as seen in many patients, a tubularized urethral plate urethroplasty is the most common repair done in a single stage or sometimes in two stages. Lately, Bhat et al. [19] reported single-stage urethroplasty in both flap and TIPU with scrotoplasty in severe hypospadias. Koyanagi [20] repair has been another option in these patients with associ-

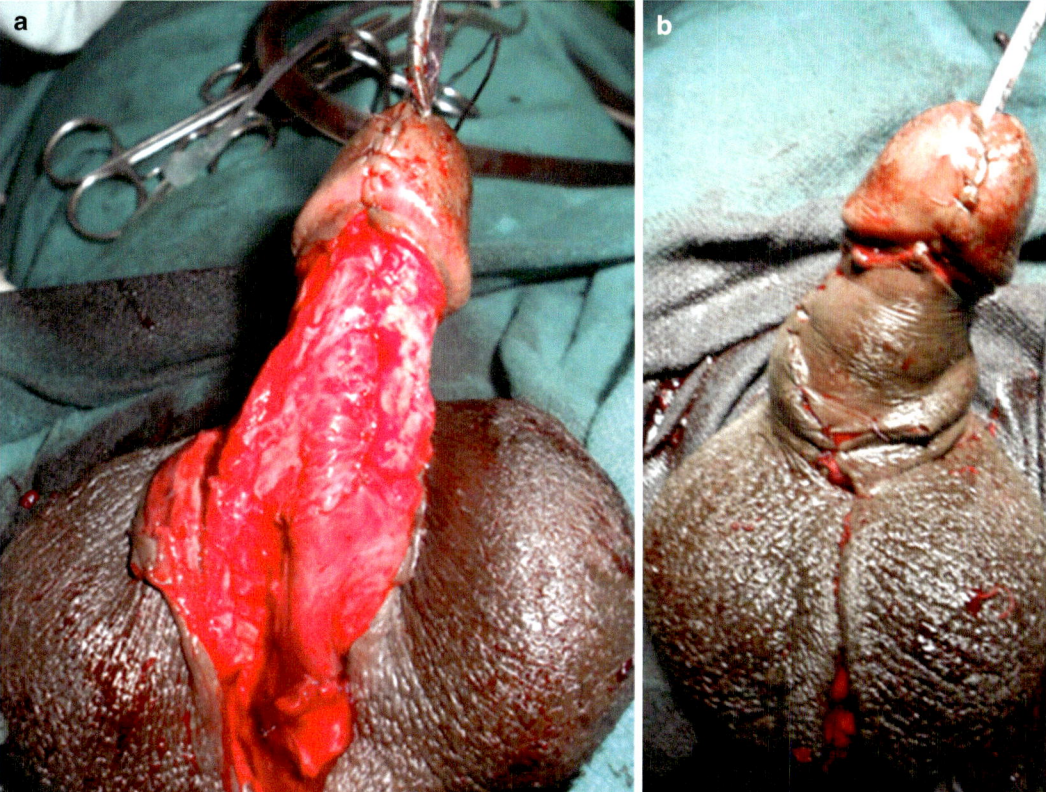

Fig. 24.7 (**a, b**) Urethroplasty and scrotoplasty

ated hypospadias. The modifications in scrotal skin closure are Z-plasty, multiple Z-plasties, V-Y-based rotational flaps, and Singapore flap repairs. Bladder mucosa or buccal mucosa has also been used during urethroplasty with satisfying results. Z-plasty involves creating two triangular flaps of equal dimensions created using an angle of 60 degrees which theoretically can lengthen a contracted scar by about 75%. These flaps are transposed to improve the functional and cosmetic appearance of scars.

Lately, pudendal-based thigh flap repairs have been used in cases with deficient penile skin and tethering of penile skin with quite satisfying cosmetic and functional results.

Complications after surgery include urethral fistula, flap necrosis, penile oedema, and rarely a testicular injury. Though Glenn–Anderson [21] popularized the circular incision at the root of the penis, it is likely to compromise lymphatic drainage leading to lymphoedema partially. In addition, the patient's transposition correction by the Glenn–Anderson technique witnessed gross oedema that persists for long periods. Even after resolution it leaves the penile skin dusky and darkly pigmented scrotal skin.

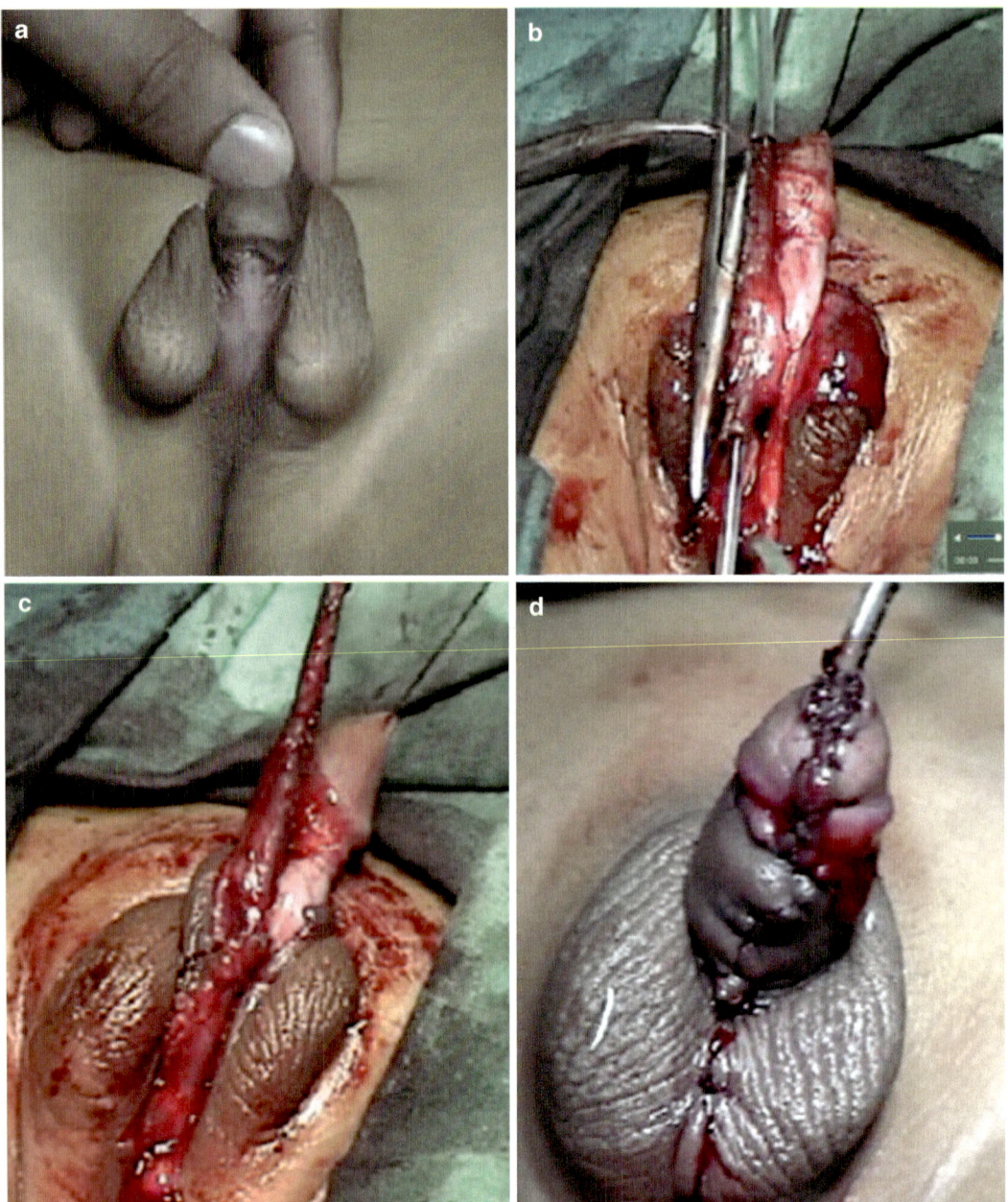

Fig. 24.8 Scrotoplasty in perineoscrotal hypospadias with bifid scrotum. (**a**) Perineoscrotal hypospadias with bifid scrotum; (**b** & **c**) Tubularized inner preputial flap to reconstruct the neourethra. (**d**). Scrotoplasty

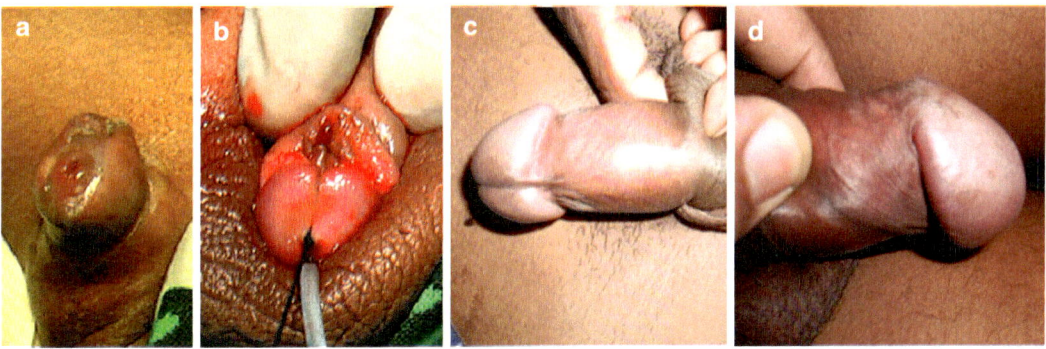

Fig. 25.1 Dorsal and ventral frenulum. (**a**). Dorsal prepucial hood with bifurcation, (**b**). Dorsal frenulum, (**c**). Ventral frenulum and (**d**) Dorsal prepuce in adult

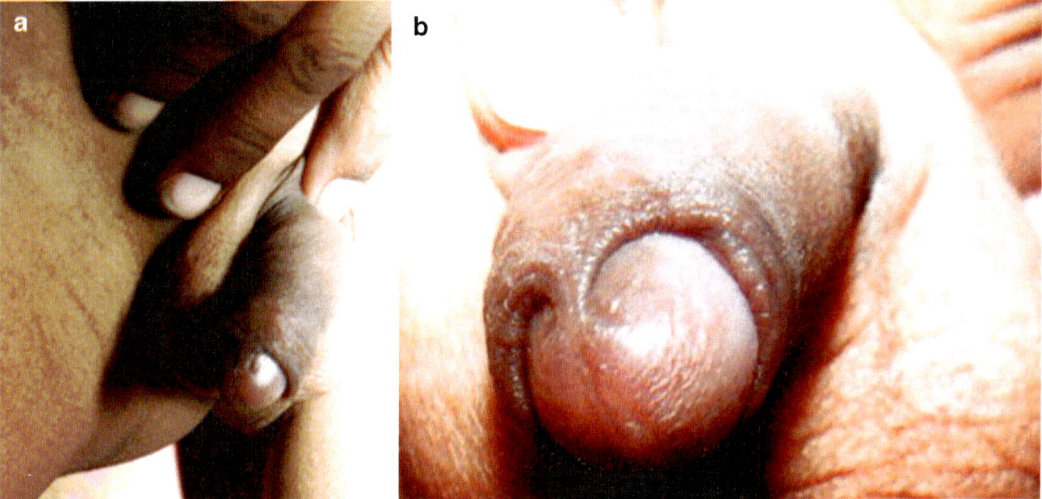

Fig. 25.2 (a & b) Well-formed tight dorsal frenulum attached to mid-glans

median raphe shows the site of bifurcation of spongiosum and length of the hypoplastic urethra (Fig. 25.4a & b).

25.5 Hooded Foreskin or Prepuce

The terminology of the hooded foreskin is used where the foreskin of a boy is wide open. It is the mildest form of hypospadias and is mainly a cosmetic defect. This is also called hooded prepuce without hypospadias (Fig. 25.5), but in a real sense, it is the hooded prepuce with glanular hypospadias. Usually, the disfigurement of the penis in the baby is noted at birth. Still, sometimes it may be diagnosed in elder boys or even routine medical examinations at service entry or during examination for other reasons.

Treatment options for hooded foreskin are:

1. No intervention: As the condition is of cosmetic concern only, it may be left as such in childhood. This will allow the child to decide if he wants treatment for the hooded foreskin at adulthood. The downside is that if he decides that he wants surgery when he is older, the operation will take more out of him.
2. Prepucioplasty: Penile disfigurement is not acceptable in modern-day hypospadiology. Foreskin reconstruction creates an aestheti-

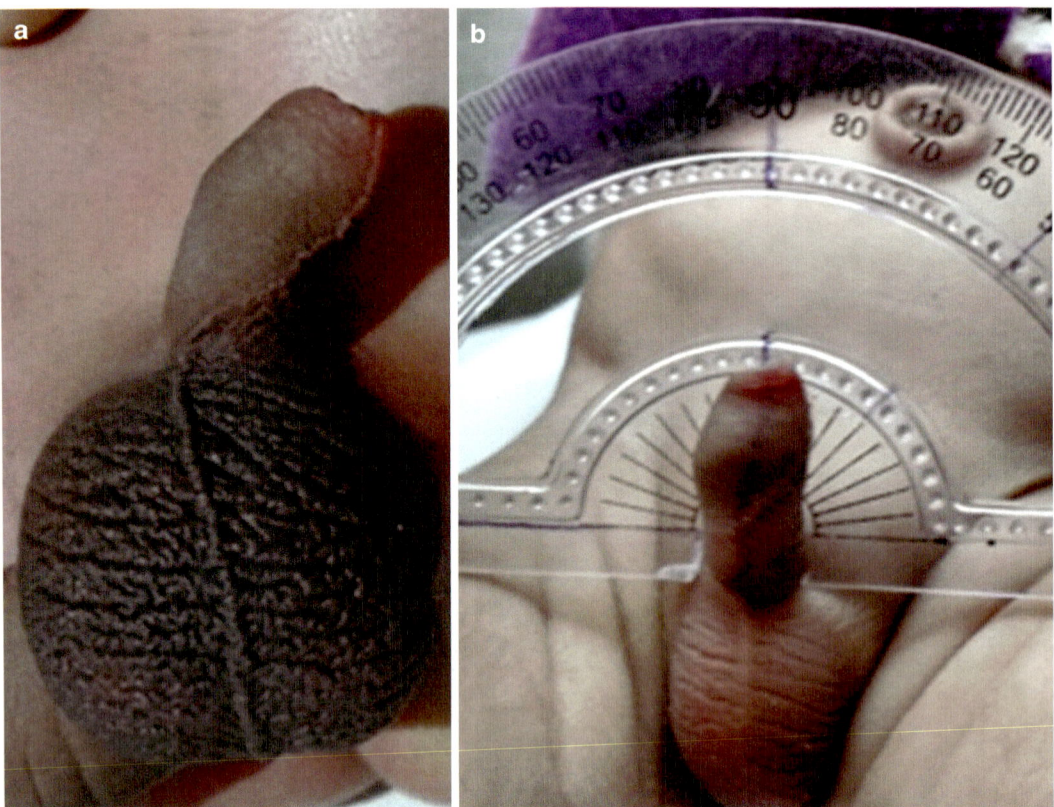

Fig. 25.3 Median raphe. (**a**). Deviance of median raphe towards left, (**b**). measuring the degree of torsion by at the point of ending median raphe on prepuce

cally normal penis and gives the chance to decide for circumcision later in life. The technique of prepucioplasty is the same as in cases of hypospadias.

3. Complete circumcision: If chosen by the parents, the circumcision is a simple daycare surgery. The choice technique for circumcision in infants with preputial defects remains uncertain and usually is performed by conventional dissection technique. It can still be done with the Plastibell method based on the usual manner or with minor modification. The disadvantage with the Plastibell approach is the incomplete coverage of bell by foreskin but does not alter the results. However, there is a theoretical risk of urethral injury if the ventral shaft skin is manipulated. The corpus spongiosum is not well developed, and the urethra may be close to the skin. There are more chances of injury with this technique if a patient has a chordee. So the Plastibell is only safe in a child with hooded prepuce without hypospadias or mild hypospadias if chordee has been ruled out. This technique is the choice of circumcision in infants and children if parents prefer their son to be circumcised without glanuloplasty.

25.6 Classification of the Prepuce in Hypospadias

The dorsal hood is the incompletely developed prepuce in hypospadias. Morphology of prepuce can have an impact on hypospadias repair. There are different types of prepuce with a difference in

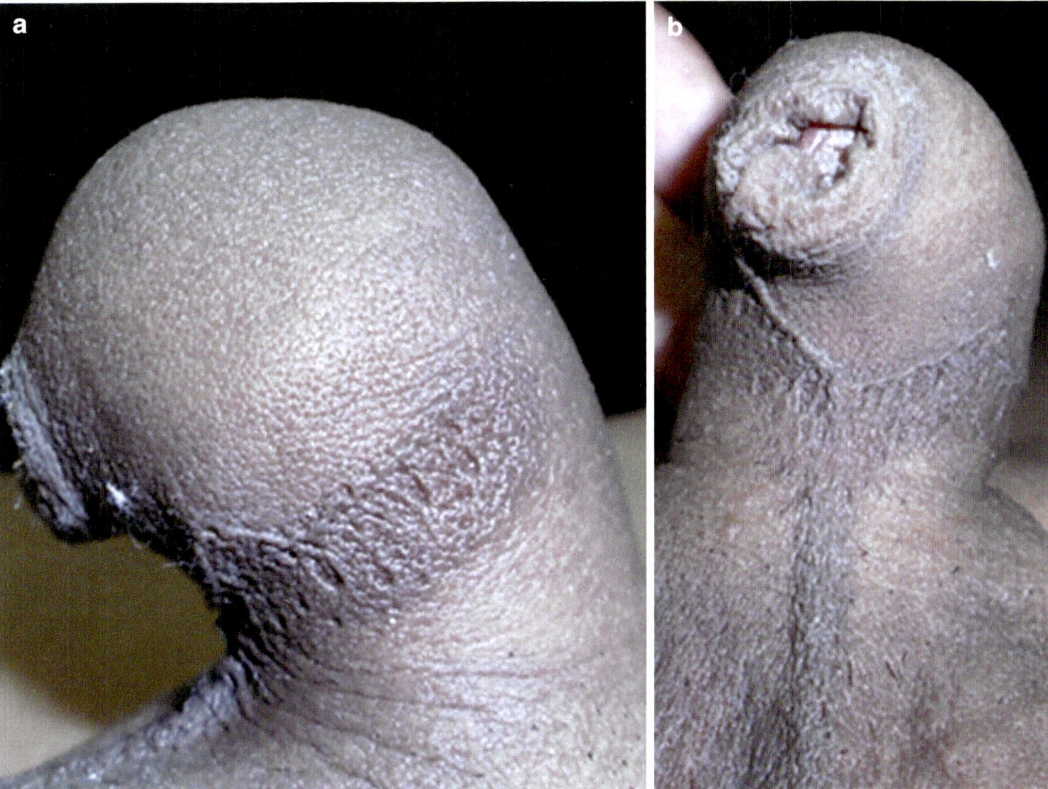

Fig. 25.4 (a & b) Intact prepuce with the deviance of median raphe starting point embryological abnormality

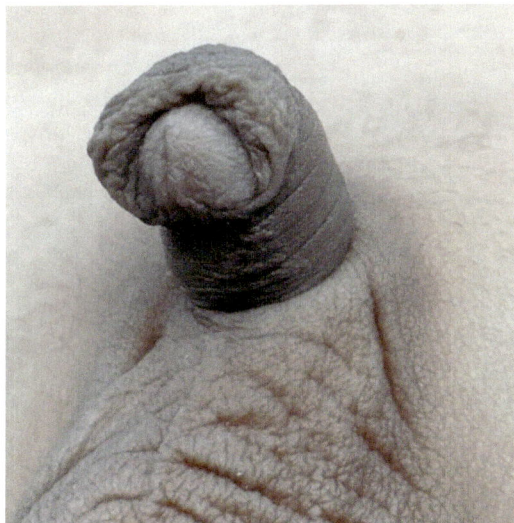

Fig. 25.5 Typical appearance of a hooded foreskin

the pattern of blood supply of the prepuce [3]. Based on length, the prepuce is divided into (Fig. 25.6):

1. Very small.
2. Small.
3. Adequate.
4. Normal length.
5. Normal prepuce.

25.7 Morphology of Prepuce in Hypospadias

The prepuce is usually utilized for the neourethra and penile body skin reconstruction in severe hypospadias, but where prepuce can be spared, it is used for prepucioplasty. There is a definite

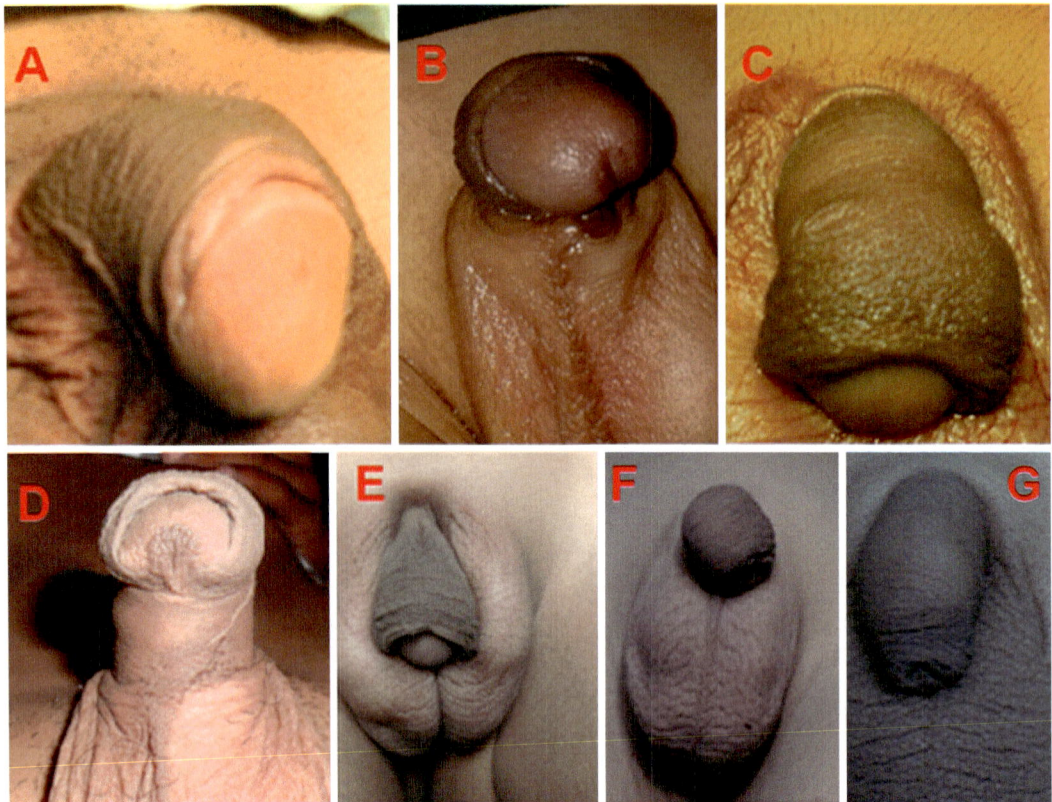

Fig. 25.6 Various sizes of the prepuce. (**a** & **b**). Small prepuce, (**c**). Adequate, (**d**). Collar-scarf. (**e**). Normal length, (**f** & **g**). Normal prepuce

correlation between the morphological and vascularization types of prepuces. Therefore, the morphological types may be a guide to see the preputial skin's adequacy for the longitudinal island flap and prepucioplasty. Furthermore, the morphology of the prepuce and correlated vascular pattern helps us to predict complications and, thus, to select the best operative technique of 1- or 2-stage surgery.

Based on the morphology and abnormalities of the prepuce in hypospadias are classified as.

A. "Monk's hood" or "1 humped": There is an area raised on the dorsal called hump, and this may range from being flat to big hump. A typical hypospadiac prepuce is shaped like a hood or hump. This deformity is the result of ventrodorsal disproportion. Depending on the connection between the prepuce ridges during embryogenesis, one (Fig. 25.7a–f) or two humps (Fig. 25.8a–f) appear on the prepuce. This may be seen distal at the site over the glans (Fig. 25.7a–c) and proximal to the corona (Fig. 25.7d–f). The location of the hump gives a clue of the severity of hypospadias as this is the site of starting of the embryological abnormality, and a large hump (as shown in Fig. 25.7f) may give problem in skin closure if we resect the hump and disfigurement if we keep the hump. The hump may be small or large, and patients with a large hump (Fig. 25.7e & f) may not be suitable for prepucioplasty.

B. "Cobra eyes" or Two humps: This is more common in distal hypospadias. These again can be divided into distal seen in distal hypospadias (Fig. 25.8a–c) and proximal in severe hypospadias (Fig. 25.8d–f). Site of the hump is directly correlated with the severity of hypospadias (Fig. 25.9a & b). Double Bull prepuce may also be present in chordee without hypospadias with

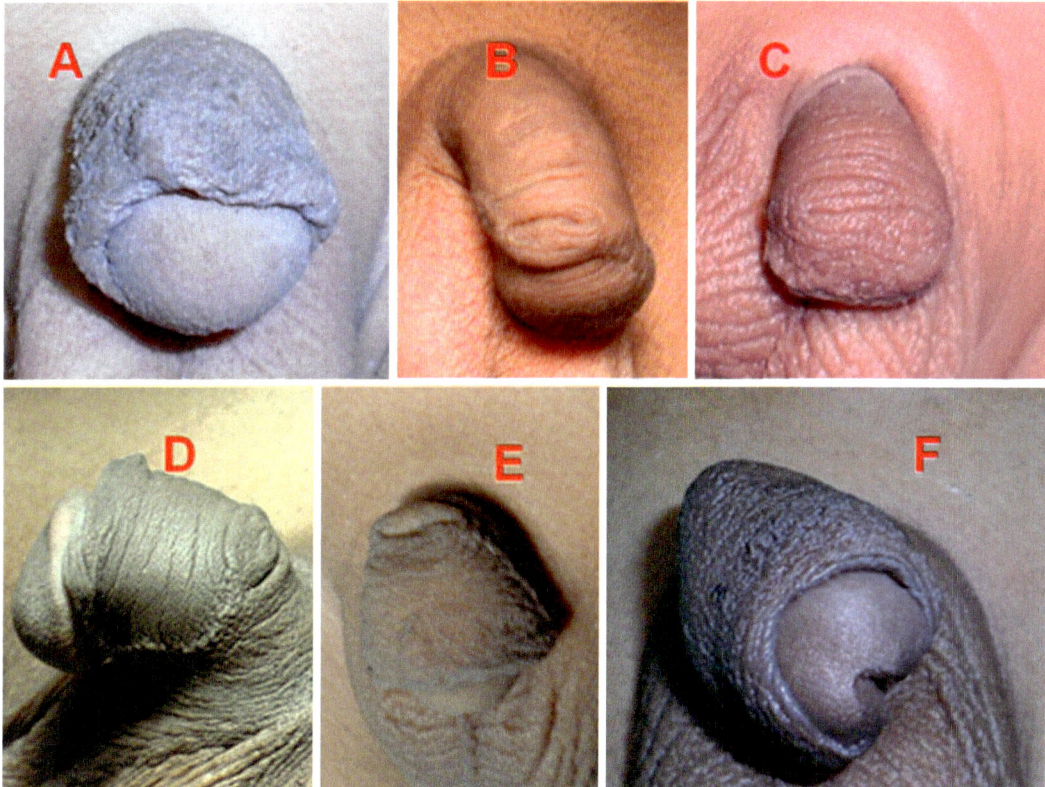

Fig. 25.7 Monks hood/single hood. (**a, b** & **c**). Distal one distal hypospadias, (**d, e** & **f**). Proximal one with severe hypospadias

intact prepuce (Fig. 25.6f). Patients with big humps may not be suitable for preputioplasty as Bull's eye may be seen on prepuce postoperatively, leading to disfigurement (Fig. 25.10a & b).

C. Triple Hump: This anomaly is very rare, not reported in the literature. The embryology of this is not known. There are three humps, two on the distal shaft and the third is seen at the margin of the prepuce (Fig. 25.11). Prepucioplasty in such cases is not feasible, but since the hump has an adequate blood supply of inner prepuce, these cases are suitable for inner prepucial flap urethroplasty; otherwise, they need circumcision for cosmesis.

D. "Flat" and E-"V"-shaped: The flat and V-shaped (Fig. 25.6e) prepuces often occur in severe hypospadias. This results from a higher degree of ventral hypoplasia and arrests the development of the prepuce. The V-shaped prepuce is usually present with penoscrotal transposition. Prepucioplasty is not feasible in these cases, and hypospadias surgery is even more complicated because the underdeveloped preputium is not appropriate to correct the ventral deficiency. In addition, there may be difficulty in covering the ventral surface skin. Therefore, in such patients, two-stage hypospadias repair is a better choice.

F. "Collar-scarf": Such a prepuce resembles a collar with an adequate size (Fig. 25.6d) and is commonly seen in distal hypospadias. The collar-scarf prepuce has a close connection on the ventral side with pillars of the hypoplastic corpus spongiosum at the open glans base. These prepuces are best suited for prepucioplasty. Prepucial hood is adequate, and margins can easily be approximated to create a frenulum and sizeable prepucial orifice. Care is taken while raising the glanular and prepucial flap not to injure the inner

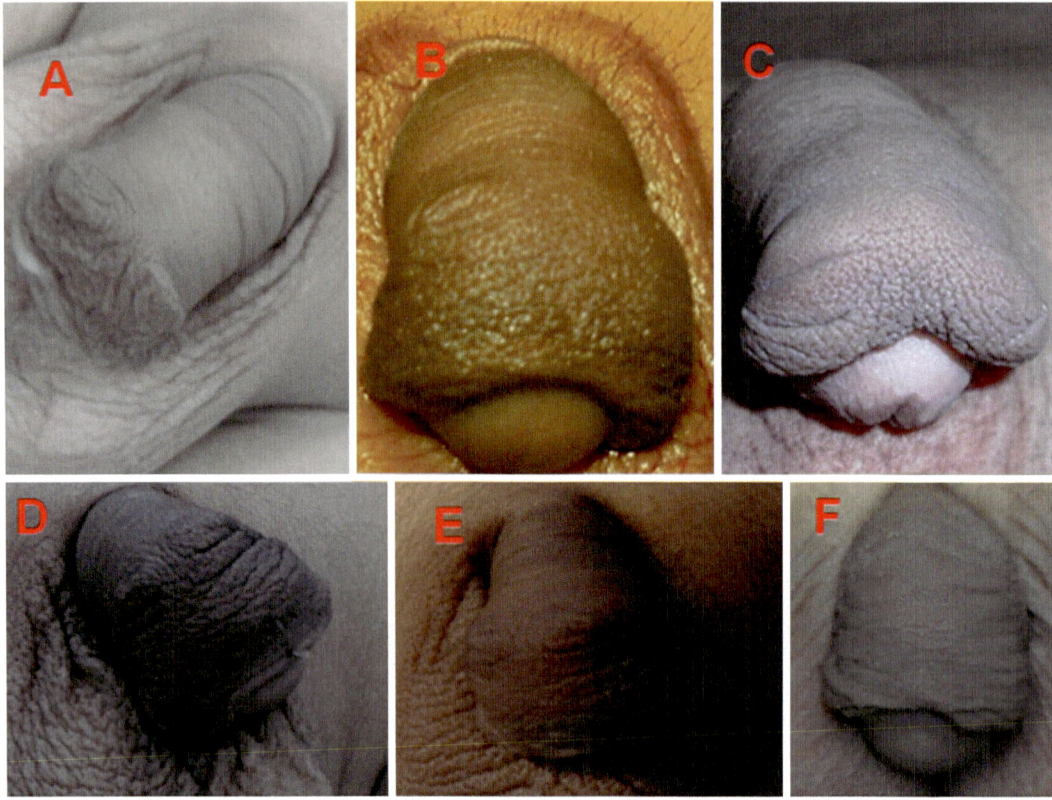

Fig. 25.8 (**a, b**, & **c**). Cobra eyes or double hump with distal hypospadias, (**d, e** & **f**). Showing hump with proximal hypospadias

prepucial skin. Operative preparation of this structure is difficult and may result in injury and defect of the ventral part of the internal preputial skin, making reconstruction of the sub-glanular part of the penile skin difficult, i.e. formation of the mucosal collar. This type of prepuce is suitable for inner prepucial flap urethroplasty also.

G. "Normal" (intact): The normal prepuce may be found in cases of variants of hypospadias like mega meatus intact prepuce and chordee without hypospadias. Single or double hump be seen on the shaft's dorsal surface, and the site of the hump indicates the severity of chordee without hypospadias (Fig. 25.6f).

Prepuce may be classified based on the vascular pattern of the prepuce

I. One blood vessel is predominant.
II. Two blood vessels are predominant.
III. Numerous blood vessels (≥ 3) are presented (Fig. 25.12).
IV. No dominant blood vessel was presented (e.g. no definite axial vessel displayed a network distribution).

All predominant vessels were axially distributed and then showed a transverse distribution and formed numerous reticular lateral branches at the junction of the inner and outer prepuce. The same pedicle's dominant vessels displayed no noticeable difference in their development, and a majority was symmetrically distributed along the middle line of the pedicle. The prepuce of type 1 with the single prominent vessel and type IV without apparent vessel blood supply of margins of the dorsal hood may be compromised. Hence, these patients may not be suitable for prepucioplasty.

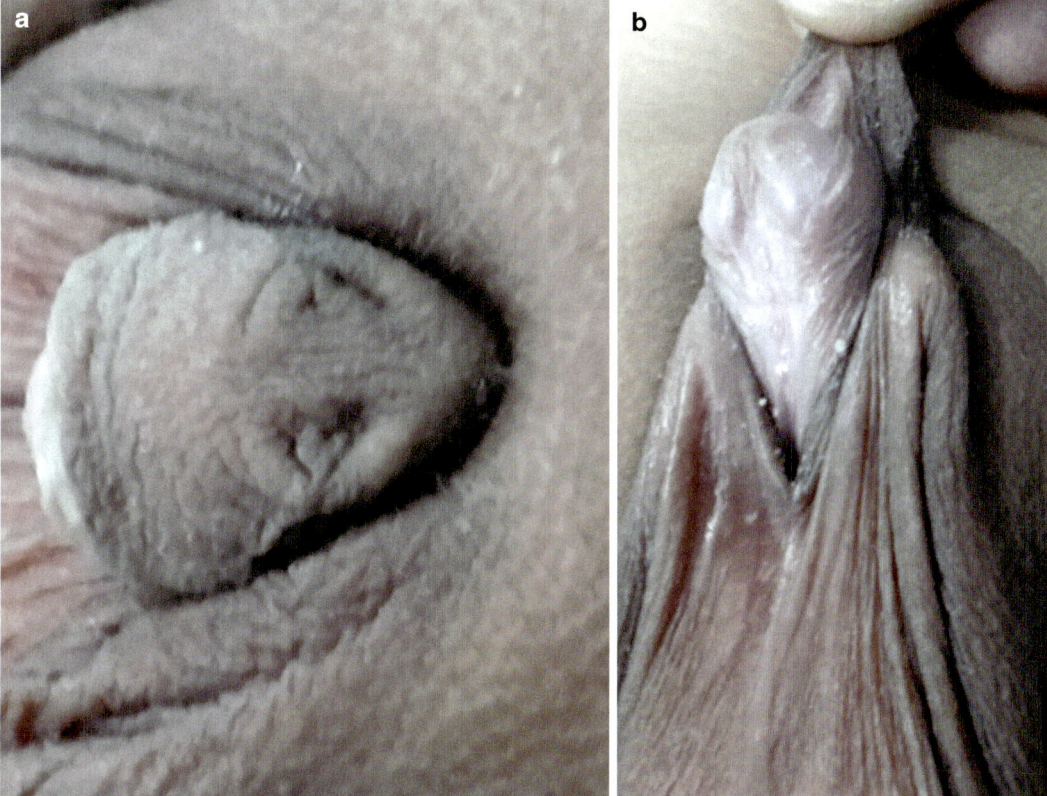

Fig. 25.9 Co-relation of the hump and severity of hypospadias. (**a**). Hump at proximal penile region. (**b**). Penoscrotal hypospadias

25.8 Prepucioplasty in Hypospadias

Hypospadias is one of the most common congenital anomalies, having an incidence of 1 in 300 male newborns [4]. With a common goal to achieve normal or near-normal penile anatomy and good functional outcome, numerous techniques have been described in the literature for hypospadias repair. The most common procedure is TIP (Tubularized Incised Plate) urethroplasty, wherein the prepuce is used as a dorsal dartos cover to form a waterproof covering over the neourethra. This results in a circumcised penis [5, 6]. But in recent times, circumcision has become less acceptable to both the parents/patients and the treating physician. Hence, the number of prepucioplasty has increased significantly, along with hypospadias repair. The prepuce can be preserved when spongioplasty is done adequately, and ventral/scrotal dartos or tunica vaginalis is used to cover the neourethra.

Initially, the only cases where prepucioplasty was done were distal, coronal or glandular hypospadias without penile curvature and did not require complete penile de-gloving [7]. With the advent of TIP repair, the number of patients undergoing prepucioplasty has increased significantly. It is now being done for both mid and proximal hypospadias with acceptable success. We had a well-formed retractable prepuce with 88.9% satisfaction rate regarding the outcome of surgery and cosmesis in the patients. The incidence of complications was also similar to the complication rate in proximal hypospadias repair cases without preputial reconstruction, i.e. 11.10%.

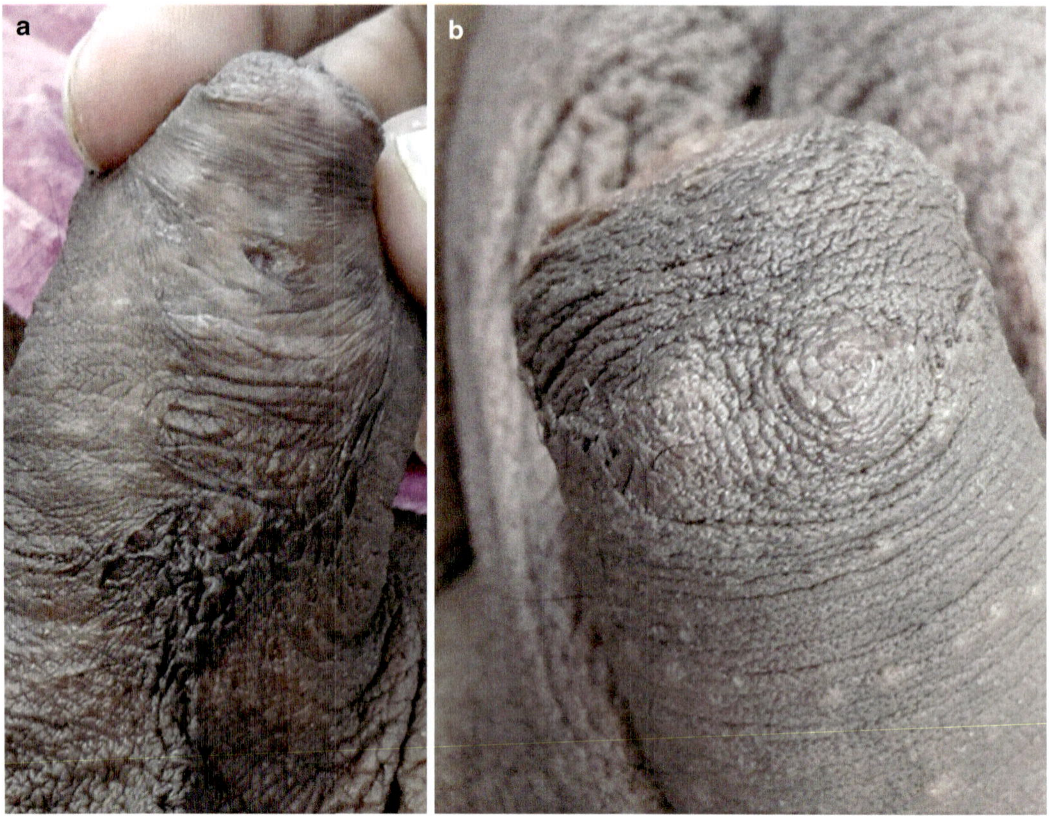

Fig. 25.10 Postoperative disfigurement in patients with prepucioplasty in double Bull prepuce. (**a**). preputial fistula, (**b**). Double Bull's eye deformity

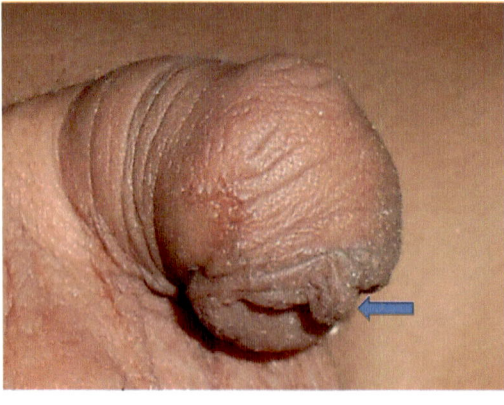

Fig. 25.11 Triple hump two humps on the dorsal surface, an arrow is marking the third hump at the margin of the prepuce

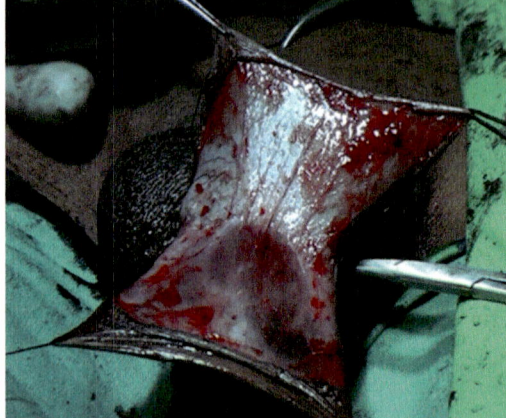

Fig. 25.12 Numerous vessels on the outer prepucial skin

Why Prepucioplasty? The human foreskin is a highly innervated and vascularized sensitive erogenous tissue. It plays a vital role in normal human sexual response and is vital for normal copulatory behaviour [8]. An understanding of this role is now emerging in the scientific literature. Removal of the foreskin (circumcision) may interfere with normal sexual function. In hypospadias management, objectives are positioning the meatus on the tip with a straight penis, normalization of erection and projectile stream in voiding, reconstructing the urethra of adequate and uniform calibre, symmetry in the appearance of glans and shaft and decreasing the complications. The basic principle in managing any congenital anomaly is to restore the normal or near-normal anatomy with the existing tissue or tissue supplementation. Many of the patients/parents want to preserve the prepuce because of their religious sentiments. Prepucial reconstruction gives the child the psychological benefit of feeling equal to his colleagues for the shape of his penis. Thirdly, the foreskin is highly innervated and vascularized and plays a vital role in normal sexual intercourse [8]. The dorsal dartos can be preserved by utilizing spongioplasty as a healthy tissue cover and then covering the neourethra with ventral dartos. Besides, a preserved prepuce can serve as a reserve of tissue if the hypospadias repair is unsuccessful. The preserved prepuce can be utilized in failed hypospadias as onlay flap urethroplasty, flap urethroplasty for stricture urethra and healthy interposing tissue single or double dorsal dartos cover.

25.9 Technqiue of Preputioplasty

25.9.1 Measuring Adequacy of the Prepuce

Preputial reconstruction should be attempted in only those whose prepuce can be approximated in the midline without any tension at the coronal groove level. If the ventral defect is large, reconstruction should not be attempted. There are different techniques to measure the adequacy of the prepuce for prepucioplasty. The ideal one is to measure the glans breadth at corona and midglans (Fig. 25.13), and the prepuce's length and width (Fig. 25.14a & b) with the Vernier callipers then decide to undergo for the prepucioplasty.

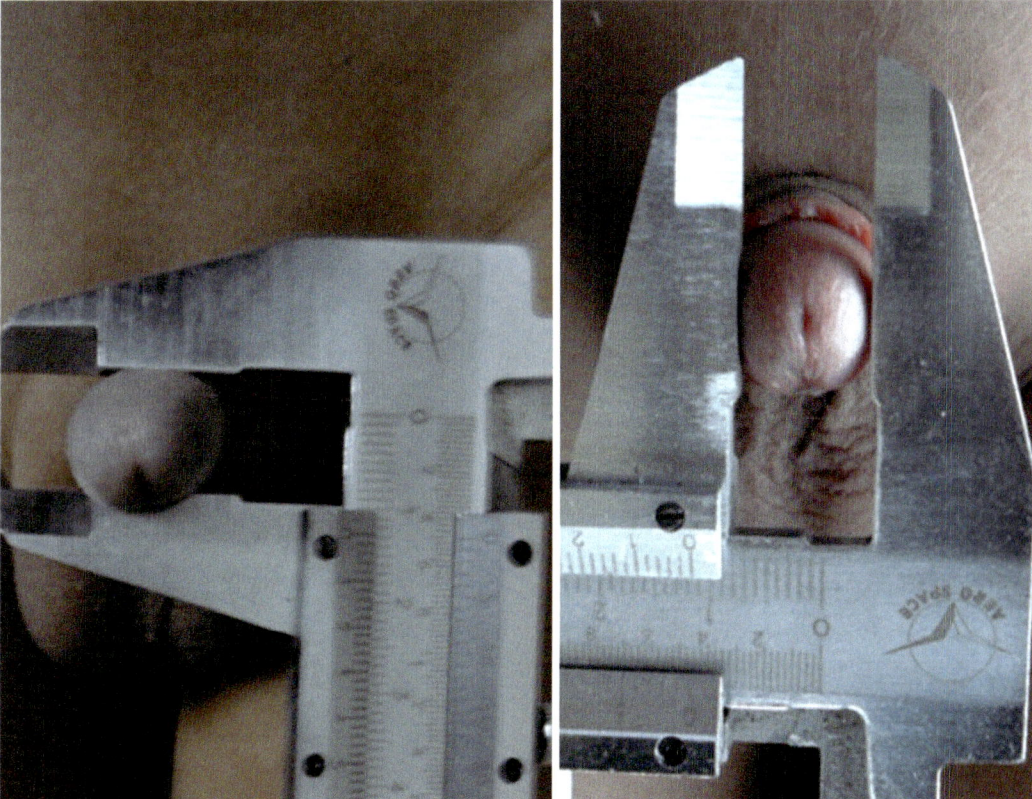

Fig. 25.13 Measuring the width of the glans using Vernier callipers

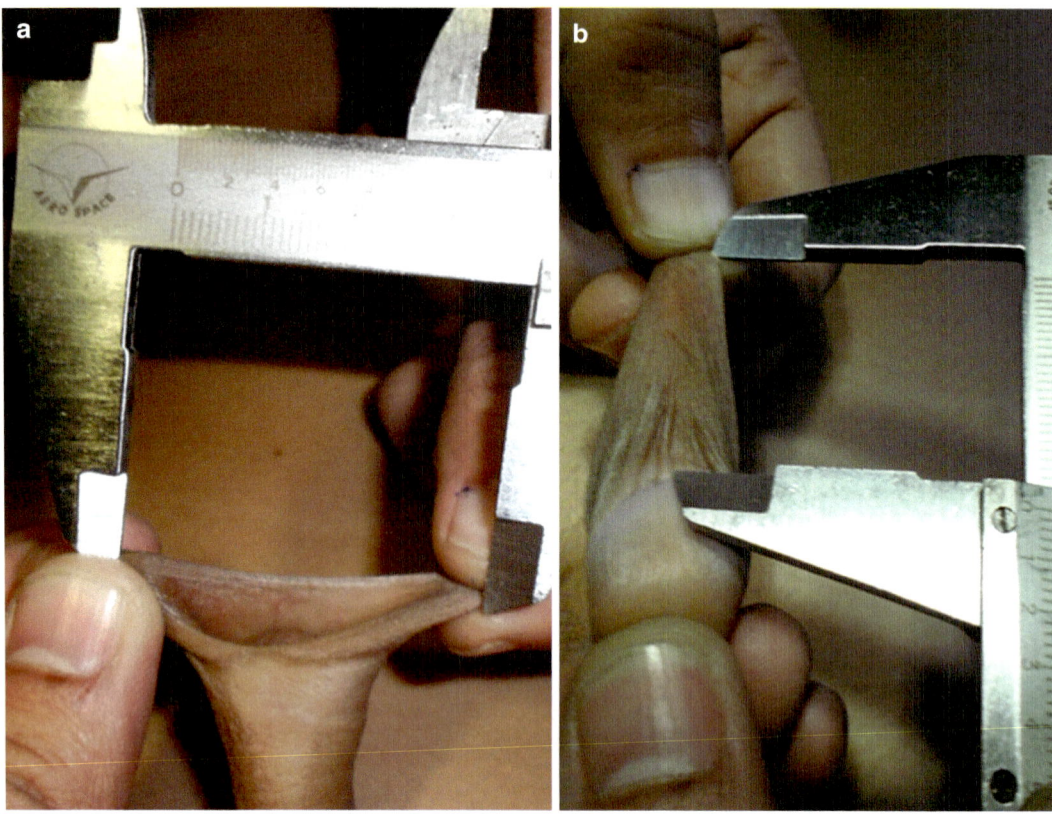

Fig. 25.14 Measuring the prepuce dimensions using Vernier callipers, (**a**). Measuring the width of prepuce. (**b**). Measuring the length of the prepuce

These dimensions also help in the estimation of the distal limit of preputial reconstruction. Though we can measure the exact length, it is cumbersome to measure with the callipers in a child. Other methods are measuring by approximation of edges of the preputial hood with finger and thumb or forceps (Fig. 25.15a & b) and three stay sutures. These are easy methods and can be done on the table before proceeding for prepucioplasty.

25.9.2 Three Stay Suture Techniques

The method to assess prepucial width is by applying three stay sutures, one at the corona level, the distal end of prepucial hood at the junction of inner and outer prepucial skin and the penile shaft skin at the level of corona after completion of the urethroplasty (Figs. 25.16 and 25.17). The second suture preputial skin is pulled over the glans after fixing the inner prepucial skin at the corona by the first stay suture (Fig. 25.17b & c). Then the prepuce is retracted by the third stay suture. When the skin can be pulled over the glans and retracted easily, the prepucial hood is considered adequate. After that, suturing the inner preputial skin between the first and second stay suture will reconstruct the prepuce's frenulum and inner layer; suturing outer prepucial skin between stay suture second and third will reconstruct the outer skin layer of the prepuce.

Surgical Techniques Three-layer closure after three stay suture technique for tissue estimation is the most common technique used for preputial reconstruction. It can be performed in either general or regional anaesthesia. General anaesthesia is preferable as it avoids the difficulty caused by

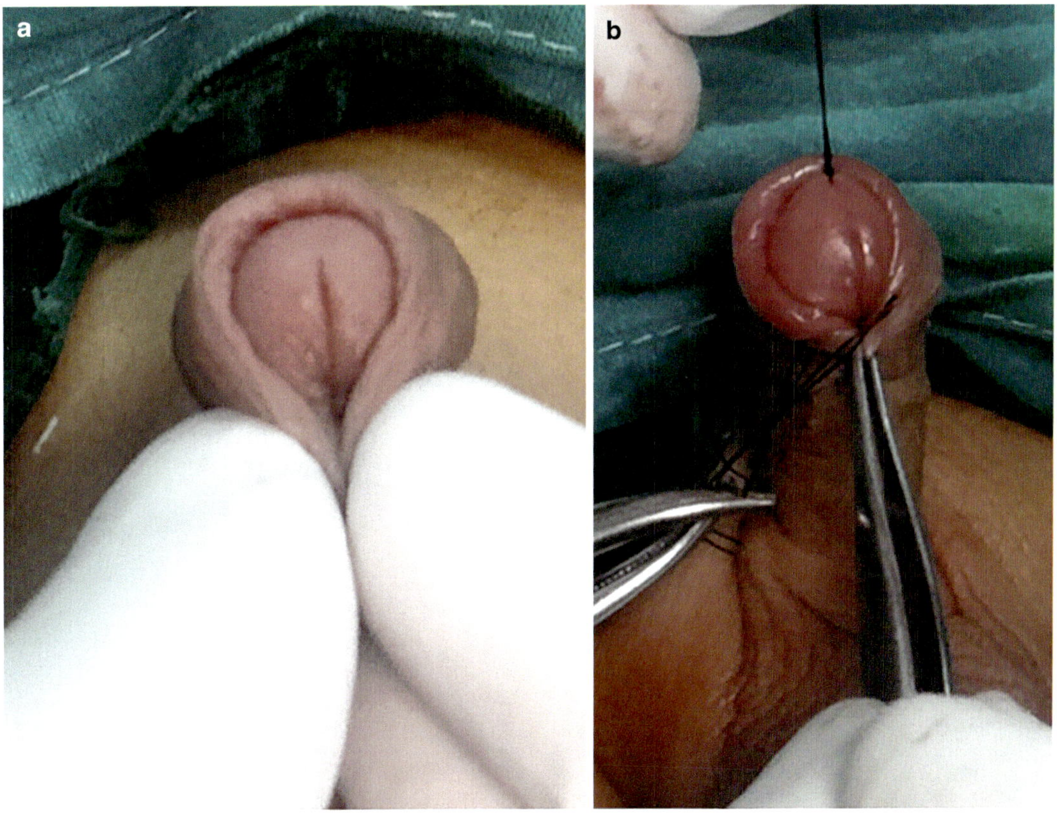

Fig. 25.15 Measurement of skin adequacy for prepucial reconstruction. (**a**). approximation with thumb and finger; (**b**). with forceps

Fig. 25.16 Sketch showing the site of three stay sutures for the three stay suture technique

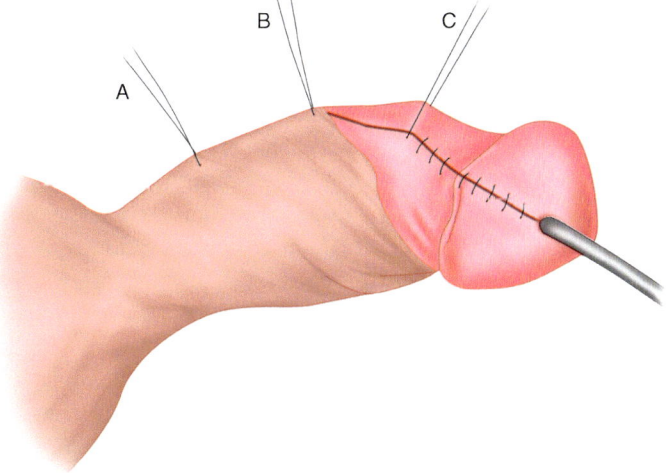

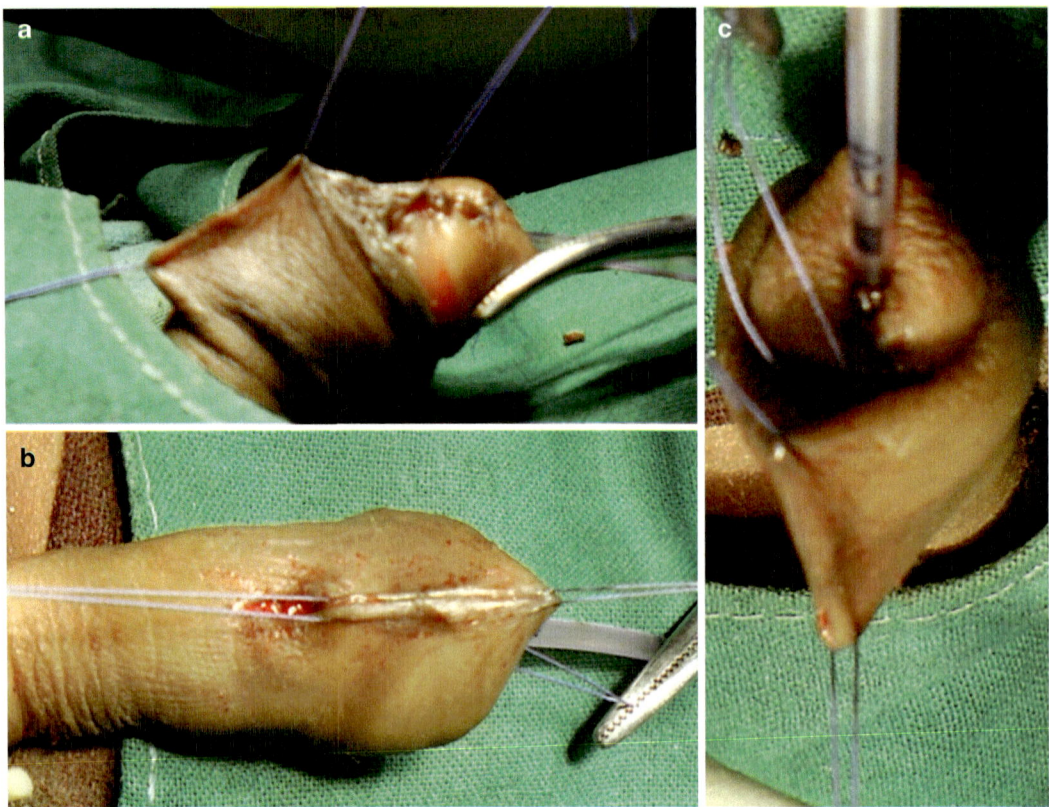

Fig. 25.17 Adequacy of prepuce for prepucioplasty. (**a**). Photograph showing three sites of stay sutures. (**b** & **c**). Middle suture pulled up to see the adequacy of the prepuce

penile engorgement occurring in regional anaesthesia. After injecting 1 in 100,000 solutions of adrenaline at the incision site, a "Y" shaped incision is given encircling the urethral plate (Fig. 25.18a). The incision is continued into the prepuce hood up to the junction of inner and outer prepucial skin (Fig. 25.18b). The next step is partial penile de-gloving (Fig. 25.18c). Those patients with chordee/torque incision are extended circumferentially in the circumcoronal region and complete penile de-gloving (Fig. 25.19a & b).

The prepuce is reconstructed after the neourethra is created by tubularization of the urethral plate and spongioplasty (Figs. 25.18d and 25.19c & d). Waterproofing of neourethra with tunica vaginalis or ventral/scrotal dartos can be done if needed. The preputial edges are freshened, and then the repair is performed in three layers. To begin, the first suture is placed at the corona (where the first stay suture is applied at the inner prepucial skin) and then sutured distally up to the second stay suture, thus reconstructing the frenulum (Fig. 25.18d) and inner prepucial layer of the prepuce (Figs. 25.18d & e and 25.19d). Next, Dartos is sutured as the second layer (Figs. 25.18e & f and 25.19e & f). Then the outer skin sutures are applied from second to third stay suture to complete the prepucioplasty (Figs. 25.18g and 25.19g). This procedure can be performed even in proximal hypospadias. First inner prepucial skin closure is done, and then circumcoronal sutures are applied when complete penile de-gloving is done. This is followed by the closure of the dartos layer and skin closure (Figs. 25.18h & i and 25.19g & h). The suture material used is 5–7/0 polydioxanone according to the child's age with interrupted sutures. Satisfactory results have been achieved.

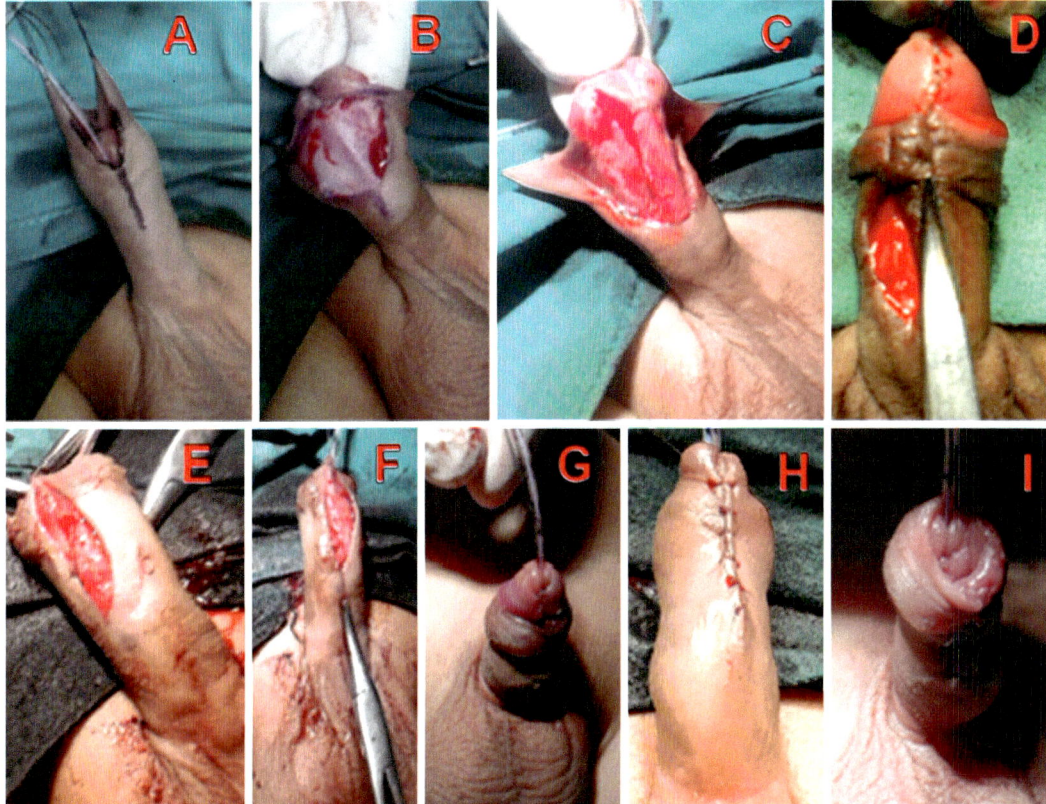

Fig. 25.18 Technique of prepucioplasty in the case of distal hypospadias. (**a**). Inverted U-shaped incision, (**b** & **c**). Partial penile de-gloving, (**d**). Glansplasty and frenuloplasty, (**e**, **f** & **g**). Prepucioplasty, (**h** & **i**). Final postoperative appearance

Gilpin et al. described an alternative technique to close the prepuce's outer skin layer by utilizing Z-plasty to decrease the tension on the suture line and its complications [9].

Follow-up A regular religious follow-up after prepucioplasty is essential to assess the cosmetic and functional outcome and diagnose complications. Our protocol involved follow-up at two weeks, one month, three months, six months, 12 months postoperatively and then annually. Prepucial oedema may last 2–3 weeks postoperatively (Fig. 25.20a). It is essential to counsel patients/parents strictly not to try retraction of prepuce by themselves. Retraction is best done for the first time by the operating surgeon when he considers it appropriate after examination in 6–8 weeks. After that, the patient/parents are advised for daily gentle retraction. Glans may remain partially or wholly covered according to the size of the prepucial hood. Klijn et al. reported a higher complication rate when they advised the parents/patients to start retraction from postoperative day ten [10].

25.10 Complications

Prepucioplasty is a technically simple procedure that requires only 15–20 min of extra time during surgery. Postoperative oedema (Fig. 25.20a, b) is usually seen in most cases but can easily be managed with conservative treatment. Phimosis/tight prepuce is a common complication and is directly

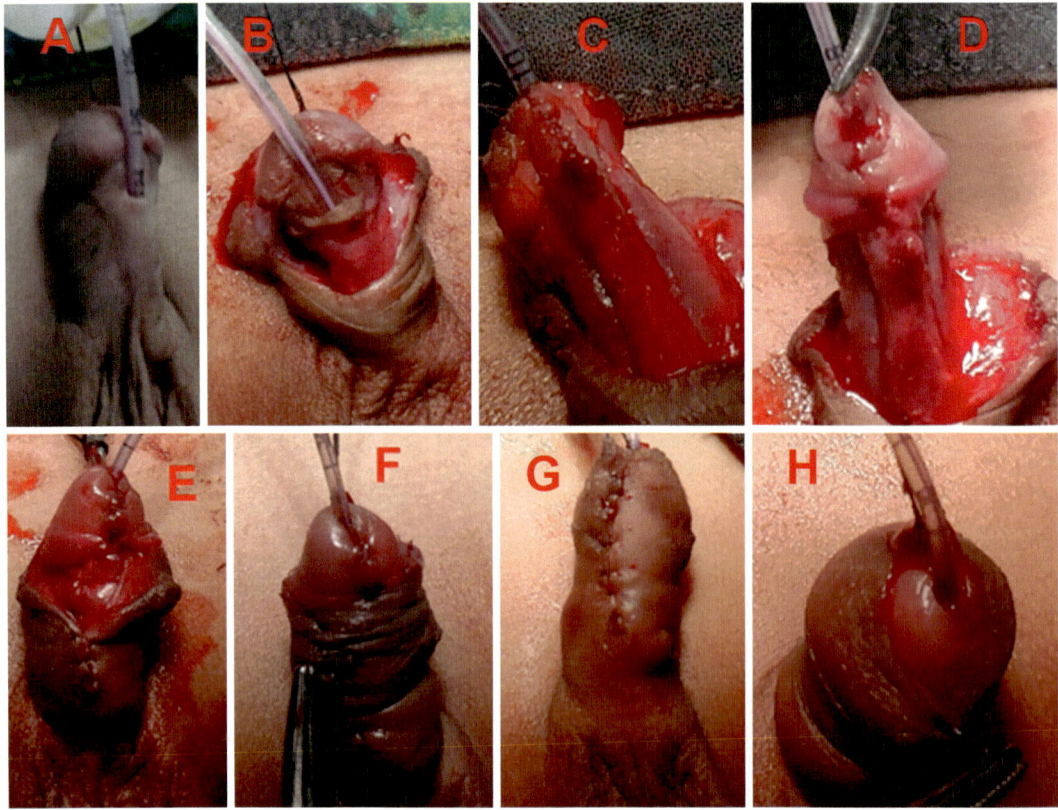

Fig. 25.19 Technique of prepucioplasty in the case of distal penile hypospadias. (**a**). Pre-operative appearance showing distal penile hypospadias, (**b**). Complete penile de-gloving, (**c**). TIP with spongioplasty, (**d**). Glansplasty. (**e**). Repair of penile shaft skin, (**f**). Reconstruction of the prepuce, (**g** & **h**). Final postoperative appearance after prepucioplasty

related to the procedure. It may get resolved with the local application of corticosteroids or eventually require circumcision if conservative management fails. Incidence of phimosis requiring circumcision ranged from 0.2 to 3.9% across various studies [11–13]. Other complications include partial dehiscence or preputial fistula (Fig. 25.21a), complete preputial dehiscence (Fig. 25.21b & c) and urethrocutaneous fistula. The incidence of prepucial dehiscence ranges from 4.5 to 7.4% [11–13]. Proximal hypospadias with penile de-gloving has a higher incidence of complications. The authors found acceptable complication rates, even in proximal hypospadias cases. We had about 11% complications in proximal hypospadias with prepucioplasty, which was similar to without prepucioplasty [14]. In a recent review (Castagnetti M et al. 2016), the prepucioplasty specific complication secondary phimosis needing circumcision and dehiscence of reconstructed prepuce was seen in 8% but does not seem to increase the risk of urethroplasty complications, and the overall reoperation rate of hypospadias repair [15].

25.11 Conclusions

Prepuce is the mirror of the urethral and penile shaft anomaly. Anomaly is seen in all three parts of prepuce median raphe, fraenulum and prepuce body. The deviation of the median raphe and its

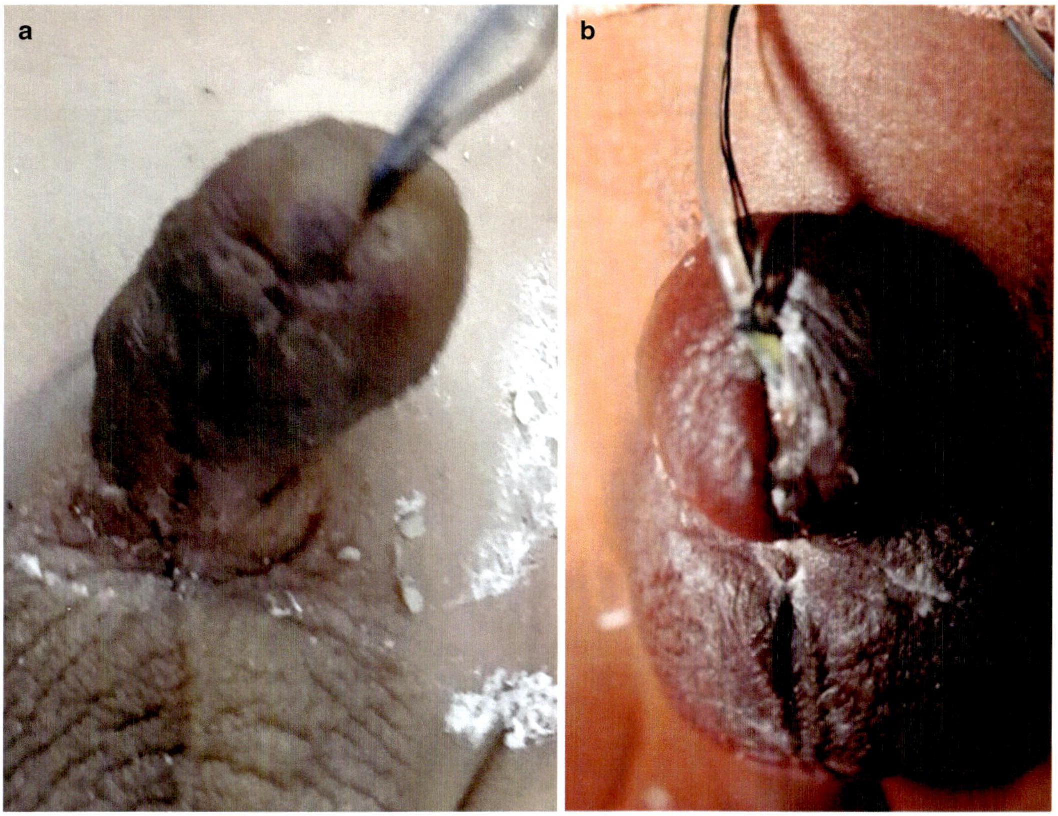

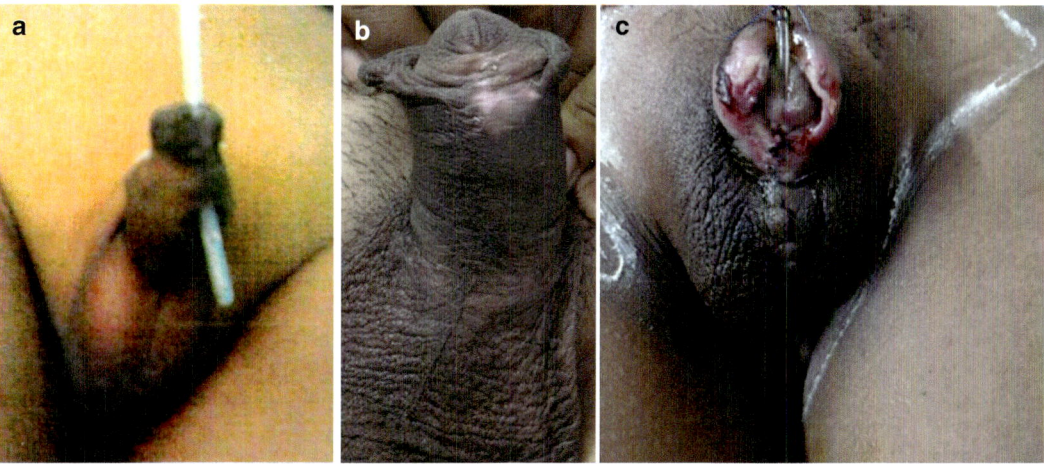

Fig. 25.20 Complications of preputioplasty. (**a** & **b**). Preputial oedema

Fig. 25.21 Complications of prepucioplasty. (**a**). Preputial fistula/partial dehiscence, (**b**). complete preputial dehiscence. (**c**). Dehiscence of the prepuce

ending on the prepuce gives information about the degree of torque. Bifurcation of median raphe and site dorsal hump offer clues regarding the severity of hypospadias. Preputial reconstruction and TIP are possible in both distal and proximal hypospadias and even cases with penile curvature and torsion. It does not increase complications associated with urethroplasty. Prepucioplasty with urethroplasty and spongioplasty reconstructs an aesthetically normal looking penis and hence, is more acceptable to the patient and/or parents of the patient with hypospadias. Type of prepuce in hypospadias is a crucial variable to predict postoperative results in prepucioplasty. The complications of prepucioplasty are postoperative oedema, phimosis and dehiscence, which may be partial or complete. Oedema can be managed conservatively with anti-inflammatory drugs and phimosis with the application of steroid cream. Phimosis can be prevented by measuring the prepuce's adequacy and marking the margins of the prepucial flaps. Circumcision is rarely required for phimosis and partial or complete prepucial dehiscence.

References

1. Liu X, Liu G, Shen J, Yue A, Isaacson D, Sinclair A, et al. Human glans and preputial development. Differentiation. 2018;103:86–99.
2. Radojicic ZI, Perovic SV. Classification of the prepuce in hypospadias according to morphological abnormalities and their impact on hypospadias repair. J Urol. 2004;172(1):301–4.
3. Zhao Z, Sun N, Mao X. Vascularization of vessel pedicle in hypospadias and its relationship to near-period complications. Exp Ther Med. 2018;16(3):2408–12.
4. Murphy JP, Ashcraft KW, Sharp RJ. Philadelphia hypospadias. In: Pediatric surgery. 2nd ed. Philadelphia: WB Saunders; 1993. p. 694.
5. Mustafa M. The concept of tubularized incised plate hypospadias repair for different types of hypospadias. Int Urol Nephrol. 2005;37(1):89–91.
6. Snodgrass WT, Koyle MA, Baskin LS, Caldamone AA. Foreskin preservation in penile surgery. J Urol. 2006;176(2):711–4.
7. Erdenetsetseg G, Dewan P. Reconstruction of the hypospadiac hooded prepuce. J Urol. 2003;169(5):1822–4.
8. Taylor JR, Lockwood AP, Taylor A. The prepuce: specialized mucosa of the penis and its loss to circumcision. Br J Urol. 1996;77(2):291–5.
9. Gilpin D, Clements W, Boston V. GRAP repair: single-stage reconstruction of hypospadias as an outpatient procedure. Br J Urol. 1993;71(2):226–9.
10. Klijn AJ, Dik P, de Jong TP. Results of preputial reconstruction in 77 boys with distal hypospadias. J Urol. 2001;165(4):1255–7.
11. Barber N, Chappell B, Carter P, Britton J. Is preputioplasty effective and acceptable? J R Soc Med. 2003;96(9):452–3.
12. Esposito C, Savanelli A, Escolino M, Giurin I, Iaquinto M, Alicchio F, et al. Preputioplasty associated with urethroplasty for correction of distal hypospadias: a prospective study and proposition of a new objective scoring system for evaluation of esthetic and functional outcome. J Pediatr Urol. 2014;10(2):294–9.
13. van den Dungen I, Rynja S, Bosch J, de Jong T, de Kort L. Comparison of preputioplasty and circumcision in distal hypospadias correction: long-term follow-up. J Pediatr Urol. 2019;15(1):47.e1–9.
14. Bhat A, Gandhi A, Saxena G, Choudhary GR. Preputial reconstruction and tubularized incised plate urethroplasty in proximal hypospadias with ventral penile curvature. Indian J Urol. 2010;26(4):507.
15. Castagnetti M, Gnech M, Angelini L, Rigamonti W, Bagnara V, Esposito C. Does preputial reconstruction increase complication rate of hypospadias repair? 20-year systematic review and meta-analysis. Front Pediatr. 2016;4:41. https://doi.org/10.3389/fped.2016.00041. e Collection 2016.PMID: 27200322

Dressing in Hypospadias Repair

Arun Chawla and Anupam Choudhary

26.1 Introduction

Dressing in hypospadias surgery is an essential aspect of management, yet it is the most controversial topic. There are several different techniques of hypospadias dressing, like different surgical approaches. Over the years, many kinds of dressing materials were used with no consensus on one over the other. The rationale for post hypospadias repair dressing is to prevent postoperative bleeding and haematoma formation, prevent bacterial contamination, hold the penis in an upright position, improve lymphatic flow, avoid formation oedema, and avoid urine and faecal soiling [1].

26.2 Difficulties Associated with Hypospadias Dressing

The degree of compression required for the repaired penis is difficult to define. The dressing should be tight enough to prevent haematoma formation with minimal pain and loose enough to allow adequate blood supply to augmented tissues [2]. Flexible dressings tend to fall off prematurely. Dressings adherent to wound cause painful episodes of undressing for the child, which may require anaesthesia [2]. The most concerning difficulty lie in stabilising the graft tissue on a mobile, soft, and boneless organ, subjected to dynamic changes in all dimensions of erection. There is a concern of frequent urine and faecal soiling of the wound and the dressing. Dressing application becomes challenging when the urethral catheter or splint is placed. In an anxious and active child, anchorage of the dressing is not easy and challenging to manage practically [3]. Immobilisation of the child has been tried with fibreglass pantaloons spica cast but has not shown to be beneficial in either preventing complications or ease of home care [4].

26.3 Ideal Hypospadias Dressing

An ideal hypospadias repair dressing should be easy to apply and to remove, non-adherent to wound, non-allergic, cost-effective, it should effectively absorb the wound leakage, produce adequate compression of the penis, should not compromise on the blood supply, and should allow regular child activity without changing its shape. There is no one dressing which satisfies all the idealistic criteria [5].

A. Chawla (✉) · A. Choudhary
Department of Urology and Renal Transplant,
Kasturba Medical College, Manipal Academy of
Higher Education, Manipal, Karnataka, India

26.4 Dressing Types

Hypospadias repair dressings can be divided into three main categories; totally concealing, partially concealing, and non-concealing dressings [6]. The most frequently used type is the partially concealing dressing and its many variations. In partially concealing, the top end towards meatus is left open to inspect the glans better and to have space for urethral catheter or splint.

In general, hypospadias dressings have 2 to 3 layers of penile coverings, with the first layer is usually a gauze around the wound. The gauze is either dry or soaked with a disinfectant agent (e.g. Betadine), antibacterial ointments, wound non-adhesive agents (e.g. Paraffin), haemostatic agents (e.g. Gelatin sponge), agents help in wound healing (e.g. oxygen-enriched oil-based gel). Adhesive strips, adhesive tapes, adhesive membranes or splints are used as second and sometimes as the third layer, to support the first layer, penile shaft, or catheter/splint. Hence, hypospadias dressings can also be broadly classified as conventional dressings, supportive splint dressings, and adhesive band/membrane dressings. The traditional dressings involve a layer of gauze which is fixed with adhesive strips. The traditional dressing has the disadvantage of premature fall and inadequate penile support. Splint dressings give good penile support; it includes silicon foam dressing, polyurethane foam dressing, or cock-up splint dressings. Adhesive band/membrane dressings are easy to apply post repair.

26.5 Dressing Techniques

Various dressing techniques have been described in the literature over the years; it includes:

- *The X-shaped elastic dressing (1980).* It is a totally concealing dressing. It consists of a flexible tape compression in X-shaped pattern in the perineum. It had a broad-spectrum of application in paediatric and adult urologic surgery. A documented complication was flexible tape burns due to allergy to the adhesive material [7].
- *Adhesive membrane dressing using OpSite (1982).* It is an adhesive, semi-permeable, translucent, hypo-allergenic membrane (OpSite). It is applied with ease directly over the wound and does not require any additional dressing. Any collected fluid under the membrane is evacuated by needle puncture. The dressing was kept in place for seven days, and undressing was easy [8].
- *Silicon foam elastomer dressing (1982).* It is a supportive splint dressing for complex hypospadias repair. Silicon foam is a popular dressing material, commercially available as an unpolymerised base and a catalyst. The mixture was poured into a cup mould or X-ray cylinder tube around the stretched penis. The mixture expands four times its original volume and sets into a soft foam in 3 minutes. The dressing is removed on day 4–6 with scissors or manually tearing it [2, 9].

The mixture preparation and adequate distribution around the penis were improvised using a special syringe with two applicators for injection of the mixture [10]. Undressing was made simpler by keeping the silk thread laid along the penis before applying the foam, and this silk thread was used to cut the foam like a cheese wire [9].

- *Transparent double Tegaderm sheet dressing (1989).* Transparent two Tegaderm sheets applied over a Telfa gauze wrap. Dressing left in place for seven days and was advised to use a hair-dryer on the dressing twice a day to avoid foul odour and skin maceration [11].
- *Sticking the gauze to the penis, catheter, and skin of the lower abdomen with adhesive spray (1990).* The Mastizoil, OpSite, or Nobecutane adhesive spray technique was defined in 1990 as new ideas and innovations. The gauze is supported on the stretched penis by digital pressure until the adhesive spray is dry. The penile support is provided without any circum-

ferential dressings and thereby reducing the risk of vascular compromise [12].

- *Outpatient hypospadias surgery dressing technique using tincture benzoin, Elastoplast, and Dermolite II tape (1991).* Tincture benzoin used for Telfa strip adhesion to penile skin, followed by application of two circles of surgical gauze and one and half-circle of Elastoplast. All three layers have maximum compression at the tip of the penis and minimum at the base. The fourth layer of Dermolite II strip encircles the penis shaft and fixes to scrotal and pubic skin after applying tincture benzoin. If urethral tubes are placed, they are also painted with benzoin and fixed with two strips of Dermolite II tapes [13].
- *Pantaloon spica cast (1997).* The idea is to immobilise the child postoperatively. The cast was used with a combination of transparent biomembrane and silicone foam dressing. This immobilisation strategy was conceptualised for better uptake of preputial graft and early discharge of child on postoperative day one, thereby reducing the total hospital cost [4].
- *SANAV dressing using plastic OpSite drape (2001).* It is a totally concealing dressing. It was designed to limit the need for specialist nursing care and has "Saved A Nurse A Visit". Two betadine gauze (Inadine) made Y cut, one applied behind and other anterior to the penis. A gauze pad placed over this. A sizeable 15 × 28 cm OpSite cut into Y. The two cut end lateral limbs are placed behind each thigh. The dressing was left behind for 7–10 days (Fig. 26.1). Undressing was much more comfortable than those that surround the penis [14].
- *Glove finger dressing (2002).* It is used for mid and distal penile hypospadias repair. Concept of glove finger for compression derived from condom dressings in adults, which is large for the paediatric group. A betadine gauze and a dry gauze wrapped around the shaft of the penis over which a cut finger of the glove is rolled over the penis from the tip

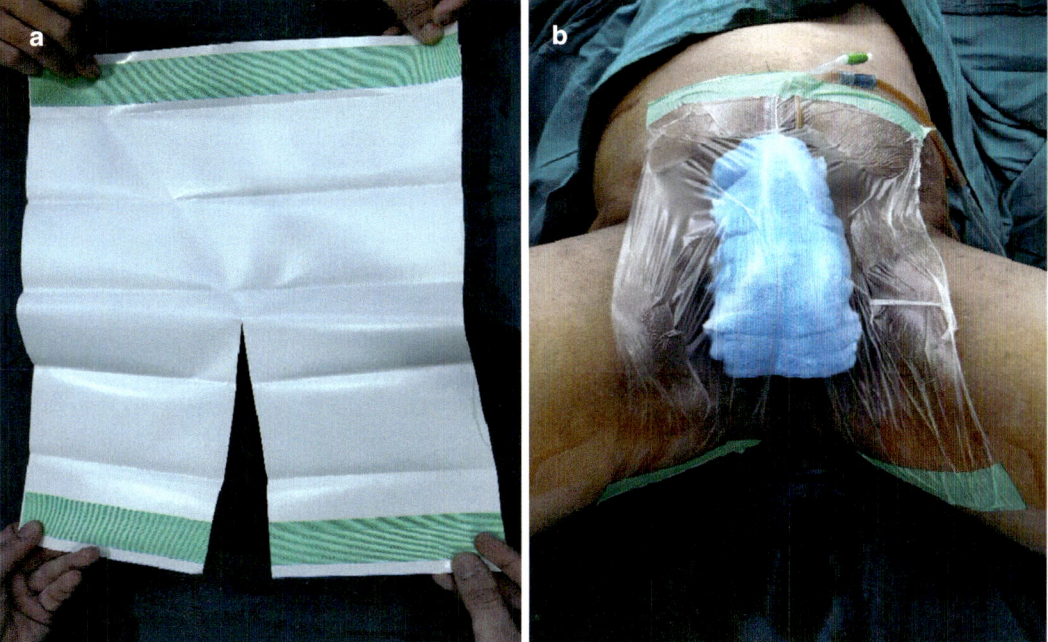

Fig. 26.1 Totally concealing plastic OpSite drape dressing. (**a**) 15 × 30 cm size OpSite made Y cut, (**b**) the two lateral limbs of OpSite adhere to the back of each thigh

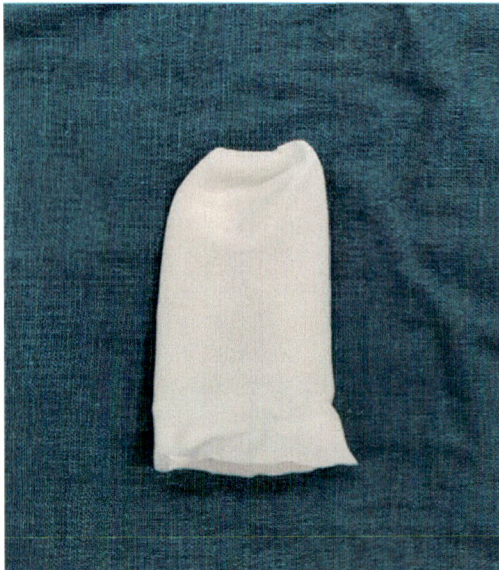 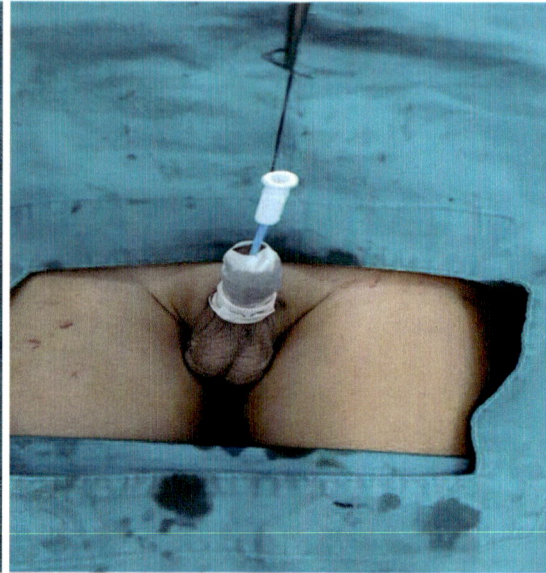

Fig. 26.2 Glove finger with rent for catheter, rolled over the penis from tip to base direction

to the base, with rent at the tip of the glove (Fig. 26.2). It has the advantage of being universally available, cost-effective, provide uniform compression, easy to inspect for wound soakage, easy to apply, and easy to remove with comparative less pain [15].

- *Elastic and Velcro dressing (2004)*. It is custom-made, cost-effective dressing material consisting of elastic strip and stitched Velcro with hook and loop fasteners. Width of the strip corresponds to the distance between the penoscrotal angle, and the corona of the stretched penis and length is one and a half to two times the penile girth. The technique includes application of antibiotic ointment over which multilayer gauze and Velcro are wrapped. The drainage tube is sandwiched between the hook and loop of Velcro. Dressing changed on 5th, 10th, and 15th postoperative day with a new set or wash-dry reused [16].
- *Non-adherent Trilaminate (Allevyn) dressing (2009)*. Dressing material is a triple-layered foam dressing consisting of inner non-adherent, middle absorbent, and outer water and microbial proof layers. The technique involves splitting the lower end onto two lateral flaps which are fixed to scrotal and pubic skin with adhesive tape and the upper end wrapped around the penile shaft with closure on the dorsal aspect with sutures. Dressing removed at 2 to 5 postoperative day [17, 18].
- *Cyanoacrylate glue dressing (2012)*. Cyanoacrylate glue is an acrylic resin, which polymerises when in contact with water forming long, strong chains. Adequate compression is achieved by applying several layers of glue on a stretched penis wound (Fig. 26.3). It is impermeable to urine and faeces. The patient is discharged in 24 h, dressing peels off by 7–10 days [19].

- *Wet dressing using multi-perforated sugarcane biopolymer membrane (2013)*. The sugarcane biopolymer membrane produced by bacterial action over sugarcane molasses. It is an inert material. Even when left in-situ for long-duration, it maintains its characteristics without the need for replacement. The dressing does not loosen due to its natural adhesive nature [20].
- *Haemostatic Gelatin sponge dressing (2014)*. Gelatin is a readily available haemostatic

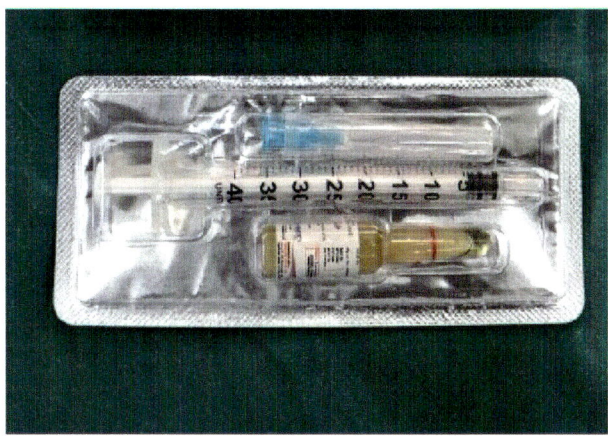
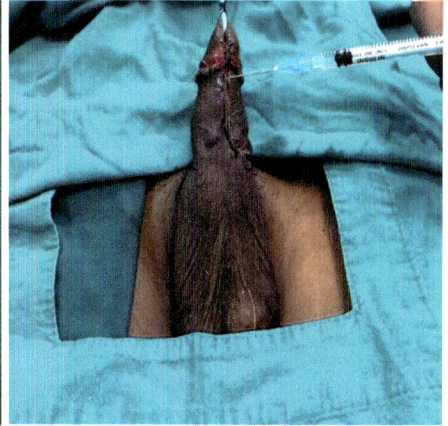

Fig. 26.3 Cyanoacrylate glue poured directly over the wound in multiple layers

agent for minor ooze used in internal cavity. The gelatin sponge is placed over gauze and wrapped around the penis for compression. It has the advantage of the ease of availability and no wound adhesion [21].

- *Tubular elastic silicon mesh netting bandage (2015).* It is an "elastic silicon mesh netting" which is placed onto the penile shaft with the help of a patented metal device. It has the advantage of gentle compression due to its elasticity and at the same time patient can void with the bandage in place. Wound inspection is possible through a bandage network. Undressing done on the fifth postoperative day [22].
- *Mepilex Border foam dressing (2017).* Mepilex Border is a self-adherent, soft, silicone foam dressing applied as a single layer with ease [23].
- *Cock-up splint dressing (2019).* It was designed for proximal penoscrotal hypospadias repair. It is a layered foam splint consisting of an aluminium shield which is hand moulded to the size of penile girth to keep the graft in position. The splint is fixed with an adhesive tape. It is fast, adjustable, easy to apply, prevent secondary contracture, and cheap, as reused during subsequent changes in the same patient [24].
- *Oxygen-enriched oil-based gel dressing (2020).* It is based on the concept of the ozone effect on wound healing. It is described for distal hypospadias repair. A wet gauze, impregnated with oxygen-enriched oil-based gel is wrapped around the penis and gauze is covered by an elastic net bandage. Faster wound healing was observed (Fig. 26.4) [5].

The author uses partially concealing dressing technique using Coban self-adherent bandage for mid and distal penile hypospadias (Fig. 26.5). For proximal penoscrotal hypospadias or hypospadias repairs with extensive tissue dissection, use Dynaplast elastic adhesive bandage technique similar to Redman et al. (Fig. 26.6).

26.6 Undressing

The wound healing process starts within hours after wound closure and deeper structures are completely sealed from the external environment by 48 hours. The dressing can be removed on postoperative day three or four, and some dressing technique removal is extended even up to postoperative day fifteen. A survey suggested that most surgeons keep the dressing for more than three days [6]. Dressing removal timing mainly depends on tissue dissection, hypospadias repair technique, and type of dressing. Some centres use anaesthesia for undressing or change of dressing. Conventional dressing auto falls off prematurely, while dressings like silicon foam and single-layer adhesive spray are easily removed in the ward setting without discomfort to the child. The dressing should be removed

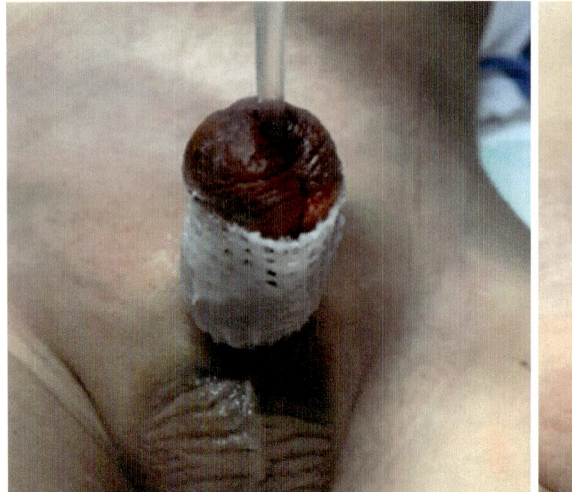 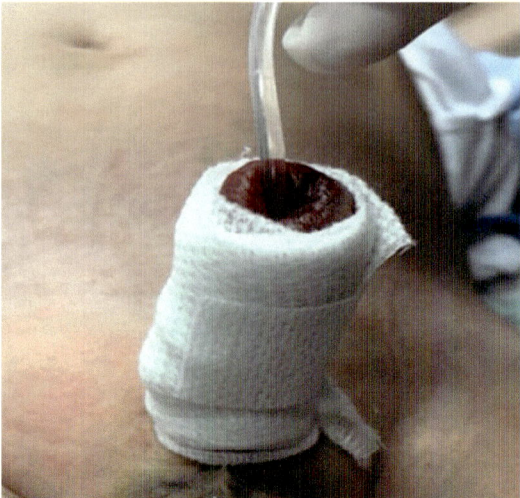

Fig. 26.4 Oxygen-enriched oil-based gel dressing (with permission Esposito et al. 2020 [5] @ copyright Springer Nature)

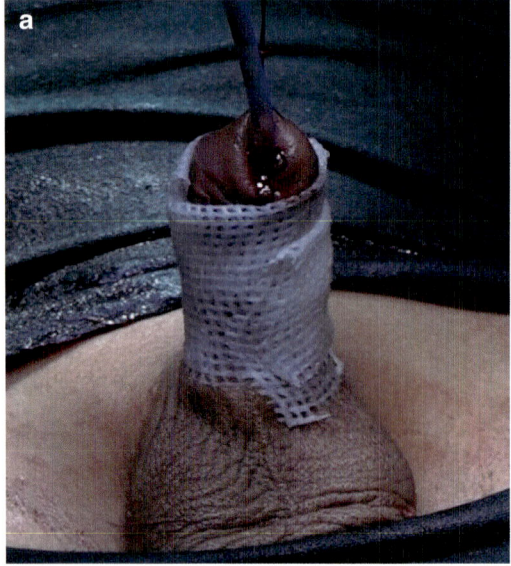 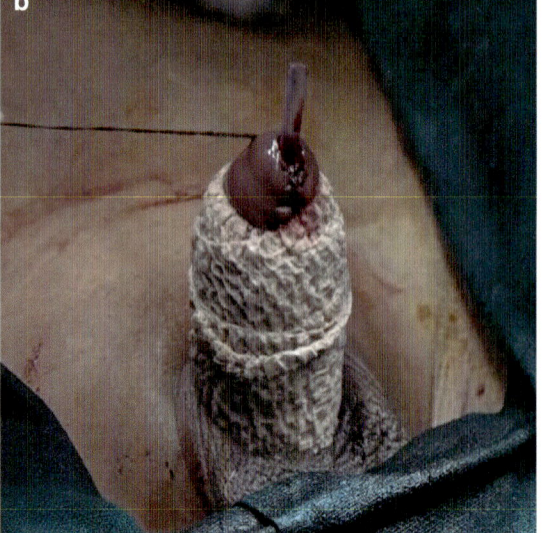

Fig. 26.5 Partially concealed dressing technique using Coban self-adherent bandage at our institute; (**a**) showing Bactigras (chlorhexidine with paraffin gauze) as a first layer covering, (**b**) Penis fixed by Coban self-adherent bandage from the base to corona keeping glans and meatus open with splint in-situ

early if soiled by urine or faecal matter, due to bacterial contamination risk.

26.7 Dressing v/s No Dressing

The role of dressing following hypospadias surgery is still controversial. Dressing in hypospadias repair is used to limit the degree of oedema, as there is concern that postoperative oedema could cut through the repair and stitches. However, compression from a dressing may also hamper the blood flow to the penis.

In a questionnaire survey study on the opinion of surgeons managing hypospadias repair by Cromie et al. in 1981, strongly suggested the need for dressing, mainly for penile immobilisation and reduction of oedema [6]. Van Savage

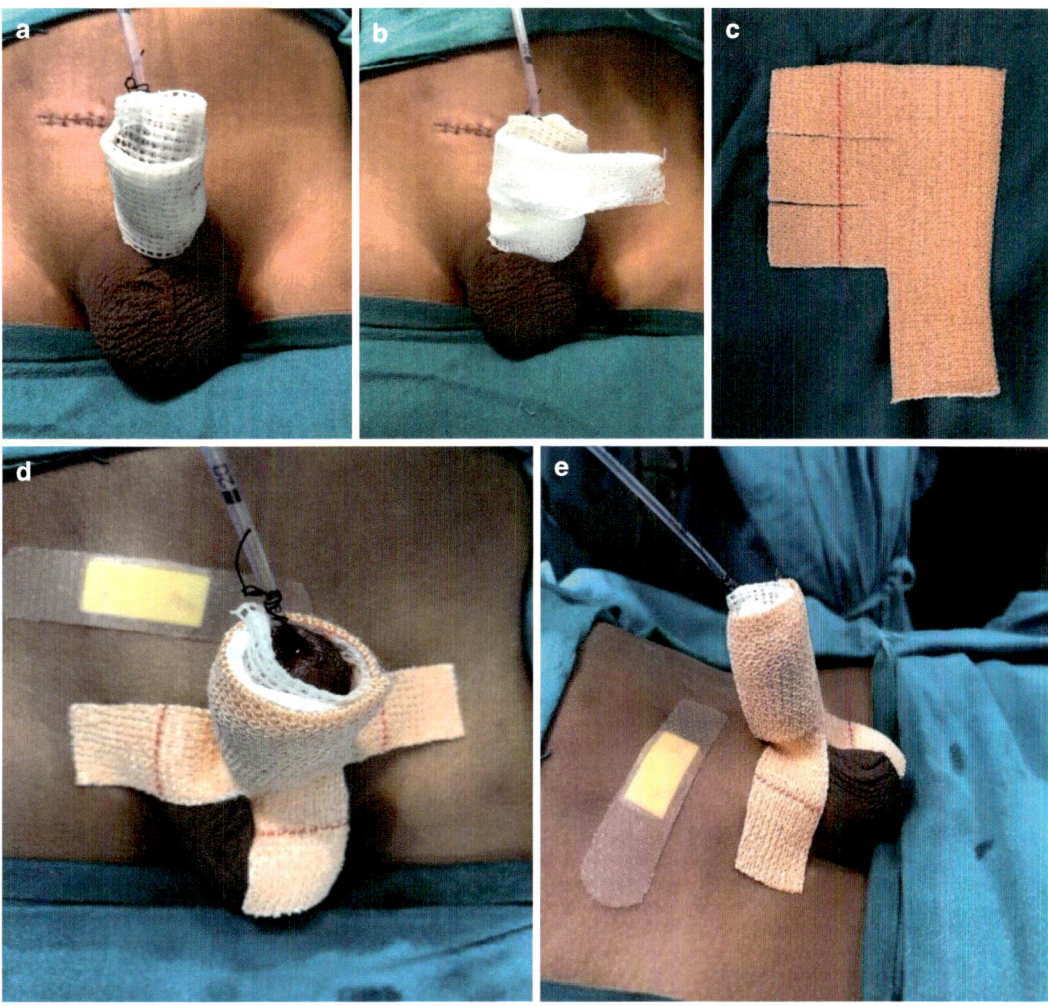

Fig. 26.6 Partially concealed dressing technique using Dynaplast elastic adhesive bandage at our institute; (**a**) showing Bactigras (chlorhexidine with paraffin gauze) as a first layer covering, (**b**) dry gauze second layer covered over the first layer, (**c**) Dynaplast elastic adhesive bandage is cut into "reverse-F" fashion with three arms, and (**d** & **e**) Penis fixed in erect position from the base at three points with the three sleeves of Dynaplast

et al. (2000) concluded that dressings might not be indicated for all types of hypospadias repair in a randomised controlled trial. McLorie et al. (2001) in a prospective study, concluded that absent dressing simplified postoperative parents delivered home care and recommended omission of routine dressing. Hadidi et al. (2003) in a randomised trial, said that results of hypospadias repair without dressing are statistically better [6]. These studies supported Herman's (1965) theory that very few bacteria retain their vitality on an exposed dry wound [6].

26.8 Conclusions

There are several different techniques with different dressing materials due to the unique challenges posed by hypospadias repair wounds. There is no consensus on the superiority of one technique over the other. The rationale behind the hypospadias dressing is for haematoma and oedema prevention, but this has been challenged in a few randomised studies. However, these results need further high volume studies, as most centres practise dressing after hypospadias surgery.

References

1. Sanders C, Rscn RGN, Enb A. A review of current practice for boys undergoing hypospadias repair: from pre-operative work up to the removal of dressing post-surgery. J Child Heal Care. 2002;6:60–9.
2. De Sy WA, Oosterlinck W. Silicone foam elastomer: A significant improvement in postoperative penile dressing. J Urol. 1982;128:39–40.
3. Fletcher J. A practical approach to dressing wounds under challenging positions. Br J Nurs. 1999;8:779–86.
4. Cilento BG, Stock JA, Kaplan GW. Pantaloon spica cast: an effective method for postoperative immobilization after free graft hypospadias repair. J Urol. 1997;157:1882–3.
5. Esposito C, Del Conte F, Cerulo M, Coppola V, Esposito G, Ricciardi E, Crocetto F, Castagnetti M, Calignano A, Escolino M. Evaluation of efficacy of oxygen-enriched oil-based gel dressing in patients who underwent surgical repair of distal hypospadias: a prospective randomised clinical trial. World J Urol. 2020;39(6):2205–15. https://doi.org/10.1007/s00345-020-03419-1.
6. Hadidi AT, Azmy AF. Hypospadias surgery. 1st ed. London: Springer; 2004. https://doi.org/10.1007/978-3-662-07841-9.
7. Falkowski WS, Firlit CF. Hypospadias surgery: the X-shaped elastic dressing. J Urol. 1980;123:904–6.
8. Vordermark JS. Adhesive membrane: a new dressing for hypospadias. Urology. 1982;20:86.
9. Whitaker RH, Dennis MS. Silastic foam dressing in hypospadias surgery. Ann R Coll Surg Engl. 1987;69:59–60.
10. Amir AZ, Isaac JP, Menachem RW. Further improvement in a dressing for hypospadias. Ann Plast Surg. 1987;18:81–2.
11. Patil UB, Alvarez J. Simple effective hypospadias repair dressing. Urology. 1989;34:49.
12. Tan KK, Reid CD. A simple penile dressing following hypospadias surgery. Br J Plast Surg. 1990;43:628–9.
13. Redman JF. A dressing technique that facilitates outpatient hypospadias surgery. Urology. 1991;37:248–50.
14. Searles JM, Mackinnon AE. The "SANAV" hypospadias dressing. BJU Int. 2001;87:531–3.
15. Singh RB, Khatri HL, Sethi R. Glove-finger dressing in paediatric hypospadias. Pediatr Surg Int. 2002;18:218–9.
16. Singh RB, Pavithran NM. Elastic and Velcro dressing for penis. Pediatr Surg Int. 2004;20:389–90.
17. Fathi K, Tsang T. A technique for applying a non-adherent, tri-laminate dressing for hypospadias repair. Ann R Coll Surg Engl. 2009;91:164–5.
18. Narci A, Embleton DB, Boyaci EÖ, Mingir S, Çetinkurşun S. A practical offer for hypospadias dressing: Allevyn®. African J Paediatr Surg. 2011;8:272–4.
19. Hosseini SMV, Rasekhi AR, Zarenezhad M, Hedjazi A. Cyanoacrylate glue dressing for hypospadias surgery. N Am J Med Sci. 2012;4:320–2.
20. Martins AGS, Lima SVC, de Araújo LAP, de Vilar FO, Cavalcante NTP. A wet dressing for hypospadias surgery. Int Braz J Urol. 2013;39:408–13.
21. Menon P, Rao KLN. Novel use of gelatine sponge as a primary dressing in hypospadias surgery. J Indian Assoc Pediatr Surg. 2014;20:54.
22. Wang Y, Li S. The tubular elastic net bandage: a useful penile dressing in Pediatric hypospadias. Indian J Surg. 2015;77:1425–7.
23. Méndez-Gallart R, García-Palacios M, Rodríguez-Barca P, Estévez-Martínez E, Carril AL, Bautista-Casasnovas A. A simple dressing for hypospadias surgery in children. Can Urol Assoc J. 2017;11:E58–9.
24. Hsieh MKH, Lai MC, Azman NM, Cheng JJSH, Lim GJS. The cock-up splint: a novel malleable, rigid, and durable dressing construct for the post-hypospadias repair. Plast Reconstr Surg - Glob Open. 2019;7:10–1.

Psychosocial, Sexual Function, and Fertility in Hypospadias

Sudhindra Jayasimha and J. Chandrasingh

27.1 Introduction

Hypospadias has several implications for a child which extend beyond those of a structural abnormality, due to the myriad functions of the penis [1]. These include abnormal appearance of genitalia, spraying of urinary stream, potential inability to void standing, the psychological impact of genital abnormality, and multiple corrective operations as a child [2]. The goal of reconstructive surgery in hypospadias is to achieve a cosmetically and functionally normal penis. This includes a normal position as well as the shape of the meatus, glans, and shaft, ability to stand and void with a stream directed forwards and normal erections without penile curvature that enables satisfactory sexual intercourse [3]. Despite repair, a large proportion continues to experience negative genital perception and desire corrective surgery as adults [4].

Long-term follow-up studies on body image, psychological and sexual function are riddled with problems such as lack of periodic review, loss to follow-up, the use of diverse techniques, and lack of a control group. These limitations make comparison difficult [5]. Many long-term studies may not be applicable today due to improvements in surgical technique and better outcomes. Most reports on psychosexual outcomes are retrospective and based on questionnaires administered to patients. Drawbacks of this approach include loss to follow-up, recall bias, representation bias (those who had better psychosexual outcomes may be over-represented as they may be more willing to participate) [6] and misunderstanding of questions. Information obtained from interviews with patients may not be completely accurate as the patients may not be forthcoming with sensitive personal information. However, mailed questionnaires allow patients to respond to delicate questions in the privacy of their homes and are more likely to elicit accurate replies [7]. These aspects emphasize the need for long-term follow-up to build trust with the patient and to understand the sequelae of hypospadias repairs carried out in childhood [2].

We aim to summarise the available evidence on psychological, sexual, and fertility outcomes after hypospadias repair.

27.2 Psychosocial and Sexual Development

27.2.1 Psychosexual Development and Gender Identity

Psychosexual development refers to the attainment of psychological and sexual maturity that enables people to have satisfactory relationships and sexual lives [8]. The term psychosexual

S. Jayasimha · J. Chandrasingh (✉)
Division of Adolescent and Pediatric Urology, Department of Urology, Christian Medical College, Vellore, Tamilnadu, India
e-mail: chandrasingh@cmcvellore.ac.in

development is used because it is believed that sexual development is not merely a physical process but is influenced by psychological factors. It encompasses multiple aspects such as gender identity, gender-related behavior, body image, and sexual habits [9]. These can be accurately assessed only after puberty which is the earliest when psychosexual maturity is achieved [10]. Studies differ in their reports of the effect of hypospadias on psychosexual development. Some suggest that boys with hypospadias had a more uncertain gender identity and more feminine traits than controls [11–13]. However, contrary results were reported in other series [14] where gender-appropriate behavior was seen in spite of hypospadias. In adolescent boys, it was found that masculine gender role was predicted by younger age at surgery [9].

27.2.1.1 Age at Surgery and Personality

Blotchsky reported that genitourinary surgery in childhood resulted in more emotional disturbances, compared to other forms of surgery [15]. In addition to personal stress, these patients also face the stress of parental anxiety and multiple operations in childhood [6]. Bracka believed that hospitalization between 18 months and 3 years of age was more stressful and preferred to perform a two-stage repair after 3 years of age [16]. However, contemporary reports have shown that adults treated for hypospadias were comfortable with surgery as a child as there was less recollection and mental trauma [3, 17]. About 10% reported decisional regret [17]. Men that were interviewed said that they did not often receive adequate information on follow-up and were reluctant to seek medical attention for problems. They were often anxious about intimate relationships and sexual performance due to which they grew up into reserved adults [13, 17, 18]. This indicates that periodic follow-up with psychological counseling may be indicated [19].

27.2.1.2 Behavior and Relationships

There was a higher prevalence of behavioral problems and worse psychosocial outcomes especially in those with proximal hypospadias, older age at surgery, and a greater number of operations, in some studies [12, 17, 20, 21]. However, others reported that there was no difference in psychosexual outcome between patients and the general population [5, 6, 8, 22]. In spite of a poorer genital image, the psychosexual satisfaction levels were similar between hypospadiacs and the general population [8]. Their education levels and professional achievement were also similar [6, 19] contrary to a few earlier reports [23]. The rates of stable relationships/marriage and biological children among those with hypospadias were no different from those in the general population in most studies [24, 25]. In a study from India, Bhat et al reported that the rate of marriage was 40.62% in those with hypospadias and 70% in controls (Fig. 27.1). This was higher than those reported by Bubanj (37.23% in cases and 33.33% in controls) [26] and Kenawi (36.6% in those treated for hypospadias) [27]. This may be attributed to earlier marriage in keeping with societal customs in India. The age at marriage was similar in the two groups (26 years in cases vs. 24.71 years in controls).

27.2.1.3 Sexual Activity and Quality of Life

Some authors have reported delayed sexual milestones, fewer partners, and less frequent sexual activity in those with hypospadias [28], especially if the genital image was poor [16, 23, 29–31]. Avellan et al showed that sexual debut was delayed in those who underwent hypospadias repair later than 13 years of age [32]. However, these findings have not been echoed by others. Milestones such as falling in love, erotic kiss, fondling, masturbation, age at ejaculation, and intercourse were not delayed in boys with hypospadias. Sexual behavior including libido, frequency of masturbation, number of partners, and intercourse, were also similar. However, they were more inhibited in seeking sexual contact due to decreased confidence of sexual performance, were reluctant to discuss topics related to sex, and feared the ridicule of genital appearance. This was more prevalent in proximal than distal hypospadias [5, 22, 30, 33, 34]. A trend towards better psychosocial function was seen with better

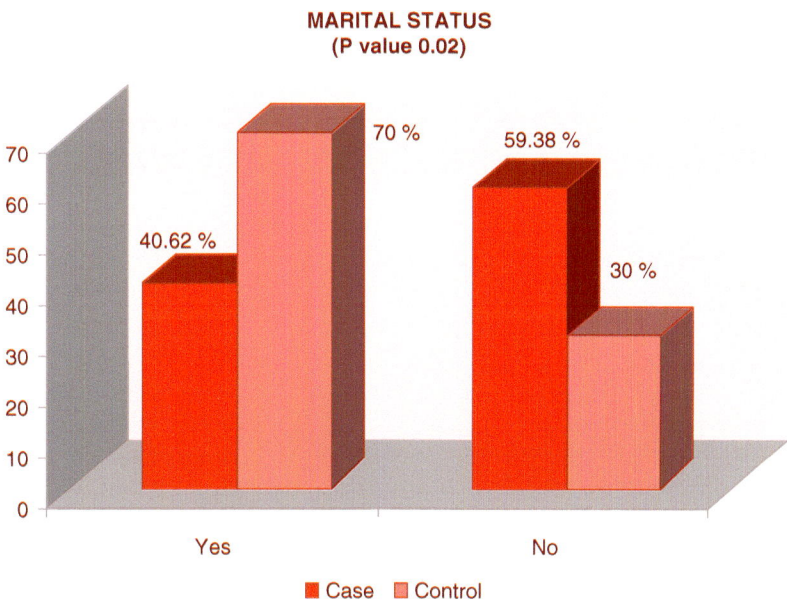

Fig. 27.1 Rates of marriage in cases and controls [Courtesy Dr. Amilal Bhat]

body/ genital perception, counseling, and higher levels of education [6, 22, 35]. Up to 50% avoided situations involving exposure of genitalia and did not prefer to change clothes in public or use communal showers and washrooms [3, 19, 36]. However, more recent series have reported that the majority of those with hypospadias had a more positive body image and did not fear adverse genital appraisal by a partner [3]. In a study on health-related quality of life (HRQoL) in young adults who had undergone hypospadias repair, it was shown that low genital perception and decreased orgasmic function directly correlated with lower HRQoL. There is a need for timely diagnosis and psychological support in these individuals [37]. Up to 50% of the patients and their parents were anxious about sexual activity and fertility in the future. This further reinforces the need for periodic counseling and prolonged follow-up [17].

27.2.1.4 Objective Assessment of Psychosexual Function

Multiple objective tools for assessment of psychosocial well-being have been used for assessment after hypospadias repair. These include Psychological general well-being index (PGWBI) [13], Minnesota Multiphasic Personality Inventory Test [22], TNO AZL Child Quality of Life Questionnaire, Child Behaviour Checklist [38], Gender Role Questionnaire [9], Child Behaviour Checklist, Youth Self Report, Self-Perception profile for adolescents [21], Psychological General Well-Being Index, Body-Esteem Scale for Adolescents and Adults [39] and Global Sexual Functioning questionnaire [10]. However, there is a need for a unique validated tool to assess psychosexual outcomes with elements such as genital image, genital ridicule, social function, behavioral problems, self-confidence, inhibition to establishing sexual contact, and the various aspects of sexual behavior.

The salient features of psychosexual development in hypospadias are summarized in Table 27.1.

27.2.2 Genital Perception

27.2.2.1 Associated Anomalies

Congenital anomalies associated with hypospadias include micropenis, penoscrotal transposition, undescended testes, inguinal hernia, ectopic kidney, and disorders of sexual differentiation [28, 40]. These are more prevalent in proximal hypospadias [13]. Reported non-urogenital

Table 27.1 Features of psychosexual development after hypospadias repair

Psychological, scholastic, and professional development is normal after hypospadias repair [14, 18]
There is a reluctance to discuss sexual issues, avoidance of intimate relationships [13, 30]
They are socially withdrawn, inhibited in seeking sexual partners [5, 30]
There is fear of genital ridicule, avoidance undressing in public [3, 19]
Sexual milestones are normal: Erotic kiss, masturbation, ejaculation, intercourse [5, 34]
Proximal hypospadias: Low genital image, delayed sexual milestones [30, 33]
There is a need for prolonged follow-up and periodic counseling [17, 19]

abnormalities are congenital heart disease, musculoskeletal anomalies, anorectal malformation, cleft palate, cerebral palsy, and psychological disorders [33, 40]. These may negatively affect genital perception and this, in turn, has been reported to influence psychological and sexual outcomes [29].

Satisfaction with Cosmesis

Older studies that reported on the cosmetic outcomes of operative techniques such as Denis Browne, Ombrédanne, van der Meulen, Broadbent, and Mustarde which are not in common use today [27, 41]. Most patients had undergone two or more operations in these series. Most (38–80%) recognized that the appearance of the repaired penis differed from normal. This was more pronounced for older techniques such as Denis-Browne, van der Meulen, and Browne dorsal meatoplasty. Cultural differences such as circumcision being less prevalent in the population also contribute to this difference [4]. Patients were often dissatisfied with the appearance of the penis due to scars, fistulae, chordee, penile torsion, flat shape of glans, and redundant distal penile skin. The reported rates of dissatisfaction with cosmesis range from 13 to 53.5% [27, 31] and were higher than that in controls [42]. A third considered their penis to be small and 40–60% wished that they had a larger penis [4]. Objective measurement of penile length showed smaller length and girth of the penis after hypospadias repair when compared to controls [30, 43]. Penile size was the single most important aspect that influenced genital perception [4]. Up to 44% requested revision surgery for poor flow, spraying of stream, fistulae, residual chordee, or poor overall cosmesis [19, 36].

More recent studies reported improved cosmetic outcomes (80–90%) with techniques such as TIP, Mathieu, MAGPI, preputial flap, and staged repairs [4]. In redo operations, the satisfaction rate was 60% [44]. Aho et al reported that dissatisfaction was higher with Denis Browne than Mathieu repair (46% vs 13%) [24]. The use of Testosterone pre-operatively did not affect genital perception or penile length [45]. Those with proximal hypospadias were less satisfied with appearance and size and were likely to be embarrassed by the same. They were also more likely to have poor flow and were thrice as likely to seek corrective surgery [24, 31, 39].

27.2.2.2 Meatal Position

Reports of the influence of the position of the meatus after repair, on body image were inconsistent. Bracka et al reported that more than two-third patients felt that a terminal meatus led to a better body image [19]. However, in other series, patients were not too concerned by a slightly proximal meatus [36] and the position of meatus and chordee did not influence satisfaction [8].

27.2.2.3 Age and Genital Perception

Flynn et al believed that children with a successful operation were satisfied till adolescence after which, growth of the neourethra failed to keep up with that of the penis [41]. However, it is more likely that pre-pubertal children have a more positive genital perception as the penis has not acquired functions other than micturition and that with the onset of sexual activity and heightened body image, adolescents have higher expectations [4]. Even after surgical correction, many patients faced ridicule from peers for the abnormal appearance of the penis [5].

Patients were more satisfied with cosmesis if they had been treated before the age of three, were younger than 12 years of age, and had more knowledge about hypospadias [5, 9]. Those who had complications after hypospadias repair and a greater number of operations were more likely to be dissatisfied [35, 46].

27.2.2.4 Patients Versus Surgeons

There is often a mismatch between the perception of results by patients and surgeons. The patient compares results with his peers whereas the surgeon uses prevailing surgical standards for a particular severity of hypospadias [4]. Mureau et al, in the first such study, showed that there was no correlation between the rates of satisfaction of surgeons and patients. Surgeons tended to rate cosmesis after hypospadias repair higher than their patients [5]. However, other studies showed that that surgeons rated penile appearance as abnormal more frequently than patients or their parents [17, 47].

Validated scores for genital perception include the following:

- Genital perception score [5]
- Hypospadias Objective Score Evaluation [48]
- Pediatric Penile Perception Score and Penile Perception Score [49]
- Hypospadias Objective Penile Evaluation [50]
- Glans Meatus Shaft Score [51]

Objective records of cosmetic outcomes postop and on follow-up and the use of validated questionnaires may improve the quality of reporting and enable objective comparison [4, 44].

27.2.2.5 Perception of Genitalia by Women and Healthy Men

In a novel study, Ruppen-Greef et al showed 105 women standard photographs of ten adults circumcised and an equal number of repaired hypospadiac genitalia. Women considered general appearance, public hair, and penile skin to be important to cosmesis. Penile length, position, and shape of meatus were not important. Distal hypospadias was graded similar to a circumcised penis while proximal forms were considered to be abnormal in appearance. Similar results were found in a study with 70 men with normal genitalia where the appearance of distal hypospadias was considered no different from that of a circumcised penis. Older age and higher sexual interest led to more favorable genital perception [52, 53].

27.2.2.6 Untreated Hypospadias

Scholmer et al. reported that untreated hypospadias, especially if proximal led to a more negative genital image, greater difficulty in voiding, and a more pronounced chordee [54].

27.2.2.7 Follow-up

The majority wished that they had a longer follow-up because of reasons such as anxiety arising from poor genital image, prior operations, and their complications and lack of understanding of their problem. There is often a reluctance to seek medical attention due to shame, ignorance, fear, or resignation [19]. This emphasizes the need for long-term periodic follow-up till adulthood in these patients [13].

The salient features of genital perception in hypospadias are summarized in Table 27.2.

Table 27.2 Genital perception in hypospadias

Most are satisfied with cosmesis with TIP, MAGPI, preputial tube [4]
More dissatisfaction seen with older repairs like Denis Browne and Ombrédanne [27, 41]
Genital perception is better in the young [5, 38]
Children face ridicule from peers even after surgical correction [5]
Negative genital perception is associated with disorders of sexual differentiation [29]
Penile length may be important for genital perception [4]
Patients request revision surgery for poor flow, spraying of stream, fistulae, residual chordee, cosmesis [19, 36]
There is a mismatch between genital perception of patients and surgeons [4, 5, 47]
Repaired distal hypospadias and circumcision appear similar for laypersons [52]
Patients are reluctant to seek medical attention due to shame, ignorance, or fear [19]

27.2.3 Erectile Function and Sexual Satisfaction

27.2.3.1 Factors Affecting Intercourse

Most studies on sexual function in hypospadias are on adolescents and data in adults is scarce. They focus on the short-term cosmetic and functional results. However, the repercussions of corrective surgery are felt a decade or two later in adolescence, with the onset of sexual activity. Patients may idealize their performance, be lost to follow-up and those who did not participate in interviews, maybe more dissatisfied with sexual life due to which the results may not be generalizable. Problems with erections in hypospadias may be due to correctable or non-correctable problems. The size of the penis cannot be corrected whereas chordee, scars, and torsion may be corrected [1]. Difficulty with sexual intercourse may be due to residual chordee, painful scars, decreased glans turgidity, or small size of penis [19, 27, 36]. Decreased glans sensation is rare [19].

27.2.3.2 Sexual Behavior

Erectile dysfunction may be seen in up to a third to half of the patients with proximal hypospadias [33, 35]. Libido, ability to have penetrative intercourse and achieve orgasm were unaffected in most reviews, [19, 27, 55] even after prior failed repairs necessitating staged reconstruction with buccal mucosal grafts [7]. In other published series, there was greater difficulty with erections, intercourse, and ejaculation with decreased satisfaction, especially in proximal hypospadias [13, 26, 31]. In a study from India, Bhat et al observed that the incidence of erectile dysfunction among hypospadiacs was greater than that in controls (Fig. 27.2).

Patients tended to masturbate less, have shorter foreplay, less frequent intercourse, and fewer partners [26]. In contrast, Majstorovic et al showed that desire, arousal, frequency of intercourse, erections, and orgasm was higher in proximal hypospadias than controls [10]. Rynjah et al reported delayed sexual milestones, lower orgasmic function, and weak ejaculation in patients with proximal hypospadias who underwent transverse preputial island tube reconstruction when compared to controls [56]. Problems with achieving orgasm may be due to shame from negative genital perception and lesser arousal [57]. However, it was also noted that the IIEF is inconsistently answered in adolescents and these results need to be interpreted with caution [58].

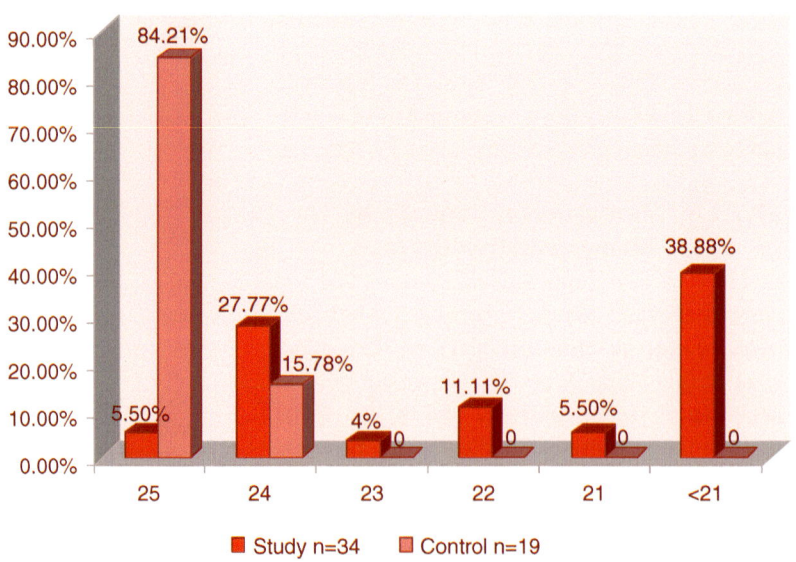

Fig. 27.2 Shim scores among patients and controls. [Courtesy Dr. Amilal Bhat]

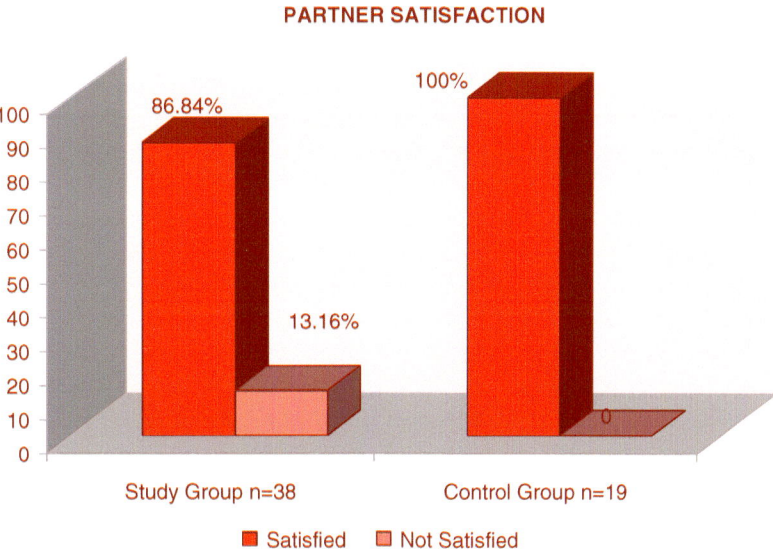

Fig. 27.3 Partner satisfaction among cases and controls. [Courtesy Dr. Amilal Bhat]

The extent of flexibility in the erect penis was more important than the degree of chordee for satisfactory intercourse [19]. A few studies reported that the size of the penis correlated with the ability to have normal intercourse [31, 57] while others showed that the overall cosmesis and not the penile length, determined sexual satisfaction [13]. Those who were dissatisfied with surgical outcomes reported poor genital image and lower sexual satisfaction. Patients, therefore, require long-term follow-up and appropriate counselling starting early in life [24]. The number of operations and occurrence of complications were not reported to influence erectile function, ejaculation, or sexual satisfaction in some series [7, 30, 35]. Bhat et al. reported a higher incidence of partner dissatisfaction among those with hypospadias due to the small size of the penis and poor erections (Fig. 27.3) which emphasizes the need for counselling of the partner in addition to that of the patient.

27.2.3.3 Ejaculation

Most series report dribbling on ejaculation: 33% overall [19] and up to 75% in proximal hypospadias [34], the need to milk out the ejaculate in up to 43% [59] or anejaculation in up to 20% [13], especially in proximal hypospadias [30]. These may be due to inadequate spongiosal and muscular support to the reconstructed skin tube, failed urethral peristalsis, abnormal bladder neck, large utricle, as well as complications such as stricture/diverticulum [7, 19, 31, 57]. Split ejaculation from urethrocutaneous fistulae, was another unique problem reported in the hypospadias group [17].

27.2.4 Hormonal Status and Fertility

Literature on hormonal levels and fertility in hypospadias is scant [1]. Associated genital anomalies (17–30%) include micropenis, penoscrotal transposition, undescended testes, inguinal hernia, and disorders of sexual differentiation. These are more prevalent in proximal hypospadias and may affect hormonal levels and fertility to varying degrees [40, 60]. Association with undescended testes, disorders of sexual differentiation, and reduced anogenital distance suggest androgen deficiency as a possibility during embryogenesis. Endocrine-disrupting chemicals were shown to influence the development of hypospadias in animals. However, this is not proven in humans. The constellation of hypospadias, undescended testes, subfertility, and testicular cancer is believed to be a result of testicular dysgenesis [61]. Defects in androgen signaling such as decreased receptor concentration and mutation in the second Zinc finger element of the

DNA binding domain, have been described in patients with ambiguous genitalia associated with hypospadias [33].

Testicular volume, Testosterone, and semen parameters were normal unless there were associated undescended testes or chromosomal abnormalities [19, 62]. In those with proximal hypospadias, hypogonadism was noted in 15% [63]. FSH and LH were high while Testosterone and semen quality were low in hypospadiacs when compared to controls [64]. However, FSH was found to be elevated only in the presence of undescended testes in another study. The confounder was that undescended testes were more commonly noted with proximal hypospadias [65]. Dihydrotestosterone was also noted to be lower among those with hypospadias. The presence of raised LH with normal Testosterone may indicate relative androgen insensitivity [66]. The incidence of oligozoospermia in hypospadias ranged from 4 to 29% [19, 27].

Fertility in hypospadias may be affected by multiple factors. These include testicular dysgenesis, mechanical factors that affect semen delivery (stricture, diverticulum, non-terminal meatus, micropenis, lack of spongiosal support resulting in dribbling on ejaculation), and reduced semen quality in proximal hypospadias [67, 68]. Fertility and paternity were both found to be lower in hypospadias, especially if proximal, even when those with undescended testes were excluded [13, 69]. This suggests that hypospadias in isolation, even without hormonal and familial factors, predisposes to lower fertility. Anatomical or surgical factors may be responsible for this finding [69]. In a population register-based study, it was noted that both hypospadias and undescended testes were associated with a 21% decrease in paternity compared to the general population. The decreased paternity rates were higher in proximal hypospadias (54%). Assisted reproduction techniques were used by 0.4% of those with hypospadias which was comparable to the general population [70]. Similarly, Asklund reported a lower paternity rate in hypospadiacs (24%) when compared with the general population (29%) [62]. Patients who underwent reoperation for obstructive causes had lower paternity (0%) when compared with those who had reoperation for non-obstructive causes and controls (80%) [71]. Bhat et al showed that paternity was similar among hypospadiacs and controls (50% in each group) which was in keeping with other published reports [13, 29].

The salient features of sexual function and fertility in hypospadias are summarized in Table 27.3.

27.3 Conclusions

Long-term follow-up studies after hypospadias repair have several drawbacks. These include their retrospective nature, small sample size, loss to follow-up, use of non-validated questionnaires with the attendant biases, lack of valid controls, and obsolete surgical techniques with late age at repair. Typically, they involved multiple operations with higher complication rates. Currently, most children undergo surgery at a much younger age (1–2 years) and the implications of this are unknown. With the advances in surgical technique, it is expected that the cosmetic, functional, and psychosexual outcomes will also improve. However, after the repair, there is a lag period of more than a decade for the subjects to become sexually active. Proximal hypospadias, especially if associated with undescended testes may be associated with low testosterone levels, decreased semen quality and subfertility [13, 64]. The development and use of validated questionnaires, appro-

Table 27.3 Sexual activity and fertility in hypospadias

Chordee, pain, scars, soft glans, and short penis hinder intercourse [19, 27]
Normal desire, erections, intercourse, and satisfaction seen in distal hypospadias [10]
Erectile dysfunction, difficult and infrequent intercourse is seen in proximal hypospadias [56]
Lower sexual satisfaction if genital perception is poor [24]
Dribbling of ejaculate may be due to poor spongiosal/muscular support or urethral stricture [7, 19]
Testicular volume, testosterone, and semen are normal unless testes are undescended [19, 62]
Fertility and paternity lower in proximal hypospadias [13, 69]

priate psychological counseling after corrective surgery, and extended follow-up till adulthood may offer the necessary support to these patients and also improve our understanding of this often neglected aspect of hypospadias [42, 72].

References

1. Singh JC, Jayanthi VR, Gopalakrishnan G. Effect of hypospadias on sexual function and reproduction. Indian J Urol. 2008;24:249–52.
2. Hoag CC, Gotto GT, Morrison KB, et al. Long-term functional outcome and satisfaction of patients with hypospadias repaired in childhood. Can Urol Assoc J. 2008;2:23–31. https://doi.org/10.5489/cuaj.521.
3. Jones BC, O'Brien M, Chase J, et al. Early hypospadias surgery may lead to a better long-term psychosexual outcome. J Urol. 2009;182:1744–9. https://doi.org/10.1016/j.juro.2009.02.089.
4. Adams J, Bracka A. Reconstructive surgery for hypospadias: a systematic review of long-term patient satisfaction with cosmetic outcomes. Indian J Urol. 2016;32:93–102. https://doi.org/10.4103/0970-1591.179178.
5. Mureau MA, Slijper FM, Nijman RJ, et al. Psychosexual adjustment of children and adolescents after different types of hypospadias surgery: a norm-related study. J Urol. 1995;154:1902–7.
6. Mureau MA, Slijper FM, Slob AK, Verhulst FC. Psychosocial functioning of children, adolescents, and adults following hypospadias surgery: a comparative study. J Pediatr Psychol. 1997;22:371–87. https://doi.org/10.1093/jpepsy/22.3.371.
7. Nelson CP, Bloom DA, Kinast R, et al. Patient-reported sexual function after oral mucosa graft urethroplasty for hypospadias. Urology. 2005;66:1086–9.; discussion 1089-1090. https://doi.org/10.1016/j.urology.2005.05.057.
8. Kiss A, Sulya B, Szász AM, et al. Long-term psychological and sexual outcomes of severe penile hypospadias repair. J Sex Med. 2011;8:1529–39. https://doi.org/10.1111/j.1743-6109.2010.02120.x.
9. Schönbucher VB, Landolt MA, Gobet R, Weber DM. Psychosexual development of children and adolescents with hypospadias. J Sex Med. 2008;5:1365–73. https://doi.org/10.1111/j.1743-6109.2007.00742.x.
10. Majstorovic M, Bizic M, Nikolic D, et al. Psychosexual functioning outcome testing after hypospadias repair. Healthcare (Basel). 2020;8:32. https://doi.org/10.3390/healthcare8010032.
11. Berg R, Berg G, Edman G, et al. Androgens and personality in normal men and men operated for hypospadias in childhood. Acta Psychiatrica Scandinavica. 1983;68:167–77. https://doi.org/10.1111/j.1600-0447.1983.tb06996.x.
12. Sandberg DE, Meyer-Bahlburg HF, Aranoff GS, et al. Boys with hypospadias: a survey of behavioral difficulties. J Pediatr Psychol. 1989;14:491–514. https://doi.org/10.1093/jpepsy/14.4.491.
13. Örtqvist L, Fossum M, Andersson M, et al. Sexuality and fertility in men with hypospadias; improved outcome. Andrology. 2017;5:286–93. https://doi.org/10.1111/andr.12309.
14. Sung JY, Han SW, Chung K-M, et al. Investigation of gender role behaviors in boys with hypospadias: comparative study with unaffected boys and girls. J Pediatr Psychol. 2014;39:1061–9. https://doi.org/10.1093/jpepsy/jsu055.
15. Blotcky MJ, Grossman I. Psychological implications of childhood genitourinary surgery: an empirical study. J Am Acad Child Psychiatry. 1978;17:488–97. https://doi.org/10.1016/S0002-7138(09)62303-7.
16. Bracka A. Sexuality after hypospadias repair. BJU Int. 1999;83(Suppl 3):29–33. https://doi.org/10.1046/j.1464-410x.1999.0830s3029.x.
17. Tack LJW, Springer A, Riedl S, et al. Psychosexual outcome, sexual function, and long-term satisfaction of adolescent and young adult men after childhood hypospadias repair. J Sex Med. 2020;17(9):1665–75. https://doi.org/10.1016/j.jsxm.2020.04.002.
18. Mureau MA, Slijper FM, Slob AK, Verhulst FC. Psychosocial functioning of children, adolescents, and adults following hypospadias surgery: a comparative study. J Pediatr Psychol. 1997;22:371–87. https://doi.org/10.1093/jpepsy/22.3.371.
19. Bracka A. A long-term view of hypospadias. Br J Plast Surg. 1989;42:251–5. https://doi.org/10.1016/0007-1226(89)90140-9.
20. van der Werff JF, Ultee J. Long-term follow-up of hypospadias repair. Br J Plast Surg. 2000;53:588–92. https://doi.org/10.1054/bjps.2000.3395.
21. Vandendriessche S, Baeyens D, Van Hoecke E, et al. Body image and sexuality in adolescents after hypospadias surgery. J Pediatr Urol. 2010;6:54–9. https://doi.org/10.1016/j.jpurol.2009.04.009.
22. Mondaini N, Ponchietti R, Bonafè M, et al. Hypospadias: incidence and effects on psychosexual development as evaluated with the Minnesota Multiphasic Personality Inventory test in a sample of 11,649 young Italian men. Urol Int. 2002;68:81–5. https://doi.org/10.1159/000048423.
23. Svensson J, Berg R, Berg G. Operated hypospadiacs: late follow-up. Social, sexual, and psychological adaptation. J Pediatr Surg. 1981;16:134–5. https://doi.org/10.1016/s0022-3468(81)80338-7.
24. Aho MO, Tammela OK, Somppi EM, Tammela TL. Sexual and social life of men operated in childhood for hypospadias and phimosis. A comparative study. Eur Urol. 2000;37:95–100.; discussion 101. https://doi.org/10.1159/000020107.
25. Chertin B, Natsheh A, Ben-Zion I, et al. Objective and subjective sexual outcomes in adult patients after hypospadias repair performed in childhood. J Urol. 2013;190:1556–60. https://doi.org/10.1016/j.juro.2012.12.104.

26. Bubanj TB, Perovic SV, Milicevic RM, et al. Sexual behavior and sexual function of adults after hypospadias surgery: a comparative study. J Urol. 2004;171:1876–9. https://doi.org/10.1097/01.ju.0000119337.19471.51.
27. Kenawi MM. Sexual function in hypospadiacs. Br J Urol. 1975;47:883–90. https://doi.org/10.1111/j.1464-410x.1975.tb04072.x.
28. Bhat AL, Sabarwal KV, Singhla M, Saran RK. 1149 A prospective study of sexual functions in hypospadiacs operated in adulthood. J Urol. 2012;187:e466. https://doi.org/10.1016/j.juro.2012.02.1259.
29. Berg R, Svensson J, Aström G. Social and sexual adjustment of men operated for hypospadias during childhood: a controlled study. J Urol. 1981;125:313–7. https://doi.org/10.1016/s0022-5347(17)55019-3.
30. Wang W-W, Tu X-A, Deng C-H, et al. Long-term sexual activity status and influencing factors in men after surgery for hypospadias. Asian J Androl. 2009;11:417–22. https://doi.org/10.1038/aja.2008.60.
31. Jiao C, Wu R, Xu X, Yu Q. Long-term outcome of penile appearance and sexual function after hypospadias repairs: situation and relation. Int Urol Nephrol. 2011;43:47–54. https://doi.org/10.1007/s11255-010-9775-y.
32. Avellán L. The development of puberty, the sexual début and sexual function in hypospadiacs. Scand J Plast Reconstr Surg. 1976;10:29–44. https://doi.org/10.1080/02844317609169744.
33. Eberle J, Uberreiter S, Radmayr C, et al. Posterior hypospadias: long-term followup after reconstructive surgery in the male direction. J Urol. 1993;150:1474–7. https://doi.org/10.1016/s0022-5347(17)35814-7.
34. Miller MA, Grant DB. Severe hypospadias with genital ambiguity: adult outcome after staged hypospadias repair. Br J Urol. 1997;80:485–8. https://doi.org/10.1046/j.1464-410x.1997.00348.x.
35. Liu G, Yuan J, Feng J, et al. Factors affecting the long-term results of hypospadias repairs. J Pediatr Surg. 2006;41:554–9. https://doi.org/10.1016/j.jpedsurg.2005.11.051.
36. Sommerlad BC. A long-term follow-up of hypospadias patients. Br J Plast Surg. 1975;28:324–30. https://doi.org/10.1016/0007-1226(75)90044-2.
37. Ruppen-Greeff NK, Weber DM, Gobet R, Landolt MA. Health-related quality of life in men with corrected hypospadias: an explorative study. J Pediatr Urol. 2013;9:551–8. https://doi.org/10.1016/j.jpurol.2013.04.016.
38. Schönbucher VB, Landolt MA, Gobet R, Weber DM. Health-related quality of life and psychological adjustment of children and adolescents with hypospadias. J Pediatr. 2008;152:865–72. https://doi.org/10.1016/j.jpeds.2007.11.036.
39. Andersson M, Sjöström S, Wängqvist M, et al. Psychosocial and sexual outcomes in adolescents following surgery for proximal hypospadias in childhood. J Urol. 2018;200:1362–70. https://doi.org/10.1016/j.juro.2018.06.032.
40. Wu W-H, Chuang J-H, Ting Y-C, et al. Developmental anomalies and disabilities associated with hypospadias. J Urol. 2002;168:229–32.
41. Flynn JT, Johnston SR, Blandy JP. Late sequelae of hypospadias repair. Br J Urol. 1980;52:555–9. https://doi.org/10.1111/j.1464-410x.1980.tb03114.x.
42. Moriya K, Kakizaki H, Tanaka H, et al. Long-term cosmetic and sexual outcome of hypospadias surgery: norm related study in adolescence. J Urol. 2006;176:1889–92.; discussion 1892-1893. https://doi.org/10.1016/S0022-5347(06)00600-8.
43. Ciancio F, Lo Russo G, Innocenti A, et al. Penile length is a very important factor for cosmesis, function and psychosexual development in patients affected by hypospadias: results from a long-term longitudinal cohort study. Int J Immunopathol Pharmacol. 2015;28:421–5. https://doi.org/10.1177/0394632015576857.
44. Baskin L. Hypospadias: a critical analysis of cosmetic outcomes using photography. BJU Int. 2001;87:534–9. https://doi.org/10.1046/j.1464-410x.2001.00092.x.
45. Rynja SP, de Jong TPVM, Bosch JLHR, de Kort LMO. Testosterone prior to hypospadias repair: postoperative complication rates and long-term cosmetic results, penile length and body height. J Pediatr Urol. 2018;14:31.e1–8. https://doi.org/10.1016/j.jpurol.2017.09.020.
46. Aho MO, Tammela OK, Tammela TL. Aspects of adult satisfaction with the result of surgery for hypospadias performed in childhood. Eur Urol. 1997;32:218–22.
47. Weber DM, Schönbucher VB, Gobet R, Landolt M. Self perception of genitalia after hypospadia repair. J Pediatr Urol. 2007;3:S52. https://doi.org/10.1016/j.jpurol.2007.01.085.
48. Holland AJ, Smith GH, Ross FI, Cass DT. HOSE: an objective scoring system for evaluating the results of hypospadias surgery. BJU Int. 2001;88:255–8. https://doi.org/10.1046/j.1464-410x.2001.02280.x.
49. Weber DM, Schönbucher VB, Landolt MA, Gobet R. The Pediatric Penile Perception Score: an instrument for patient self-assessment and surgeon evaluation after hypospadias repair. J Urol. 2008;180:1080–4.; discussion 1084. https://doi.org/10.1016/j.juro.2008.05.060.
50. van der Toorn F, de Jong TPVM, de Gier RPE, et al. Introducing the HOPE (Hypospadias Objective Penile Evaluation)-score: a validation study of an objective scoring system for evaluating cosmetic appearance in hypospadias patients. J Pediatr Urol. 2013;9:1006–16. https://doi.org/10.1016/j.jpurol.2013.01.015.
51. Merriman LS, Arlen AM, Broecker BH, et al. The GMS hypospadias score: assessment of inter-observer reliability and correlation with post-operative complications. Journal of Pediatric Urology. 2013;9:707–12. https://doi.org/10.1016/j.jpurol.2013.04.006.
52. Ruppen-Greeff NK, Weber DM, Gobet R, Landolt MA. What is a good looking penis? How women rate the penile appearance of men with surgically corrected hypospadias. J Sex Med. 2015;12:1737–45. https://doi.org/10.1111/jsm.12942.

53. Ruppen-Greeff NK, Landolt MA, Gobet R, Weber DM. Appraisal of adult genitalia after hypospadias repair: Do laypersons mind the difference? J Pediatr Urol. 2016;12:32.e1–8. https://doi.org/10.1016/j.jpurol.2015.09.012.
54. Schlomer B, Breyer B, Copp H, et al. Do adult men with untreated hypospadias have adverse outcomes? A pilot study using a social media advertised survey. J Pediatr Urol. 2014;10:672–9. https://doi.org/10.1016/j.jpurol.2014.01.024.
55. Chertin B, Prat D, Shenfeld OZ. Outcome of pediatric hypospadias repair in adulthood. Open Access J Urol. 2010;2:57–62. https://doi.org/10.2147/rru.s6523.
56. Rynja SP, de Jong TPVM, Bosch JLHR, de Kort LMO. Proximal hypospadias treated with a transverse preputial island tube: long-term functional, sexual, and cosmetic outcomes. BJU Int. 2018;122:463–71. https://doi.org/10.1111/bju.14234.
57. Rynja SP, Wouters GA, Van Schaijk M, et al. Long-term followup of hypospadias: functional and cosmetic results. J Urol. 2009;182:1736–43. https://doi.org/10.1016/j.juro.2009.03.073.
58. Rynja S, Bosch R, Kok E, et al. IIEF-15: unsuitable for assessing erectile function of young men? J Sex Med. 2010;7:2825–30. https://doi.org/10.1111/j.1743-6109.2010.01847.x.
59. Lam PN, Greenfield SP, Williot P. 2-stage repair in infancy for severe hypospadias with chordee: long-term results after puberty. J Urol. 2005;174:1567–72.; discussion 1572. https://doi.org/10.1097/01.ju.0000179395.99944.48.
60. Mieusset R, Soulié M. Hypospadias: psychosocial, sexual, and reproductive consequences in adult life. J Androl. 2005;26:163–8. https://doi.org/10.1002/j.1939-4640.2005.tb01078.x.
61. van der Horst HJR, de Wall LL. Hypospadias, all there is to know. Eur J Pediatr. 2017;176:435–41. https://doi.org/10.1007/s00431-017-2864-5.
62. Asklund C, Jensen TK, Main KM, et al. Semen quality, reproductive hormones and fertility of men operated for hypospadias. Int J Androl. 2010;33:80–7. https://doi.org/10.1111/j.1365-2605.2009.00957.x.
63. Moriya K, Mitsui T, Tanaka H, et al. Long-term outcome of pituitary-gonadal axis and gonadal growth in patients with hypospadias at puberty. J Urol. 2010;184:1610–4. https://doi.org/10.1016/j.juro.2010.04.022.
64. Kumar S, Tomar V, Yadav SS, et al. Fertility Potential in Adult Hypospadias. J Clin Diagn Res. 2016;10:PC01-05. https://doi.org/10.7860/JCDR/2016/21307.8276.
65. Moriya K, Nakamura M, Kon M, et al. Risk factors affecting post-pubertal high serum follicle-stimulating hormone in patients with hypospadias. World J Urol. 2019;37:2795–9. https://doi.org/10.1007/s00345-019-02687-w.
66. Berg G, Berg R. Castration complex. Evidence from men operated for hypospadias. Acta Psychiatr Scand. 1983;68:143–53. https://doi.org/10.1111/j.1600-0447.1983.tb06994.x.
67. Kanematsu A. Response and rebuttal to editorial comment regarding "multivariate analyses of the factors associated with sexual intercourse, marriage, and paternity of hypospadias patients.". J Sex Med. 2016;13:1497. https://doi.org/10.1016/j.jsxm.2016.08.009.
68. Spinoit A-F, Waterschoot M, Sinatti C, et al. Fertility and sexuality issues in congenital lifelong urology patients: male aspects. World J Urol. 2021;39(4):1013–9. https://doi.org/10.1007/s00345-020-03121-2.
69. Skarin Nordenvall A, Chen Q, Norrby C, et al. Fertility in adult men born with hypospadias: a nationwide register-based cohort study on birthrates, the use of assisted reproductive technologies and infertility. Andrology. 2020;8:372–80. https://doi.org/10.1111/andr.12723.
70. Schneuer FJ, Milne E, Jamieson SE, et al. Association between male genital anomalies and adult male reproductive disorders: a population-based data linkage study spanning more than 40 years. Lancet Child Adolesc Health. 2018;2:736–43. https://doi.org/10.1016/S2352-4642(18)30254-2.
71. Kanematsu A, Tanaka S, Hashimoto T, et al. Analysis of the association between paternity and reoperation for urethral obstruction in adult hypospadias patients who underwent two-stage repair in childhood. BMC Urol. 2019;19:88. https://doi.org/10.1186/s12894-019-0512-2.
72. Deibert CM, Hensle TW. The psychosexual aspects of hypospadias repair: a review. Arab J Urol. 2011;9:279–82. https://doi.org/10.1016/j.aju.2011.10.004.

28

Current Status Evaluation of Hypospadias Repair Results

M. A. Baky Fahmy

Abbreviations

AYA	Adolescents and Young Adults
DSD	Disorders of Sex Development
GMS	Glans–Meatus–Shaft
HOPE	Hypospadias Objective Penile Evaluation
HOSE	Hypospadias Objective Scoring Evaluation
IIEF	International Index of Erectile Function
PPPS	Paediatric Penile Perception Score
TIP	Tubularized Incised Plate

28.1 Introduction

The imagination and creativity of surgeons for centuries dealing with hypospadias have been challenged to create a functional and cosmetically acceptable phallus. Numerous new operations and techniques have been developed to achieve improved aesthetic results with fewer complications over the last 30 years. The current goals of hypospadias surgery are creating a straight penis with the meatus at the glans tip, creating a urethra of adequate and uniform calibre, symmetrical appearance of the glans and shaft, and possible normalization of erections and voiding [1].

The postoperative complications rate of hypospadias repair are still high, vary from 12 to 24% in the first years after surgery, and may go up to 60% in the long-term follow-up [2]. The incidence of late complications is directly related to the assemblage of other associated anomalies and the complexity of the repair; it is globally different from centre to centre, with a wide spectrum of presentations, previously it was around 24% in tertiary care centres [3], and the most common complication is a fistula, followed by meatal stenosis, penile curvature, and micturition related problems.

However, recent shreds of evidence suggest that complication rates for hypospadias repair may be greater than reported, approaching 50% for proximal hypospadias [4].

Some of these complications can be treated easily, like meatal stenosis, and some may need repetitive surgeries like fistula complications. End-stage renal affection may follow simple meatal stenosis or urethral stricture if it is not recognized early or not managed properly, especially if an inexperienced surgeon does urethroplasty or if the child is not precisely followed up.

A meticulously designed meatus during commences of hypospadias repair and a simple postoperative technique like meatal dilation may preserve renal function in a considerable number of cases. It may improve the future quality of life for those children.

Proper evaluation of hypospadias repair is crucial for both the operating surgeons and the affected children. Therefore, global standardiz-

M. A. Baky Fahmy (✉)
Pediatric Surgery, Al-Azhar University, Cairo, Egypt

ing the evaluating scores for different follow-up aspects is the main core for auditing this common anomaly.

28.2 Preoperative Evaluation and Scoring

Proper evaluation of the hypospadias repair results should be extended to include an early precise preoperative assessment, as the different types of hypospadias and chordee degrees require various operations, have diverse complication rates, and different prognoses. On the other hand, some researchers may still argue that the complication rate may not correlate exactly with the degree of hypospadias nor the preoperative symptoms.

To improve treatment and comparison across centres and surgeons, a clear and consistent classification is necessary to standardize the hypospadias terminology. Though there are many classifications for hypospadias, the first, simplest, and practical classification was described a long time ago in 1886 by Kaufmann [5].

Later on, Duckett [6] classified hypospadias depending on the exact site of the meatus and presence or absence of chordee into eight subgroups (glanular, coronal, subcoronal, distal penile, mid-penile, proximal penile, penoscrotal, and perineal). Accordingly, one may choose the techniques designed for either distal or proximal hypospadias. But children with hypospadias associated with penile and gonadal anomalies should be classified under DSD (Fig. 28.1).

Microphallus is common in severe hypospadias. Gender assignment, endocrinal measurement, and the possibility of proper endocrinal treatment should be evaluated before the decision of surgical correction in such cases, especially when bilateral impalpable undescended testicles are associating the case. The hypospadias repair is warranted only after assigning the gender as male. Underdeveloped scrotum with bilateral cryptorchidism usually limits hypospadias reconstruction, so orchidopexy and properly staged hypospadias reconstruction are the best choice, preceding endocrinal management and orchidopexy are helpful for local tissue augmentation and decrease the rate of complication risk [7].

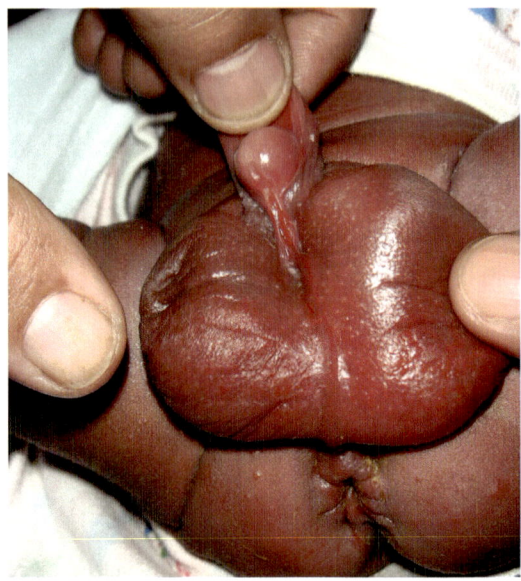

Fig. 28.1 Neonate with proximal hypospadias "scrotal", small phallus, severe chordee, and scrotal transposition, such case should be categorized as DSD

At 2004 Hadidi and Azmy [8], suggested that preoperative evaluation could be completed at the first operation for proper assessment by considering glans configuration, urethral opening, and quality of the penile skin. However, a two-stage procedure may be necessary in some cases, and this assessment may not be valid. The surgeon should evaluate the patient under good illumination with magnification and perception of the following features:

1. Glans configuration (cleft, incomplete cleft, or flat).
2. Urethral opening (if narrow, it should be dilated or incised).
3. Quality of the skin on the ventral aspect of the penis distal to the urethral meatus.
4. Quality of the skin proximal to the urethral opening (sometimes it is very thin and requires incision).
5. The scrotum (ensure that both testes are in the scrotum and exclude bifid scrotum and penoscrotal transposition).

A simple sheet including these items could be used for this unpretentious preoperative evaluation, even by junior staff (Fig. 28.2).

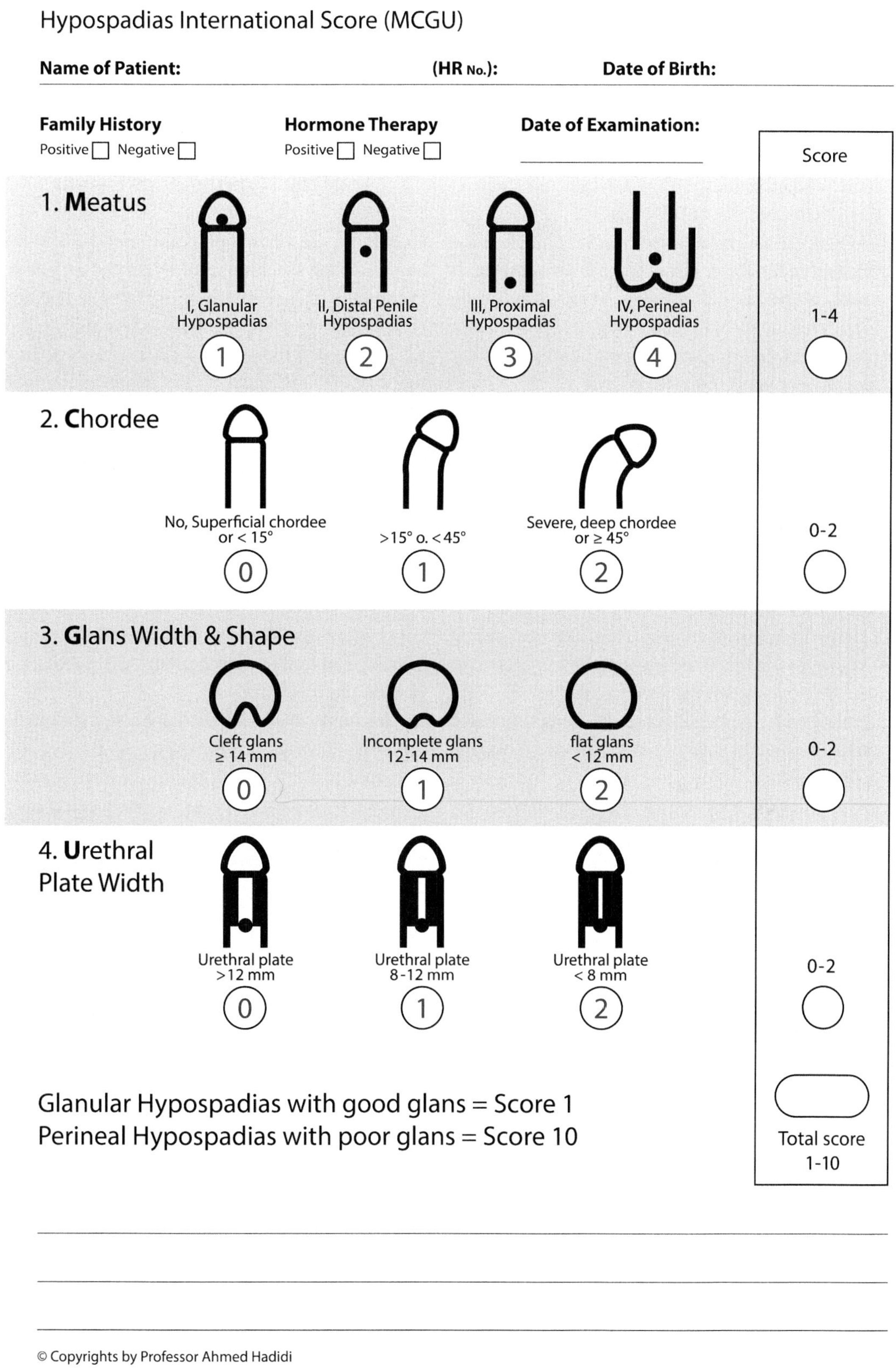

Hypospadias International Score (MCGU)

Name of Patient: **(HR No.):**   **Date of Birth:**

Family History   **Hormone Therapy**   **Date of Examination:**
Positive ☐ Negative ☐   Positive ☐ Negative ☐

Score

1. Meatus

I, Glanular Hypospadias	II, Distal Penile Hypospadias	III, Proximal Hypospadias	IV, Perineal Hypospadias
1	2	3	4

Score: 1-4

2. Chordee

No, Superficial chordee or < 15°	>15° o. <45°	Severe, deep chordee or ≥ 45°
0	1	2

Score: 0-2

3. Glans Width & Shape

Cleft glans ≥ 14 mm	Incomplete glans 12-14 mm	flat glans < 12 mm
0	1	2

Score: 0-2

4. Urethral Plate Width

Urethral plate >12 mm	Urethral plate 8-12 mm	Urethral plate < 8 mm
0	1	2

Score: 0-2

Glanular Hypospadias with good glans = Score 1
Perineal Hypospadias with poor glans = Score 10

Total score 1-10

© Copyrights by Professor Ahmed Hadidi

Fig. 28.2 Hypospadias score sheet [8]

Importantly though, the surgeon has to consider the preoperative anatomic assessment of the glans–meatus–shaft (GMS) scoring, and recently a multivariate binary logistic regression analysis found the urethral plate, glandular groove, and glans shape were proved to be a more predictive factor for the fistula and stenosis complications [9].

Difficulty in classification will occur when the scrotum is distally transposed or when a different grade of penile curvature is present; ignoring these two items will end with a non-aesthetic penile look and may result in an inappropriately functioning penis (Fig. 28.3).

Radojicic and Perovic [10] found the correlation between morphology and vascularization of the prepuce and their impact on results of hypospadias repair, they reported morphological characteristics and their correlation with hypospadiac prepuce vascularization. The underdeveloped foreskin with an unfavourable vascular pattern, when used for urethroplasty, had higher complications. The severe hypospadias, the anatomical features of the prepuce have a greater influence in deciding one or two stages of repair.

However, in the absence of comprehensive paediatric penile anthropometry nomograms, the assessments are often subjective and are prone to have an interobserver variation. Furthermore, few studies describe penile anthropometry in children beyond neonatal age, and most of the publications have consider only the penile length and diameter [11]. In addition, there is a scarcity of data on normal glans concerned anthropometry, normal penile angles, and penoscrotal orientation, although similar ethnicity of study population poses another limitation.

28.3 Postoperative Evaluation of the Hypospadias Repair

Generally, measurement is the core of any science. But the assessment of hypospadias surgery is confined only to redo surgery rates and postoperative complications such as fistula and stenosis during the previous two decades. However, from the start of this century, the advances in techniques in specialist centres had consistently lowered complication rates. This has led to focus more on the subjective measures of voiding function, aesthetic look, psychosexual outcomes, and patient or parental satisfaction. In addition, the urinary flow rate assessment after hypospadias repair has been recently prompted with the availability of simpler equipment and theoretical concerns of an increased risk of neourethral stricture, which is mainly complicating the tubularized incised plate (TIP) repair.

Cosmetic result assessment of hypospadias repair is inherently a subjective one. But recently, several researchers tried to introduce an objective criterion by the participation of healthcare professionals and also the parents. They are asked to share in the score evaluation of the aesthetic outcome of hypospadias repair by evaluating a series of standardized postoperative photographs. In one of such studies: the aesthetic result of the TIP repair was rated significantly better than the Mathieu repair for evaluation of the meatus, glans, shaft, and the overall penile appearance [12].

A validated scheme for the hypospadias repair evaluation was missing in the literature until the publication of the hypospadias objective scoring evaluation (HOSE) system score in 2001 [13]. Unfortunately, the uniformly recorded data in all repairs globally is missing. Applying the HOSE scoring system at all centres worldwide will help to compare the outcome of various techniques and decision-making, this will allow to counsel the parents preoperatively before deciding to consent for surgery.

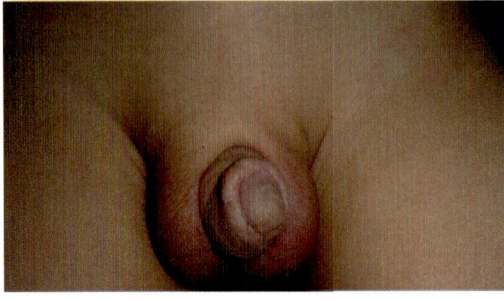

Fig. 28.3 Despite a well-formed hypospadias repair, and this child still had unrecognized scrotal transposition, which reduces the actual functioning penile length

The shortcoming of the scoring system is that it does not assess relevant cosmetic variables like scrotal position, the shape of the glans, or the penile skin. Also, about the psychometric properties of the HOSE-score, only the interobserver reliability was tested.

So latter on (Hypospadias Objective Penile Evaluation), HOPE scoring system was developed to incorporate all surgically correctable variables: meatus position, meatus shape, glans shape, penile skin shape, and penile axis objectivity with standardized photographs, and anonymously coded patients, independent assessment by a panel, standards for a "normal" penile appearance, reference pictures, and assessment of abnormality degree [14].

In 2006, Toorn et al. [15] developed and presented the Hypospadias Penile Perception Score (HPPS), which incorporated all relevant surgically correctable variables through a set of standardized photographs and a panel assessing anonymous patients.

Validating instruments is painstaking work that requires meticulously following the highest methodological and technical standards, so other research projects went through this process to improve the instruments.

As the HOPE score solely reports the aesthetic outcome assessed by a physician, it must be supplemented with additional tools that evaluate the patient or caregiver satisfaction. So the Paediatric Penile Perception Score (PPPS) assesses patient or parental satisfaction of the genital appearance, which has been shown to differ from the surgeons' opinion regarding the aesthetic outcome [16].

PPPS instrument proved to be practical to use, and the good internal consistency indicates its reliability. However, the high patient satisfaction similar to the control group was not anticipated and may contradict some of the few publications available. Good self-perception could reflect the improvement of surgical results that have been achieved with contemporary techniques. However, it seems unlikely that this is the main reason for the parents and the surgeon evaluation, and other factors must be meditated.

More recently, the attention to assessing the chordee and its correction (orthoplasty) emerged, especially after a long-term follow-up. Penile curvature may be evaluated in the infant or child who has an erection at the time of examination; intraoperative assessment after penile shaft skin degloving by artificial erection which is usually achieved by injection of normal saline with a fine needle into the corpora directly or by insertion of the needle through the lateral aspect of one or the other corpora cavernosa [17].

Severe ventral curvature of the penis of 30° or more may impede normal sexual intercourse later on. Usually, it has a negative impact on the psychosexual functions in adulthood (Fig. 28.4). As a result, various techniques for straightening the penis has come into existence. However, on the other hand, preserving the neurovascular bundle remains precarious to maintain the glans sensitivity and thus avoid potential sexual dysfunction in the future.

In my opinion, the use of photography is neither a reliable nor an objective tool for judgement of the proper penile appeal; comparison between different photos by different cameras, with various resolutions and the varied focal distance, is extremely difficult or impossible, so using the digital callipers, measuring scale, and calibrated angle metre should be popularized and standardized for both anthropometry nomograms and evaluation of the results of penile reconstructive surgeries (Fig. 28.5).

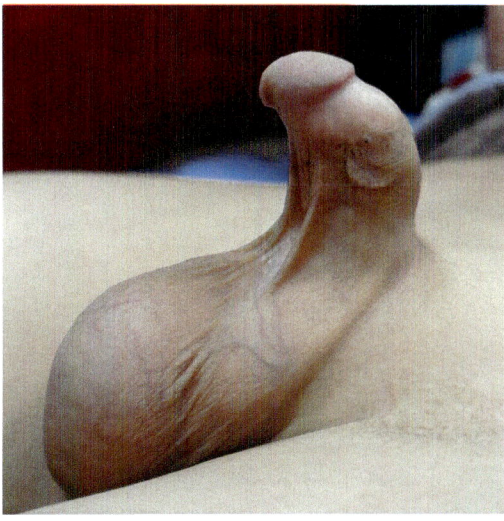

Fig. 28.4 Severe residual penile chordee after a repaired distal hypospadias

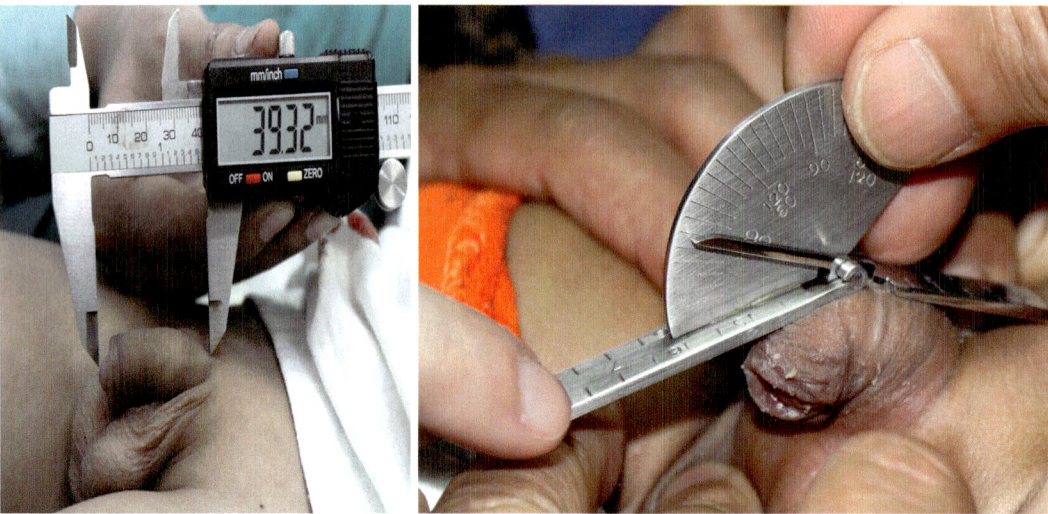

Fig. 28.5 Digital measuring scale and calibrated angle metre for precise penile anthropometric assessment

28.4 Psychosexual Outcome

Long-term psychological and psychosexual sequelae of hypospadias and their management are the most difficult aspects hypospadias repair to be quantified. The surveys and psychological tests in the 1990s inevitably reflect the unsatisfactory results achieved by outdated multistage procedures repair, and the surgery was generally undertaken at an older age. For example, Mureau et al. [18] reported that semi-structured interview studies in the Netherlands were conducted in men who had previously undergone hypospadias surgery, showed normal sexual adjustment, and experienced a normal adult sexual life. However, they expressed a more negative genital appraisal. Moreover, 37% sought further penile surgery to improve their functional or cosmetic outcome.

More recently, Mondiani et al. [19] compared variables of psychosexual adjustment in 42 men previously treated for hypospadias with a random sample of 500 unaffected men and found no differences in sexual function between the groups.

Most of the time, sexual function is normal or with minimal deviation after a successful correction of hypospadias. An erection should be obtainable, and fertility should not be affected unless the patient had associated undescended or atrophic testicles or some forms of severe DSD. There has been considerable concern about these men's psychosocial and sexual outcomes, but a recent psychosocial study appears to refute this concern. A study used standardized questionnaires to compare psychosocial function in 189 children and adults who had undergone hypospadias surgery. They were compared with an age-matched set of controls who had undergone an inguinal herniotomy. There was no difference in psychosocial functioning between the groups [20]. The rate of sexually active cases increased with age. Still, it was consistently lower than in controls, which agrees with other studies showing a slightly delayed period at sexarche and masturbarche [21].

The erectile and sexual functions were suboptimal in approximately 10% of cases. Only mild erectile dysfunction was found, but no factors could be identified that could underlie the occurrence of erectile dysfunction. Diverse ejaculation problems were reported by a small number of participants in many studies. However, the lack of a standardized screening tool for ejaculation problems makes the comparison between studies more or less ponderous. Therefore, milking of the ejaculate, anejaculation, and other issues have been inconsistently reported. Still, if specifically asked for, such problems seem to affect a significant proportion of men who had a previous hypospadias repair [22].

Generally, a respectable number of adolescents and young adults (AYA) who underwent hypospadiac surgeries were afraid to be mocked when naked compared to controls (20%). The most reported reasons mentioned by cases were shame, their genitals look different from their peer, smaller penis, and most of them being circumcised after hypospadias surgeries.

The International Index of Erectile Function (IIEF-5) is an abbreviated screening tool for erectile dysfunction based on the IIEF-15 questionnaire, which may be more accurate for assessing sexuality for hypospadiac cases [23].

Generally, men born with hypospadias have a good long-term outcome concerning sexual function and fertility than older reports. This indicates that surgical results and medical care have improved over the last decades, reflecting on the beneficent results for most hypospadias cases. But men with proximal forms are still present with lower fertility and are less satisfied with their sexual life. Of course, satisfaction with genital cosmetics is also essential for sound sexual life satisfaction. However, the acceptance of the cosmetic result is even more important. Clinical and psychological follow-up into adulthood is substantial, especially in boys born with proximal hypospadias [21].

The overall psychosexual outcome of a male suffering from hypospadias is unsteady but not comparable to normal healthy male peers. The most important factors associated with an impaired outcome were frequent penile surgeries and dissatisfaction regarding their penile aesthetic look. Importantly, these factors also seem involved in their satisfaction regarding hypospadias repair. Furthermore, most men were satisfied with their penile appearance, although the treating physicians may not perceive the final penile look after repeated surgeries as normal. Thus, accepting a more or less suboptimal aesthetic outcome as a physician could ultimately prove is more important for psychosexual well-being.

28.5 Fertility

Several studies have reported that severe hypospadias patients are more at risk of reduced fertility. Fertility issues and worry were most common in proximal cases of hypospadias and with more penile surgeries than controls (25.9% vs 12.0%, respectively) [24].

Nowadays, most of the hypospadiologists are facing a considerable number of new cases of hypospadias born to a father who had a previous hypospadiac surgery, and such cases are challenging for the operating surgeon to convince the family about the surgical and functional outcomes, where usually there is a decision regret after healthcare decisions.

References

1. Spinout AF, Poelaert F, Groen L, Van Laecke E, Hoebeke P. Hypospadias repair at a tertiary care center: long-term follow-up is mandatory to determine the real complication rate. J Urol. 2013;189(6):2276–81.
2. Winberg H, et al. The complication rate after hypospadias repair and correlated preoperative symptoms. Open J Urol. 2014;4:155–62. http://www.scirp.org/journal/oju. https://doi.org/10.4236/oju.2014.412027.
3. Retik AB, Atala A. Complications of hypospadias repair. Urol Clin N Am. 2002;29:329–39.
4. Pohl HG, Rana S, Sprague BM, Beamer M, Rushton HG. Discrepant rates of hypospadias surgical complications: a comparison of U.S. News & World Report and Pediatric Health Information System! Data and published literature. J Urol. 2020;203:616–23. https://doi.org/10.1097/JU.0000000000000554.
5. Kaufmann C. Verletzungen und Krankenheiten der männlichen Harnröhre und des Penis. In: Bilrothe T, Luecke A, editors. Deutsche Chirurgie. Lieferung 50a. Stuttgart: Verlag von Ferdinand Enke; 1886., Chap 5. p. 18–39.
6. Duckett JW. Hypospadias. In: Gillenwater JY, Grayhack JT, Howards SS, Duckett JW, editors. Adult and pediatric urology. 3rd ed. St. Louis: Mosby Year Book; 1996. p. 2550.
7. Spinoit A-F, Poelaert F, Van Praet C, et al. Grade of hypospadias is the only factor predicting for re-intervention after primary hypospadias repair: a multivariate analysis from a cohort of 474 patients. J Pediatr Urol. 2015;11(70):e1–6.
8. Hadidi AT, Azmy AF, editors. Hypospadias surgery: an illustrated guide. 1st ed. London: Springer Verlag; 2004. Reproduced with the kind permission of Springer Verlag

9. Güler Y. TIPU outcomes for hypospadias treatment and predictive factors causing urethrocutaneous fistula and external urethral meatus stenosis in TIPU: clinical study. Andrologia. 2020;52(9):e13668. https://doi.org/10.1111/and.13668.
10. Radojicic ZI, Perovic SV. Classification of the prepuce in hypospadias according to morphological abnormalities and their impact on hypospadias repair. J Urol. 2004;172:301–4. https://doi.org/10.1097/01.ju.0000129008.31212.3d.
11. Puri A, Sikdar S, Prakash R. Pediatric penile and glans anthropometry nomograms: an aid in hypospadias management. J Indian Assoc Pediatr Surg. 2017;22:9–12.
12. Gough DCS, Ververidis M, Dickson AP. An objective assessment of the results of hypospadias surgery. BJU Int. 2003;91(Suppl. 1):62.
13. Holland AJ, Smith GH, Ross FI, Cass DT. HOSE: an objective scoring system for evaluating the results of hypospadias surgery. BJU Int. 2001;88:255–8. https://doi.org/10.1046/j.1464-410x.2001.02280.
14. van der Toorn F, Scheepe JR, Essnk-Bot ML, Borsboom GJJM, Wolffenbuttel KP, van den Hoek J. HPPS: a validated scoring system for evaluating cosmetic result after hypospadias surgery. J Ped Urol. 2006;2:135.
15. Toorn F, de Jong T, de Gier RE, et al. Introducing the HOPE (hypospadias objective penile evaluation)-score: a validation study of an objective scoring system for evaluating cosmetic appearance in hypospadias patients. J Pediatr Urol. 2013;9:1006–17.
16. Haid B, Becker T, Koen M, et al. Penile appearance after hypospadias correction from a parent's point of view: comparison of the hypospadias objective penile evaluation score and parents penile perception score. J Pediatr Urol. 2016;12(33):e1–7.
17. Menon V, Breyer B, Copp HL, et al. Do adult men with untreated ventral penile curvature have adverse outcomes? J Pediatr Urol. 2016;12:31.e1ee7.
18. Mureau MA, Slijper FM, van der Meulen JC, Verhulst FC. Psychosexual adjustment of men who underwent hypospadias surgery; a norm–related study. J Urol. 1995;154:1351–5.
19. Mondiani N, Ponchietti R, Bonafe M, et al. Hypospadias. Incidence and effects on psychosexual development as evaluated with the Minnesota multiphasic personality inventory test in a sample of 11,649 young Italian men. Urol Int. 2002;68:81–5.
20. Wilcox DT, Ransley PG. Medicolegal aspects of hypospadias. BJU Int. 2000;86:327–13.
21. Örtqvist L, Fossum M, Andersson M, Nordenström A, Frisén L, Holmdahl G, Nordenskjöld A. Sexuality and fertility in men with hypospadias; improved outcome. Andrology. 2017;5:286–93. https://doi.org/10.1111/andr.12309.
22. Tack LG, Springer A, Riedl S, et al. Psychosexual outcome, sexual function, and long-term satisfaction of adolescent and young adult men after childhood hypospadias repair. J Sex Med. 2020;17:1–11.
23. Rosen RC, Cappelleri JC, Smith MD, et al. Development and evaluation of an abridged, 5-item version of the international index of erectile function (IIEF-5) as a diagnostic tool for erectile dysfunction. Int J Impot Res. 1999;11:319–26.
24. Kumar S, Tomar V, Yadav SS, et al. Fertility potential in adult hypospadias. J Clin Diagn Res. 2016;10:PC01–5.

Radiological Evaluation of Hypospadias Patients

Aparna Prakash, Mahakshit Bhat, and Amilal Bhat

Abbreviation

CECT	Contrast Enhanced Computerized Tomogram
CT	Computerized Tomogram
DSD	Disorders of Sexual Differentiation
MRI	Magnetic Resonance Imaging
RGU	Retrograde Urethrogram
USG	Ultrasonography
VCUG	Voiding Cysto-Urethrogram

A. Prakash
OK Diagnostic and Research Centre,
Jaipur, Rajasthan, India

Department of Radiology, SMS Medical College,
Jaipur, Rajasthan, India

M. Bhat (✉)
Department of Urology, National Institute of Medical Sciences Medical College, Jaipur, Rajasthan, India

A. Bhat
Bhat's Hypospadias and Reconstructive Urology Hospital and Research Centre,
Jaipur, Rajasthan, India

Department of Urology, Jaipur National University Institute for Medical Sciences and Research Centre, Jaipur, Rajasthan, India

Department of Urology, Dr. S.N. Medical College, Jodhpur, Rajasthan, India

Department of Urology, S.P. Medical College, Bikaner, Rajasthan, India

P.G. Committee Medical Council of India,
New Delhi, India

Academic and Research Council of RUHS, Jaipur, Rajasthan, India

29.1 Introduction

Hypospadias is the most common congenital urogenital anomalies in a male child, with an incidence of 3–5 in 1000 live births [1]. Hypospadias is mainly a clinical diagnosis, and imaging has a limited role to play. VCUG and RUG can be used to demonstrate prostatic utricle in hypospadias. However, in the prenatal period, diagnosis is increasingly being made using ultrasonography. Further, MRI and elastography are being used in patients with hypospadias to demonstrate the adequacy of spongiosum, neurovascular bundles, and associated anomalies such as an enlarged prostatic utricle and disorders of sexual differentiation.

29.2 Fetal USG in the Diagnosis of Hypospadias

While human genitalia can be visualized in the antenatal first-trimester scan at 10–11 weeks, it is impossible to differentiate sex until later. The external genitalia can be seen in 60% of the cases at 14 weeks and 80–100% at 20 weeks. Visualization of the external genitalia can be improved by three-dimensional and four-dimensional ultrasound scans [2]. Thus, the second-trimester scans can be used as a window for the prenatal diagnosis of hypospadias and other congenital anomalies.

The sonographic markers for prenatal diagnosis of hypospadias include [3]:

(i) Change of the normal conical shape of the penile shaft to a blunt expanded tip, which has also been named a "squashed cone." This corresponds to the dorsal hooded prepuce.
(ii) Varying degree of chordee can be visualized as bowstringing of the penile shaft.
(iii) A small penile shaft can also be seen. This is not a diagnostic marker but is highly suggestive of hypospadias.
(iv) Often, two parallel echogenic lines corresponding to the dorsal hood's lateral folds can be seen in the second trimester. Depending on the meatus' location and the penile curvature, these oblique raphes end at the apex of a small skin cone or peaks of a Cowl-shaped Monk's hood. They have been described to have an appearance similar to "Cobra eyes."
(v) The urinary stream may be visualized to be ventrally deflected due to the abnormal location of the urethral meatus. The stream is often fan-shaped. Abnormal micturition can also be delineated with the help of color Doppler studies.

The "tulip sign" describes the appearance of the penis similar to a tulip flower with excessive downwards angulation of the penile shaft, with or without chordee [3]. This shape is formed by a downwardly bent penile shaft which is seen between the scrotal folds.

The "tulip sign" represents the severe curvature of the penis in association with the penoscrotal transposition of a bifid scrotum. Thus, this sign is pathognomic of severe hypospadias. The anatomy is similar to what is seen in females during embryonal development. The ventral bending of the penile shaft is identical to the appearance of the clitoris as it is folded between the two labia. Therefore, the anatomy of severe hypospadias is difficult to distinguish from the normal female phenotype. However, the "tulip sign" may help differentiate between severe penoscrotal hypospadias and other genital abnormalities, especially in some conditions of ambiguous genitalia.

29.3 Fetal MRI in the Evaluation of Hypospadias

Fetal MRI is used as a complementary investigation to fetal USG to confirm the in-utero diagnoses and illustrate associated abnormalities such as renal anomalies and other syndromic malformations. Various authors have reported fetal MRI's efficacy in genitourinary abnormalities, especially congenital renal anomalies [4–6]. However, only a few studies in the literature describe the use of fetal MRI in diagnosing congenital urogenital anomalies such as hypospadias [7]. Nemec et al. demonstrated penile anomalies and associated urogenital abnormalities on fetal MRI, providing important information for perinatal management. The "tulip sign" of posterior hypospadias could be seen on MRI as well and be found to be the main finding similar to that described by Meizner et al. on USG [8]. Further research can be done using a fetal MRI to elucidate the disputed embryology of hypospadias better.

29.4 Role of USG in the Evaluation of Hypospadias

Ultrasound is an excellent modality for penile anatomy evaluation [9]. The penis is highly amenable to an ultrasound scan as it is located superficially [10]. Ultrasound of the penis is done with real-time B-mode scanning, utilizing a linear probe [11]. High-frequency (7.5 MHz or more) transducers are used to obtain high-resolution images of the penis. The penile Ultrasound should be performed in a dark and warm room to be comfortable during the study. Both flaccid and erect states provide good quality scans. The high-frequency probe is placed perpendicular to the penis on the ventral aspect and moved from proximal to distal (Fig. 29.1a–b). If the penis is too short and the chordee is severe, the study can be conducted by placing the probe on the dorsal

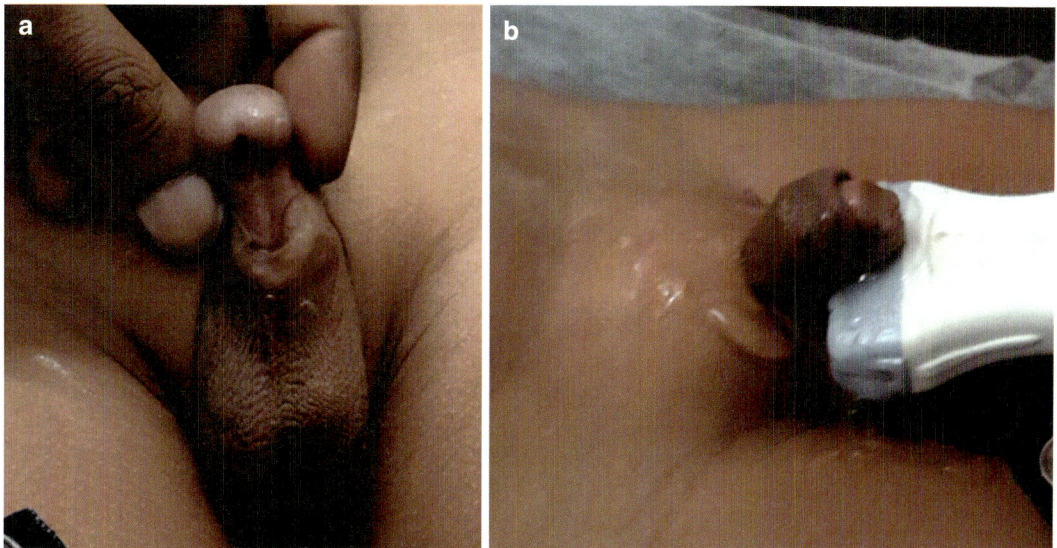

Fig. 29.1 The technique for penile Ultrasound and sonoelastography. (**a**). Clinical photograph of the patient showing proximal penile hypospadias. (**b**). Position of the probe to evaluate penile anatomy in a case of hypospadias

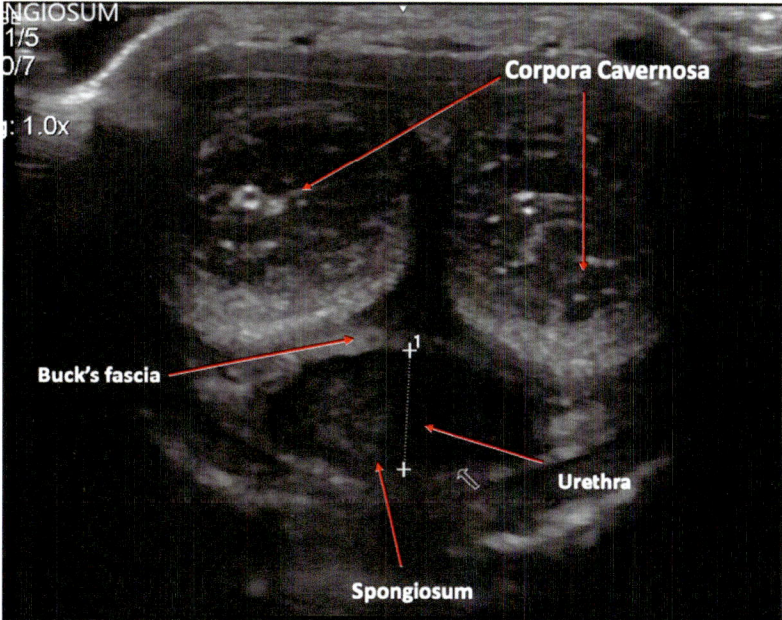

Fig. 29.2 Ultrasound anatomy of the normal penis (probe on the dorsal aspect) with the two cylindrical corpora cavernosa and the urethra surrounded by the corpus spongiosum

aspect of the penis. The cross-section images proximal, at the level, and distal to the meatus are recorded. In addition, the dimensions of the urethral plate and the spongiosum are measured.

The corpora cavernosa are visualized as homogeneous and relatively hypoechoic cylindrical structures [12] lined with a relatively hyperechoic tunica albuginea (Fig. 29.2). The tunica albuginea is approximately 2 mm thick in the flaccid state and 0.25 mm in an erect penis [13]. The spongiosum is hyperechoic compared to the corpora cavernosa and is also surrounded by Buck's fascia. The urethra is visualized as a central hypoechoic structure within the spongio-

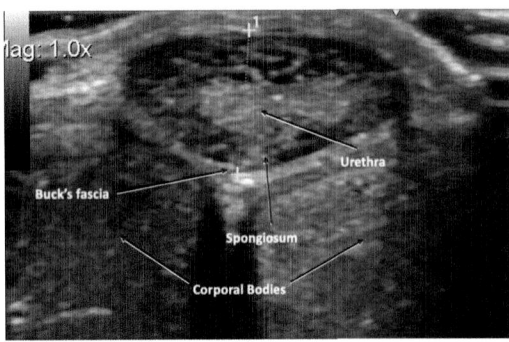

Fig. 29.3 Penile Ultrasound with the probe on the ventral aspect showing corpus spongiosum surrounding the central hyperechoic urethra. Bilateral corpora cavernosa can be seen deep to the urethra and spongiosum

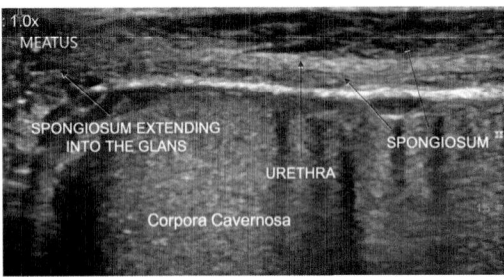

Fig. 29.4 Longitudinal view of a hypospadiac penis showing extension of the urethra beyond the meatus into the glans

sum (Fig. 29.3). The spongiosum is expanded in its proximal segment, the bulb, and distally expands into the glans [12].

The visualization of the internal penile anatomy is especially useful in the evaluation of the hypospadiac penis. The ultrasonographic anatomy of the hypospadiac penis reveals that the spongiosum splits open at the meatus and extends into the glans distal to the meatus (Fig. 29.4). The thickness of the spongiosum can be visualized proximal (Fig. 29.5a), at the level (Fig. 29.5b), and distal to the meatus (Fig. 29.5c). At the opposite end of the spectrum are the rare cases where the urethral meatus is at the tip, but the spongiosum is absent on the ventral aspect of the penis. These cases are known as absent spongiosum leading to the anterior urethral diverticulum. A similar condition with absent ventral spongiosum is chordee without hypospadias type I.

The only classification of spongiosum to date has been given by Bhat et al. [14] and is as follows:

- Well developed.
- Moderately developed.
- Poorly developed.

This classification, however, is subjective and may vary from observer to observer. Therefore, the measurement of spongiosal dimensions by Ultrasound is a better evaluation of the spongiosum.

In unpublished data from our institute, we found that the spongiosum and the urethral plate dimensions remained fairly consistent across the penis in the nine cases (Table 29.1). Therefore, this thickness might provide the urologist with a clue regarding the feasibility of spongioplasty during hypospadias repair and the patient's prognosis and may help in objective preoperative classification of the spongiosum in the future.

Penile curvature and chordee are multifactorial in origin. The cause may lie in one or more of the following: the penile skin, dartos, spongiosum, the urethra itself, and corporal disproportion. Chordee can be seen in around 35% of cases of hypospadiac penis, and its severity increases with the severity of hypospadias [15]. Sonoelastography is a useful imaging technique to evaluate tissue elasticity. It can be interpreted qualitatively on a color scale, where green indicates pliable tissues and blue denotes tissues with increased stiffness. Red represents medium stiffness in standard depiction. This imaging technique allows the determination of tissue characteristics in real-time and can be focussed on specific tissues [16] (Fig. 29.6). Elastosonography showed that the corpus spongiosum in the hypospadiac penis has a higher tissue stiffness and reduced elasticity, and the corpora cavernosa are more pliable.

Sonoelastography can also be used for a quantitative assessment of the stiffness of the spongio-

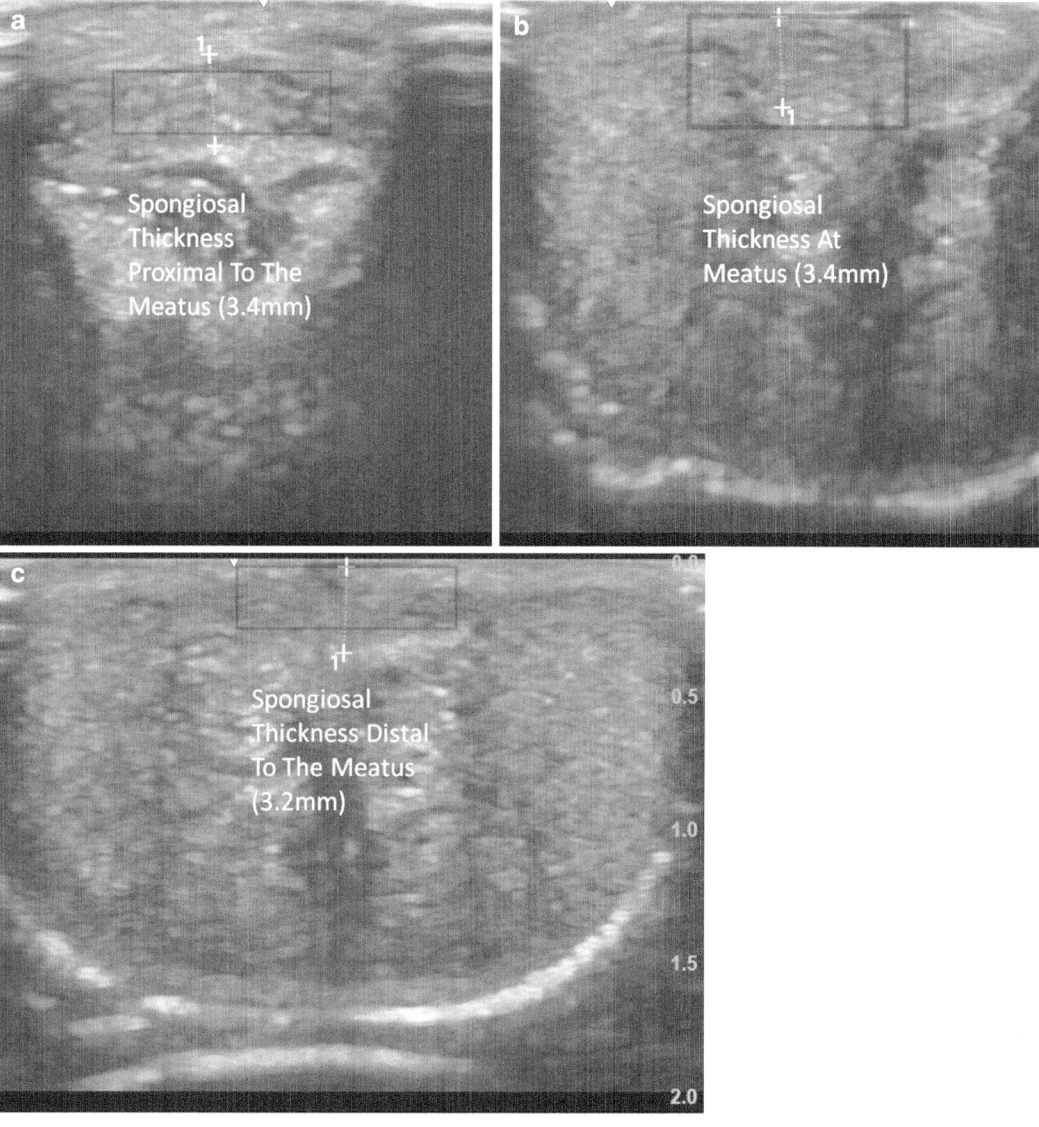

Fig. 29.5 Ultrasound images showing thickness of the spongiosum. (**a**). proximal, (**b**). at the level, and (**c**). distal to the meatus

sum. In future, these can be correlated with the operative findings to determine the feasibility of spongioplasty in hypospadias repair preoperatively. We assessed nine patients in our institute, three with mild chordee, five with moderate chordee, and one with severe chordee. We found that the stiffness of the spongiosum in cases with moderate and severe chordee was considerably higher than the cases with mild chordee (unpublished data) (Fig. 29.7).

Thus, Ultrasound and Sonoelastography can be used for more appropriate preoperative counseling and as a prognostic marker for the success of the repair. Unfortunately, no such standard has yet been established, but with future research, penile ultrasound and strain elastography may

Table 29.1 Data on spongiosal and urethral plate dimensions on nine patients of hypospadias

S. No.	Age (yrs)	Spongiosal dimensions (mm)			Urethral plate dimensions (mm)	
		Proximal	At meatus	Distal to meatus	Thickness at meatus	Distal to meatus
1.	18	17 × 3.4	16 × 3	19 × 3.4	9 × 1.7	12 × 2
2.	3	8.4 × 2	5.3 × 1.9	4.9 × 1.3	3.2 × 1.3	2.2 × 0.8
3.	3	8 × 1.5	7.4 × 2.1	8.5 × 1.8	6.8 × 2.6	3.8 × 1.6
4.	4	4.2 × 1.4	4.9 × 1.2	6.4 × 1.9	2.8 × 0.6	1.9 × 0.8
5.	5	8.9 × 3	14 × 3	14.1 × 2.7	7.5 × 4.4	7.7 × 2.5
6.	4	6.9 × 1.3	7.5 × 1.8	6.3 × 0.8	2.4 × 0.5	2.7 × 0.7
7.	2	5.0 × 2.4	6 × 1.1	5 × 1.3	3 × 0.7	2 × 0.7
8.	6	7.3 × 2.2	5.0 × 1.4	6.2 × 0.9	1.4 × 0.5	4.6 × 0.7
9.	2	10.0 × 3.0	9.5 × 1.4	11 × 1.8	4.9 × 0.8	3.7 × 1.0

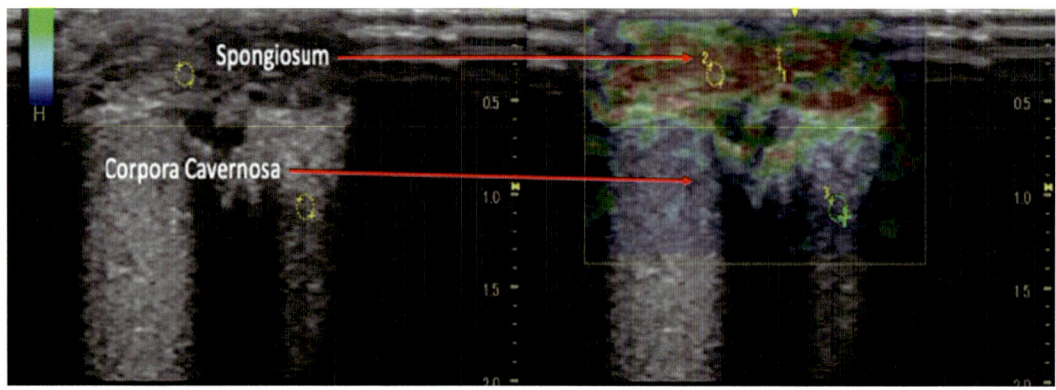

Fig. 29.6 Sonoelastography images are showing the stiffness of the tissues in a hypospadiac penis. The corpora cavernosa are blue and green suggestive of greater stiffness, and the spongiosal tissue is green and red suggestive of lesser stiffness

become a part of the evaluation of the hypospadiac patient.

29.5 Role of RUG and VCUG in Pre and Postoperative Evaluation of Hypospadias

Fluoroscopic imaging is usually performed in severe cases of hypospadias before surgery. It can characterize the size and position of the prostatic utricle. The utricle regresses, accompanied by the migration of the urethral plate. The pathophysiologic phenomenon that inhibits the migration of the urethral plate also inhibits the regression of the utricle. Typically, the more severe the hypospadias, the larger and more distal the utricle. Imaging of hypospadias is generally performed using modalities such as RUG and VCUG. If a retrograde study cannot delineate the entire urethra, a VCUG can be performed in conjunction.

The pathologic urethra grows disproportionately to the penis, and the tubularized tissue is implanted with a certain amount of redundancy. As a result, a postoperative VCUG or RUG usually demonstrates patent proximal anastomosis, a moderate-caliber, often redundant neourethra, and a widely patent neomeatus [17].

Complications of hypospadias can be early, occurring in the immediate postoperative period or late, occurring years after the surgery. For example, an anastomotic leak in early postoperative complications might lead to an urethrocutaneous fistula, the most common complication. Therefore, RUG should be performed to rule out a stricture as the causative factor if a fistula occurs in the late postoperative period.

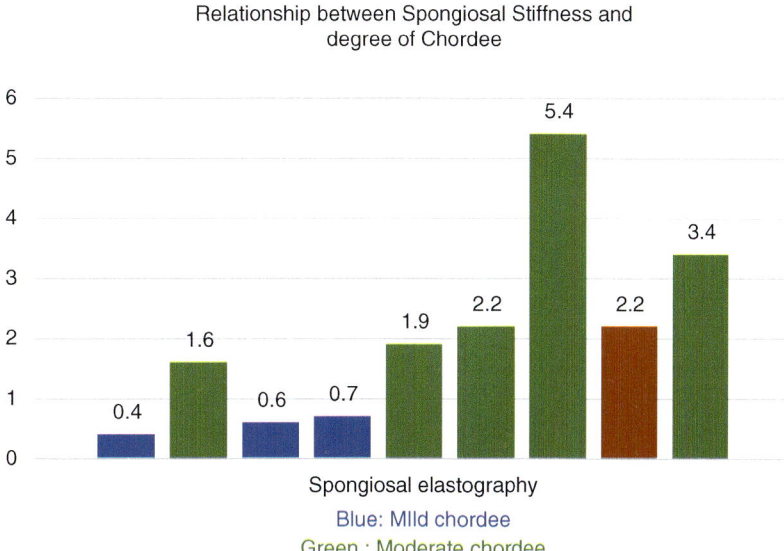

Fig. 29.7 The bar graph compares stiffness values on elastography of cases with mild, moderate, and severe chordee

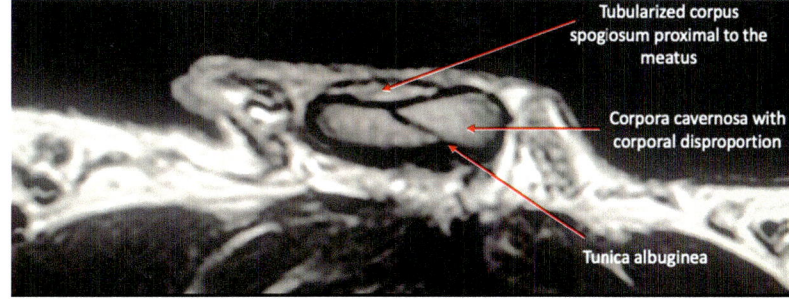

Fig. 29.8 T2-weighted image (with penis lying on the abdomen) showing tubularized corpus spongiosum proximal to the urethral meatus

Aneurysmal dilation of the reconstructed urethra is also a common complication. The tissue of the neourethra is flimsy and lacks the normal tensile strength and elasticity of the normal urethra. Aneurysmal dilation of the neourethral tissue can occur without stricture and is known as the urethral diverticulum [18].

29.6 Role of MRI in Hypospadias

MRI is the gold standard investigation for the visualization of soft tissue anatomy. The penile anatomy has been well described in various studies [19, 20], and MRI is used extensively to study the pathophysiology of urethral strictures and malignant penile lesions [21]. In addition, one study has described the MR anatomy of a hypospadiac penis in detail [22].

The corpora cavernosa and the corpus spongiosum encasing the urethra are visualized (Figs. 29.8 and 29.9). Distal to the ventrally displaced meatus, a bifurcated and flattened corpus spongiosum parallel to the flattened and open urethral plate is seen. This corpus spongiosum merges into the glans distally (Fig. 29.10). The corpus spongiosum is thus continuous with the glans penis (Fig. 29.11).

At the base of the glans, the Buck's fascia extending into the glans merges with the lamina propria. The lamina propria extends proximally from the glans base as the lamina propria of the laid open corpus spongiosum. Dorsal to the lamina propria of the laid open and bifurcated corpus spongiosum, the Buck's fascia lies deep to the lamina propria of the spongiosum and extends across the midline to the merger with the lamina propria of the contralateral side.

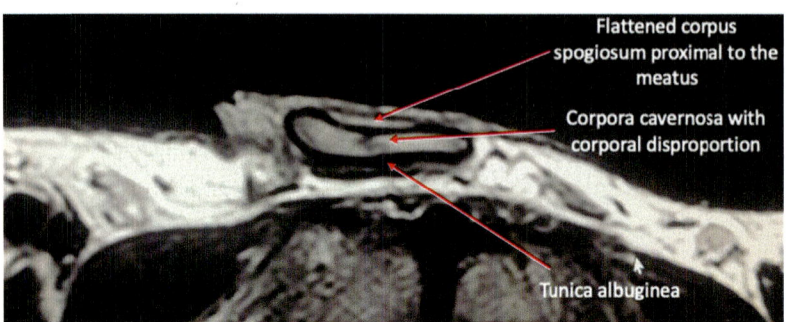

Fig. 29.9 T2-weighted image (with penis lying on the abdomen) showing flattening of the corpus spongiosum proximal to the meatus

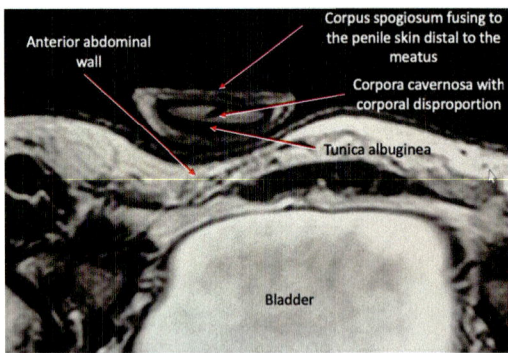

Fig. 29.10 T2-weighted image (with penis lying on the abdomen) showing the corpus spongiosum flattening and fusing to the urethral plate distal to the meatus

Tunica albuginea surrounding the corpora cavernosa is seen as a low signal density layer all around (Figs. 29.12 and 29.13). It is visualized as a bilaminar structure forming two layers of the tunica albuginea, an outer longitudinal and an inner circular layer. Only a unilaminar layer of tunica albuginea can be seen at the apex of the corpora cavernosa.

The Buck's fascia was seen as a bright, distinct layer surrounding the corpora cavernosa and the corpus spongiosum. Visualizing the penile anatomy in axial sections, we can observe two layers of Buck's fascia split to enclose the corpus spongiosum but continue laterally as a single layer. Next, Buck's fascia splits again on the dorsal aspect of the penis to surround the dorsal neurovascular bundles. This bundle contains the dorsal vein of the penis and nerves.

In the T2-weighted images superficial to the Buck's fascia, the dartos fascia is visualized as an intermediate signal density layer. The dartos is thick on the dorsal aspect and extends up to the dorsal hooded prepuce. However, the dartos is thin and extends only until the midline's meatus and up to the corona laterally on the ventral aspect.

Kureel et al., in a landmark study, concluded that (1) The penile vascularity is well developed dorsally on the penile shaft as axially distributed vessels can be seen on the dorsal aspect. The ventral surface, however, shows the paucity of superficial vessels with a relatively avascular plane seen on the ventral midline, (2) the ventral penile artery arising from the anterior scrotal vessels is seldom seen in the hypospadiac penis, (3) the lamina propria of the glans fuses with the glanular extension Buck's fascia and protects the lateral branches of the dorsal penile artery; these form the intraglanular arcade which supplies the glans, and (4) a plane of dissection can be created between the tunica albuginea of the corpora cavernosa and the fused deep layer of Buck's fascia and the lamina propria of the glans. Creating space in this plane prevents injury to the intraglanular arcade of vessels and preserves the blood supply to the glans [22].

MRI anatomy of the hypospadiac penis provides a clue to the pathophysiology of hypospadias and the distribution of the various neurovascular bundles and the various tissue layers. While the choice of technique of hypospadias repair remains an intraoperative decision, the MRI may arm the urologist with additional information to make a more informed choice. MRI can especially be used to evaluate the adequacy of the spongiosum

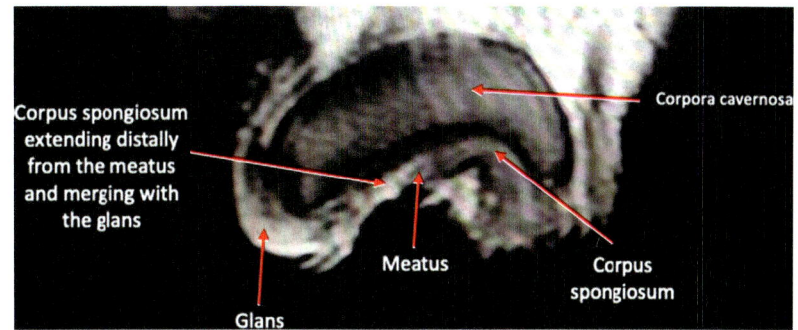

Fig. 29.11 T2-weighted image showing corpus spongiosum extending into the glans distal to the meatus

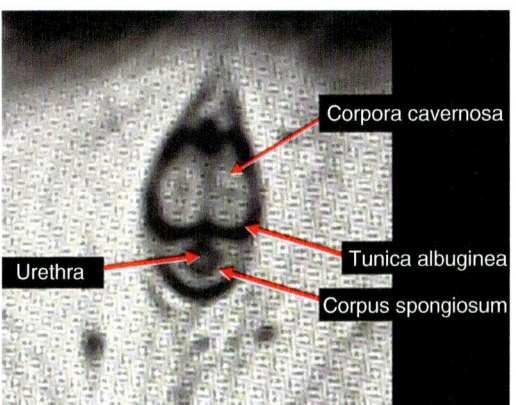

Fig. 29.12 Urethra surrounded by the spongiosum proximal to the hypospadiac meatus

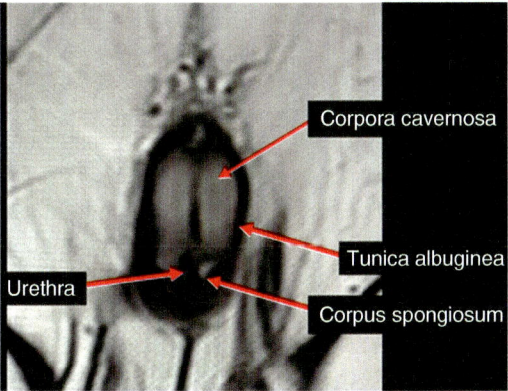

Fig. 29.13 T2-weighted image showing thinning of the corpus spongiosum ventrally proximal to the level of the meatus

and the width of the urethral plate. Bhat et al. have classified the spongiosum based on thickness and vascularity to predict the efficacy of spongioplasty in hypospadias repair. A similar approach can be taken preoperatively using MRI to classify and assess the spongiosum for adequacy.

29.7 Radiology of Associated Abnormalities

Hypospadias is an anomaly frequently associated with other congenital anomalies. While the diagnosis of hypospadias primarily remains clinical, radiological investigations play an important role in diagnosing anomalies associated with hypospadias. The commonest congenital anomaly associated with hypospadias is congenital inguinal hernia [23]. Other common urogenital anomalies seen in association with hypospadias are undescended testes, hypoplastic testes, bifid scrotum, concurrent urethral strictures, micropenis, and VACTERL anomalies which portend a more severe hypospadiac abnormality [24].

29.8 Imaging of DSD

Radiological investigations play a crucial role in the cases of ambiguous genitalia and DSD. They are the primary mode of assessing the child's internal anatomy and play a critical role in the final gender assignment. Ultrasonography is the investigation of choice as it is easily accessible and non-invasive [25]. However, it is operator-dependent and requires expertise and may need to

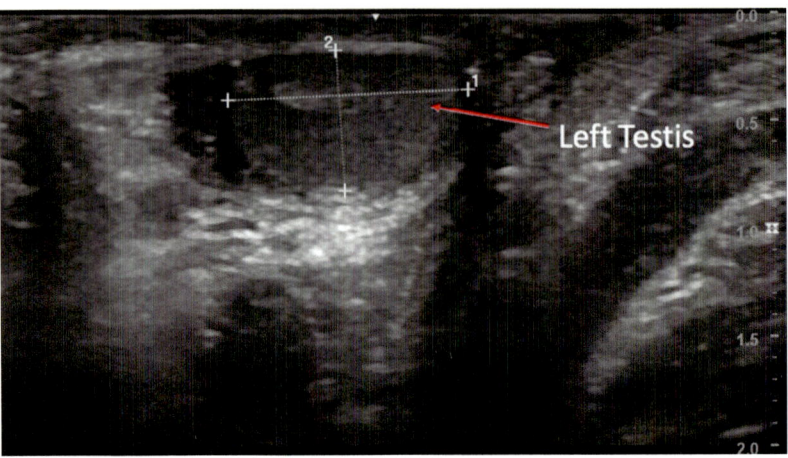

Fig. 29.14 Ultrasound image of a DSD patient showing left testis as an isoechoic structure

be supplemented with investigations such as MRI, genitography, and voiding cystourethrography.

Ultrasonography: It is the primary investigation in evaluating DSD and involves imaging the abdominal organs such as kidneys, adrenal glands, and pelvis and screening inguinal, perineal, and anal regions. The primary aim is to visualize the gonads and secondary sexual organs. The ovaries and the uterus can be visualized quite easily in the neonatal period. Neonatal ovaries show gradually disappearing follicles, and the uterus is visualized as a tubular structure [25]. Identification of only one ovary in 40% and neither ovary in 16% of cases has been seen in normal patients [26]. The neonatal testes are seen as homogenous iso to hyperechoic structures (Fig. 29.14) [25]. The anatomical situation, number, and echotexture of the gonads should also be observed during the study.

Both kidneys should be screened for congenital anomalies such as hydronephrosis. Special attention should be paid to the adrenal glands, and the gland should be screened for space-occupying lesions, alterations in echotexture, and abnormalities on the gland surface. Congenital adrenal hyperplasia is characterized by hyperplastic adrenal glands showing normal corticomedullary differentiation with a single-limb length > 20 mm and width > 4 mm [27]. Normal-sized adrenal glands do not exclude the diagnosis of CAH [28, 29]. "Cerebriform appearance" is reportedly specific for CAH [30].

Ambiguous genitalia can also be diagnosed prenatally on fetal Ultrasound with further evaluation using fetal MRI and postnatal studies. Ambiguous genitalia can be diagnosed and classified by using the diagnostic algorithm given in (Fig. 29.19).

29.9 Genitography

Genitography delineates the internal anatomy of the urethra, vagina, cervix, and urethrovaginal confluence [25]. The patient is positioned on the X-ray table in a lateral position. The patient's hips are flexed at 90°; separate catheters are inserted into each perineal orifice, and contrast is injected gently in a retrograde fashion. The catheters should be placed as proximally as possible to maintain native anatomy. The urogenital tract is visualized, and the size and capacity of the vagina, if present, must be documented. If observed, any urogenital fistula must be documented in length, relation to the perineum and external sphincter. It can demonstrate the configuration of the urethra, whether female or male and document any anomalous communication between the urethra, vagina, and rectum. Any fistula can be visualized by opacification of contrast. A urogenital sinus malformation is characterized by hydrocolpos or hydrometocolpos associated with ambiguous genitalia and two orifices in the perineum [27]. An opaque perineal marker

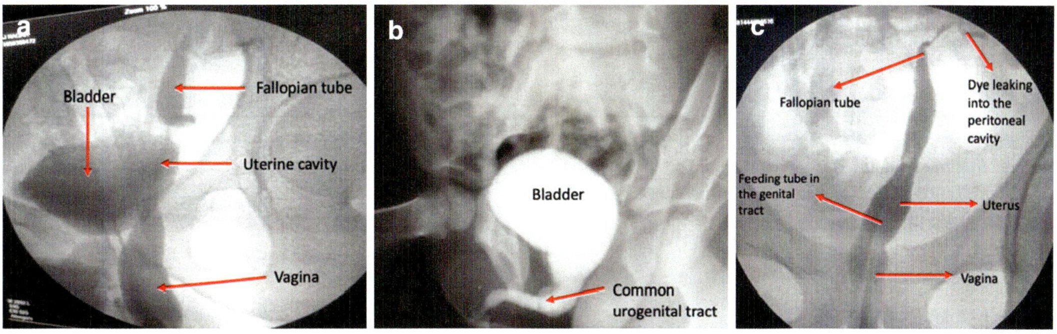

29 Radiological Evaluation of Hypospadias Patients

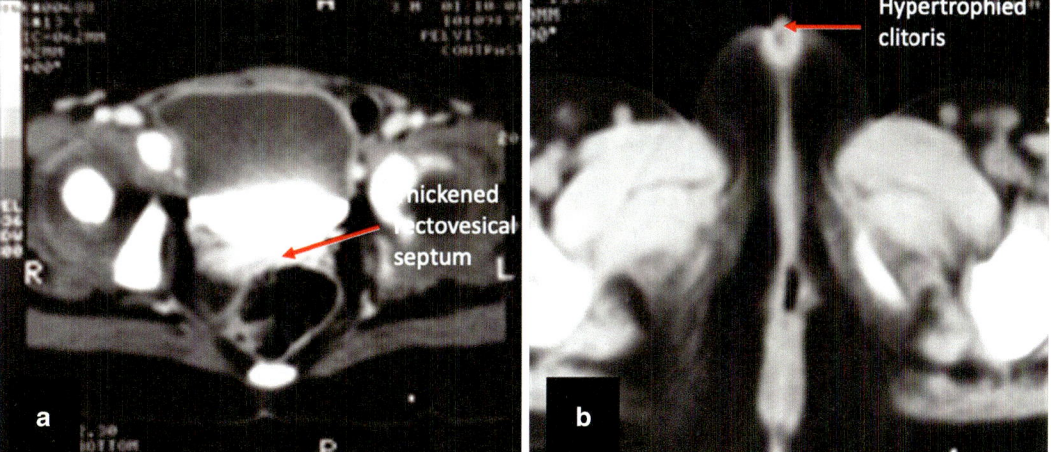

Fig. 29.15 Genitography. (**a**). showing separate bladder and vagina. (**b**). showing a common urogenital tract. (**c**). Showing genitogram with a well-developed uterine cavity with the dye in the fallopian tube and leaking into the peritoneum via the fimbriae

Fig. 29.16 CECT abdomen showing (**a**) absence of testes, prostate, and seminal vesicles with the presence of a thick rectovesical septum and (**b**) a hypertrophied clitoris with labia on either side

should be placed to allow for subsequent measurements. The degree of virilization is assessed by the ratio of the horizontal part to the vertical part (H/V) of the urethra. In the normal male H/V = 1.6 ± 0.2. Verumontanum presence should also be recorded as a distinctive feature of the male urethra [31]. The urogenital confluence is measured in relation to the perineum and characterized in relation to the external sphincter, determining the timing and the type of surgery to be performed [31]. The presence and size of the vagina and the presence of a cervical impression in the contrast material column should be noted [25] (Fig. 29.15a–c).

29.10 Computed Tomography

Computed tomography is the modality of choice for evaluating DSD-associated malignancies and staging of germ cell tumors. CT can also be used to detect the anatomy (Fig. 29.16) and plan the management of DSD. CT is also useful for evaluating postoperative complications such as hematoma and

Fig. 29.17 Axial T2-weighted image at the level of pubic symphysis showing undescended testes at the level of the superficial inguinal ring and a vaginal remnant between the bladder and the rectum

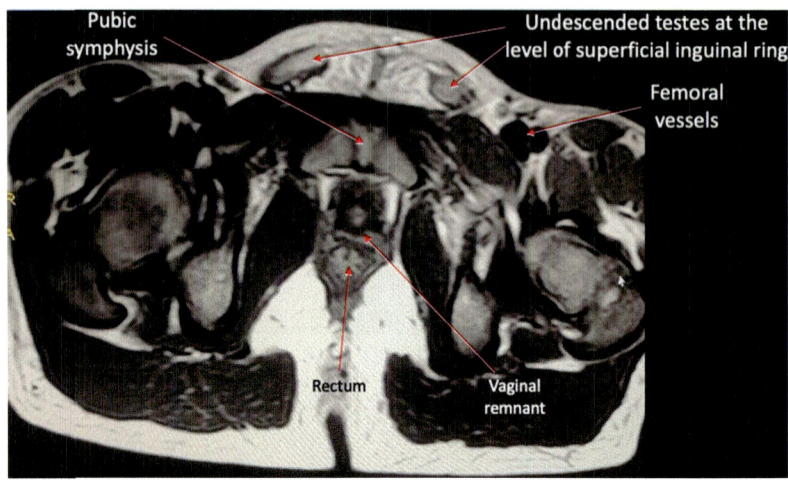

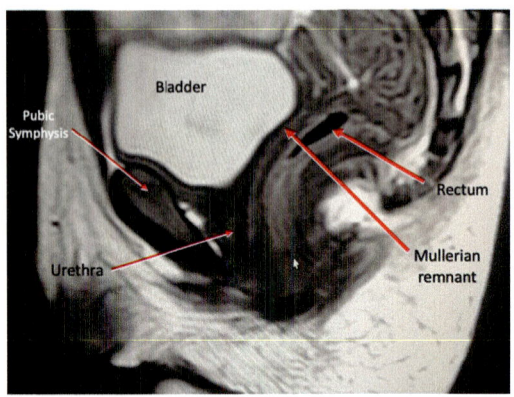

Fig. 29.18 Coronal T2-weighted image of the same patient showing a vaginal remnant between the bladder and the rectum

abscesses that arise because of sex reassignment procedures or tumor resection [32].

29.11 MRI

Magnetic resonance imaging is the gold standard modality for soft tissue imaging and can be used as an adjunct to ultrasonography when the anatomy is unclear. MRI is useful in evaluating ambiguous genitalia, with MR depiction of uterus possible in 93%, vagina in 95%, penis in 100%, testes in 88%, and ovary in 74% cases [33] (Figs. 29.17 and 29.18).

It can also be used to localize testes (Fig. 29.17). A study by Kanemoto et al. documented the sensitivity and specificity of the MRI as 86% and 79%, respectively, for the detection of intraabdominal testes [34]. Newer studies, however, report a sensitivity of 85% and a specificity of 87.5%. The addition of diffusion-weighted improved the sensitivity to 89.5%, but the specificity was unchanged. Interobserver variability was also observed [35] (Fig. 29.19).

29.12 Conclusion

Hypospadias is mainly a clinical diagnosis. However, with the increasingly better resolution of the ultrasonography machines, prenatal diagnosis is emerging as a possibility, especially in severe cases. MRI remains the imaging modality of choice because of objectivity and a detailed assessment of penile anatomy. Still, with the advancement of ultrasonographic modalities such as sonoelastography, ultrasound assessment has a promising future in evaluating hypospadias. The detection and classification of spongiosum can become norms in the future and may provide the urologist with additional information regarding the case-specific anatomy and may aid in decision-making regarding the technique of hypospadias repair be utilized. DSD is a disease

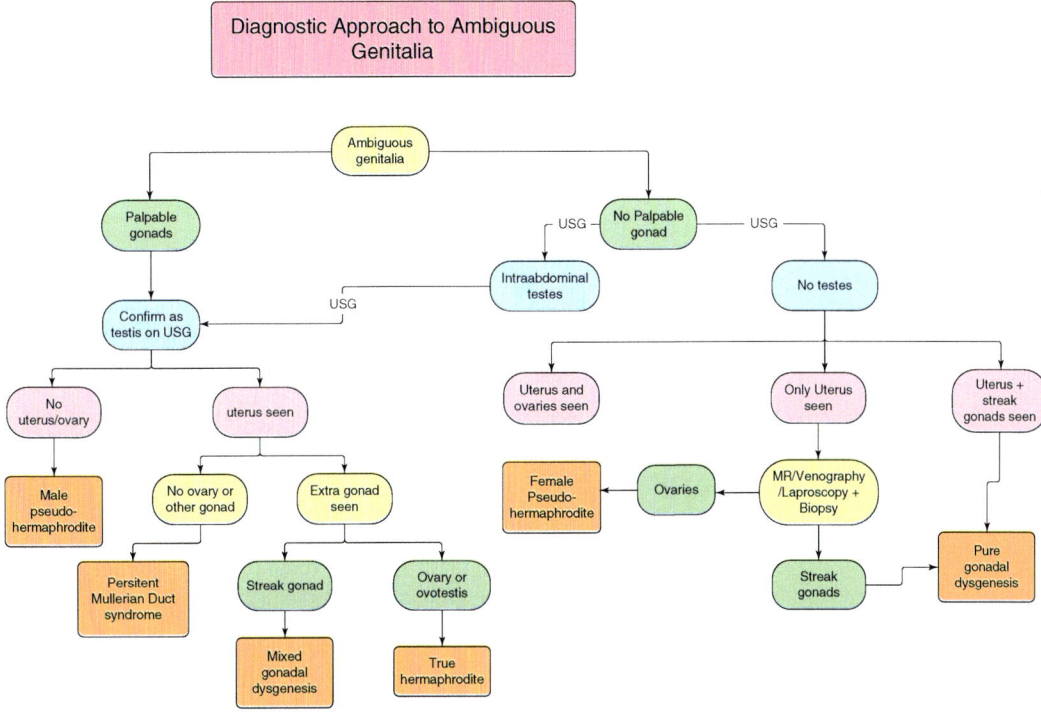

Fig. 29.19 Algorithm showing the diagnostic approach to ambiguous genitalia

complex with various presentations, and ultrasonography plays a critical role in DSD classification. Radiology in hypospadias is a developing field with rapidly evolving protocols and in future may become a strong tool in the evaluation of hypospadias.

References

1. Bhat A, Kumar V, Bhat M, Kumar R, Patni M, Mittal R. The incidence of apparent congenital urogenital anomalies in North Indian newborns: a study of 20,432 pregnancies. Afr J Urol. 2016;22(3):183–8.
2. Hackett LK, Tarsa M, Wolfson TJ, Kaplan G, Vaux KK, Pretorius DH. Use of multiplanar 3-dimensional ultrasonography for prenatal sex identification. J Ultrasound Med. 2010;29(2):195–202.
3. Meizner I, Mashiach R, Shalev J, Efrat Z, Feldberg D. The 'tulip sign': a sonographic clue for the in-utero diagnosis of severe hypospadias. Ultrasound Obstet Gynecol. 2002;19(3):250–3.
4. Hörmann M, Brugger PC, Balassy C, Witzani L, Prayer D. Fetal MRI of the urinary system. Eur J Radiol. 2006;57(2):303–11.
5. Lissauer D, Morris RK, Kilby MD. Fetal lower urinary tract obstruction. Semin Fetal Neonatal Med. 2007;6. Elsevier:464–70.
6. Alamo L, Laswad T, Schnyder P, Meuli R, Vial Y, Osterheld M-C, Gudinchet F. Fetal M.R.I. as a complement to the U.S. in the diagnosis and characterization of anomalies of the genito-urinary tract. Eur J Radiol. 2010;76(2):258–64.
7. Nakamura Y, Jennings RW, Connolly S, Diamond DA. Fetal diagnosis of penoscrotal transposition associated with perineal lipoma in one twin. Diag Ther. 2010;27(3):164–7.
8. Nemec SF, Kasprian G, Brugger PC, Bettelheim D, Nemec U, Krestan CR, Rotmensch S, Rimoin DL, Graham JM, Prayer D. Abnormalities of the penis in utero–hypospadias on fetal MRI. J Perinat Med. 2011;39(4):451–6.
9. Fernandes MAV, Souza LRMFD, Cartafina LP. Ultrasound evaluation of the penis. Radiol Bras. 2018;51(4):257–61.
10. Wilkins C, Sriprasad S, Sidhu P. Colour doppler ultrasound of the penis. Clin Radiol. 2003;58(7):514–23.
11. Medicine AIoUi, Association A.U. A.I.U.M. practice guideline for performing an ultrasound examination in urology practice. J Ultrasound Med. 2012;31(1):133–44.
12. Avery LL, Scheinfeld MH. Imaging of penile and scrotal emergencies. Radiographics. 2013;33(3):721–40.

13. Bhatt S, Kocakoc E, Rubens DJ, Seftel AD, Dogra VS. Sonographic evaluation of penile trauma. J Ultrasound Med. 2005;24(7):993–1000. quiz 1001
14. Bhat A, Sabharwal K, Bhat M, Saran R, Singla M, Kumar V. Outcome of tubularized incised plate urethroplasty with spongioplasty alone as additional tissue cover: a prospective study. Indian J Urol. 2014;30(4):392.
15. Schultz JR, Klykylo WM, Wacksman J. Timing of elective hypospadias repair in children. Paediatrics. 1983;71(3):342–51.
16. Camoglio FS, Bruno C, Zambaldo S, Zampieri N. Hypospadias anatomy: elastosonographic evaluation of the normal and hypospadic penis. J Pediatr Urol. 2016;12(4):199:1–5.
17. Milla SS, Chow JS, Lebowitz RL. Imaging of hypospadias: pre-and postoperative appearances. Pediatr Radiol. 2008;38(2):202–8.
18. Cimador M, Vallasciani S, Manzoni G, Rigamonti W, De Grazia E, Castagnetti M. Failed hypospadias in paediatric patients. Nat Rev Urol. 2013;10(11): 657.
19. Satragno L, Martinoli C, Cittadini G. Magnetic resonance imaging of the penis: Normal anatomy. Magn Reson Imaging. 1989;7(1):95–100. https://doi.org/10.1016/0730-725X(89)90329-9.
20. Vossough A, Pretorius E, Siegelman E, Ramchandani P, Banner M. Magnetic resonance imaging of the penis. Abdom Radiol. 2002;27(6):640.
21. Kirkham AP, Illing RO, Minhas S, Minhas S, Allen C. M.R. imaging of nonmalignant penile lesions. Radiographics. 2008;28(3):837–53.
22. Kureel SN, Gupta A, Sunil K, Dheer Y, Kumar M, Tomar VK. Surgical anatomy of the penis in hypospadias magnetic resonance imaging study of the tissue planes, vessels, and collaterals. Urology. 2015;85(5):1173–8.
23. Wu W-H, Chuang J-H, Ting Y-C, Lee S-Y, Hsieh C-S. Developmental anomalies and disabilities associated with hypospadias. J Urol. 2002;168(1):229–32.
24. Kulkarni B, Oak S, Patel M, Merchant S, Borwankar S. Developmental anomalies associated with hypospadias. J Postgrad Med. 1991;37(3):140.
25. Moshiri M, Chapman T, Fechner PY, Dubinsky TJ, Shnorhavorian M, Osman S, Bhargava P, Katz DS. Evaluation and management of disorders of sex development: a multidisciplinary approach to a complex diagnosis. Radiographics. 2012;32(6):1599–618.
26. Cohen H, Shapiro M, Mandel F, Shapiro M. Normal ovaries in neonates and infants: a sonographic study of 77 patients 1 day to 24 months old. Am J Roentgenol. 1993;160(3):583–6.
27. Wright N, Smith C, Rickwood A, Carty H. Imaging children with ambiguous genitalia and intersex states. Clin Radiol. 1995;50(12):823–9.
28. Sivit C, Hung W, Taylor G, Catena L, Brown-Jones C, Kushner D. Sonography in neonatal congenital adrenal hyperplasia. Am J Roentgenol. 1991;156(1):141–3.
29. Bryan P, Caldamone A, Morrison S, Yulish B, Owens R. Ultrasound findings in the adreno-genital syndrome (congenital adrenal hyperplasia). J Ultrasound Med. 1988;7(12):675–9.
30. Davis DM. Surgical treatment of hypospadias, especially scrotal and perineal. J Urol. 1951;65(4): 595–602.
31. Garel L. Abnormal sex differentiation: who, how and when to image. Pediatr Radiol. 2008;38:508.
32. Sohaib S, Cook G, Koh D-M. Imaging studies for germ cell tumours. Hematol Oncol Clin. 2011;25(3):487–502.
33. Secaf E, Hricak H, Gooding C, Ho V, Gorczyca D, Ringertz H, Conte F, Kogan B, Grumbach M. Role of M.R.I. in the valuation of ambiguous genitalia. Pediatr Radiol. 1994;24(4):231–5.
34. Kanemoto K, Hayashi Y, Kojima Y, Maruyama T, Ito M, Kohri K. Accuracy of ultrasonography and magnetic resonance imaging in diagnosing non-palpable testis. Int J Urol. 2005;12(7):668–72.
35. Kantarci M, Doganay S, Yalcin A, Aksoy Y, Yilmaz-Cankaya B, Salman B. Diagnostic performance of diffusion-weighted M.R.I. in the detection of nonpalpable undescended testes: comparison with conventional M.R.I. and surgical findings. Am J Roentgenol. 2010;195(4):W268–73.

30

Evolutions in Hypospadiology and Current Status of Tissue Engineering

Priyank Yadav and Martin A. Koyle

Abbreviations

ECM	Extracellular matrix
P(LLA-CL)	Poly(L-lactide-co-caprolactone)
PCL	Polycaprolactone
PGA	Poly(glycolic acid)
PLA	Poly(lactic acid)
PLGA	Poly(lactic-co-glycolic acid)
SIS	Small intestine submucosa

30.1 Introduction

Hypospadias is characterized by a deficiency in the development of all the layers of the urethra and the surrounding corpus spongiosum and occurs due to incomplete fusion of the urethral folds, typically between 8 and 20 weeks of gestation. The term "hypospadiology" was introduced by John W. Duckett Jr. 4 decades ago, during a renaissance in urethral reconstruction and hypospadias surgery [1]. It is a broad term that incorporates all the available knowledge in the field and the long list of techniques over more than a century of continuous development. The sheer number of procedures described for hypospadias points towards the challenges in achieving perfect reconstruction and also reminds hypospadias surgeons that every case of hypospadias is unique. Surgical success is dependent upon accurate correction of penile curvature, tubularization of the urethra, reconstruction of the glans, and adequate skin coverage, ultimately aiming towards cosmetic and functional normalcy. Attempts to restore the anatomy of the urethra and correct the curvature of the penis have progressed through transitions in the philosophies of treatment, from single stage to multi-stage repairs and from use of local tissues to distant autologous grafts. While in distal hypospadias, representing at least 70% of all hypospadias cases, the urethral plate is usually amenable to single stage repairs, proximal hypospadias and re-do hypospadias repairs present a challenge for even experienced hypospadiologists. When preputial tissue is available, flaps or grafts of this skin might be used for the urethroplasty. When penile skin is inadequate, skin from non-hair bearing areas and buccal mucosa represent the most common sources of autologous graft tissue used to form the neourethra, almost invariably involving multi-stage surgery. However, even staged repairs are associated with significant complications and reoperations are necessary in >50% of boys undergoing surgery [2]. Furthermore, a urethra constructed from buccal mucosa or non-genital

P. Yadav (✉)
Division of Pediatric Urology, The Hospital for Sick Children, University of Toronto,
Toronto, ON, Canada

M. A. Koyle
University of Toronto & Hospital for Sick Children,
Toronto, ON, Canada

skin grafts may not develop in the same way as a native urethra over longer period of follow-up. In boys with severe hypospadias, particularly those who have undergone multiple repairs using autologous tissue, the options for urethral replacement are limited, especially for long defects. Additionally, in other boys who have less severe varieties of hypospadias, use of extragenital skin or mucosa may not be desirable due to donor site morbidity.

Concepts in hypospadiology are evolving constantly with the ultimate aim of the "perfect" technique, that is, the right operation for the right patient at the right time. Tissue engineering is emerging as an attractive solution to the conundrum where there is a paucity of ideal local tissue for urethral reconstruction. It eliminates the need of harvesting autologous tissues and the associated morbidity related to donor site harvesting. Further, it has the potential to offer readymade, prefabricated constructs that can be used for urethral replacement directly. Importantly, tissue-engineered grafts can also be designed to reproduce the structural, mechanical, and biological characteristics of the urethra by adjusting their composition. They can be made to bear the stretch during passage of urine and erection as well as avoid overdistension that may compromise their integrity and barrier function. An ideal tissue-engineered urethra has the following characteristics—(a) biocompatible, (b) multilayered, consisting of different type of cells (epithelial cells, fibroblasts, and smooth muscle cells), (c) effective barrier against the metabolites present in urine, (d) elastic to allow distension during voiding and stretching during erection, and (e) resistant to manipulative forces and during surgery, particularly suturing. Mimicking the native urethra, a tissue-engineered urethra should be fairly adaptable to voiding pressures, thus avoiding deformation and the potential for overdistension and diverticulum formation. Tissue engineering has progressed over the last three decades, with much research having been focused on finding suitable biomaterials and cells that can be tailored to meet the properties of the native urethra.

30.2 Biomaterials for Urethral Tissue Engineering

Three types of biomaterials are used to tissue engineer the urethra: (a) autologous cells, (b) acellular biomaterials or scaffolds (polymeric or extracellular matrix derived), and (c) autologous cells seeded on the scaffolds. The cell-only constructs are too fragile to bear transportation or handling and therefore are impractical for surgical use. So, acellular and cell-seeded scaffolds have undergone the most testing in animal and clinical studies for urethral regeneration. Scaffolds provide a mechanical framework for tissue regeneration. They promote three-dimensional movement of cells and may be degraded in the process. They can be classified as per their origin (natural or synthetic) and biodegradability (biodegradable and non-biodegradable).

30.2.1 Acellular Synthetic Polymeric Scaffolds

Scaffolds derived from synthetic polymers are easy to construct and may be biodegradable or non-biodegradable. The biodegradable scaffolds are synthesized from polymers such as poly(glycolic acid) (PGA), poly(lactic acid) (PLA), polycaprolactone (PCL), and poly(lactic-co-glycolic acid) (PLGA). The ester bonds in these polymers degrade by nonenzymatic hydrolysis, and their nontoxic degradation products are eliminated from the body in the form of carbon dioxide and water. Their rate of degradation depends on their crystallinity, molecular weight, and copolymer ratio which is useful for tailoring them to suit the needs of the tissue being reconstructed. Non-biodegradable scaffolds such as polytetrafluoroethylene and poly(ethylene terephthalate) are mainly used as temporary supports and hence have limited application as they frequently undergo calcification, shortening, and migration. A disadvantage of all synthetic polymers whether biodegradable or not, is that they lack the specific proteins on their surface that interact with cells and facilitate adhesion. Hence, they require surface treatment to promote cell attachment.

30.2.2 Acellular Natural Polymeric Scaffolds

The natural polymers that have been used to make scaffolds are collagen, alginate, chitosan, hyaluronic acid, and silk fibroin. Collagen is the most abundant protein and forms a major part of the extracellular matrix (ECM). It is usually derived from animal sources (such as bovine or porcine skin) although recombinant human collagen is also available. However, it is antigenic and has a fast degradation rate limiting its use in urethral regeneration. Silk fibroin, on the other hand, is an excellent biomaterial which has low immunogenicity and hence generates less inflammatory response. When compared with small intestine submucosa (SIS) grafts or urethrotomy in male rabbits, silk fibroin scaffolds had a lower inflammatory response though the growth of epithelial cells and smooth muscle cells was the same [3]. Furthermore, it has a hydrophobic structure with strong intramolecular and intermolecular interactions, and is hydrolyzed by proteolytic enzymes. Its elasticity and shape memory are good for urological application and blending it with synthetic polymer can impart cell adhesion property to the latter. A composite scaffold of silk, keratin, gelatin, and calcium peroxide film allows high continuous oxygen delivery and also has antimicrobial activity while having similar regenerative capacity as SIS [4]. Natural polymers have integrin-binding peptide sequences and a surface topography that promotes cell adhesion as well as angiogenesis. The rate of degradation of difficult to control and transfer of pathogens is possible during their use.

30.2.3 Acellular Extracellular Matrix Scaffolds

Decellularization of allogenic and xenogenic tissues yields acellular ECM scaffolds that retain the biomechanical properties and structural integrity as well as bioactive growth factors. They degrade rapidly once implanted and the degradation products stimulate regeneration by *constructive tissue remodelling*. When the scaffolds have an optimized degradation that is synchronous with the growth of the cellular component, the resultant tissue has layered epithelia, organized smooth muscle cells, and better vascularization. On the other hand, non-degradable synthetic biocompatible scaffolds are associated with a nonfunctional remodeling that is associated with complications such as migration, calcification, and narrowing. The most common acellular ECMs used in urethral repair are SIS. It is obtained by mechanical removal of tunica mucosa and muscularis, and serosa from porcine small intestine. When used for urethral replacement, the results are similar to those obtained with skin and buccal mucosal grafts, achieving high rates of cell growth and angiogenesis. The degradation time is four to eight weeks and the degradation components are eliminated in urine. SIS has been used successfully during corporal incision and grafting for correction of chordee and demonstrates low tendency to break. However, the regenerative potential of SIS depends on age of donor and the part of small intestine used to derive it resulting in batch-to-batch variability. Another acellular ECM is bladder acellular matrix which has shown encouraging results in animal studies on urethral regeneration. All acellular ECM scaffolds have potential to cause inflammatory reactions due to residual nucleic acids and xeno-antigens.

30.2.4 Cell-seeded Scaffolds

For urethral defects up to 0.5 cm, acellular scaffolds promote healing and facilitate repair but for larger lesions, cells are required on the scaffolds. These cells may be harvested from the urinary tract or other sources. Both urothelial cells and oral mucosal cells can produce a stratified epithelium for urethral reconstruction, although, urine-derived stem cells can differentiate into urothelial as well as smooth muscle cells. The cells for seeding may be obtained by invasive or non-invasive methods. Invasive methods including open bladder biopsy harvest a small number of cells only and additionally require general anesthesia besides causing donor site morbidity. Bladder washings is a non-invasive method that is safe and easily reproducible. When seeding cells on a scaffold, it must be remembered that the proliferation of cells is greatly affected by the mechanical properties of the scaffold. Multiple cell types can be cultured at the same time. In fact, coculture is found superior to the culture of individual cell types highlighting the importance of paracrine signaling. The cell-seeded scaffolds can be fabricated to form tubular constructs that look like urethra and are lined on the inside by urothelial cells. They can be bio-functionalized using exogenous trophic factors and suitable microenvironment in a bioreactor to stimulate differentiation of the construct for functional maturation.

30.3 Approach to Urethral Tissue Engineering

30.3.1 Selecting the Type of Construct

Cell-only constructs are not suitable for urethral reconstruction due to lack of mechanical strength. So, tissue-engineered urethra must be derived from either acellular matrices or cell-seeded matrices. For acellular matrices to be successfully epithelized, the defect must be small and the urethral bed must be vascular. They are not suitable for patients with extensive spongiofibrosis, recurrent strictures, and long defects. Autologous cell-seeded matrices are useful in these situations. The cells are harvested from a tissue biopsy and then expanded in a culture after which they are seeded into the matrix. Urothelial as well as non-urothelial cells such as keratinocytes may be used for seeding. The matrix in then implanted to replace the urethral defect.

SIS is unsuitable for use as a tubularized construct and is associated with fibrosis and luminal obstruction [5]. When used as an onlay patch, four-layer SIS has less shrinkage than single-layer SIS although they have similar re-epithelization and neovascularization [6]. For long and complex urethral defects, tubular cell-loaded constructs are superior to onlay grafts. Bladder acellular matrix when combined with silk fibroin has excellent revascularization, a property that is desired in patients with failed hypospadias repair [7].

30.3.2 Natural vs Synthetic Biomaterials

The structure and properties of a synthetic scaffold can be altered based upon the site of implantation. Such precise tuning is not possible for natural polymeric and ECM based scaffolds because of the variability of the source. However, the ECM proteins that facilitate adhesion and ingrowth of cells are absent in synthetic scaffolds, so, they cannot be used without surface treatment. Recently, hybrid or composite scaffolds have been developed, which combine a synthetic polymer with a natural matrix [8]. PLGA microfibers can be attached onto the abluminal surface of bladder acellular matrix to produce a hybrid scaffold.

30.3.3 Electrospinning

Electrospinning is one of the latest techniques that has evolved in the last few years and helps to design, produce, and characterize the 3D scaffolds for in vitro as well as in vivo culturing. It can produce biomaterials with nanoscale properties. Such materials have a high porosity and spatial interconnectivity suitable for tissue engineering. Using electrospinning, it is possible to add cells and proteins within the scaffold with high efficiency. Natural as well as synthetic materials can be electrospun. Zhang et al. fabricated a nanofiber scaffold of collagen type I and poly(L-lactide-co-caprolactone) (P(LLA-CL)) using coaxial electrospinning technique and reported satisfactory programmed biodegradation and tensile strength [9]. Wei et al. prepared nanofiber scaffolds of polycaprolactone (PCL), collagen, and silk fibroin which allowed adhesion and proliferation of oral mucosal cells to produce a seeded scaffold for urethral reconstruction [10].

30.3.4 3D Bioprinting

3D Bioprinting deposits cells and biomaterials in a manner similar to an inkjet printer to prepare a construct with predefined architecture. The deposited substances are called bioink. 3D Bioprinting was used to produce a spiral scaffold in which urothelial cells and smooth muscle cells were applied on the inner and outer layer of the scaffolds to produce a urethral construct with mechanical properties of the native rabbit urethra [11]. Recently, multichannel coaxial extrusion system has been developed, which allows bioprinting of circumferential multilayered tubular structures [12]. Using this technique, tubular constructs of urethra have been developed using human urothelial cells and human bladder smooth muscle cells.

30.4 Clinical Results of Tissue-Engineered Grafts

Both animal and human studies have assessed the feasibility of using tissue-engineered grafts for urethral regeneration. The results of these studies have been encouraging; however, it was noted by Versteegden et al. in a recent meta-analysis of preclinical and clinical studies that the results obtained in animal models did not translate into the human subjects [13]. This difference is likely due to the design of preclinical studies. The animal models usually had a healthy urethra which provided a suitable environment for the uptake of the graft whereas most of the patients who require such grafts usually have a scarred and fibrotic region where the graft is placed.

Most of the clinical studies on the use of tissue-engineered grafts for urethral replacement have been performed in adults with urethral strictures. The use of tissue-engineered urethra in children is still considered experimental. The earliest studies were performed in the early 1990s and involved use of autologous urethral epithelial cells mounted on petroleum gauze or polytetrafluoroethylene tube and had dismal results [14, 15]. In 1999, Atala et al. reported the use of bladder submucosal, collagen-based inert matrix for urethral repair in four boys with history of failed hypospadias surgery [16]. The collagen matrices were obtained from cadaver bladders after processing to render them noncellular and nonimmunogenic. They were used in an onlay fashion over the urethral plate and the length of the neo-urethra ranged from 5 to 15 cm. At 22 months, except for one boy who had a subglanular fistula, the remaining three boys had a successful outcome. Much later, in 2009, Li et al. used gelatin sponge in combination with tissue from prepuce or urethral plate to reconstruct the urethra, supported by a local flap [17]. The mean repaired length was smaller, about 3.4 cm and over a follow-up period of 2–24 months, none had a fistula or a stricture although slight penile curvature was noted in one patient.

Raya-Rivera et al. reported use of cell-seeded tubularized PGA:PLGA scaffolds in five boys with posterior urethral defects [18]. Autologous epithelial and muscle cells were obtained from a tissue biopsy and were expanded in culture before being seeded. After posterior urethroplasty, urethral biopsies at 3 months revealed a normal appearing architecture in the engineered grafts which remained functional for up to 6 years of follow-up. Long-term results of this type of graft are not yet known. In the next year, Fossum et al. reported long-term follow-up of 8 boys with severe hypospadias, who underwent urethroplasty with autologous urothelial cell-seeded acellular dermis [19]. At 7.25 years of follow-up, all had a good cosmetic appearance and all but one had bell shaped uroflowmetry curve. Though this study lacked a control group and had a small sample size, it indicated that the cell-seeded matrices have a good long-term outcome. Subsequently, Orabi et al. performed a pilot study of 12 patients with hypospadias (distal in six, mid-shaft in four, and proximal in two) who underwent a repair with four-layer prefabricated SIS as an onlay graft [20]. These boys were either circumcised or had a failed previous repair. After a mean follow-up of 23 months, six patients had a successful repair, three had urethrocutaneous fistula requiring closure, and remaining three had complete disruption or stricture. The authors identified graft infection as the main cause of graft failure.

Till now, there is lack of well-designed studies with a control group on use of engineered urethra. The series reported thus far are retrospective reviews with a small sample size. The results are no better than those with the current techniques of repair which underline the need for further refinement in technology.

30.5 Future Outlook

The evolution of biomaterials for urethral regeneration began with non-biodegradable materials which were very soon replaced by biodegradable scaffolds. However, the transition of biodegradable materials from preclinical to clinical studies failed the expectations. Composite materials involving natural and synthetic components improved the mechanical and biological properties suited for urethral regeneration. As the technology evolved further, the last decade saw a rise in "smart" biomaterials which respond reversibly to temperature, pH, light, and ionic strength. These responses include gelation, reversible adsorption, collapse, and alteration between hydrophobic and hydrophilic states. Further, incorporation of peptides into the structure of the smart biomaterials can create 3D scaffolds for synthesizing scaffolds that closely mimic the native ECM.

Thermo-responsive polymers change volume or phase with change in temperature. They are precipitated above a lower critical solution temperature, becoming hydrophobic while they remain hydrated and hence hydrophilic below the critical temperature. Shape-memory polymers change shape in response to a stimulus such as heat. Similarly, electroconductive polymers may be useful to regenerate electrically active tissue such as muscle. A collaborative effort between the clinics and the laboratory will pave way for the advent of biomaterials with successful bench-to-beside application.

References

1. Duckett JW. The current hype in hypospadiology. Br J Urol. 1995;76(Suppl 3):1–7.
2. Pippi Salle JL, Sayed S, Salle A, et al. Proximal hypospadias: a persistent challenge. Single institution outcome analysis of three surgical techniques over a 10-year period. J Pediatr Urol. 2016;12(1):28.e1–7.
3. Chung YG, Tu D, Franck D, et al. Acellular bi-layer silk fibroin scaffolds support tissue regeneration in a rabbit model of onlay urethroplasty. PLoS One. 2014;9(3):e91592.
4. Lv X, Li Z, Chen S, et al. Structural and functional evaluation of oxygenating keratin/silk fibroin scaffold and initial assessment of their potential for urethral tissue engineering. Biomaterials. 2016;84:99–110.
5. El-assmy A, El-hamid MA, Hafez AT. Urethral replacement: a comparison between small intestinal submucosa grafts and spontaneous regeneration. BJU Int. 2004;94(7):1132–5.
6. Kawano PR, Fugita OE, Yamamoto HA, Quitzan JG, Padovani C, Amaro JL. Comparative study between porcine small intestinal submucosa and buccal mucosa in a partial urethra substitution in rabbits. J Endourol. 2012;26(5):427–32.
7. Cao N, Song L, Liu W, et al. Prevascularized bladder acellular matrix hydrogel/silk fibroin composite scaffolds promote the regeneration of urethra in a rabbit model. Biomed Mater. 2018;14(1):015002.
8. Horst M, Madduri S, Milleret V, Sulser T, Gobet R, Eberli D. A bilayered hybrid microfibrous PLGA--acellular matrix scaffold for hollow organ tissue engineering. Biomaterials. 2013;34(5):1537–45.
9. Zhang K, Guo X, Zhao W, Niu G, Mo X, Fu Q. Application of Wnt pathway inhibitor delivering scaffold for inhibiting fibrosis in urethra strictures: in vitro and in vivo study. Int J Mol Sci. 2015;16(11):27659–76.
10. Wei G, Li C, Fu Q, Xu Y, Li H. Preparation of PCL/silk fibroin/collagen electrospun fiber for urethral reconstruction. Int Urol Nephrol. 2015;47(1):95–9.
11. Zhang K, Fu Q, Yoo J, et al. 3D bioprinting of urethra with PCL/PLCL blend and dual autologous cells in fibrin hydrogel: an in vitro evaluation of biomimetic mechanical property and cell growth environment. Acta Biomater. 2017;50:154–64.
12. Pi Q, Maharjan S, Yan X, et al. Digitally Tunable microfluidic bioprinting of multilayered cannular tissues. Adv Mater Weinheim. 2018;30(43):e1706913.
13. Versteegden LRM, De Jonge PKJD, Inthout J, et al. Tissue engineering of the urethra: a systematic review and meta-analysis of preclinical and clinical studies. Eur Urol. 2017;72(4):594–606.

14. Romagnoli G, De Luca M, Faranda F, Franzi AT, Cancedda R. One-step treatment of proximal hypospadias by the autologous graft of cultured urethral epithelium. J Urol. 1993;150(4):1204–7.
15. Romagnoli G, De Luca M, Faranda F, et al. Treatment of posterior hypospadias by the autologous graft of cultured urethral epithelium. N Engl J Med. 1990;323(8):527–30.
16. Atala A, Guzman L, Retik AB. A novel inert collagen matrix for hypospadias repair. J Urol. 1999;162(3 Pt 2):1148–51.
17. Li P, Li S, Zhao M, et al. Urethral reconstruction using gelatin sponge and micro-mucosa graft combined with local flap. Zhongguo Xiu Fu Chong Jian Wai Ke Za Zhi. 2009;23(3):313–5.
18. Raya-rivera A, Esquiliano DR, Yoo JJ, Lopez-bayghen E, Soker S, Atala A. Tissue-engineered autologous urethras for patients who need reconstruction: an observational study. Lancet. 2011;377(9772):1175–82.
19. Fossum M, Skikuniene J, Orrego A, Nordenskjöld A. Prepubertal follow-up after hypospadias repair with autologous in vitro cultured urothelial cells. Acta Paediatr. 2012;101(7):755–60.
20. Orabi H, Safwat AS, Shahat A, Hammouda HM. The use of small intestinal submucosa graft for hypospadias repair: pilot study. Arab J Urol. 2013;11(4):415–20.

Variables in Hypospadias Repair

31

Amilal Bhat

31.1 Introduction

Hypospadias is one of the most common congenital anomalies of external genitalia. There are more than 300 techniques and their modifications. Still, the results of hypospadias surgery remain challenging to idealize. Modern-day hypospadiology is emerging as a super-speciality. Despite the advances in surgical procedures, complication rates after hypospadias repair remain high. Patient-related variables of hypospadias surgery are the hypospadias type, patient age, chordee severity, penis and glans size, the width of the urethral plate and spongiosum development, and length, presence, and length of the hypoplastic urethra, preputial reconstruction, and suture material used. These factors affect the outcome in isolation or combination. The effect of suture material, sutures, and general considerations are described in Chap. 5 on general considerations in hypospadias. The variables related to the patients and surgical skills are of immense importance in the outcome of the repair. Knowing these variables will guide the surgeon to choose the type of repair, planning of surgery, anticipated difficulties during surgery, and measures to improve the results.

31.2 Variables

31.2.1 Surgical Experience

Every surgical procedure has a learning curve. Most surgeries have a short learning curve, but it is a long journey in hypospadias surgery. The workload of hypospadias surgery is insufficient in most of the training centers during the fellowship program. The surgeon must handle the tissue with the viable vessels, manipulate the tissue very exquisitely, suture without tension, and use fine suture materials and obtain careful hemostasis to increase the hypospadias repair success rate. The trainees have a more number and a better exposure in the high-volume training centers and hospitals, which shortens the learning curve. But the low volume hypospadias centers trained fellows needing a specialized training program after completing the fellowship. In general, most of the residents and attending physicians have limited assess and participation in hypospadias

A. Bhat (✉)
Bhat's Hypospadias and Reconstructive Urology Hospital and Research Centre,
Jaipur, Rajasthan, India

Department of Urology, Jaipur National University Institute for Medical Sciences and Research Centre,
Jaipur, Rajasthan, India

Department of Urology, Dr. S.N. Medical College,
Jodhpur, Rajasthan, India

Department of Urology, S.P. Medical College,
Bikaner, Rajasthan, India

P.G. Committee Medical Council of India,
New Delhi, India

Academic and Research Council of RUHS,
Jaipur, Rajasthan, India

surgery. The pediatric urologists and trainee fellows believe that a specialized training program is needed to perform an independent hypospadias surgery [1]. Ansari et al. (2016) reported that the consultant has to spend about two years reaching the learning curve with at least 50 cases [2]. Rompre et al. in 2013 reported that it takes about 50–75 cases in TIPU repair to stabilize the learning curve. It became a predictable negative exponential curve, suggesting that the surgical outcome improved constantly and did not rapidly reach a plateau. This indicates that even after intensive fellowship training and exposure to many different hypospadias procedures under the supervision of experienced surgeons, the urologists may still experience a steep learning curve at the beginning of independent practice and had to face a significantly higher rate of complications [3]. Mohammed M et al. (2020) reported lower complications in the patients operated by an experienced surgeon than a less experienced surgeon and a significant impact on reducing long-term complications from 35% to 9% [4]. Fewer complications by experienced surgeons are due to improved learning curve and hand skills, having a better judgment in choosing the best technique for the individual case. Authors believe that the decision-making, planning, execution, and outcome of the hypospadias surgery improve with the surgeon's experience.

31.2.2 Age

Based on a review of psychological, aesthetic, and surgical factors, the current recommendation of the American Academy of Paediatrics primary hypospadias repair age is 6–12 months. Higher complication rates in older patients with hypospadias repair have been reported in several studies. In our study, we grouped the patients into (i) the children before toilet training, (ii) toilet trained children who had and started going to school, (iii) school-going children with a rebellious attitude, (iv) pubertal boys with a penile growth spurt with rising testosterone level leading to increased vascularity of penile tissues and (v) adolescents and adults with problems of nocturnal and day time erections. The complications increased statistically significant with age. Age becomes an important independent factor in patients of more than 15 years (Tables 31.1 and 31.2). Poor results may be due to increased susceptibility to infection, differences in vascularity, wound healing, and postoperative erections in adolescents and adults [5–7]. Lu W et al. (2012) reported an inverse relationship between the age at surgery and operation memory; patients less than two years are less likely to remember the surgical procedure. There have been reports of greater satisfaction and cosmetic outcome with younger age of hypospadias repair. Performing hypospadias surgery at later ages may predispose patients to a greater likelihood of post-surgical complications, the most common being urethral fistulas [8]. Yildiz et al. (2013) analyzed the data of 307 patients and found the highest fistula rate in the age group of 10–14 years. They recommended the age and surgical technique variable in the hypospadias surgery planning [9]. Perlmutter et al. (2006) reported a complication rate of 2% in 102 cases of age <6 months and 10.3% in 223 cases of hypospadias > 6 months of age. They concluded that the complications could be minimized by performing hypospadias repair surgery at 4–6 months [10]. Bush et al. (2013) found no correlation of complications with age in 669 consecutive hypospadias surgery and recommended that the surgery can be undertaken any time after three months of age [11]. The authors believe that age is an independent variable in hypospadias repair, and childhood surgery has better results than adulthood.

31.2.3 Hypospadias Severity

Hypospadias severity is the single most pertinent factor in its surgical outcome. The severity of the hypospadias and the degree of chordee guides the surgeon to decide the type of urethroplasty; single-stage or two-stage repair and plate preservation or transaction urethroplasty. The plate preservation procedures have a better outcome than plate transection techniques. In one of our studies of 125 cases, we classified the severity of the hypospadias by the location of meatus after

Table 31.1 Showing various variables, complications, and statistical significance in TIPU (with permission Bhat et al. [5] © copyright Bhat et al. IBIMA Publishing)

Age (in years)	0.5–2 years	2–5 Years	5–10 Years	10–15 Years	<15 Years	Total No.125	Complications	p-value
No of Patients	30 (24)	28(22.4)	22(17.6)	20(16)	25 (20)	(100.0)		
Complications	1(3.3)	1(3.6)	3(13.6)	3(15)	5(20)	13 (100)		0.001
Degree of Hypospadias No. Patients (%)								0.001
Distal Penile	20(66.7)	18(64.3)	15(68.2)	15(75)	19 (76)	87(69.6)	5(5.7)	
Mid Penile	4(13.3)	6(21.4)	3(13.6)	2(10)	3(12)	18(14.4)	2(11.1)	
Proximal	6(20)	4(14.3)	4(18.2)	3(15)	3(12)	20(16)	6(30)	
Penile Chordee 55/125 (44%) (Mean = 30.0°) No. Patients (%)								0.0001
Nil	17(56.7)	13(46.4)	10(45.5)	14(70)	16(64)	70(56)	3(4.3)	
Mild	6(20)	8(28.6)	8(36.4)	2(10)	4(16)	28(22.4)	1(3.6)	
Moderate	4(13.3)	4(14.3)	2(9.1)	2(10)	1 (4)	13(10.4)	4(30.8)	
Severe	3(10)	3(10.7)	2(9.1)	2(10)	4(16)	14(11.2)	5(35.7)	
Quality of Spongiosum No. Patients (%)								0.0001
Well Developed	8(26.7)	18(64.3)	13(59.1)	11(55)	16 (64)	66(52.8)	3(4.5)	
Mod. Developed	20(66.7)	8(28.5)	8(36.4)	7(35)	5(20)	48(38.4)	3(6.4)	
Poorly Developed	2(6.7)	2(7.14)	1(4.5)	2(10)	4(16)	11(8.8)	7(63.6)	
Urethral Plate No. Patients (%)								0.0001
Wide	13(43.3)	18(64.3)	10(45.5)	10(50)	9(36)	60(48)	2(3.3)	
Average	15(50)	8(28.6)	8(36.4)	7(35)	10(40)	48(38.4)	4(8.3)	
Narrow	2(6.7)	2(7.14)	4(18.2)	3(15)	6(24)	17(13.6)	7(41.2)	
Penile Torsion 25/125 (20%) (Mean = 18°) No. Patients (%)								
Nil	15(50)	15(53.6)	11(50)	9(45)	10(40)	60(48)	3(5)	
Mild	12(40)	10(35.7)	8(36.4)	9(45)	10(40)	49(39.2)	7(14.3)	
Moderate	2(6.7)	2(7.1)	2(9.1)	1(5)	3(12)	10(8)	3(30)	
Severe	1(3.3)	1(3.6)	1(4.5)	1(5)	2(8)	6(4.8)	0(0)	
Size of Penis in cm (small penis-Length of penis G I <3.5, G II <4.5, GIII <5, GIV <5.5, G V <11.5) No. Patients (%)								0.43
Average	28(93.3)	27(96.4)	20(90.9)	20(100)	25 (100)	120(96)	13(10.8)	
Small	2(6.7)	1(3.5)	2(9.1)	0	0	5(4)	0(0)	
Size of Glans in mm (Small glans Diameter G I <8.0, G II <11.3, GIII <12.6, GIV <13.9, G V <21.5) No. Patients (%)								0.39
Average	27(90)	27(96.2)	20(90.9)	20(100)	25(100)	119(95.2)	13(10.9)	
Small	3(10)	1(3.6)	2(9.1)	0	0	6(4.8)	0(0)	

Table 31.2 Comparative analysis of the variables affecting surgical outcome in TIPU {with permission Bhat et al. [6] @ copyright Elsevier}

Variables	Group A (Adult)		Group B (Pediatric)	
	Cases	Complications	Cases	Complications
Type of Hypospadias				
Distal	43(71.67%)	4(9.3%)	41(68.33%)	0
Mid	07(11.67%)	2(28.5%)	10(16.67%)	1(10%)
Proximal	10(16.67%)	4(40%)	09(15%)	3(33.33%)
Total	60	10(16.67%)	60	4(6.67%)
Quality of Spongiosum				
Well developed	38(63.33%)	2(5.26%)	37(61.66%)	0
Moderately developed	11(18.33%)	2(18.18%)	11(18.33%)	0
Poorly developed	11(18.33%)	6(54.54%)	12(20%)	4(33.33%)
Width of the urethral plate				
Wide	22(36.66%)	0	24(40%)	0
Average	26(43.33%)	4(15.38%)	22(36.66%)	1(4.54%)
Narrow	12(20%)	6(50%)	14(23.33%)	3(21.43%)
Presence of Chordee				
Distal	2(4.65%)	1(50%)	3(7.32%)	0
Mid	2(28.5%)	1(50%)	3(30%)	0
Proximal	10(100%)	4(40%)	9(100%)	3(33.33%)
Presence of Torque				
Distal	9(20.93%)	0	7(17%)	0
Mid	1(14.28%)	0	2(20%)	0
Proximal	0	0	0	0

penile degloving. The hypospadias was distal penile in 69.6%, mid penile in 14.4%, and proximal penile hypospadias in 26% of the patients. There was a statistically significant (p-value = 0.001) correlation of hypospadias severity with complications rate; 30% was seen in proximal (proximal penile 11, penoscrotal 6, and perineal 3) compared to 5.7% in distal hypospadias and 11.1% in mid penile hypospadias (Tables 31.1, 31.2 and 31.3 and Fig. 31.1) [5–7]. Complications in relation to the severity of hypospadias were statistically significant with the severity of the curvature, the width of the urethral plate, and the development of spongiosum [5]. Hansson et al. (2007) analyzed 184 patients and remarked that hypospadias severity was the most decisive risk factor in predicting complications [12]. Sarhan et al. (2009) studied 500 patients operated by five surgeons and, in a multivariate analysis, concluded that proximal location of the meatus is an independent risk factor in the occurrence of complication, and the other significant factors were neourethra not covered with intervening tissue and learning curve [13]. Bush et al. evaluated the risk factors in prospectively collected data of 669 consecutive patients and concluded that meatal location (i.e., the severity of hypospadias) and reoperation were the only two independent risk factors for increased complications in the study [14]. Pfistermuller et al. al (2015) conducted a meta-analysis of studies that discussed complications following TIP repair of hypospadias and concluded that the incidence rate of complication was greater in proximal hypospadias than distal hypospadias [15]. Silva et al. reported 36.96% complications in proximal hypospadias in a study of 300 patients [16] Long et al., in a meta-analysis of 11 studies, concluded that only 13% of the patients had severe hypospadias and the incidence of complication after hypospadias repair is greater in proximal hypospadias (45%) which was significantly higher than the overall complication rate (17%) [17]. Mohamad M et al. (2020) reported that the proximal type of hypospadias has a 29% higher chance of developing long-term complications than the middle and distal types. Urethrocutaneous fistula was observed in 66% proximal, 51% middle, and 20% distal, espe-

Table 31.3 Correlation of variables with the type of hypospadias in TIPU {with permission Bhat et al. [5] @ copyright Bhat et al. IBIMA Publishing}

Variables		Type of hypospadias			Complications	p-value
		Distal	Mid penile	Proximal		
Age of patients	Group I 6 m–2 years	20 (0)	4 (0)	6 (1)	1	0.126
	Group II 2–5 years	18 (0)	6 (1)	4 (0)	1	0.149
	Group III 5–10 years	15 (1)	3 (0)	4 (2)	3	0.064
	Group IV 10–15 years	15 (1)	2 (0)	3 (2)	3	0.024
	Groups III & IV (Combine)	30 (2)	5 (0)	7 (4)	6	0.0017
	Group V >15 years	19 (3)	3 (1)	3 (1)	5	0.645
Quality of spongiosum	Well developed	49	12	5	3	$P = 0.0001$
	Moderately developed	32	7	9	3	
	Poorly developed	6	0	5	7	
Width of Urethral Plate	Wide	41	11	8	2	$P = 0.0018$
	Average	35	8	5	4	
	Narrow	11	0	6	7	
Penile Torsion	Mild (<45)	12	2	2	6	$P = 0.823$
	Moderate (45–90)	4	2	1	3	
	Severe (>90)	2	0	0	0	
Degree of Penile curvature	Mild (<30)	24	3	1	2	$P = 0.0004$
	Moderate (30–60)	6	3	4	3	
	Severe (>90)	3	2	9	5	
Size of penis	Average	84	17	19	13	$P = 0.929$
	Small	3	1	1	0	
Size of glans	Average	83	17	19	13	$P = 0.876$
	Small	4	1	1	0	

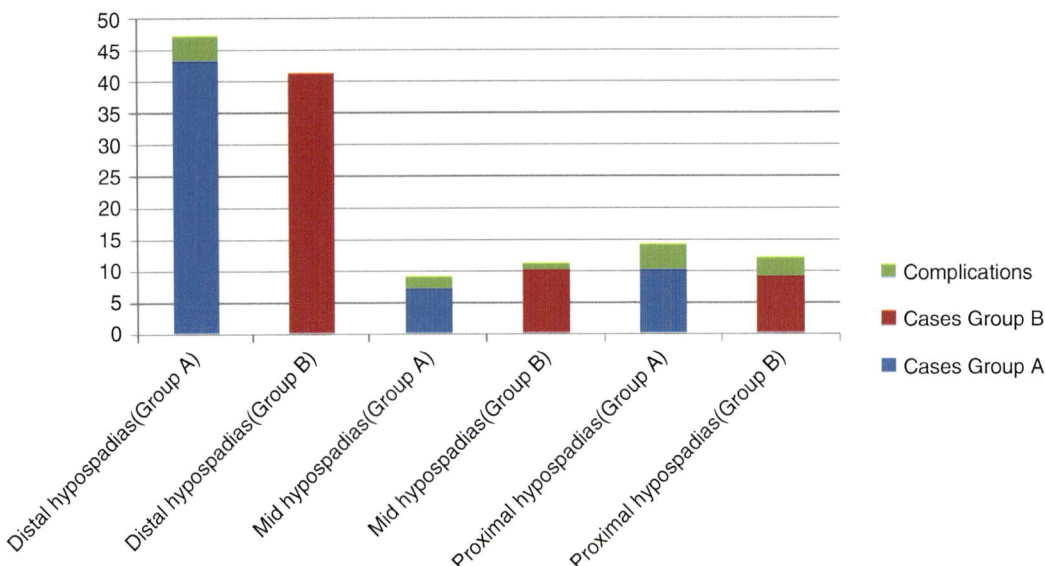

Fig. 31.1 Showing the effect of type of hypospadias on surgical outcome in TIPU (Group A – Adults; Group B – Pediatric cases) {with permission Bhat et al. [6] @ copyright Elsevier}

cially if it was associated with severe chordee [4]. Chung et al. (2013) reported a significantly better outcome in distal hypospadias. Only the severity of hypospadias has a statistically significant impact on urethrocutaneous fistula development, but the type of hypospadias repair, suture materials, and technique had no significant effect on the outcome [18].

31.2.4 Chordee

Chordee is divided into mild, moderate, and severe. Chordee is an independent variable in the outcome of hypospadias repair. Depending upon the severity of the chordee and its correction, the urethroplasty is decided. Chordee may be mild to severe in all types of hypospadias (Fig. 31.2a–j). Most of the moderate to severe chordee cases require transection of the urethral plate. So, these patients are managed either by replacing urethroplasty or two-stage repairs with poor results compared to plate preservation procedures. A detailed description of etiology and methods of chordee corrections is described in Chap. 6 on chordee correction. A step-by-step approach is better to preserve the urethral plate, increase the chances of TIPU having better results (Fig. 31.3a–i), and decrease the dorsal plication rate (Fig. 31.4a–f). In one of our studies of 125 cases 3.6% of mild, 38.8% moderate, and 35.7% of severe cases had complications ($p = 0.0001$) (Tables 31.1, 31.2 and 31.3). The degree of curvature was directly proportional to the severity of hypospadias; 50% of cases of proximal hypospadias had severe curvature, while in distal hypospadias, 62.06% did not have curvature at all (Table 31.1) [5]. Bhat et al. (2016), in a prospective study of 60 pediatric and 60 adult patients undergoing TIPU, analyzed factors influencing the outcome of hypospadias repair. They had a significantly higher complication rate in patients with severe chordee when compared to mild chordee in both adult and pediatric patients (Fig. 31.5) [6]. Uygur et al. (2002) performed a retrospective analysis of 422 cases who underwent a single-stage hypospadias repair. They reported complication rates with each technique: MAGPI (8%), meatal advancement (10%), Allen-Spence (24%), Mathieu (21%), onlay island flap (40%), and double-faced island flap (17%). They found that the complication rates were higher if the meatus was proximal with moderate chordee [19]. Snodgrass and Bush (2020) evaluated the out-

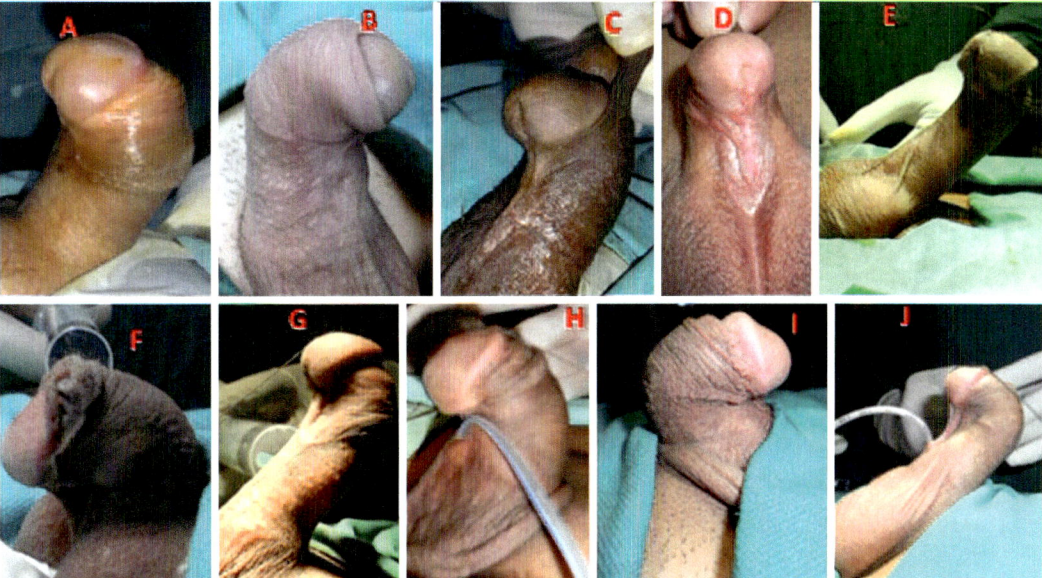

Fig. 31.2 (**a–j**) Showing a different degree of chordee (**a** and **b**) Distal penile hypospadias with Moderate chordee. (**d–h**) Mid-penile hypospadias with moderate to severe chordee. (**i** and **j**) Proximal penile hypospadias with severe chordee

come of 77 patients who had undergone TIP for proximal hypospadias and concluded that TIP should be performed only when the ventral curvature after degloving is <30 degrees. So, chordee is an independent variable in the outcome of hypospadias repair [20].

31.2.5 Urethral Plate

The commonest technique used in hypospadias repair is TIPU, so the urethral plate's width and characteristics impact the outcome of hypospadias surgery. The narrow urethral plate is commonly defined as a width less than 8 mm [13]. But this criterion does not hold true in all cases, as the penile length and the urethral size vary with the child's age. So in our study, we took the urethral plate size compared with the proximal healthy urethra size. The urethral plate was classified into wide, average, and narrow. It was labeled wide when the urethral plate could be easily tubularized without incision (on the largest size catheter accepted by the normal proximal urethra). If it required a superficial incision for this purpose, it was taken as average. If a deep incision of the plate was needed, it was considered a narrow one [5–7]. The width of the urethral plate and its development are also very important variables in the outcome of the hypospadias repair. Most of the literature is on the effect of the width of the urethral plate on hypospadias repair and that too in distal hypospadias. Therefore, we included the width and other characteristics of the urethral plate and divided it into three groups.

- Favorable: The urethral plate is wide enough to tubularize without incision, underlying spongiosum is healthy, tissue is pliable (Fig. 31.6a–j).
- Intermediate: Another important observation in distal hypospadias is an intervening skin or breach in the continuity of the meatus with the urethral plate (Fig. 31.7a–j), which, after incision, can adversely affect the epithelization and may increase the chances of stricture. Average width can be tubularized after incision, and moderately developed urethral plate

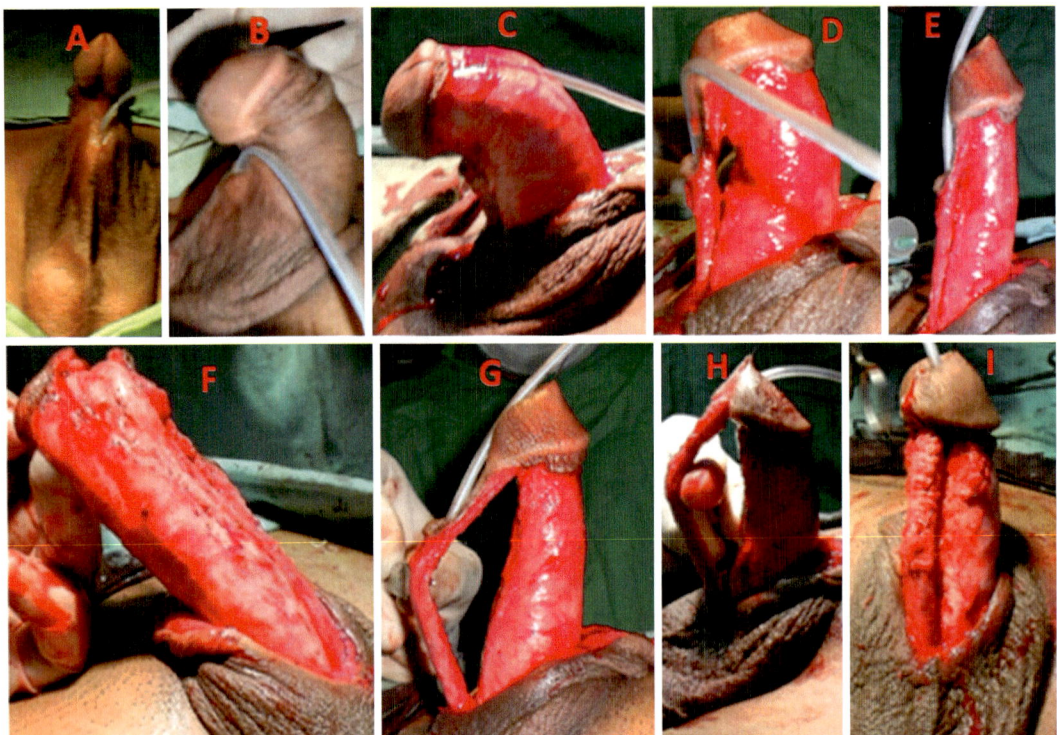

Fig. 31.3 Showing step-by-step correction of curvature in plate preserving procedure. (**a** and **b**) Mid-penile hypospadias with severe chordee. (**c**) Penile degloving and chordee persisting. (**d** and **e**) Urethral plate with spongiosum mobilisation (**f**) Resection of tethering tissue and midline dissection of Buck's fascia, (**g**) Proximal mobilization of urethra up to penoscrotal junction (**h**) Urethral plate mobilization into glans and urethral plate tubularization. (**i**) Glansplasty and spongioplasty and chordee corrected

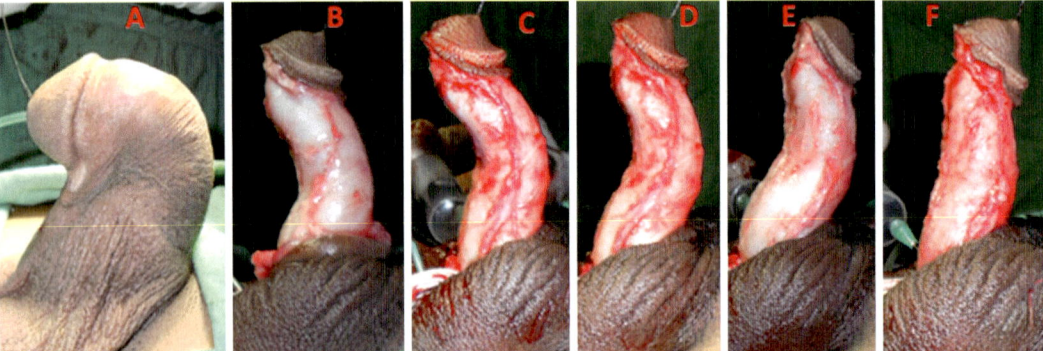

Fig. 31.4 Showing step-by-step correction of curvature in plate transecting procedure. (**a**) Proximal penile hypospadias with severe chordee (**b**) Penile degloving chordee persisting, (**c**) Midline dissection of Bucks fascia (**d**) Lateralization of Buck's fascia, (**e**) Superficial corporotomies. (**f**) Release of glanular chordee and chordee corrected

31 Variables in Hypospadias Repair

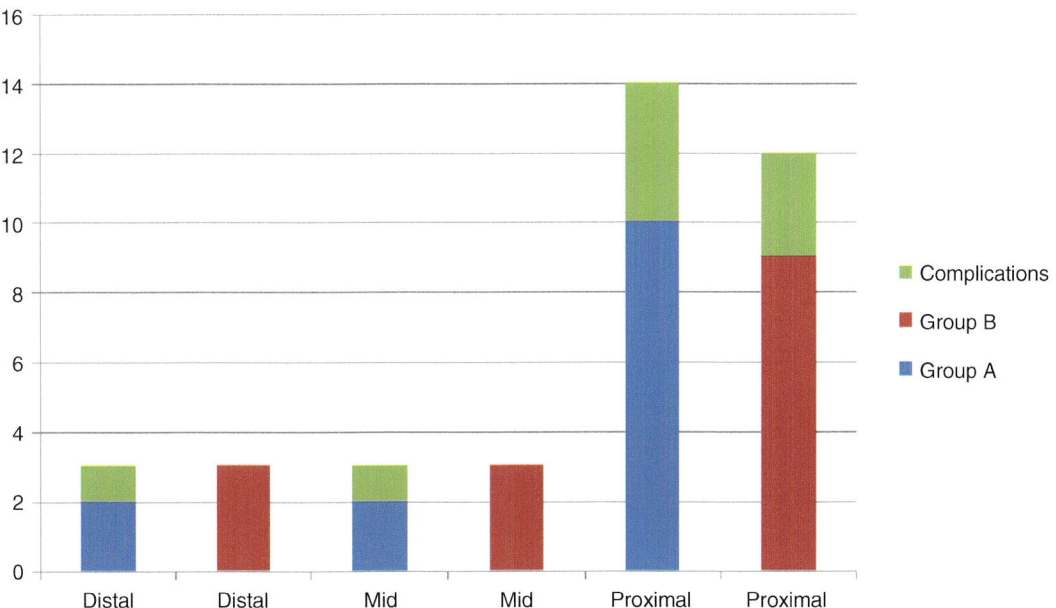

Fig. 31.5 Showing the effect of Chordee on surgical outcome in TIPU (Group A – Adults; Group B – Pediatric cases) {with permission Bhat et al. [6] @ copyright Elsevier}

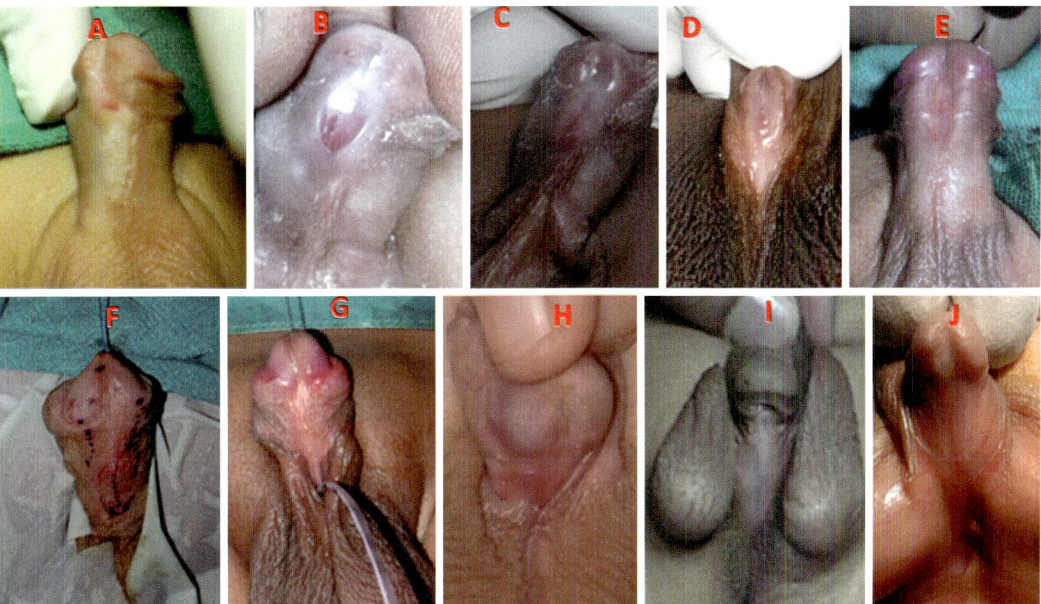

Fig. 31.6 Showing the various type of hypospadias with a favorable urethral plate (**a** and **b**) distal Penile hypospadias. (**c–e**) Mid -Penile hypospadias. (**f–h**) Proximal Penile hypospadias (**i** and **j**) Perineal hypospadias

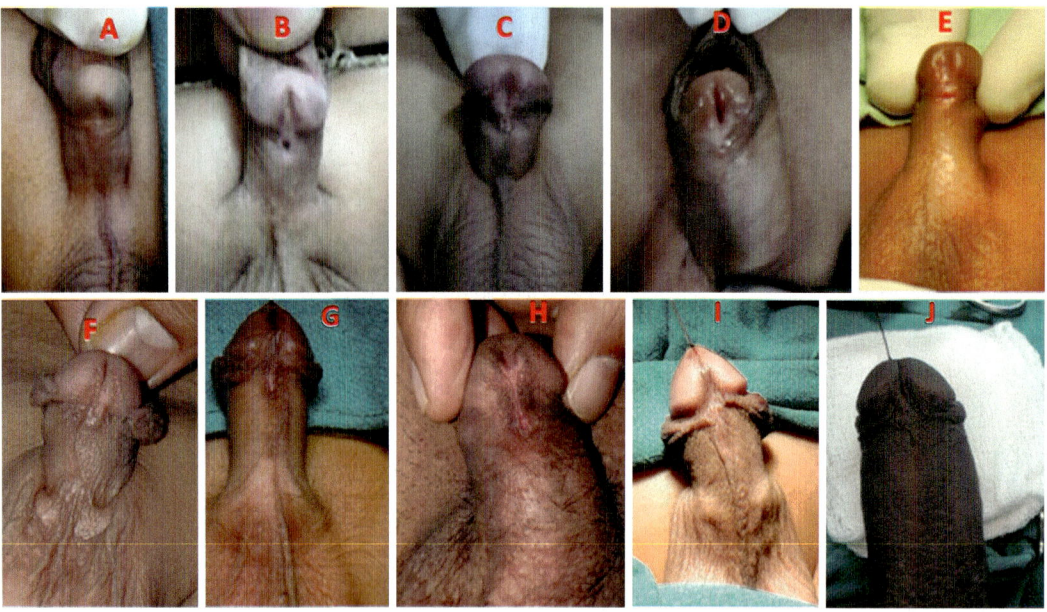

Fig. 31.7 (**a–j**) Showing the various type of urethral plate in the favorable group with intervening tissue between the meatus and urethral plate

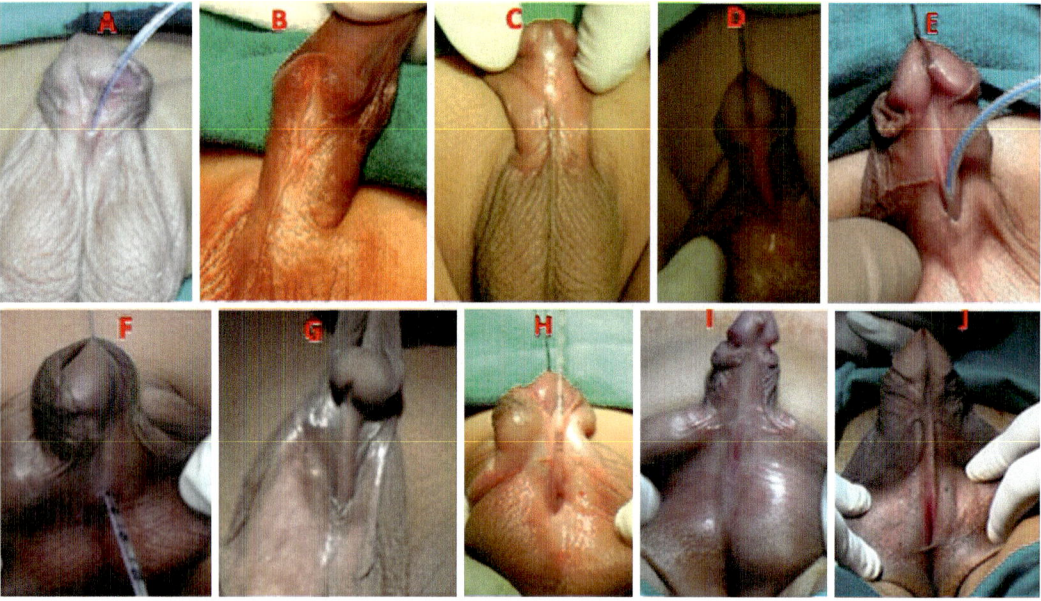

Fig. 31.8 Showing the various type of Narrow urethral plate with an intermediate urethral plate (**a–c**) Mid penile hypospadias (**d** and **e**) proximal penile hypospadias (**f–i**) Scrotal hypospadias (**j**) Perineoscrotal hypospadias

may also have an increased likelihood of complication (Fig. 31.8a–j). These intermediate urethral plate patients are the most difficult ones to choose the type of repair. Depending on the surgeon's choice, experience & preference, both plate preservation and plate transection procedures may be chosen. It is advisable to augment the urethral plate with dorsal inlay grafts in plate preservation procedures.

31 Variables in Hypospadias Repair

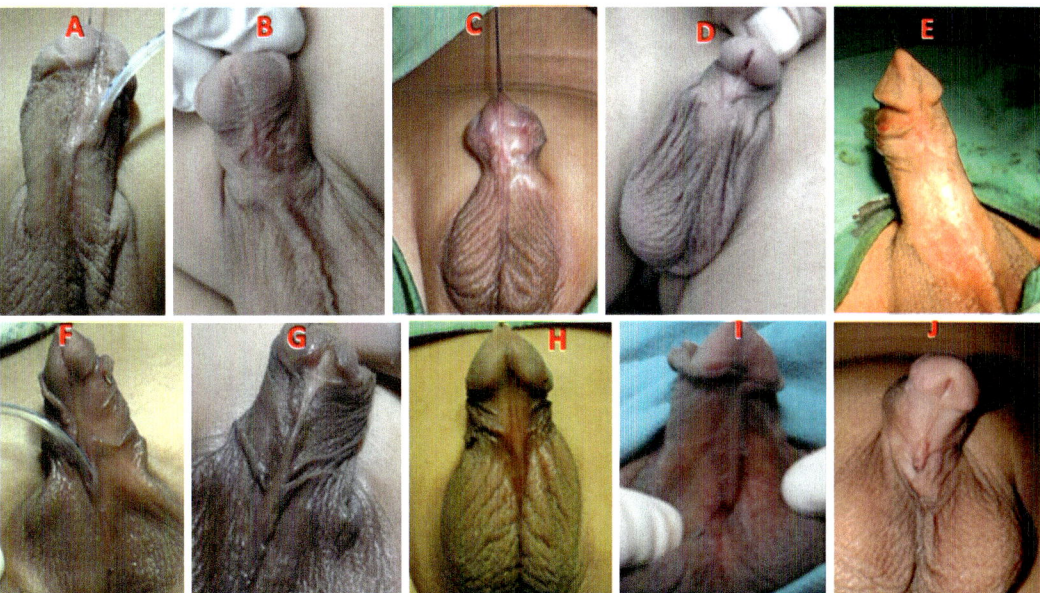

Fig. 31.9 Showing hypospadias with Unfavorable Poorly developed urethral plate (**a–e**) Mid-penile hypospadias with the poor urethral plate. (**f–i**) Scrotal hypospadias with poor urethral plate

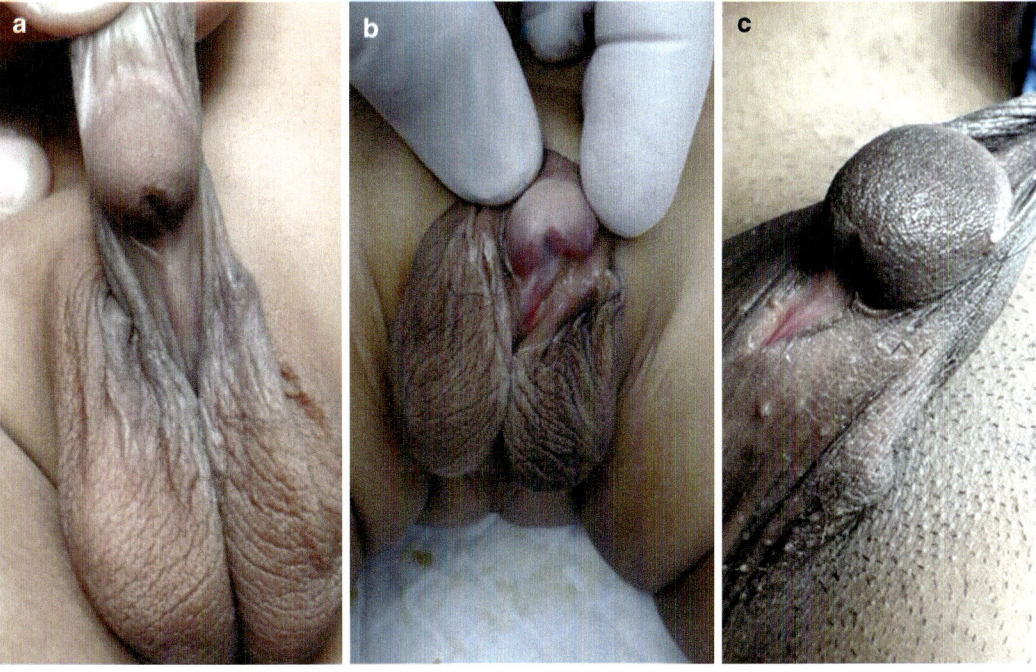

Fig. 31.10 (**a–c**) Showing wide urethral plate with moderate to severe curvature

- Unfavorable: This group of cases has hardly any urethral plate identifiable (Fig. 31.9a–j) or severe hypospadias with moderate to severe curvature (Fig. 31.2a–j). These urethral plates usually require excision and the replacement urethroplasty. But a wide urethral plate in severe hypospadias (Fig. 31.10a–c) can be mobilized and preserved to be used to cover the anastomosis in single-stage repair and two-stage repair.

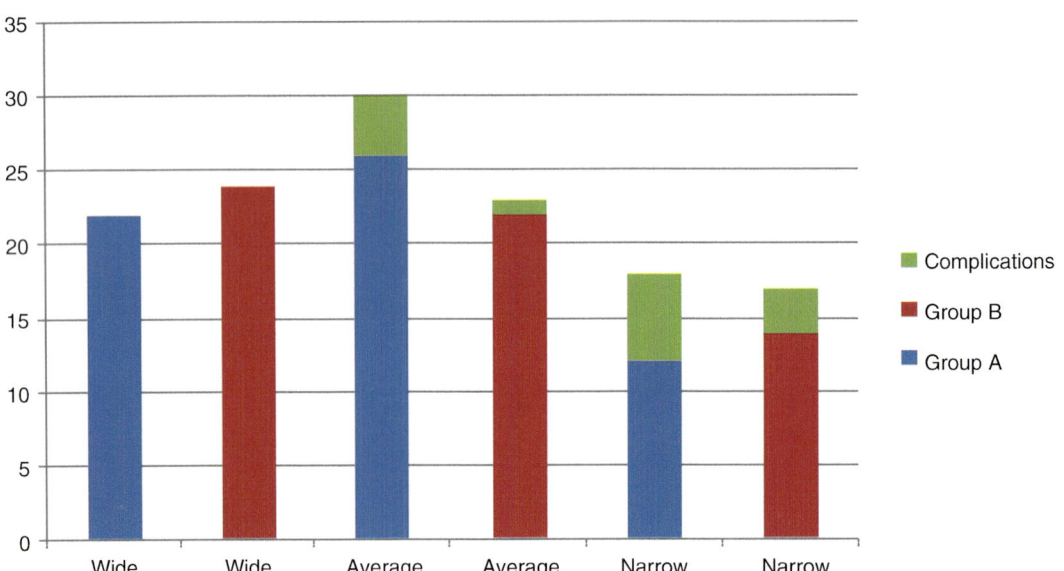

Fig. 31.11 Showing the effect of width of urethral plate on surgical outcome in TIPU (Group A – Adults; Group B – Pediatric cases) {with permission Bhat et al. [6] @ copyright Elsevier}

We reported in our study that the urethral plate was wide in 48%, average in 38.4%, and narrow in 13.6% of patients. Complications were found in 41.2% of narrow urethral plate cases and 8.3% of average width cases. None of the patients with wide urethral plate had any complications, which again was statistically significant (Table 31.2 and Fig. 31.11) (p-value = 0.0001) [6].

Nguyen et al.al (2004) analyzed TIPU outcomes in a patient with distal hypospadias with respect to urethral plate characteristics. They found no significant difference in the complication rates in cases with urethral plate width greater and lesser than 8 mm [21]. But Sarhan et al. (2009) evaluated urethral plate depth, length, and width before and after incision. They found that the width of the urethral plate was significantly associated with the incidence of complications [13].

Moshrafa et al. (2009) analyzed the outcome of 117 patients undergoing hypospadias repair regarding urethral plate. They reported a high complication rate in the 8 Fr group, 18.45% in comparison, the 10 Fr group had a complication rate of only 6.32% [p.08] [22].

Chukwubuike et al. (2019) analyzed the outcome of two groups of patients undergoing urethroplasty with urethral plate greater and lesser than 8mm. They found that the cosmetic outcomes were similar in both groups. However, they found that the urinary stream was better in patients with urethral plate width greater than 8 mm. They concluded that the width of the urethral plate does not influence the cosmetic outcomes. But it plays a significant role in the functional outcome of hypospadias repair [23]. As per the author's view, the width and development urethral plate is a key factor in deciding the type of repair and results of hypospadias repair.

31.2.6 Development of Spongiosum and Spongioplasty

Spongiosum is vascular tissue spread over the corporal bodies under and by the side of the urethral plate. The spongiosum development affects the characteristics of the urethral plate. Spongiosum is infrequently used as a healthy tissue cover in hypospadias repair. We classified the spongiosum into well-developed, moderately developed, and poorly developed depending on the thickness and vascularity of the spongiosal tissue and recently [24–27]. Details of classification with figures are described in Chap. 11 on

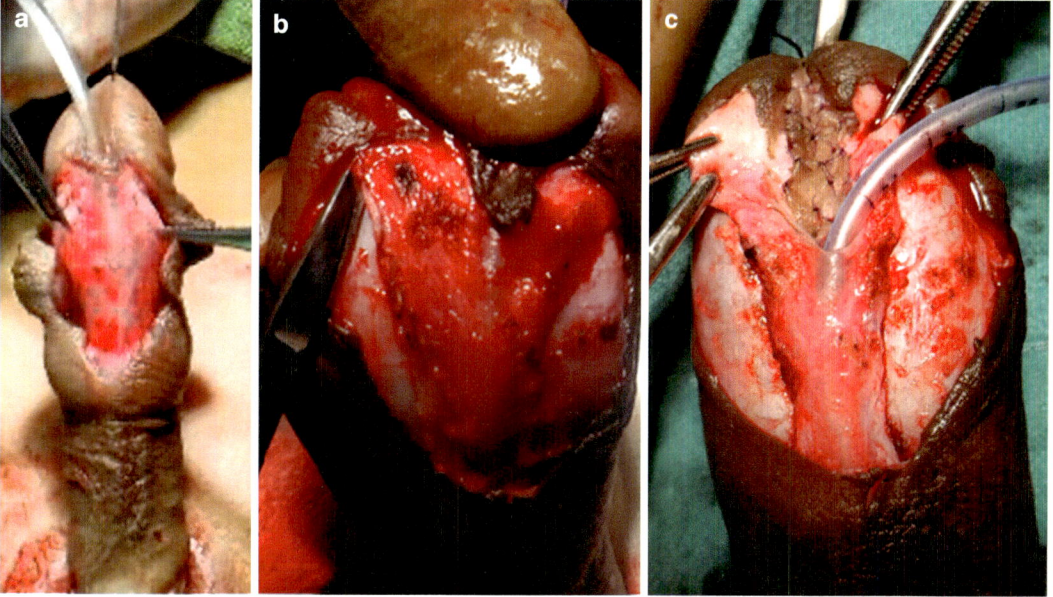

Fig. 31.12 Showing prominent pillar of spongiosum. (**a**) Distal hypospadias bifurcarion of spongiosum pillar Just proximal to meatus. (**b**) Distal meatus with hyposplastic urethra bifurcarion of spongiosum pillar proximal to hpoyplastic urethra. (**c**) Proximal Hypospadias and bifurcarion of spongiosum pillar Just proximal to meatus. (**d**) Midpenile hypospadias with bifurcarion of spongiosum pillar Just proximal to meatus. (**e**) Distal penile hypospadias with wide meatus urethral plate and bifurcarion of spongiosum pillar Just proximal to meatus

Fig. 31.13 showing the Development of the spongiosum (**a**) Poorly developed. (**b**) Moderately developed. (**c**) Well developed

Spongioplasty. Zhang et al. (2020) divided the spongiosum into well-developed with light fibrosis and poorly developed with severe fibrosis [28]. Well-developed healthy spongiosum can be identified during clinical examination of the patient (Fig. 31.12a–e) and can be classified during surgery (Fig. 31.13a–c). Spongiosum can be used to interpose the healthy issues over the tubularized urethral as alone and along with other tissues like dartos and tunica vaginalis. Spongioplasty has the edge over the other interposing layers as it reconstructs a near-normal functional urethra; it is available locally and is very vascular. It maintains the vascular supply of the urethral plate and corrects curvature by adding length in a Y to I spongioplasty. The quality of spongiosum has a definite correlation with complications (Tables 31.1, 31.2 and 31.3 and Fig. 31.14). In our study, the adult group had 5.2%, and pediatric had 0% complications when

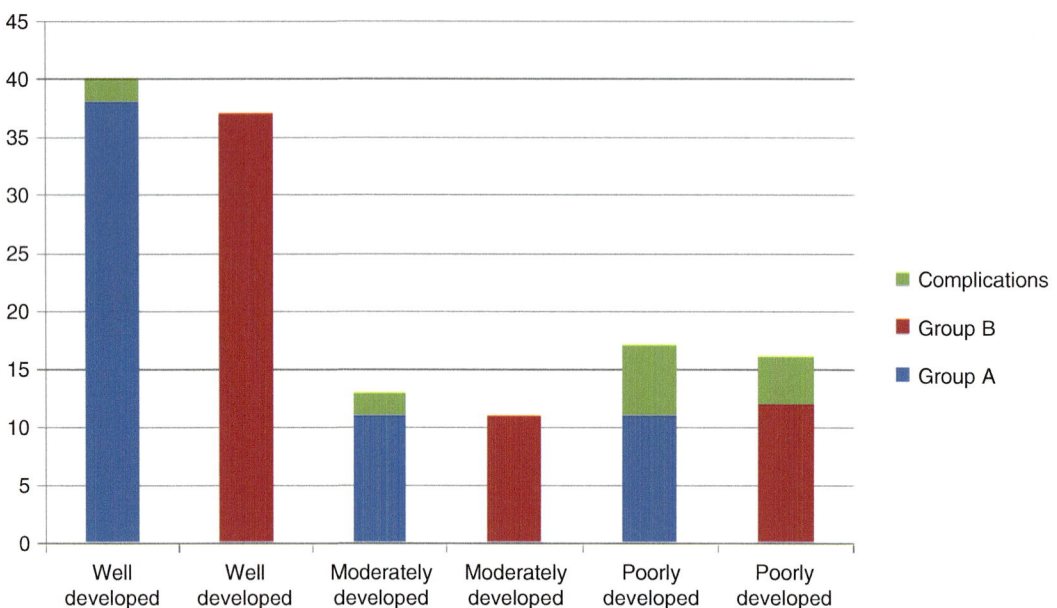

Fig. 31.14 Showing the effect of quality of spongiosum on surgical outcome in TIPU (Group A – Adults; Group B – Pediatric cases) {with permission Bhat et al. [6] @ copyright Elsevier}

the spongiosum was well developed compared with 54.5% and 33.3% in adults and pediatric patients, respectively when poorly developed. Spongioplasty was only performed as a waterproofing layer without the addition of dorsal dartos in all cases. Still, others have used the tunica vaginalis to reduce the complications in proximal hypospadias [6]. Additional dorsal dartos or tunica vaginalis is recommended to prevent complications in poorly developed spongiosum cases. Additionally, the shape of the neourethra after spongioplasty is conical. Double-breasting spongioplasty overcomes all these pitfalls, and Bhat et al. reported their results with this technique in 2017 with a significantly reduced complication rate (1.66%) than reported earlier [27]. The spongioplasty in flap repairs to cover the anastomosis was reported by Bhat et al. in 2017 with good results [29]. Cooper et al. (2001) reported the outcomes of onlay island flap urethroplasty with preservation of the spongiosum and its incorporation as a covering layer of the proximal anastomosis. They documented a complication rate of 13.8% and had no urethrocutaneous fistulae in any of the 36 patients. They concluded that the spongiosum could be readily preserved in all cases with meticulous dissection and provides a healthy vascular tissue cover over the suture lines, and reduces the incidence of urethrocutaneous fistula formation. [30]

Lyu et al. (2020) compared the outcomes of proximal hypospadias with and without spongioplasty. They found that spongioplasty patients had a significantly lower incidence of coronal fistula, glans dehiscence, and urethral strictures. [31]

Zhang et al. (2020) reviewed their experience in correcting the glans droop or glanular chordee by reconstructing forked spongiosum or spongioplasty. They operated on 85 consecutive patients in which they approximated the spongiosum in the midline in a technique similar to Yerkes Y to I spongioplasty. They reported a complication rate of 5.9% and no case of residual chordee or stricture [28].

Zhang et al. (2021) reported the efficacy of reconstructing forked corpus spongiosum in distal or midshaft hypospadias repair. They reported significantly lower complication rates in patients where spongiosum was reconstructed against the patients in the non-reconstructive group (6.8% vs 18.8%) [32]. In the author's experience, spongio-

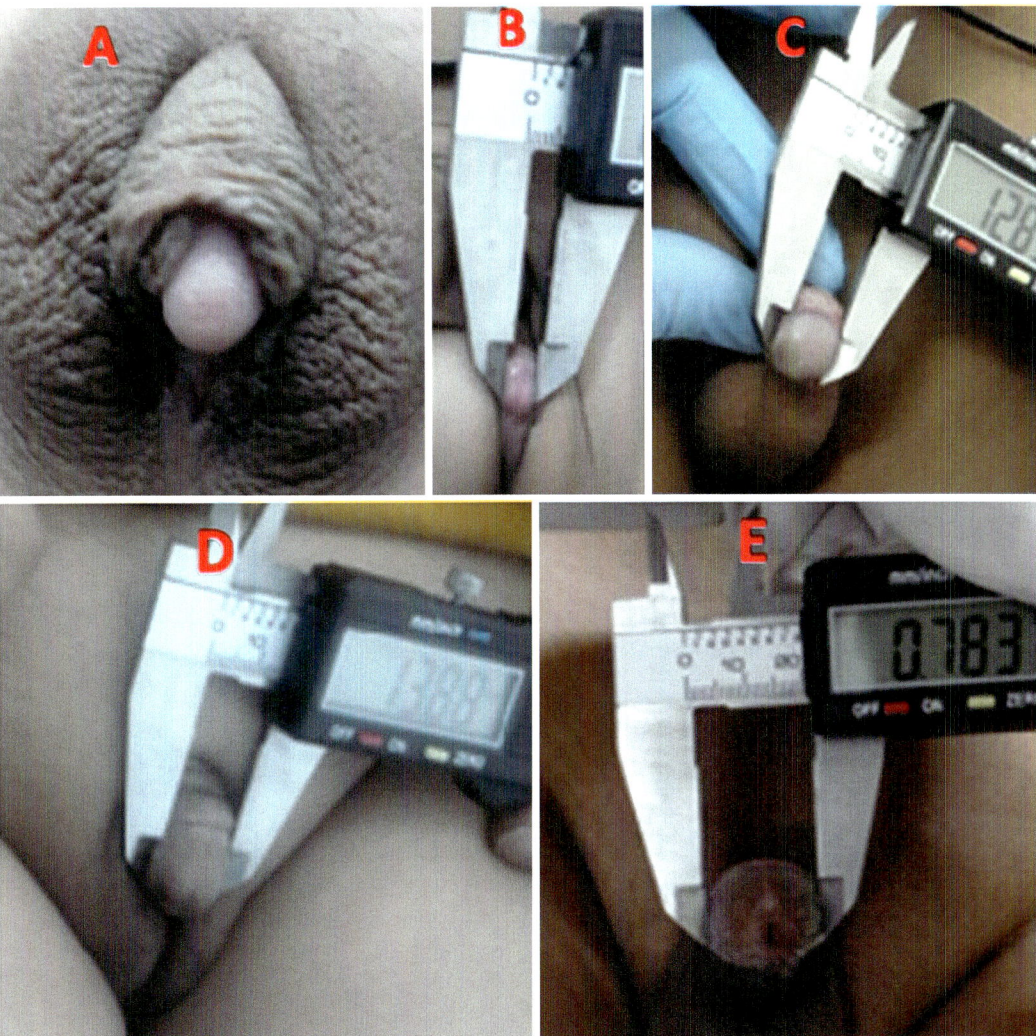

Fig. 31.15 Showing the difference in the size of glans at the same age. (**a** and **b**) 2 year child with glans size of 8 mm. (**c**) 2 year male with normal size glans 12.8 mm. (**d**) 6 years small glans 13.8 mm. (**e**) Normal 20 mm

plasty reconstructs a near-normal urethra in TIPU and reduces fistula and other complications.

31.2.7 Penis and Glans Size

The penis and glans size shows the extent of virilization. Smaller penis and glans may pose difficulties in handling the penis during surgery, and the size of suture material has to be chosen accordingly. Size may also vary with the weight of the child. Nomogram of the penile length and size of the glans is described in detail in Chap. 4, Penile anthropometry. In our study, penis and glans size was normal in more than 90% of the cases (Fig. 31.15e). At the same time, the remaining had a smaller penis (Fig. 31.15a–d). There was no statistically significant correlation between the penis and glans size and the complication rate (p-value for the size of penis 0.43 and the size of glans 0.39). No patient with the small size of the penis and glans had complications [5, 6].

Bush et al. (2013) compared glans width between 217 hypospadiacs and 240 normal male children and found that the children suffering from hypospadias had smaller glans than normal controls [33]. Bush et al. (2015), in the study of 490 continuous patients undergoing hypospadias repair, concluded that small glans size, defined as glans width <14 mm, was an independent risk factor predicting the increased incidence of complications. The complication rate was 25% in patients with a small glans and 10% in patients with a glans width >14 mm. Analyzing glans width as a continuous variable, each 1 mm increase in glans width leads to decreased odds of complications [34].

Merriman et al. (2013) introduced the GMS score, which took into account factors about the glans, meatus, and the shaft and demonstrated an adverse complication rate in cases with a GMS score less than 6 (5.6%) vs those with a score greater than 6 (25%). They, however, did not analyze the role of individual factors in complication rates following hypospadias repair [35].

Arlen et al. (2015) evaluated the performance of the GMS score in 262 boys undergoing hypospadias repair in a prospective study. They found a significant correlation between the total GMS score and postoperative complications. They described a substantial difference in fistula rates in patients with low GMS scores (2.4%) versus the patients with moderate (11.1%) and severe (22.6%) scores. They also found an independent correlation between the degree of chordee and fistula rate in a multivariate analysis. They also describe the limitations of the GMS score, the major among them being non-inclusion of the type of repair and various tissue characteristics such as tissue quality, urethral hypoplasia, and penoscrotal transposition [36]. The author shares the view that the smaller penis and glans size pose difficulty in bringing the meatus at the glans tip and affects the results of hypospadias surgery.

31.2.8 Hypoplastic Urethra

The Hypoplastic urethra is devoid of corpus spongiosum as spongiosum spreads laterally in a "Y" manner and is attached to the glans. Sometimes it is adherent to the skin as seen in chordee without hypospadias type I of Devine Horton or a few millimeters proximal to the hypospadiac meatus (Fig. 31.16a–f). Resecting more than 1cm urethra may change the location of hypospadiac meatus from distal penile to mid-penile, mid-penile to proximal penile and increases the chances of complications. Preserving the hypoplastic urethra enlarges the scope of the urethral preservation procedures like TIP, having better results than replacement urethroplasty. Since the skin adheres to the hypoplastic urethra, care is taken during mobilization, as damage to the hypoplastic urethra is likely to cause the urethral fistula. If the hypoplastic urethra is damaged during mobilization, it should be resected and replaced. Skin mobilization can be facilitated by saline injection at the site of the hypoplastic urethra to create the plane of dissection and prevent damage. The hypoplastic urethra is also resected in proximal hypospadias with chordee or middle hypospadias with severe chordee where chordee correction is required urethral plate transection. The anastomosis of the skin flap/tube increases the chances of anastomotic fistula because of poor vascularity of the hypoplastic urethra. The hypoplastic urethra should be resected up to healthy urethra covered with corpus spongiosum, and anastomosis is done with the healthy, well-vascularized urethra [37–40]. The patients with hypoplastic urethra are not suitable for the urethral mobilization technique in distal hypospadias [41]. In a study by Wong et al. (2019), Twenty-nine of 31 patients needed cutting back of the hypoplastic urethra in 6.5%, 22.6%, and 70.9% in distal, midshaft, and proximal repairs, respectively. They reported 19.4% complication in a median follow-up of 30 months and advised complex hypospadias repair to be treated by experienced surgeons [40]. In the author's opinion, the length of the hypoplastic urethra impacts decision-making and the outcome of hypospadias repair.

31.2.9 Pre-Operative Hormone Stimulation

Pre-operative hormonal treatment is used by many pediatric urologists and is usually limited to proximal hypospadias, a small penis glans, and

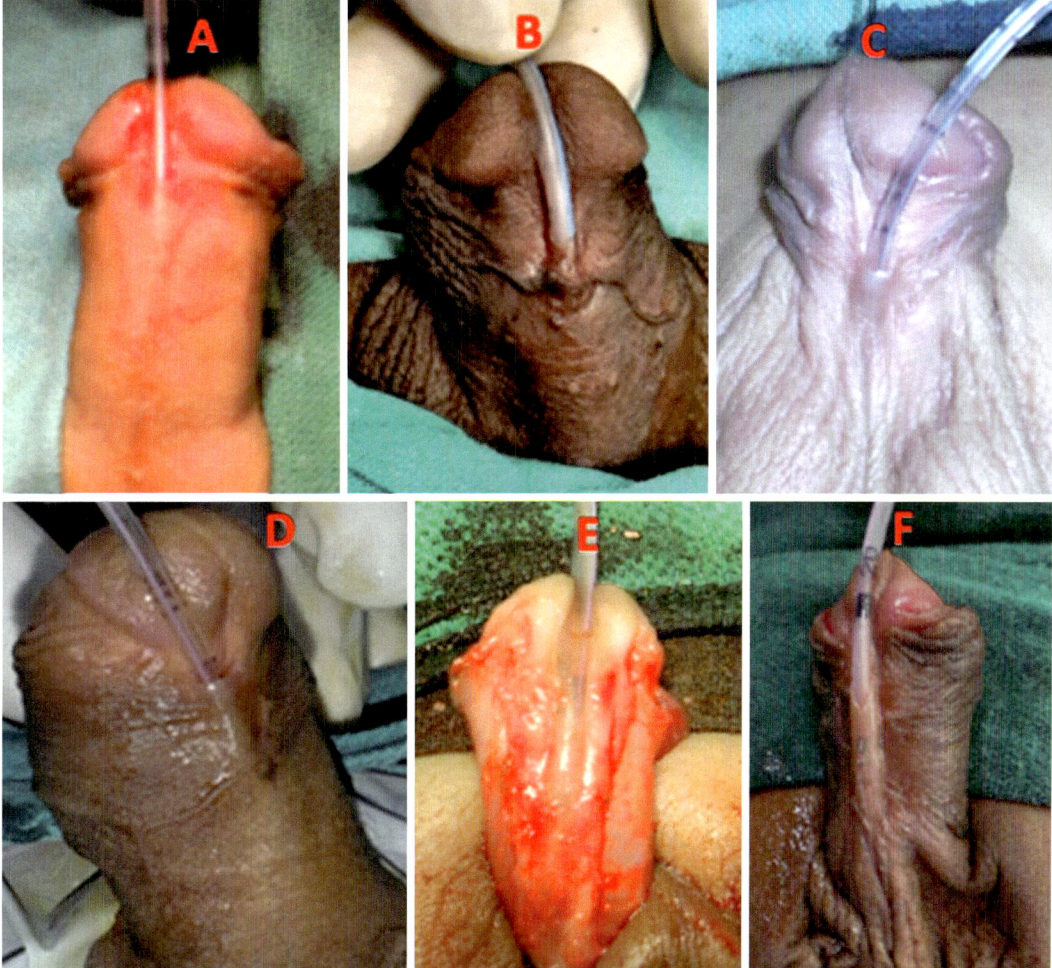

Fig. 31.16 (a–f) Showing the increasing length of the hypoplastic urethra

a narrow urethral plate. It is well tolerated and leads to significant enlargement of the glans and shaft of the penis without an increase in complication rate. Noted transient side effects are child's behavior change, genital pigmentation, the pubic hair appearance, penile skin redness and irritation, more frequent erections, and perioperative bleeding. But no persistent side effects related to hormonal stimulation have been reported in the literature and no evidence of possible effects on bone maturation. Moderate quality evidence from three randomized studies demonstrates significantly lower urethrocutaneous fistulae and reoperation rates in patients who received preoperative hormonal treatment [42].

Wright et al. (2013) in a meta-analysis of 11 studies with 622 patients, reported persistent side effects after androgen stimulation [43]. Gorduza et al. (2011) 30% complication rate with androgen stimulation vs 17% without testosterone stimulation, if <3 months of age complication rate was 57%. They reported that although the numbers were too small to reach statistical significance, dermatologists report on the tissue interactions of androgens in the healing process alert the Hypospadiologists. This demands a further prospective study to define the optimal protocol for stimulating the penis in specific cases without affecting the outcome [44]. A meta-analysis by Kaya and Radmayr concluded a significant increase in penile length and glans circumference in hypospadiac children after hormonal stimulation before repair and improved the functional and cosmetic results [45]. In the author's experience, testosterone use increases the size and vascularity of the glans and urethral plate and improves hypospadias repair in distal and middle hypospadias.

31.2.10 Penile Torsion

Penile torsion rarely gets cognizance in hypospadias surgery and is underreported. The reported incidence of isolated penile torsion is 1.7–27.0%, and severe torsion is 0.7%. Torsion is reported on both the right and left sides (Fig. 31.17a–b). Torsion is more common on the left side than on the right side [3:1]. The torsion in our study was seen in 20% of the cases. Torsion was more common as well as severe in distal hypospadias and chordee without hypospadias (Table 31.1). Etiology details and management with complications are described in Chap. 18. Zeid and Soliman reported the torque of 32% in distal hypospadias and nil proximal hypospadias [46]. In our study, the overall incidence of penile torsion associated with hypospadias was 31.6%, was commoner in distal (68.9%) than proximal (10.34%) hypospadias. Torsion is possible with chordee correction by with mobilization technique, and if required, the dorsal dartos wrap is done to correct torsion by counter-torque. There was no increase in the urethroplasty-related complications after correction of torsion [5, 47, 48]. Authors view penile torsion does not increase the complications in hypospadias repair and should be corrected with hypospadias repair.

31.2.11 Caudal Analgesia

General anesthesia is commonly used in hypospadias repair. Many centers add caudal analgesia and local penile block for a pain-free and comfortable postoperative period. Kundra et al. (2012) reported better analgesia with penile block than caudal epidural in primary hypospadias repair. The postoperative urethral fistula was more in children who received the caudal epidural [49].

In a retrospective case–control study, Zaidi et al. (2015) included 45 patients with and 90

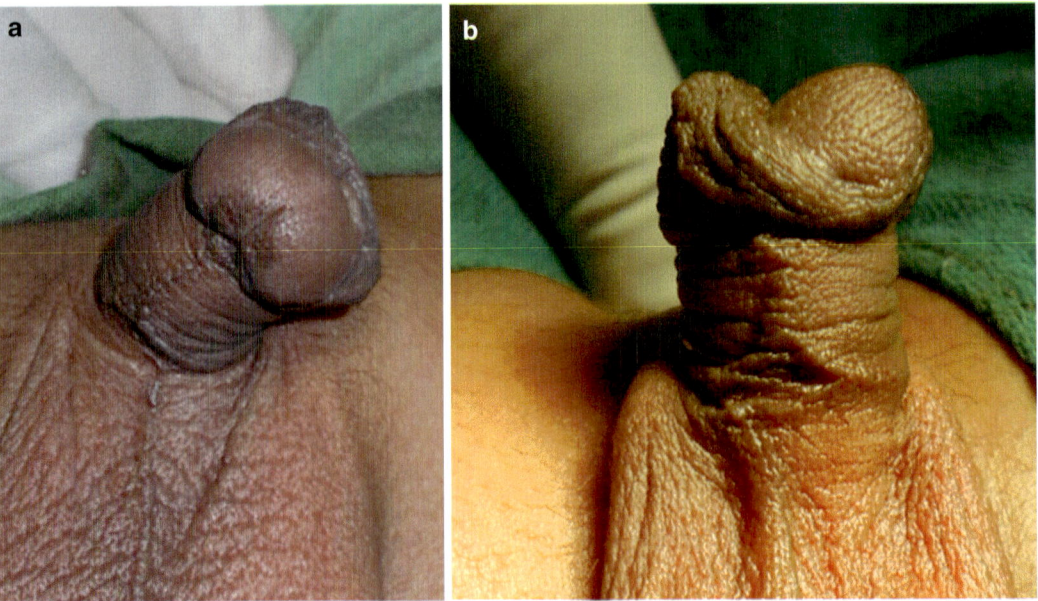

Fig. 31.17 Showing torsion with hypospadias. (**a**) Right-side torsion 45 degrees. (**b**) Left side torsion more than 90 degree

patients without urethrocutaneous fistula, did not find any causative association between administration of caudal analgesia urethrocutaneous fistula [50]. Goel et al. al (2019), in a meta-analysis of seven studies with 1706 patients, found the caudal block analgesia is associated with a significantly higher risk (12% vs 5.8%) of urethrocutaneous fistula formation and other complications (14.6% vs 6.4%) [51]. Zhu et al. (2019) performed a meta-analysis of comparative studies of caudal block versus peripheral nerve block or no caudal block. They included data from 298 patients in four randomized clinical trials and 1726 patients in observational studies. They found that in both randomized clinical trials and observational studies, the administration of caudal block analgesia was not associated with a higher risk of post-operative complication, including urethrocutaneous fistula and glans dehiscence [52]. In our experience, it does not alter the results of urethroplasty and be used safely.

31.2.12 Application of Tourniquet

Hemostasis during surgery is necessary for proper dissection and tissue handling. The tourniquet and adrenaline solution are used for the bloodless field in hypospadias surgery. The duration of the tourniquet is 30–40 min, and the adrenaline solution used is 1:100000 solution. Do these methods of hemostasis have any effect on the outcome of the study? Kaseem et al. (2017) carried out a prospective study to compare the results of hypospadias repair with the application of a tourniquet (rolled rubber glove) against the adrenaline administration. They found no significant difference in complication rates in the two groups but the operative time was significantly higher when the adrenaline was used [53].

Helmy et al. (2020), in their study of 110 cases of TIPU, found penile tourniquet application reduces operative time, diathermy need and improves junior surgeons' satisfaction with intra-operative hemostasis without adversely affecting success rates of patient-reported outcomes [54]. In our experience, the adrenaline solution and tourniquet use are safe and do not increase hypospadias repair complications.

31.2.13 Type of Repair

Mainly, repair choice is according to chordee severity, urethral plate and spongiosum development, and the length of the hypoplastic urethra. The details about the choice of the repair are described in the chapters "management of anterior and middle hypospadias", and "flaps in hypospadias repair" in Chaps. 7 and 12. Two-stage repair in hypospadias. Choice of repair in anterior and middle hypospadias are TIPU, augmented TIPU, onlay flap urethroplasty, and replacement urethroplasty. And in severe hypospadias is flap repairs, modified flap repairs, Long TIPU, and two-stage repair. Snodgrass et al. (1996) reported TIP results in distal hypospadias in a multicenter study involving 148 patients. They documented a complication rate of 7% [55]. The complication reported by Braga (2008) et al. performed a meta-analysis of studies involving TIP in distal hypospadias and documented a mean complication rate of 7.3% and ranged from 0 to 23% [56]. Pfistermullera et al (2015) in a meta-analysis complication 10.6% and re-operation rate 4.5% in 3621 patients in distal hypospadias, 16.7% & 12.5% in 625 cases of proximal hypospadias and 26.8% & 23.3% in 429 cases of re-operative cases [57].

Snodgrass et al. (2002) had 33% complication rates in TIP repair for proximal hypospadias. They corrected chordee by dorsal plication in all cases. They concluded that TIP was a feasible option for proximal hypospadias without severe curvature and if the incised urethral plate has a supple appearance. The results improved when step by step method of chordee correction was used to preserve the urethral plate [58, 59]. Bhat A (2007) reported 13% complications in proximal hypospadias in 34 patients with a follow-up of 23 months [60]. Bhat et al. (2015) reported excellent functional and cosmetic results achieved with a single-stage procedure in 85.8% of our patients, compare favorably with the results of two-stage procedures reported in the literature.

Single-stage repair in severe hypospadias with plate preservations should be preferred because of an anesthetic, safety, and economic perspective, especially in this era where cost reduction is becoming more important [61].

Since the results of TIPU are very good, augmented urethral plate urethroplasty dorsal inlay or onlay flap urethroplasty is done for better results in cases of compromised width and development urethral plate. Kolon et al. (2000) described the use of an inner preputial based dorsal inlay graft in patients with a narrow urethral plate undergoing TIP in 32 patients with coronal to the penoscrotal meatus. They reported that at a mean of 21 months of follow up no complications were observed [62]. Gundeti et al. (2005) also documented their results using the inner prepucial dorsal inlay graft and coined 'Snodgraft'. In the fourteen patients operated on, only one patient had a fistula, and in two patients, the meatus was slightly recessed. They concluded that the Snodgraft procedure enables the TIP extension TIP in small glans or shallow or narrow urethral plate patients [63].

Asanuma et al. (2006) reported the outcomes of the Snodgraft repair in 28 patients with no deep groove of the urethral plate and no severe curvature. They reported a complication rate of 3.6%, with only one patient having a urethrocutaneous fistula. No patients in the study had meatal stenosis, stricture, or urethral diverticulum [64].

Silay et al. (2012), in a study of 102 consecutive patients of Snodgraft repair for primary distal hypospadias, reported none of the patients had meatal stenosis or diverticulum at the inlay graft sit had urethral fistula in 9.8% A slit-like appearance of neo-meatus was achieved in all patients. Similarly, no obstructive urinary flow pattern was detected. The early and long-term maximum urine flow rates were comparable [65].

Eldeeb et al. (2020), in a randomized controlled trial, compared the outcomes of hypospadias repair in patients with a narrow urethral plate (8 mm) operated using the Snodgrass procedure (30 patients) and Snodgraft procedure (30 patients). They found that while the operative time was higher in patients who underwent the Snodgraft procedure, and complication rates were similar in both. They concluded that the Snodgraft procedure is not superior to the Snodgrass operation in the narrow healthy urethral plate [66].

Xu et al. (2013) compared the results of TIP and transverse island onlay flap techniques in a study. In the study, 83 patients underwent TIPU, and 93 patients were managed by TVIF onlay repair. They found complication rates of 18.1% and 21.5% in the two groups, respectively. Still, the difference was not significantly different, and there was no difference in the pediatric penile perception scores in the two groups [67].

Moursy E (2010) compared the TIP results, onlay island flap urethroplasty, and two-stage repair in a study of 194 boys. They found comparable complication rates in all groups with 13.6%, 14%, and 15%. They concluded that a single-stage procedure using either TIP or onlay island flap urethroplasty could be successfully used to repair proximal hypospadias when urethral plate preservation is possible. In cases where transection is necessary, a two-stage procedure can be performed with similar complication rates [68].

Bhat et al. (2017), in a study of 21 patients with proximal hypospadias repaired with modified Glassberg-Duckett, had success 81%. The important modification reported were covering the anastomosis with spongiosum, proximal neourethra up to the penoscrotal junction with tubularization of the urethral plate, dartos vascular pedicle was mobilized up to the root of the penis & split in the midline into equal halves, and brought ventrally each side, covering neourethra with dartos and fixing it corpora and large meatal reconstruction and glanuloplasty [69]. Daboos M. et al. (2020) compared the results of a single (80) and double-faced (80) flap urethroplasty. They reported fewer complications (15%/25%), better urinary function, and good cosmetic results in the double-faced tubularized preputial flap technique [70]. The results of single-stage flap urethroplasty and two-stage repair are similar, so the choice depends on the training and comfort of the surgeon. The author prefers a single stage in severe hypospadias and step-by-step correction of chordee and plate preservation procedures and spongioplasty in anterior and middle hypospadias.

31.2.14 Prepucioplasty

Prepucioplasty with hypospadias repair adds 15–20 min to surgery but restores normal penile anatomy [71]. It is more frequently done with hypospadias repair as it does not increase the complications. Details about prepucioplasty are described in Chap. 25 on prepucioplasty. Prepucioplasty is feasible even in proximal hypospadias with mild to moderate curvature. Bhat et al. (2010) reported an 88.88% success rate in 27 patients of proximal hypospadias in a mean follow-up of 18 months (Fig. 31.18a–h) But there may be complications like phimosis and prepucial dehiscence requiring surgery in 11.11% of cases [72]. Similar rates of re-surgery (10%) (preputial dehiscence with fistula 2%, isolated preputial dehiscence 2%, and patients requiring circumcision of disfigurement 6%) were observed by Papouis et al. in proximal hypospadias and (phimosis 3.8% and foreskin dehiscence 2.5%) in distal hypospadias [73, 74]. The results of urethroplasty with prepucial reconstruction are similar in both pediatric and adult patients. Bhat et al. 2016 reported 50.0% of the patients in the adult group and 58.3% in pediatric prepucioplasty without increasing the urethroplasty-related complications [6]. Therefore, the author's view is that prepucioplasty can be done in suitable patients without increasing the complication rate.

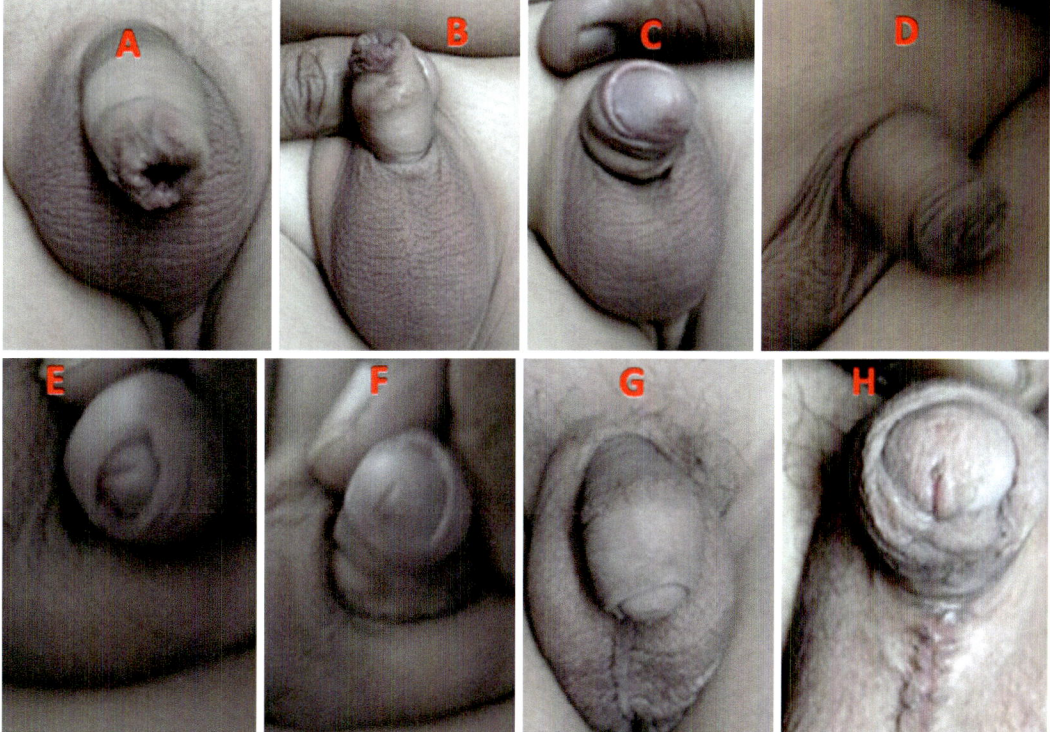

Fig. 31.18 showing postoperative results of prepucioplasty. (**a** and **b**) Normal looking prepuce and penis in distal hypospadias. (**c**) Retracted prepuce normal-looking meatus in distal hypospadias. (**d**) Normal looking penis in distal hypospadias. (**e**) Partially retracted prepuce in distal hypospadias. (**e**) Retracted prepuce in distal hypospadias. (**f**) Normal looking glans and meatus in proximal hypospadias. (**g** and **h**) Prepucioplasty in proximal hypospadias partially opened glans

Table 31.4 Details of complications in each case of TIPU {with permission Bhat et al. [5] @ copyright Bhat et al IBIMA Publishing}

Case No.	Complication	Age in years.	Type of Hypospadias	Chordee in Degree (°)	Urethral Plate	Spongiosum	No. of Risk Factors*
1	Fistula	1.5	Peno-scrotal	70	Narrow	Poor	4
2	Fistula	3	Mid Penile	35	Average	Well	1
3	Fistula	5.6	Peno-scrotal	40	Narrow	Moderate	4
4	Superficial skin necrosis	8	Proximal penile	90	Average	Well	3
5	Meatal Stenosis	9	Distal	Nil	Wide	Well	1
6	Meatal Stenosis	12	Distal penile	Nil	Narrow	Moderate	2
7	Stricture	13	Proximal	65	Wide	Poor	4
8	Fistula	15	Peno-scrotal	95	Narrow	Poor	5
9	Stricture	18	Distal penile	35	Narrow	Poor	4
10	Fistula	18	Mid penile	10	Average	Moderate	2
11	Fistula	20	Peno-Scrotal	70	Narrow	Poor	5
12	Meatal stenosis	22	Distal penile	25	Average	Poor	3
13	Disruption of urethra	23	Distal penile	Nil	Narrow	Poor	3
Total 13		Mean = 12.9	Prox. 6	Mean = 41.1	N = 8	Poor = 7	<3F = 4
							3F = 3
					A = 4	Mod = 3	4F = 4
					W = 1	Well = 3	5F = 2

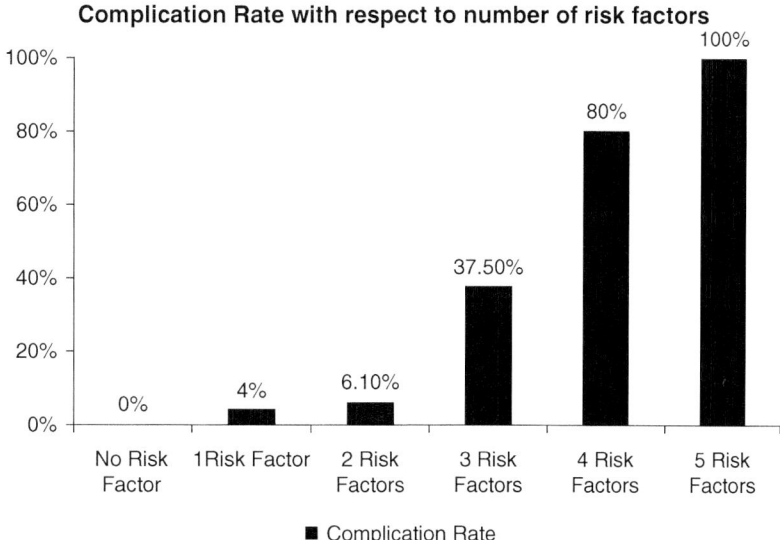

Fig. 31.19 Bar diagram showing complication with number of factors in TIPU

31.3 Discussion

The variables affecting surgical outcomes are age, hypospadias & chordee severity, the urethral plate width and spongiosum development, glans and penis size, and the length of the hypoplastic urethra. The complication rates are higher proximal hypospadias (43%), a narrow urethral plate (50%), and a poorly developed spongiosum (55%) in TIPU [7]. Our study of 125 patients of TIPU had complications in 13 cases, and variables in individual cases varied from 1 to 5 (Table 31.4). When we consider these factors into account together, any patient having more than three risk factors has a higher chance of complications (Fig. 31.19). Such patients should have additional preventive measures in TIPU like preoperative testosterone to improve the quality of the urethral plate and healthy intervening tissue tunica vaginalis/ dorsal dartos cover with spongioplasty or change a decision to replacement urethroplasty/two-stage repair. Parents/patients should be counseled about the expected complications. The overall risk score guides the new surgeons in an appropriate case selection and refers high-risk group patients to more experienced surgeons.

31.4 Conclusions

Decision-making in surgery becomes more difficult when multiple choices are available. It depends on the various variables of the patients, surgical skill, and surgical environment. The variables affecting the surgical outcome in hypospadias surgery are the hypospadias and chordee severity, width and development of urethral plate and spongiosum, length of the hypoplastic urethra, type of urethroplasty, glans and penis size, and the patient age. The number of the variables will decide the type of urethroplasty and surgical outcome. The variables which do not lead to poor results are penile torsion, hormonal stimulation, application of the tourniquet, use of caudal analgesia and anesthesia, the addition of prepucioplasty; so can be used without increasing the complication of urethroplasty. The results of single-stage flap urethroplasty and two-stage repair are similar in severe hypospadias. Hence, the choice is based on the training, experience, and comfort of the surgeon. The single-stage modified flap repair in severe hypospadias and step by step correction of chordee with plate preservation procedures, i.e. tubularization of urethral plate and spongioplasty in anterior and middle hypospadias, are the preferred procedures.

References

1. DeLair SM, Tanaka ST, Yap SA, Kurzrock EA. Training residents in hypospadias repair: variations of involvement J Urol. 2008 Mar;179(3):1102–1106. https://doi.org/10.1016/j.juro.2007.10.090. Epub 2008 Jan 18. PMID: 18206935.
2. Ansari MS, Agarwal S, Sureka SK, Mandhani A, Kapoor R, Srivastava A. Impact of changing trends in technique and learning curve on the outcome of hypospadias repair: An experience from tertiary care center. Indian J Urol. 2016 Jul–Sep;32(3):216–20.
3. Rompré MP, Nadeau G, Moore K, Ajjaouj Y, Braga LH, Bolduc S. Learning curve for TIP urethroplasty: a single-surgeon experience. Can Urol Assoc J. 2013;7:E789–94.
4. Mohammed M, Bright F, Mteta A, Mbwambo J, Ngowi BN, Mbwambo O, Yongolo S, Mganga A. Long-term complications of hypospadias repair: a ten-year experience from Northern Zone of Tanzania. Res Rep Urol. 2020;12:463–9.
5. Bhat A, Bhat M, Sabharwal K, Singla M, Saran R, Gokhroo S, et al. A prospective study to evaluate the role of different variables in TIPU results for hypospadias. Int J Res Urol. 2014;2014:1–12. https://doi.org/10.5171/2014.547185.
6. Bhat A, Bhat M, Kumar V, Kumar R, Mittal R, Saksena G. Comparison of variables affecting the surgical outcomes of tubularized incised plate urethroplasty in adult and pediatric hypospadias. J Pediatr Urol. 2016 Apr 1;12(2):108.e1-7.
7. Bhat A, Bhat M, Upadhaya R, Kumar V, Kumar R, Mittal R. Tubularized incised plate urethroplasty repair in adult hypospadias patients. Are results similar to those reported in the pediatric age group? A prospective study. Afr J Urol. 2016;22:86–91.
8. Wenli L, Tao Y, Wisniewski AB, Frimberger D, Kropp BP. Different outcomes of hypospadias surgery between North America, Europe and China: is patient age a factor? Nephrourol Mon. 2012 Autumn;4(4):609–12.
9. Yildiz T, Tahtali IN, Ates DC, Keles I, Ilce Z. Age of patient is a risk factor for urethrocutaneous fistula in hypospadias surgery. J Pediatr Urol. 2013 Dec;9(6 Pt A):900–3.
10. Perlmutter AE, Morabito R, Tarry WF. Impact of patient age on distal hypospadias repair: a surgical perspective. Urology. 2006 Sep;68(3):648–51.
11. Bush NC, Holzer M, Zhang S, Snodgrass W. Age does not impact risk for urethroplasty complications after tubularized incised plate repair of hypospadias in prepubertal boys. J Pediatr Urol. 2013 Jun 1;9(3):252–6.
12. Hansson E, Becker M, Åberg M, Svensson H. Analysis of complications after repair of hypospadias. Scand J Plast Reconstr Surg Hand Surg. 2007;41(3):120–4. https://doi.org/10.1080/02844310701228669.
13. Sarhan OM, El-Hefnawy AS, Hafez AT, Elsherbiny MT, Dawaba ME, Ghali AM. Factors affecting outcome of tubularized incised plate (TIP) urethroplasty: a single-centre experience with 500 cases. J Pediatr Urol. 2009 Oct 1;5(5):378–82.
14. Bush NC, Holzer M, Zhang S, Snodgrass W. Age does not impact risk for urethroplasty complications after tubularized incised plate repair of hypospadias in prepubertal boys. J Pediatr Urol. 2013 Jun 1;9(3):252–6.
15. Pfistermuller KL, McArdle AJ, Cuckow PM. Meta-analysis of complication rates of the tubularized incised plate (TIP) repair. J Pediatr Urol. 2015 Apr 1;11(2):54–9.
16. de Mattos e Silva E, Gorduza DB, Catti M, Valmalle AF, Demede D, Hameury F, Pierre-Yves M, Mouriquand P. Outcome of severe hypospadias repair using three different techniques. J Pediatr Urol. 2009 Jun 1;5(3):205–11.
17. Long CJ, Canning DA. Hypospadias: are we as good as we think when we correct proximal hypospadias? J Pediatr Urol. 2016 Aug 1;12(4):196–e1.
18. Chung JW, Choi SC, Kim BS, Sung Chung SK. Risk factors for the development of urethrocutaneous fistula after hypospadias repair: a retrospective study Korean. J Urol. 2012 Oct;53(10):711–5.
19. Uygur M, Ünal D, Tan M, et al. Factors affecting outcome of one-stage anterior hypospadias repair: analysis of 422 cases. Pediatr Surg Int. 2002;18:142–6.
20. Snodgrass W, Bush N. Recurrent ventral curvature after proximal TIP hypospadias repair. J Pediatr Urol. 2020;30:222–5.
21. Nguyen MT, Snodgrass WT. Effect of urethral plate characteristics on tubularized incised plate urethroplasty. J Urol. 2004 Mar;171(3):1260–2.
22. Mosharafa AA, Agbo-Panzo D, Priso R, Aubry E, Besson R. Repair of hypospadias: the effect of urethral plate configuration on the outcome of Duplay-Snodgrass repair. Progres en urologie: journal de l'Association francaise d'urologie et de la Societe francaise d'urologie. 2009 Apr 22;19(7):507–10.
23. Chukwubuike KE, Obianyo NE, Ekenze SO, Ezomike UO. Assessment of the effect of urethral plate width on outcome of hypospadias repair. J Pediatr Urol. 2019;15(6):627.e1–6.
24. Bhat A, Sabharwal K, Bhat M, Saran R, Singla M, Kumar V. Outcome of tubularized incised plate urethroplasty with spongioplasty alone as additional tissue cover: a prospective study. Indian J Urol. 2014;30:392–7.
25. Bhat AL, Bhat M, Sabharwal KV, Singla M, Saran R, Gokhroo S, et al. Comparison of results of TIPU repair for hypospadias with "Spongioplasty Alone" and "Spongioplasty with Dorsal Dartos Flap". Open J Urol. 2014;4:41e8.
26. Bhat A, Sabharwal K, Bhat M, Saran R, Singla M, Kumar V. Outcome of tubularized incised plate urethroplasty with spongioplasty alone as additional tissue cover: A prospective study. Indian J Urol IJU: Journal of the Urological Society of India. 2014;30(4):39.
27. Bhat A, Bhat M, Kumar R, Bhat A. Double breasting spongioplasty in tubularized/tubularized incise plate urethroplasty: A new technique. Indian J Urol IJU: Journal of the Urological Society of India. 2017;33(1):58.

28. Zhang B, Bi Y, Ruan S. Reconstructing forked corpus spongiosum to correct glans droop in distal/midshaft hypospadias repair. J Int Med Res. 2020 May;48(5):300060520925698.
29. Bhat A, Bhat M, Sabharwal K, Kumar R. Bhat's modifications of Glassberg–Duckett repair to reduce complications in management severe hypospadias with curvature. Afr J Urol. 2017;23(2):94–9.
30. Cooper CS, Noh PH, Snyder HM III. Preservation of urethral plate spongiosum: technique to reduce hypospadias fistulas. Urology. 2001 Feb 1;57(2):351–4.
31. Lyu YQ, Yu L, Xie H, Huang YC, Li XX, Sun L, Liang Y, Chen F. Spongiosum-combined glanuloplasty reduces glans complications after proximal hypospadias repair. Asian J Androl. 2021 Mar 12;23:1–5.
32. Zhang B, Bi YL, Ruan SS. Application and efficacy of reconstructing forked corpus spongiosum in distal/midshaft hypospadias repair. Asian J Androl. 2021 Jan;23(1):47.
33. Bush NC, Villanueva C, Snodgrass W. Glans size is an independent risk factor for urethroplasty complications after hypospadias repair. J Pediatr Urol. 2015 Dec 1;11(6):355–e1.
34. Bush NC, Da Justa D, Snodgrass WT. Glans penis width in patients with hypospadias compared to healthy controls. J Pediatr Urol. 2013 Dec 1;9(6):1188–91.
35. Merriman LS, Arlen AM, Broecker BH, Smith EA, Kirsch AJ, Elmore JM. The GMS hypospadias score: assessment of inter-observer reliability and correlation with post-operative complications. J Pediatr Urol. 2013 Dec 1;9(6):707–12.
36. Arlen AM, Kirsch AJ, Leong T, Broecker BH, Smith EA, Elmore JM. Further analysis of the Glans-Urethral Meatus-Shaft (GMS) hypospadias score: correlation with postoperative complications. J Pediatr Urol. 2015 Apr 1;11(2):71–e1.
37. Yang SS, Chen YT, Hsieh CH, Chen SC. Preservation of the thin distal urethra in hypospadias repair. J Urol. 2000;164:151–3.
38. Sarin YK, Manchanda V. Preservation of urethra devoid of corpus spongiosum in patients undergoing urethroplasty. Indian J Urol. 2006;22:326–8.
39. Bhat A. Preservation of urethra devoid of corpus spongiosum in patients undergoing urethroplasty. Indian J Urol. 2007;23:213–4.
40. Wong YS, Pang KKY, Tam YH. The hypospadias phenotype with a distal meatus in the presence of distal penile penoscrotal angle fixation. Res Rep Urol. 2019;11:255–60.
41. Hashish MS, Elsawaf MI, Moussa MA. Urethral advancement procedure in the treatment of primary distal hypospadias: a series of 20 cases. Ann Pediatr Surg. 2017;13:29–37.
42. Luo CC, Lin JN, Chiu CH, et al. Use of parenteral testosterone prior to hypospadias surgery. Pediatr Surg Int. 2003;19:82–4.
43. Wright I, Cole E, Farrokhyar F, et al. Effect of preoperative hormonal stimulation on postoperative complication rates after proximal hypospadias repair: a systematic review. J Urol. 2013;190:652–9.
44. Gorduza DB, Gay CL, de Mattos E, Silva E, et al. Does androgen stimulation prior to hypospadias surgery increase the rate of healing complications? A preliminary report. J Pediatr Urol. 2011;7:158–61.
45. Kaya C, Radmayr C. The role of pre-operative androgen stimulation in hypospadias surgery. Transl Androl Urol. 2014 Dec;3(4):340–6.
46. Zeid A, Soliman H. Penile torsion: an overlooked anomaly with distal hypospadias. Ann Pediatr Surg. 2010;6(2):93–7.
47. Bhat A, Singh V, Bhat M. Penile torsion. In: Surgical techniques in pediatric and adult urology. 1st ed. New Delhi/London: Jaypee Brothers Medical Publishers; 2020. p. 207–22.
48. Bhat A, Bhat MP, Saxena G. Correction of penile torsion by mobilization of urethral plate and urethra. J Pediatr Urol. 2009;5(6):451–7.
49. Kundra P, Yuvaraj K, Agrawal K, Krishnappa S, Kumar LT. Surgical outcome in children undergoing hypospadias repair under caudal epidural vs penile block. Pediatric Anesth. 2012 July;22(7):707–12.
50. Zaidi RH, Casanova NF, Haydar B, Voepel-Lewis T, Wan JH. Urethrocutaneous fistula following hypospadias repair: Regional anaesthesia and other factors. Paediatr Anaesth. 2015;25:1144–50.
51. Goel P, Jain S, Bajpai M, Khanna P, Jain V, Yadav DK. Does caudal analgesia increase the rates of urethrocutaneous fistula formation after hypospadias repair? Systematic review and meta-analysis. Indian J Urol IJU: Journal of the Urological Society of India. 2019 Jul;35(3):222.
52. Zhu C, Wei R, Tong Y, Liu J, Song Z, Zhang S. Analgesic efficacy and impact of the caudal block on surgical complications of hypospadias repair: a systematic review and meta-analysis. Reg Anesth Pain Med. 2019 Feb 1;44(2):259–67.
53. Kassem R, Shreef K, Eltayeb H, Gobran T, Jetley NK, Saleem M. The use of tourniquet versus bipolar cautery as hemostatic aid in distal hypospadias repair in children: a multicentric study. Egypt J Surg. 2017;36:58–61.
54. Helmy TE, Hashem A, Mursi K, AbdelHalim A, Hafez A, Dawaba MS. Does intraoperative penile tourniquet application during hypospadias repair affect the patients and surgeons reported outcomes? A randomized controlled trial. J Pediatr Urol. 2020 Oct 1;16(5):683–91.
55. Snodgrass W, Koyle M, Manzoni G, Hurwitz R, Caldamone A, Ehrlich R. Tubularized incised plate hypospadias repair: results of a multicenter experience. J Urol. 1996 Aug;156(2S):839–41.
56. Braga LH, Lorenzo AJ, Salle JL. Tubularized incised plate urethroplasty for distal hypospadias: a literature review. Indian J Urol IJU: Journal of the Urological Society of India. 2008 Apr;24(2):219.
57. Pfistermuller KLM, McArdle AJ, Cuckow PM. Meta-analysis of complication rates of the tubularized incised plate (TIP) repair. J Pediatr Urol. 2015;2:54–9.

58. Snodgrass WT, Lorenzo A. Tubularized incised-plate urethroplasty for proximal hypospadias. BJU Int. 2002 Jan;89(1):90–3.
59. Snodgrass WT, Bush N. Tubularized incised-plate urethroplasty in proximal hypospadias. Continued evolution and extended application. J Ped Urol. 2011;7:2–9.
60. Bhat A. Extended urethral mobilization in incised plate urethroplasty for severe hypospadias: a variation in technique to improve chordee correction. J Urol. 2007;178(3):1031–5.
61. Bhat A, Singla M, Bhat M, Sabharwala K, Upadhaya R, Kumara V. Incised plate urethroplasty in perineal and perineo-scrotal hypospadias. African. J Urol. 2015;21(2):105–10.
62. Kolon TF, Gonzales ET. The dorsal inlay graft for hypospadias repair. J Urol. 2000 Jun;163(6):1941–3.
63. Gundeti M, Queteishat A, Desai D, Cuckow P. Use of an inner preputial free graft to extend the indications of Snodgrass hypospadias repair (Snodgraft). J Pediatr Urol. 2005 Dec 1;1(6):395–6.
64. Asanuma H, Satoh H, Shishido S. Dorsal inlay graft urethroplasty for primary hypospadiac repair. Int J Urol. 2007 Jan;14(1):43–7.
65. Silay MS, Sirin H, Tepeler A, Karatag T, Armagan A, Horasanli K, Miroglu C. "Snodgraft" technique for the treatment of primary distal hypospadias: pushing the envelope. J Urol. 2012 Sep;188(3):938–42.
66. Eldeeb M, Nagla S, Abou-Farha M, Hassan A. Snodgrass vs Snodgraft operation to repair the distal hypospadias in the narrow urethral plate. J Pediatr Urol. 2020 Apr 1;16(2):165–e1.
67. Xu N, Xue XY, Li XD, Wei Y, Zheng QS, Jiang T, Huang JB, Sun XL. Comparative outcomes of the tubularized incised plate and transverse island flap onlay techniques for the repair of proximal hypospadias. Int Urol Nephrol. 2014 Mar 1;46(3):487–91.
68. Moursy EE. Outcome of proximal hypospadias repair using three different techniques. J Pediatr Urol. 2010 Feb 1;6(1):45–53.
69. Bhat A, Bhat M, Sabharwal K, Kumar R. Bhat's modifications of Glassberg–Duckett repair to reduce complications in management severe hypospadias with curvature. Afr J Urol. 2017 Jul 7;23(2):94–9.
70. Daboos M, Helal AA, Salama A. Five years' experience of double-faced tubularized preputial flap for penoscrotal hypospadias repair in paediatrics. J Pediatr Urol. 2020;16(5):673 e1–7.
71. Bhat A, Singh V, Bhat M. Prepucioplasty in hypospadias repair In surgical techniques in Pediatric and adult urology. 1st ed. New Delhi/London: Jaypee Brothers Medical Publishers; 2020. p. 212–6.
72. Bhat A, Gandhi A, Saxena G, et al. Preputial reconstruction and tubularized incised plate urethroplasty in proximal hypospadias with ventral penile curvature. Indian J Urol. 2010;26:507–10.
73. Snodgrass WT, Koyle MA, Baskin LA, et al. Foreskin preservation in penile surgery. J Urol. 2006;176:711–4.
74. Papouis G, Kaselas C, Skoumis K, Kaselas V. Repair of distal hypospadias and preputioplasty in one operation: risks and advantages. Urol Int. 2009;82:183–6.

Printed by Printforce, the Netherlands

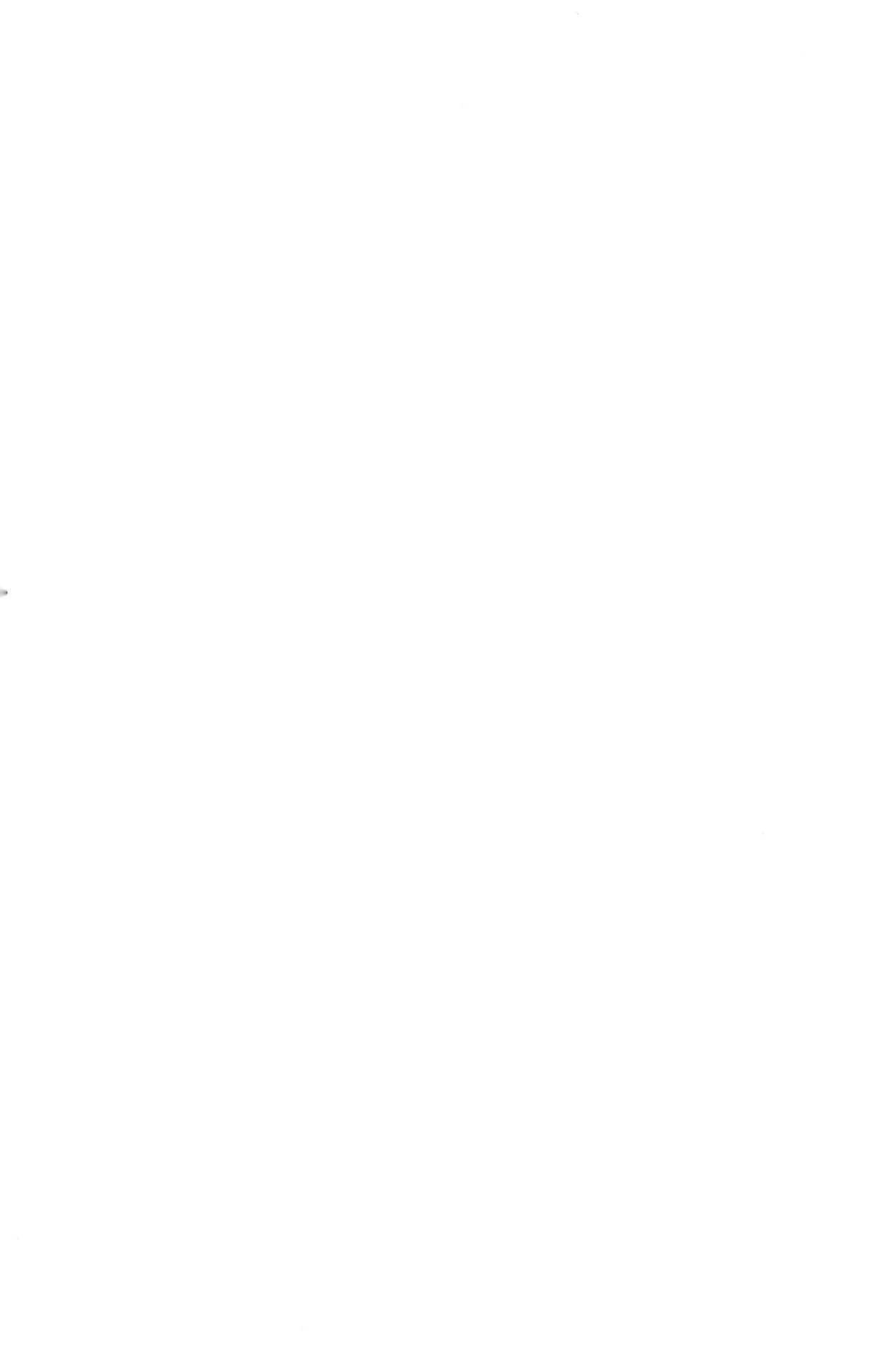